Concise Pocket
Medical Dictionary

Concise Pocket
Medical Dictionary

Second Edition

Compiled and Edited by

UN Panda MD
Senior Physician
New Delhi, India

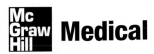

© 2011, Jaypee Brothers Medical Publishers
First published in India in 2009 by

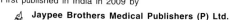

Jaypee Brothers Medical Publishers (P) Ltd.

Corporate Office
4838/24 Ansari Road, Daryaganj, **New Delhi** - 110002, India,
+91-11-43574357

Registered Office
B-3 EMCA House, 23/23B Ansari Road, Daryaganj,
New Delhi 110 002, India
Phones: +91-11-23272143, +91-11-23272703, +91-11-23282021,
+91-11-23245672, Rel: +91-11-32558559 Fax: +91-11-23276490,
+91-11-23245683
e-mail: jaypee@jaypeebrothers.com
Website: www.jaypeebrothers.com

First published in USA by The McGraw-Hill Companies, 2 Penn Plaza, New
York, NY 10121. Exclusively worldwide distributor except South Asia
(India, Nepal, Sri Lanka, Bhutan, Pakistan, Bangladesh, Malaysia).

ISBN-13: 978-0-07-175999-1
ISBN-10: 0-07-175999-9

To
My wife
and
Children

Preface to the Second Edition

This new edition of *Concise Pocket Medical Dictionary* has undergone a thorough revision process. It includes beautiful, self-explanatory diagrams and illustrations, all in four colors. More than 500 new figures and numerous new enteries have been added.

It is sincerely hoped that this concise, yet complete medical dictionary would prove as a readily available source of reference and would greatly benefit the medical students, teachers, practitioners as well as all the professionals engaged in health care. This dictionary incorporates most commonly used vocabulary and words encountered in numerous medical specialities including medicine, surgery, obstetrics and gynecology, ENT, ophthalmology, etc. The meaning of each medical terminology, its explanation and examples have been described in an easy to understand, comprehensible format.

Constructive criticism and continuing support from the readers is highly encouraged.

UN Panda

Preface to the First Edition

There is mushrooming growth of medical dictionaries in the market. Some are too big to only serve as reference books while others are too small and incomplete to be depended upon. Most dictionaries do not incorporate pharmaceutical preparations. Hence, students feel let down when they fall back on a medical dictionary for help.

This distinct gap prompted me to compile and present to our esteemed readers a compact and complete dictionary titled *Concise Medical Dictionary*. Though concise, it incorporates most commonly used words and vocabulary mentioned in any dictionary of repute. The meaning of a word, its explanation and examples are described in a simple and comprehensible form. Most pharmaceutical products presently available in the market find their rightful place in the book. However, unnecessary explanations and examples have been avoided. The book should be useful for medical students, practitioners as well as teachers and all professionals engaged in health care.

With the continuing support from the readers, I am confident to upgrade the book over coming years.

UN Panda

Plate 1

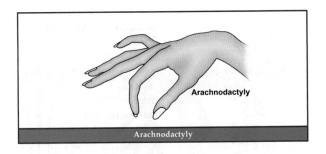

Arachnodactyly

Arachnodactyly

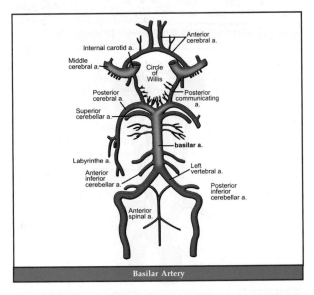

Basilar Artery

Plate 2

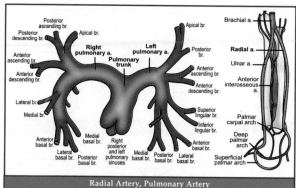

Radial Artery, Pulmonary Artery

Vertebral Artery

Plate 3

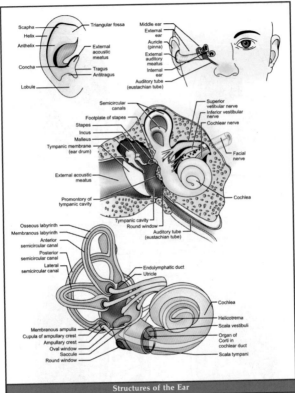

Structures of the Ear

Plate 4

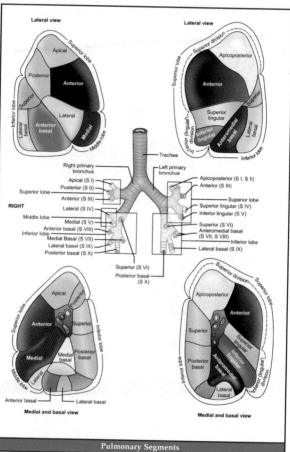

Pulmonary Segments

Plate 5

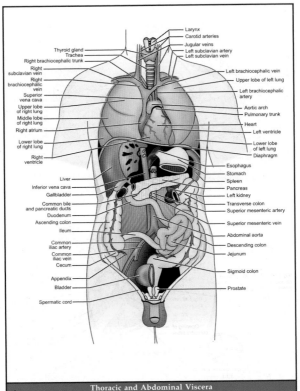

Larynx
Carotid arteries
Jugular veins
Left subclavian artery
Left subclavian vein
Thyroid gland
Trachea
Right brachiocephalic trunk
Right subclavian vein
Right brachiocephalic vein
Superior vena cava
Upper lobe of right lung
Middle lobe of right lung
Right atrium
Lower lobe of right lung
Right ventricle

Left brachiocephalic vein
Upper lobe of left lung
Left brachiocephalic vein
Aortic arch
Pulmonary trunk
Heart
Left ventricle
Lower lobe of left lung
Diaphragm

Liver
Inferior vena cava
Gallbladder
Common bile and pancreatic ducts
Duodenum
Ascending colon
Ileum
Common iliac artery
Common iliac vein
Cecum
Appendix
Bladder
Spermatic cord

Esophagus
Stomach
Spleen
Pancreas
Left kidney
Transverse colon
Superior mesenteric artery
Superior mesenteric vein
Abdominal aorta
Descending colon
Jejunum
Sigmoid colon
Prostate

Thoracic and Abdominal Viscera

Plate 6

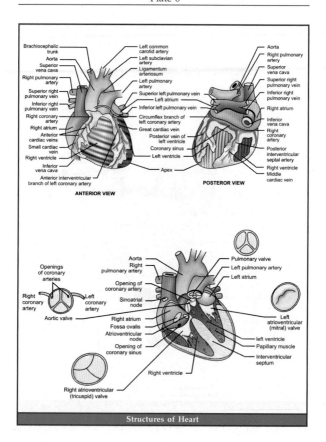

Structures of Heart

Plate 7

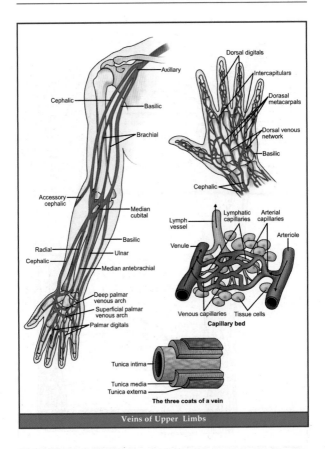

Veins of Upper Limbs

Plate 8

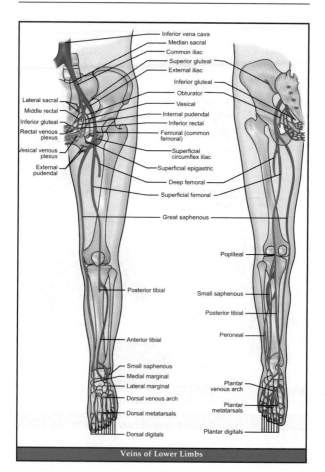

Inferior vena cava
Median sacral
Common iliac
Superior gluteal
External iliac
Inferior gluteal
Obturator
Vesical
Internal pudendal
Inferior rectal
Femoral (common femoral)
Superficial circumflex iliac
Superficial epigastric
Deep femoral
Superficial femoral

Lateral sacral
Middle rectal
Inferior gluteal
Rectal venous plexus
Vesical venous plexus
External pudendal

Great saphenous

Popliteal

Posterior tibial

Small saphenous

Posterior tibial

Peroneal

Anterior tibial

Small saphenous
Medial marginal
Lateral marginal
Dorsal venous arch
Dorsal metatarsals
Dorsal digitals

Plantar venous arch

Plantar metatarsals

Plantar digitals

Veins of Lower Limbs

Plate 9

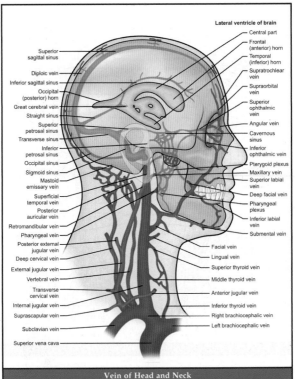

Lateral ventricle of brain

Central part
Frontal (anterior) horn
Temporal (inferior) horn
Supratrochlear vein
Supraorbital vein
Superior ophthalmic vein
Angular vein
Cavernous sinus
Inferior ophthalmic vein
Pterygoid plexus
Maxillary vein
Superior labial vein
Deep facial vein
Pharyngeal plexus
Inferior labial vein
Submental vein
Facial vein
Lingual vein
Superior thyroid vein
Middle thyroid vein
Anterior jugular vein
Inferior thyroid vein
Right brachiocephalic vein
Left brachiocephalic vein

Superior sagittal sinus
Diploic vein
Inferior sagittal sinus
Occipital (posterior) horn
Great cerebral vein
Straight sinus
Superior petrosal sinus
Transverse sinus
Inferior petrosal sinus
Occipital sinus
Sigmoid sinus
Mastoid emissary vein
Superficial temporal vein
Posterior auricular vein
Retromandibular vein
Pharyngeal vein
Posterior external jugular vein
Deep cervical vein
External jugular vein
Vertebral vein
Transverse cervical vein
Internal jugular vein
Suprascapular vein
Subclavian vein
Superior vena cava

Vein of Head and Neck

Plate 10

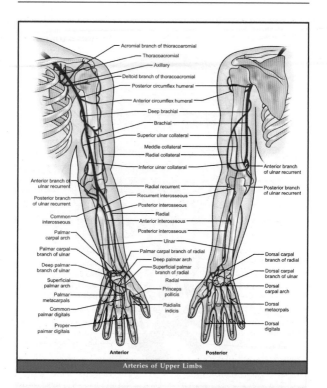

Acromial branch of thioracoaromial
Thoracoacromial
Axillary
Deltoid branch of thoracoacromial
Posterior circumflex humeral
Anterior circumflex humeral
Deep brachial
Brachial
Superior ulnar collateral
Meddle collateral
Radial collateral
Inferior ulnar collateral
Anterior branch of ulnar recurrent
Posterior branch of ulnar recurrent
Anterior branch of ulnar recurrent
Posterior branch of ulnar recurrent
Radial recurrent
Recurrent interosseous
Posterior interosseous
Common interosseous
Radial
Anterior interosseous
Palmar carpal arch
Posterior interosseous
Palmar carpal branch of ulnar
Ulnar
Palmar carpal branch of radial
Dorsal carpal branch of radial
Deep palmar branch of ulnar
Deep palmar arch
Superficial palmar branch of radial
Dorsal carpal branch of ulnar
Superficial palmar arch
Radial
Dorsal carpal arch
Palmar metacarpals
Princeps pollicis
Dorsal metacrpals
Common palmar digitals
Radialis indicis
Proper paimar digitals
Dorsal digitals

Anterior   Posterior

Arteries of Upper Limbs

Plate 11

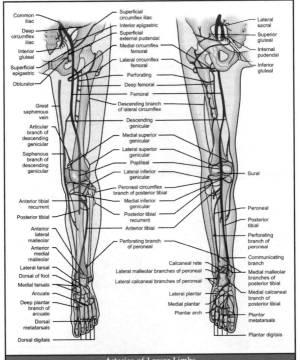

Common iliac
Deep circumflex iliac
Interior gluteal
Superficial epigastric
Obturator

Great saphenous vein
Articular branch of descending genicular
Saphenous branch of descending genicular

Anterior tibial recurrent
Posterior tibial

Anterior lateral malleolar
Anterior medial malleolar
Lateral tarsal
Dorsal of foot
Medial tarsals
Arcuate
Deep plantar branch of arcuate
Dorsal metatarsals

Dorsal digitals

Superficial circumflex iliac
Interior epigastric
Superficial external pudendal
Medial circumflex femoral
Lateral circumflex femoral
Perforating
Deep femoral
Femoral
Descending branch of lateral circumflex
Descending genicular
Medial superior genicular
Lateral superior genicular
Popliteal
Lateral inferior genicular
Peroneal circumflex branch of posterior tibial
Medial inferior genicular
Posterior tibial recurrent
Anterior tibial
Perforating branch of peroneal
Calcaneal rete
Lateral malleolar branches of peroneal
Lateral calcaneal branches of peroneal
Lateral plantar
Medial plantar
Plantar arch

Lateral sacral
Superior gluteal
Internal pudendal
Inferior gluteal

Sural

Peroneal
Posterior tibial
Perforating branch of peroneal
Communicating branch
Medial malleolar branches of posterior tibial
Medial calcaneal branch of posterior tibial
Plantar metatarsals

Plantar digitals

Arteries of Lower Limbs

Plate 12

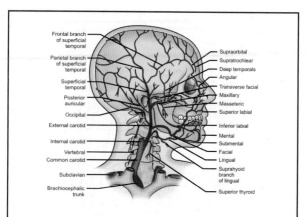

Frontal branch of superficial temporal
Parietal branch of superficial temporal
Superficial temporal
Posterior auricular
Occipital
External carotid
Internal carotid
Vertebral
Common carotid
Subclavian
Brachiocephalic trunk

Supraorbital
Supratrochlear
Deep temporals
Angular
Transverse facial
Maxillary
Masseteric
Superior labial
Inferior labial
Mental
Submental
Facial
Lingual
Suprahyoid branch of lingual
Superior thyroid

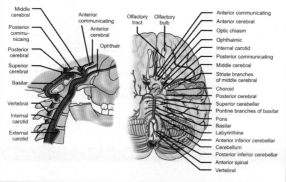

Middle cerebral
Posterior communicating
Posterior cerebral
Superior cerebral
Basilar
Vertebral
Internal carotid
External carotid

Anterior communicating
Anterior cerebral
Ophthalr

Olfactory tract
Olfactory bulb

Anterior communicating
Anterior cerebral
Optic chiasm
Ophthalmic
Internal carotid
Posterior communicating
Middle cerebral
Striate branches of middle cerebral
Choroid
Posterior cerebral
Superior cerebellar
Pontine branches of basilar
Pons
Basilar
Labyrinthine
Anterior inferior cerebellar
Cerebellum
Posterior inferior cerebellar
Anterior spinal
Vertebral

Arteries of Head, Neck and Base of Brain

Plate 13

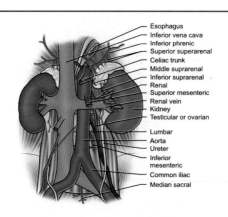

Esophagus
Inferior vena cava
Inferior phrenic
Superior superarenal
Celiac trunk
Middle suprarenal
Inferior suprarenal
Renal
Superior mesenteric
Renal vein
Kidney
Testicular or ovarian

Lumbar
Aorta
Ureter
Inferior mesenteric
Common iliac
Median sacral

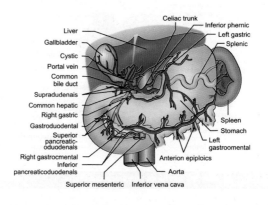

Celiac trunk
Inferior phernic
Liver
Left gastric
Gallbladder
Splenic
Cystic
Portal vein
Common bile duct
Supradudenais
Common hepatic
Right gastric
Gastroduodental
Spleen
Superior pancreatic-oduodenals
Stomach
Right gastrocmental
Left gastromental
Inferior pancreaticoduodenals
Anterion epiploics
Superior mesenteric
Aorta
Inferior vena cava

Arteries of the Abdomen and Pelvis

Plate 14

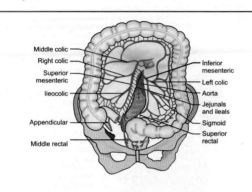

Middle colic
Right colic
Superior mesenteric
Ileocolic
Appendicular
Middle rectal

Inferior mesenteric
Left colic
Aorta
Jejunals and ileals
Sigmoid
Superior rectal

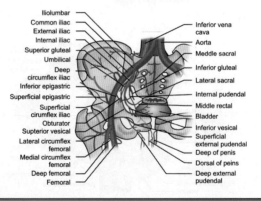

Iliolumbar
Common iliac
External iliac
Internal iliac
Superior gluteal
Umbilical
Deep circumflex iliac
Inferior epigastric
Superficial epigastric
Superficial cirumflex iliac
Obturator
Supterior vesical
Lateral circumflex femoral
Medial circumflex femoral
Deep femoral
Femoral

Inferior vena cava
Aorta
Meddle sacral
Inferior gluteal
Lateral sacral
Internal pudendal
Middle rectal
Bladder
Inferior vesical
Superficial external pudendal
Deep of penis
Dorsal of peins
Deep external pudendal

Arteries of the Abdomen and Pelvis

Plate 15

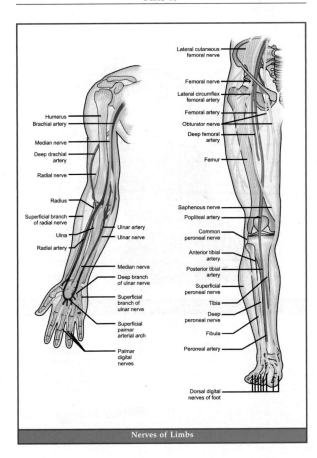

Lateral cutaneous femoral nerve
Femoral nerve
Lateral circumflex femoral artery
Femoral artery
Obturator nerve
Deep femoral artery
Femur
Saphenous nerve
Popliteal artery
Common peroneal nerve
Anterior tibial artery
Posterior tibial artery
Superficial peroneal nerve
Tibia
Deep peroneal nerve
Fibula
Peroneal artery
Dorsal digital nerves of foot

Humerus
Brachial artery
Median nerve
Deep drachial artery
Radial nerve
Radius
Superficial branch of radial nerve
Ulna
Radial artery
Ulnar artery
Ulnar nerve
Median nerva
Deep branch of ulnar nerve
Superficial branch of ulnar nerve
Superficial paimar arterial arch
Palmar digital nerves

Nerves of Limbs

Plate 16

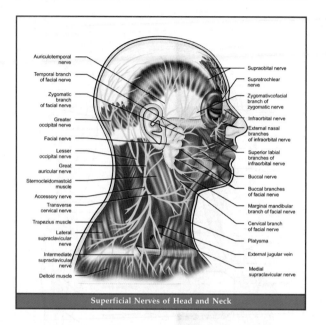

Auriculotemporal nerve

Temporal branch of facial nerve

Zygomatic branch of facial nerve

Greater occipital nerve

Facial nerve

Lesser occipital nerve

Great auricular nerve

Sternocleidomastoid muscle

Accessory nerve

Transverse cervical nerve

Trapezius muscle

Lateral supraclavicular nerve

Intermediate supraclavicular nerve

Deltoid muscle

Supraobital nerve

Supratrochlear nerve

Zygomativcofacial branch of zygomatic nerve

Infraorbital nerve

External nasal branches of infraorbital nerve

Superior labial branches of infraorbital nerve

Buccal nerve

Buccal branches of facial nerve

Marginal mandibular branch of facial nerve

Cervical branch of facial nerve

Platysma

External jugular vein

Medial supraclavicular nerve

Superficial Nerves of Head and Neck

Plate 17

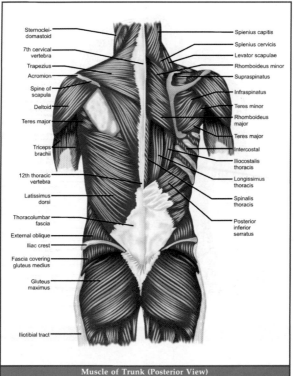

Sternoclei-domastoid

7th cervical vertebra

Trapezius

Acromion

Spine of scapula

Deltoid

Teres major

Triceps brachii

12th thoracic vertebra

Latissimus dorsi

Thoracolumbar fascia

External oblique

Iliac crest

Fascia covering gluteus medius

Gluteus maximus

Iliotibial tract

Splenius capitis

Splenius cervicis

Levator scapulae

Rhomboideus minor

Supraspinatus

Infraspinatus

Teres minor

Rhomboideus major

Teres major

Intercostal

Iliocostalis thoracis

Longissimus thoracis

Spinalis thoracis

Posterior inferior serratus

Muscle of Trunk (Posterior View)

Plate 18

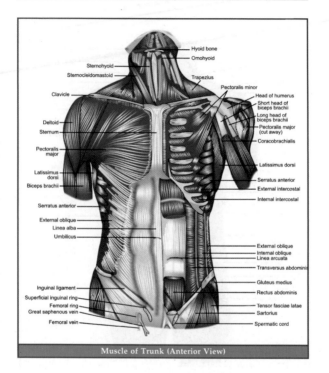

Muscle of Trunk (Anterior View)

Plate 19

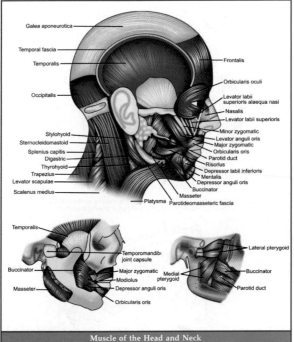

Galea aponeurotica
Temporal fascia
Temporalis
Occipitalis
Frontalis
Orbicularis oculi
Levator labii superioris alaequa nasi
Nasalis
Levator labii superioris
Minor zygomatic
Levator anguli oris
Major zygomatic
Orbicularis oris
Parotid duct
Risorius
Depressor labii inferioris
Mentalis
Depressor anguli oris
Buccinator
Masseter
Parotideomasseteric fascia
Stylohyoid
Sternocleidomastoid
Splenius capitis
Digastric
Thyrohyoid
Trapezius
Levator scapulae
Scalenus medius
Platysma

Temporalis
Buccinator
Masseter
Temporomandibular joint capsule
Major zygomatic
Modiolus
Depressor anguli oris
Orbicularis oris

Lateral pterygoid
Buccinator
Medial pterygoid
Parotid duct

Muscle of the Head and Neck

Plate 20

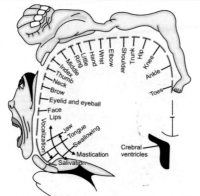

Motor homunculus demonstrating the relative somatotopical representation in the principal motor area of the brain

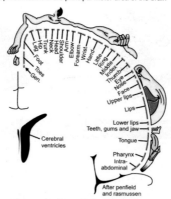

Sensory homunculus demonstrating the relative somatotopical representation in the somesthetic cortex of the brain

Motor-Sensory Homunculus

A

Abadie's sign 1. A sign in tabes dorsalis in which there is loss of pain from squeezing the calcaneal tendon 2. Spasm of the levator palpebrae superioris muscles occurring frequently in thyrotoxicosis but also seen normally especially with tension and fatigue.

Abalienation Mental deterioration or derangement.

Abampere An electromagnetic unit of current equivalent to 10 amperes.

Abapical Away from or opposite the apex.

Abaptiston A conical trephine so designed that it will not slip through the bony opening and injure the underlying dura mater or brain.

Abarognosis Loss or lack of the ability to estimate weight, bragnosis.

Abarticular Not connected with or situated near a joint.

Abarticulation 1. A diarthrodial joint 2. A dislocation of a joint.

Abasia Inability to walk because of motor incoordination; compare astasia.

Abate To lessen in force or intensity; to moderate or subside.

Abattage, abatage 1. The slaughter of animals, specifically, the slaughter of diseased animals to prevent infection of others 2. The art of casting an animal preparatory to an operation.

Abattoir A slaughter house or an establishment for the killing and dressing of animals.

Abaxial Not situated in the line of the axis of a structure.

Abderhalden reaction or test The detection of an abnormal proteolytic enzyme active against a foreign protein elaborated in the course of pregnancy, cancer, schizophrenia and various infections.

Abdomen abstipum An abdominal deformity resulting from congenitally short recti muscles.

Abdominal angina An acute attack of severe abdominal pain, commonly occurring after eating and often associated with weight loss, nausea, vomiting and diarrhoea. It is caused by narrowing or obstruction of the mesenteric arteries, primarily atherosclerotic in origin.

Abdominal aponeurosis The wide tendinous expanse by which the external oblique, internal oblique and transverse muscles are inserted.

Abdominal apoplexy Infarction of an abdominal organ, usually the small intestine, resulting from vascular stenosis or occlusion.

Abdominal dropsy Ascites.

Abdominal epilepsy A convulsive equivalent in which abdominal pain, a sense of nausea and often headache are the most prominent symptoms.

Abdominal influenza Viral gastroenteritis.

Abdominal migraine Abdominal pain, nausea, vomiting or diarrhea associated with migraine. See also convulsive equivalent.

Abdominal ptosis Visceroptosis.

Abdominal reflex Contraction of the abdominal muscles induced by stroking the overlying skin; a superficial or cutaneous reflex.

Abdominal regions The nine regions of the abdomen artificially delineated by two horizontal and two parasagittal lines. The horizontal lines are tangent to the cartilages of the ninth ribs and iliac crests, respectively, and the parasagittal lines are drawn vertically on each side from the middle of the inguinal ligament The regions thus formed are 1. Above—the right hypochondriac, the epigastric and the left hypochondriac. 2. in the middle—the right/left lateral or lumbar, umbilical and, 3. below—the right inguinal or iliac, the pubic or hypo gastric, and the left inguinal or iliac. Also called regions abdominis.

Abdominal respiration A type of respiration caused by the contraction of the diaphragm and the elastic expansion and recoil of the abdominal walls.

Abdominal ribs 1. The floating ribs. 2. Ossifications of the intersections tendineae.

Abdominoposterior In obstetrics, designating a fetal position in which the belly is forward.

Abdominovesical pouch A pouch formed by the reflection of the peritoneum from the anterior abdominal wall onto the distended urinary bladder, it contains the lateral and medial inguinal fossae.

Abducent nerve The sixth cranial nerve, whose fibres arise from the nucleus in the dorsal portion of the pons near the internal genu of the facial nerve and runs a long course to supply the lateral rectus muscle which moves the eyeball outward; also called nerves abducens.

Abducent nucleus A nucleus lying under the floor of the fourth ventricle at the junction of the pons and medulla which gives origin to the abducent nerve.

Abduct To draw away from the median line.

Abduction 1. A movement whereby one part is drawn away from the axis of the body or of an extremity. 2. In ophthalmology (a) Turning of

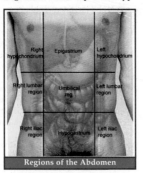

Regions of the Abdomen

the eyes outward beyond parallelism.

Abduction cap An orthopedic appliance of canvas or leather to maintain abduction in case of subdeltoid bursitis.

Abductor A muscle which on contraction, draws a part away from the axis of the body or of an extremity.

Abductor A muscle found in tailed animals corresponding to the coccygeal muscle in man.

Abductor digitiminimi The abductor muscle of the little finger or little toe. Also called musculus abductor digitiminimi.

Abductor hallucis A muscle of the medial side of the foot inserted into the base of the first metatarsal. Also called musculus abductor hallucis.

Abductor hallucis longus A muscle of the anterior region of the leg inserted into the base of the first metatarsal.

Abductor indicis The first dorsal interosseous muscle of the hand.

Abductor ossis metatarsi quinti A variant slip of the abductor digitiminimi inserted into the tuberosity of the fourth metatarsal.

Abductor paralysis Paralysis of abduction especially of the posterior cricoarytenoid muscle and, thus of the vocal cords.

Abductor pollicis brevis The short abductor muscle of the thumb. Also called musculus abductor pollicis.

Abductor pollicis longus The long abductor muscle of the thumb. Also called musculus abductor pollicis longus.

Aberrant Varying or deviating from the normal in form, structure or course.

Aberration 1. Deviation from the normal or usual. 2. Unequal refraction or focalization of a lens. *Chromatic aberration:* unequal refraction of light rays of different wavelengths, producing a blurred image with fringes of color. *Chromosomal aberration:* loss/gain/or exchange of genetic material in the chromosomes of a cell resulting in a deletion, duplication, inversion or translocation of genes.

Abetalipoproteinemia A disease entity due to almost total absence of β-lipoproteins, characterized by the predominating presence in blood of acanthocytes, hypocholesterolemia, the celiac syndrome in early childhood and later ataxia, peripheral neuropathy and frequent retinitis pigmentosa and muscular atrophy; an autosomal hereditary trait.

Abeyance 1. A cessation of activity or function 2. A state of suspended animation.

Abiochemistry Inorganic chemistry.

Abiogenesis A theory that living organisms can originate from nonliving matter; spontaneous generation.

Abionarce Lethargy due to infirmity.

Abiosis 1. Absence of life 2. Nonviability.

Abiotrophy Progressive loss of vitality of certain tissues or organs leading to disorders or loss of function applied especially to degenerative, hereditary diseases of late onset, e.g. Huntington's chorea.

Abirritant An agent such as a cream or powder, that relieves irritation.

Ablasten An antibody like substance, appearing in the blood of rats infected with trypanosomes, which inhibits reproduction of these organisms.

Ablation The removal of part of a tumor by amputation, excision or other mechanical means.

Ablatio placentae Abruptio placenate.

Ablepharia A congenital defect marked by partial or total absence of the eyelids.

Ablepsia Loss or absence of vision.

Abluent Detergent, Cleansing.

Abnormal 1. Not normal. 2. Deviating in form, structure or position, not conforming with the natural or general rule.

ABO blood group That genetically determined blood group system defined by the agglutination reaction of erythrocytes exposed to the naturally occurring antibodies anti-A and anti-B and to similar antiserums. The serum of normal individuals contains isoantibodies against the antigens lacking in their erythrocytes giving the following arrangement of antigens (isoagglutinogens) and antibodies.

Group (Land-steiner)	Erythrolyte Antigen (Agglutinogen) (Agglutinin)	Serum Antibody
0	A and B absent	Anti-A anti-B
A	A	Anti-B
B	B	Anti-A
AB	A,B	NONE

Sub Groups of A are recognised and designated by subscripts as A_1, A_2 etc.

Abort 1. To miscarry, to bring forth a nonviable fetus. 2. To terminate prematurely or stop in the early stages, as the course of a disease. 3. To check or fall short of maximal growth and development.

Aborted systole A premature cardiac systole which produces no peripheral pulse wave because of minimal venticular filling in the short preceding diastole.

Aborticide 1. The killing of an unborn fetus. 2. An agent that destroys fetus and produces abortion.

Abortifacient A drug or agent inducing expulsion of the fetus.

Abortion A broth filtrate of Brucella abortus used to elicit a reaction in patients with active brucellosis or in those who have recovered from the infection.

Abortion 1. The giving birth to an embryo or fetus prior to the stage of viability, i.e. 20 weeks of gestation (fetus weighs less than 400 gm). A distinction is made between abortion and premature birth. Premature infants are those born after the stage of viability has been reached but before full term, 2. The product of such nonviable birth. 3. The arrest of any action or process before its normal completion.

a. accidental Due to a fall, blow or other injury.

a. complete One in which the embryo including the membranes is expelled entirely and identified.

a. criminal Induced termination of pregnancy without medical or legal justification.

a. habitual A condition in which a woman has had three or more consecutive spontaneous abortions.

a. insipient Threatened or imminent or impending abortion in which there is copious vaginal bleeding, uterine contractions and cervical dilation.

a. incomplete In which part of the product of conception has been passed but part (usually the placenta) remains in uterus.

a inevitable One signalled by rupture of the membranes in the presence of cervical dilation that has advanced beyond any hope of preventing complete abortion.

a. missed One in which the fetus dies in utero but the product of conception is retained in utero for two months or longer.

Abortive poliomyelitis An early form of poliomyelitis, characterized clinically by relatively mild symptoms of upper respiratory infection, headache, gastro-intestinal disturbances, nausea, and vomiting but which does not progress to involve the central nervous system. Definite diagnosis tests upon isolation of the virus and serologic reactions.

Abrachia Armlessness.

Abrachiocephalia Congenital absence of the head and arms.

Abrachius An armless individual.

Abrasion 1. A spot denuded of skin, mucous membrane or superficial epithelim by rubbing or scraping as of corneal abrasion, an excoriation. 2. The mechanical wearing down of teeth, as from incorrect brushing, appliances or bruxism. Compare attrition, erosion.

Abreaction In psychoanalysis, the mental process by which repressed emotionally charged memories and experiences are brought to consciousness and occur in hypnosis and narcoanalysis.

Abrikosov's or Abrikosoff's tumor Granular cell myoblastoma.

Abrosia Abstinence from food, fasting.

Abruptio Abruption, a tearing away.

Abruptio placentae Premature separation of the placenta prior to delivery of the infant.

Abscess A circumscribed collection of pus.

a. amebic An abscess of the liver that contains ameba, and may follow amebic dysentery. It may occur independently also without intestinal infection.

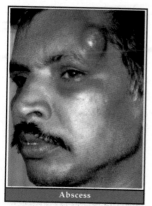

Abscess

a. anorectal One in the connective tissues about the anus.

a. bezold's A deep abscess in the neck associated with suppuration of the middle ear and purulent sinus thrombosis.

a. Brodie's A chronic inflammation, sometimes tuberculus, of the head of a bone especially of the tibia.

a. canalicular An abscess of the breast discharging into the milk ducts.

a. caseous One in which the pus has a soft cheesy consistency.

a. cold Abscess without heat or other usual signs of inflammation commonly tuberculous.

a. delpech's An abscess appearing suddenly but with slight inflammatory symptoms accompanied by marked adynamia.

a. dentoalveolar An abscess confined to the alveolar process investing a tooth's roots.

a. Douglas' Suppuration in Douglas' pouch.

a. Dubois' A cyst of the thymus caused by the growth of thymic tissue into Hassall's corpuscles.

a. epiploic Abscess in or surrounded by omentum majus.

a. glandular An abscess within any gland but especially on or around a lymph node.

a. gummatous One due to the softening and breaking down of a gumma especially in bone or in the thymus of children with congenital syphilis, e.g. Duboisa.

a. ischiorectal One involving the tissues in the ischiorectal fossa.

a. lacoinar One involving the urethral lacunae.

a. milk A mammary abscess occurring during lactation.

a. munro's A microscopic collection of leukocytes found in stratum corneum at the granular layer in psoriasis.

a. omental Abscess in or surrounded by omentum majus.

a. ossifluent Usually a cold wandering abscess originating from a focus of disease in a bone.

a. parametric One in the connective tissue of the broad ligament of the uterus.

a. Pautrier's A microscopic lesion in the epidermis seen in mycosis fungoides. It is composed of the same type of cells as those that form the infiltrate in the corium.

a. pericoronal Infection with collection of pus around the crown of a partially erupted tooth usually upper or lower third molars. Pus collects in a pocket, either distal, distobuccal and or distolingual to the tooth crown.

a. *phegmonous* Circumscribed suppuration associated with acute inflammation of the subcutaneous connective tissue.

a. Pott's Cold or tuberculous a.

a. *wandering* An abscess occurring at a distance from the primary focus of disease, pus burrowing along fascial planes or other structures.

Abscessus flatuosus Tympanitic abscess.

Abscessus perdecobitum Wandering abscess.

Abscissa 1. The horizontal of the two coordinates used in plotting the interrelationship of two sets of data The vertical line is called the ordinate. 2. In optics, the point where a ray of light crosses the principal axis.

Absence 1. Inattention to one's environment. 2. Temporary loss of consciousness, as in absence attacks or psycho motor seizures. 3. Fleeting loss of consciousness occurring in hysterical attacks or at the climax of completed or very intense sexual gratification (Freud).

Absence attack or seizure A form of epilepsy characterized by a sudden transient lapse of consciousness, by a blank stare as in a state of "Suspended animation", sometimes accompanied by minor motor activities such as blinking of the eyes, smacking of lips, stereotyped hand movements and automatism, often there is indistinct vision.

Absolute refractory period: The refractory period in which no stimulus, however strong can excite a response.

Absolute scotoma Scotoma with perception of light entirely absent.

Absolute temperature Temperature reckoned from the absolute zero estimated at approximately -273° C or-459°F.

Absolute threshold The lowest intensity as measured under optimal experimental conditions. At which a stimulus is effective or perceived.

Absolute zero A temperature of approximately-273.2° C or-459.8° F; the complete absence of heat.

Absorb 1. In physiology to suck; take, imbibe as fluids or gases through osmosis and capillarity. 2. To infiltrate into the skin as ultraviolet rays. 3. To incorporate into the body via the blood and lymph. 4. To receive radiant energy and convert it to another form often with rise of temperature.

Absorbance In applied spectroscopy the negative logarithm to the base 10 of transmittance. The term optical density has been used to express the absorbance of solutions.

Absorbable ligature A ligature composed of animal tissue such as catgut which can be absorbed by the tissues.

Absorbed dose In radiology the amount of energy imparted by ionizing particles to a unit mass of irradiated material at a place of interest.

Absorbefacient Any agent that promote absorption.

Absorbent 1. Anything capable of absorbing or sucking up fluids, faeces or light waves, 2. A drug application or dressing that promotes absorption of diseased tissues.

Absorptiometer 1. An instrument which determines the solubility of a gas or the amount absorbed. 2. An apparatus which measures the thickness of a layer of fluid between two parallel sheets of plate glass in apparent apposition.

Absorption 1. In physiology and pharmacology the passage by one or more processes of various body constituents or of medicinal agents through body membranes from one tissue compartment to another, e.g. products of digestion through gastrointestinal mucosa or of drugs through the skin. 2. In physics, and chemistry the taking up by one or more physical or chemical processes of a gas by a solid or liquid or of a liquid by a solid. 3. In physics, radiology and spectro-photometry the process whereby the intensity of a beam of any electromagnetic radiation is attenuated in passing through any material by conversion of the energy of radiation to an equivalent amount of energy which appears within the medium, the radiant energy is converted to heat or some other form of molecular energy. 4. In psychology inattention to all but a single thought or activity.

Absorption atelectasis Obstructive alelectasis.

Absorption band A region of the absorption spectrum in which the absorptivity passes through maximum or inflection.

Absorption coefficient A constant in the law of absorption for homogeneous radiations.

Absorption curve In radiobiology a curve showing variation in absorption of radiation as a function of wave length.

Absorption spectrum A spectrum of radiation which has passed through some selectively absorbing substance as white light after it has passed through a vapor.

Absorptive Absorbent.

Abstergent 1. Having cleansing or purgative properties. 2. A cleaning lotion. 3. A purgative.

Abstinence Voluntary self denial of or forbearance from, indulgence of appetites, especially from food, alcoholic drink or sex relations.

Abstinence delirium Delirium occurring on withdrawal of alcohol or of a drug from one addicted to it.

Abulia Loss or defect of the ability to make decisions.

Abulomania Mental disorder characterized by lack of will power and indecisiveness.

Acalcerosis Calcium deficiency of the diet or of the body as a result of the loss of the mineral in the excreta.

Acalculia Loss of the power to work out any mathematical problems even the simplest.

Acampsia Rigidity of a joint; ankylosis.

Acanthesthesia A form of paresthesia in which there is a sensation as of a pinprick.

Acanthion The tip of the anterior nasal spine.

Acanthocephaliasis Infestation with a species of acanthocephala.

Acanthocheilonema A genus of filaria worms parasitic in man characterised by adult forms that live chiefly in the body cavities or in skin and subcutaneous tissue.

a. perstans The 'persistent filaria', is prevalent in tropical Africa and the northern part of South America, characterised by adult forms that live in the peritoneal, pericardial cavities and by microfilaria that are not sheathed and manifest no periodicity in the circulating blood; transmitted by culioides species (biting gnats). A. perstans is usually regarded as a harmless parasite but some observers think that it may cause oedema and a condition that resembles trypanosomiasis. Formerly termed Filaria sanguinis.

a. streptocerca A species of filaria worms found only rarely and exclusively in natives of tropical Africa characterized by adult forms that live in the dermis and subcutaneous tissues and by microfilaria that are not sheathed and manifest biperiodicity in the circulating blood, may cause rare examples of chronic edema of the skin. Formerly termed Microfilaria streptocera.

Acanthocyte A throny or peculiarly spiny erythrocyte characterized by multiple spiny cytoplasmic projections.

Acanthocytosis A rare condition in which as many as 70 to 80 percent of the redblood cells are acanthocytes 'throny erythrocytes, i.e. peculiar spherocytes with irregularly placed broad or coarse pseudopodia like projections; the abnormal cells manifest a greatly increased mechanical fragility and content of lipolecithin A; is thought to result from a mutant recessive allele for a gene that controls normal structure of redblood cells.

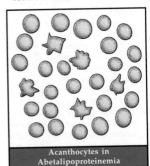

Acanthocytes in Abetalipoproteinemia

Acanthoid Spine shaped, spinous.

Acanthokeratodermia Hyperkeratosis.

Acantholysis A term used in dermal pathology to denote dissolution of the layers of the epidermis. It is seen in such conditions as pemphigus vulgaris and keratosis follicularis.

Acanthoma Well differentiated keratinizing cornifying squamous cell (or epidermoid) carcinoma, term sometimes used especially with reference to such neoplasms in the skin with little or no histologic evidence of invasion. Regarded by some observers as benign neoplasms.

a. adenoidescysticum A cutaneous disease consisting of multiple small (2 to 5 mm) pearly yellow or flesh colored nodules of neoplastic benign epithelial cells derived from basal cell of the epidermis or similar cells in hairs follicles occurring mostly on the face, at the root of the nose, temples, eyelids, cheek, forehead and chin. Also known as epithelioma adenoids cysticum or multiple benign cystic epithelioma, sometimes associated with syringoma or cylindroma.

a. acanthosis An increase in the thickness of the prickle cell layer of the epidermis. May be due to an increase in the size of the cells.

a. nigricans An eruption of warty growths and hyperpigmentation occurring in the skin of the axillae and in the groins. In adults it is indicative of abdominal malignancy. A benign type occurs in children. In the benign or juvenile type the subjects are obese and the skin condition is self limited.

Acarbia Pronounced reduction in bicarbonate of the blood.

Acardia Congenital absence of the heart, a condition sometimes present in the parasitic members of conjoined twins.

Acardiacus A conjoined twin parasitic on its mate or utilizing the placental circulation of its mate and having no heart.

Acariasis Any disease caused by an acarid.

Acarid A member of the order Acarina, a mite.

Acaroid 1. Resembling a mite 2. An acarus or mite.

Acarophobia Fear of small parasites or small particles

Acatalepsia, catalepsy 1. Mental deficiency characterized by a lack of understanding 2. Uncertainty in diagnosis or prognosis.

Acataleptic Deficient in comprehension. 2. Uncertain.

Acataphasia A loss of the power of correctly formulating a statement.

Acataposis Difficulty in swallowing liquids; strictly inability to do so.

Acathexia An abnormal loss of the secretions.

Acathexis A mental disorder in which certain objects or ideas fail to arouse an emotional response in the individual.

Accident A sudden unexpected event or injury occurring without omen or forewarning or developing in the course of a disease.

Accommodation Adjustment of the eye for various distances specifically alteration of the covexity of the crystalline lens in order to bring light rays from an external object to a focus on the retina.

Accoucheur Obstetrician.

Accretic cordis Adhesion of the pericardium to adjacent extra-cardiac structures.

Accretion 1. Increase by addition to the periphery or material of the same nature as that already present, e.g. the manner of growth of crystals. 2. In dentistry foreign material collecting on the surface of a tooth or in a cavity. 3. A growing together.

Acebutolol Betadrenergic blocking agent used in hypertension.

Aceclidine A synthetic compound resembling acecholine, used in glaucoma 0.5–4%.

Acenesthesia Absence of the normal sensation of physical existence or of the consciousness of visceral function.

Acecainide A metabolite of pro-cainamide.

Acenocoumarol (NND) An orally effective synthetic anticoagulant of the coumarin type and with similar action.

Acephalechiria Absence of head and hands.

Acephalopodus A malformed fetus without head or feet.

Acephalogastria Absence of head, thorax and abdomen as noted in a parasitic twin with pelvis and legs only.

Acephalopodia Congenital absence of head and feet.

Acephalostoamus A malformed fetus having partically no head, but with a mouth like opening in its uppermost region.

Accervuloma An intracranial tumor containing ocervulus or brain sand, psammoma.

Acervulus Brain sand.

Acescence 1. A slight degree of acidity. 2. The process of becoming sour.

Acescent Slightly acid.

Acestoma Exuberant granulations that are forming a cicatrix.

Acetal A clear liquid made by the imperfect oxidation of alcohol. Has been used as hypnotic.

Acetal dehyde 1. Acetic aldehyde 2. Elthaldehyde ethanol, CH_3CHO, a colourless liquid of irritating odor; it is polymerized into paraldehyde in presence of sulphuric acid. It is an intermediate in yeast fermentation of carbohydrate and in alcohol metabolism in man.

Acetatmide Acetic acid amide formed by the action of ethyl acetate on ammonia, occurs in colourless deliquescent crystals of a mousy odor.

Acetaminophen N-Acetyl-p-amino-phenol, P-acetamidophenol, a white odorless crystalline slightly bitter powder used as an anti-pyretic and analgesic.

Acetanilide Made from aniline by the action upon it of acetyl chloride. Occurs in the form of white scales or crystalline powder, very slightly soluble in water but soluble in 5 parts of alcohol, used as an analgesic and antipyretic Toxic, continued use causes cyanosis.

Acetarsone Acetarsol(BP) acetyl amino hydroxy phenyl arsenic acid, N acetyl-4- hydroxy-M-arsanilic acid; stovarsol, used in amebiasis and as a local application in vincents angina and in trichomonas vaginalis.

Acetate A salt of acetic acid.

Acetazolamide Diamox, the heterocyclic sulfonamide. 2. Acetylamino-1.3.4, thiadiazole 5-sulfonamide. It inhibits the action of carbonic anhydrase in the kidney causing an increase in the urinary excretion of sodium, potassium and bicarbonate, reduced excretion of ammonium, a rise in the pH of the urine and a fall in the pH of the blood. Has been used in respiratory acidosis for diuresis and control of fluid retention in epilepsy and in glaucoma.

Acetic Relating to vinegar, sour.

Acid-acetic Diacetic acid, CH_3, COOH, a product of the oxidation of alcohol and of the destructive distillate of wood, the official acid is a liquid containing 36 percent (BP 33%) of absolute acetic acid (hydrogen acetate). Used locally as a counterirritant and occasionally internally. Used also as a reagent.

Acetoacetic acid Diacetic acid, CH_3 $COCH_2$ COOH, one of the ketone bodies formed in excess and appearing in the urine in starvation or diabetes.

Acetobacter A genus of the family pseudomonadaceae, containing rodshaped organisms frequently found in elongated, branched or swollen forms, polarly flagellate when motile, energy secured by oxidation of alcohol in wine cider or beer to acetic acid.

Acetohexamide A sulfonylurea, used in diabetes.

Acetokinase An enzyme found in Escherichia coli catalyzing the formation of acetylphosphate from acetate in the presence of ATP.

Acetolactic acid An intermediate in pyruvic acid catabolism in yeast.

Acetolase An enzyme that catalyzes the oxidation of alcohol to acetic acid.

Acetomenaphthone Used in the preparative treatment of obstructive jaundice, in hemorrhagic disease of the newborn and prophylactically to prevent neonatal hemorrhage.

Acetomeroctol An organic mercurial antibacterial agent.

Acetomorphine Heroin, see diacetylmorphine.

Acetonaphthone Naphthyl methyl ketone occurs as yellow needles.

Acetone A colourless volatile inflammable liquid dimethyl ketone. Extremely small amounts are found in normal urine but large quantities occur in urine and blood of diabetic persons, it sometimes imparts an ethereal odor to urine and breath of such patient.

Acetonuria The excretion in the urine of large amount of acetone, an indication of incomplete oxidation of large amount of fat, commonly occurs in diabetic acidosis.

Acetophenazine maleate Tindal maleate, phenothiazine dimaleate, a tranquilizing agent with antiemetic hypotensive spasmolytic and antihistaminic actions.

Acetophenetidin Occurs as colourless glistening crystals usually scaly or a fine white glistening powder, antipyretic.

Acetophenone A coal tar derivative, phenylethyl ketone, a colorless liquid crystalizing to white needles at low temperatures with an odor, of bitter almond. Has been used as a hypnotic or mild depressant.

Acetrizoate A radio-opaque compound used in urography, injected intravenously.

Acetrizoic acid A radio-opaque medium.

Acetyl-p-aminophenylsalicylate Salicylic acid ester of acetyl-p-aminophenol, used as an analgesic, antipyretic, and intestinal antiseptic.

Acetylcholine The acetic acid ester of choline isolated from ergot. Also liberated from preganglionic and postganglionic, endings of parasympathetic fibers and from preganglionic fibers of the sympathetic. Causes cardiac inhibition, vasodilation, gastrointestinal peristalsis and other parasympathetic effects. It is hydrolized into choline and acetic acid by the enzyme cholinesterase that is present in blood and other tissue.

Acetylcholinesterase Cholinesterase, that breaks down acetyl choline into choline and acetic acid.

Acetylcoenzyme A Condensation product of coenzyme A and acetic acid, an intermediate in transfer of two carbon fragment notably in its entrance into the tricarboxylic acid cycle.

Acetylcysteine Mucomyst, a mucolytic agent that reduces the viscosity of mucous secretions.

Acetyldigitoxin Acylanid, same actions and uses as digitoxin but of more rapid onset and shorter duration of action.

Acetylene A colorless gas of a disagreeable odor that burns with an intense white flame. It is prepared commercially by the action of water on calcium carbide.

N-Acetylglucosamine A hydrolysis product of some mucopolysaccharides, notably of hyaluronic acid.

Acetylphenylhydrazine A crystalline powder obtained by treating phenylhydrazine with acetic anhydride, a powerful antipyretic but destructive to red blood cells. Used in polycythemia vera, also used externally in parasitic skin diseases as 10 percent ointment.

Acetylphosphate A high energy phosphate that plays the part of "active acetate" in the metabolism of various bacteria.

3-Acetylpyridine An antimetabolite of nicotinamide, produces symptoms of nicotenamide deficiency when fed to mice.

Acetylsalicylic acid An odorless white crystalline powder soluble in 300 part of water or 5% alcohol readily absorbed from mucous membranes and excreted in urine within 6 hours, widely used as an analgesic, anti-inflammatory agent and in the treatment of rheumatism.

Achalasia Failure to relax, referring especially to visceral openings such as the cardia or any other sphincter of muscles.

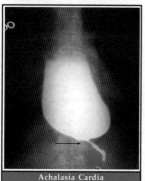
Achalasia Cardia

Acheilia Congenital absence of the lips.

Achilles A mythical greek warrior who was vulnerable only in the heel.

Achillodynia Pain due to inflammation of the bursa between the calcaneus and the tendo Achilles, (achillobursitis).

Achilliotomy Division of the tendo calcaneus.

Achiria 1. Congenital absence of the hands. 2. Anesthesia with loss of the sense of possession of one or both hands, a condition sometimes noted in hysteria. 3. A form of dyschiria in which the patient is unable to tell on which side of the body a stimulus has been applied.

Achirus A malformed individual without hands.

Achlorhydria Absence of hydro-chloric acid from the gastric juice.

Achluophobia Fear of darkness.

Acholia Suppressed secretion of bile.

Acholic Without bile.

Acholuria Absence of bile pigments from the urine in certain cases of jaundice.

Acholuric Without bile in urine.

Achondroplasia Chondrodystrophy, diaphysial aclasis, abnormality in conversion of cartilage into bone resulting in an asymmetrical dwarf.

Achondroplasty Chondrodystrophy.

Achorion A genus of parasitic fungi, proper term now Trichophyton.

Achroacytosis The occurrence of a great number of lymphocytes in the peripheral circulation; lympho-cytosis.

Achromasia 1. Cachectic pallor, pallor associated with the Hipocratic facies of extremely severe and chronic illness often heralding the moribund state 2. Absence of the ordinary staining reaction in a cell or tissue. 3. Achromatopsia.

Achromate An absolutely color blind person.

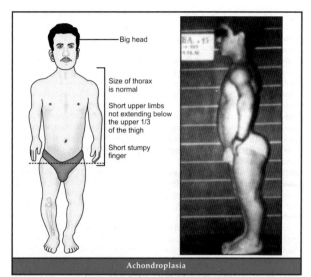

- Big head
- Size of thorax is normal
- Short upper limbs not extending below the upper 1/3 of the thigh
- Short stumpy finger

Achondroplasia

Achromatic 1. Colorless. 2. Not decomposing white light. 3. Not staining readily.

Achromatolysis Plasmalysis, protoplasmolysis, karyoplasmolysis–dissolution of the chromatic of a cell or of its nucleus.

Achromatophil 1. Not being colored by the histologic or bacteriologic stains. 2. A cell or tissue that cannot be stained in the usual way.

Achromatopsia Complete color blindness.

Achromatosis Absence of natural pigmentation as in albinism.

Achromaturia The passage of colorless or very pale urine.

Achylia 1. Absence of gastric juice or other digestive forment 2. Absence of chyle.

Achylous 1. Lacking in gastric juice or other digestive secretion. 2. Having no chyle.

Acid 1. A compound of an electronegative element or radical with hydrogen; it forms salts by replacing all or part of the hydrogen with electropositive elements or radical. An acid containing one displaceable atom of hydrogen in the molecule is called monobasic; one-containing two such atoms dibasic and one containing more than two-polybasic. 2. In popular language any chemical compound which has a sour taste.

Acidaminuria The passage of an excess of amino acid in the urine.

Acidemia An increase in the H-ion concentration of the blood–a fall below normal in pH not withstanding alterations in content of bicarbonate.

Acid-fast A term denoting bacteria that are not decolorized by mineral acids after having been stained with aniline dyes; the leprosy, tubercle and hay bacilli are examples.

Acidismus Poisoning by acids introduced from without as contradistinguished from acidosis or poisoning by acids formed in metabolism.

Acidosis Oxysis, a condition of reduced alkali reserve (bicarbonate) of the blood and other body fluids with or without an actual decrease in pH.

a. carbon dioxide Acidosis resulting from retention of CO_2, it is an exception to the definition in the main heading, for the bicarbonate of the body fluids is usually increased.

a. compensated Reduced alkali reserve in which compensatory mechanisms maintain the pH of the body fluids at the normal value; in compensated acidosis CO_2 and bicarbonate usually increases although pH remains within normal range.

a. renal tubular Inability to excrete acid urine with hyper-chloremia due to congenital defect in carbonic anhydrase. causing deficient formation of bicarbonate.

a. respiratory Reduced alkali reserve of the body fluids with a fall in pH resulting from the failure of adequate compensatory mechanisms; bicarbonate may be within normal range in uncompensated acidosis from CO_2 retention.

Acinus 1. One of the minute sac like secretory portions of an acinous gland. Some authorities use the terms acinus and alveolus interchangeably with reference to glands whereas other differentiate them by the constricted openings of the acinus into the excretory duct. 2. In the lung territory supplied by one terminal bronchiole (an absolute usage).

Acivicis A pyrimidine analog that blocks conversion of UTP to LTP.

Aclasis Pathologic tissue originating from and continuous with normal tissues thereby providing continuity of structure as in chondrodystrophy.

Aclusion Lack of contact of opposing surface of molar and bicuspid teeth when jaws are closed.

Acne The period of greatest intensity of any symptom, sign or process.

Acne A papular and pustular eruption due to inflammation with accumulation of secretion involving the sebaceous glands.

a. agminata Acnitis, an eruption of small dusky reddish papules on the face becoming pustular and followed by slight scarring.

a. artificialis Produced by external irritants such as tar or drugs internally administered such as iodine. Often self inflicted.

a. atrophica Vulgaris in which the lesions leave a slight amount of scarring.

a. ciliaris Follicular papules and pustules on the free edges of the eyelids.

a. decalvans A rare type of pustular folliculitis of scalp producing scar and then a alopecia.

a. keratosa An eruption of papules consisting of horny plugs projecting from the hair follicles accompanied by inflammation.

a. neonatorum A rare condition in infants characterized by papules and comedones on forehead and cheeks.

a. papulosa A condition that resembles chloracne in that black central comedones are present in all the lesions.

a. rosacea Erythematosa, rosacea, acne of the cheeks and nose associated with papules, pustules, dilated blood vessels in the nasolabilal folds and dilated follicles.

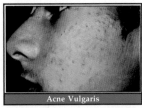
Acne Vulgaris

a. syphilitica Pustular syphilides, a rare type of secondary; syphilis.

a. telangiectodes An acneiform eruption associated with tuberculosis.

a. urticata An eruption beginning as small urticarial wheals and followed by slight scarring.

a. vulgaris Acne simplex, acne disseminata, simple uncomplicated acne, an eruption of papules and pustules on an inflammatory

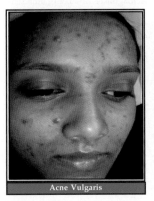
Acne Vulgaris

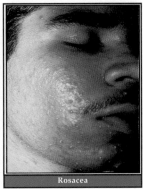
Rosacea

base; condition occurs primarily during puberty and adolescence due to overactive sebaceous apparatus, probably affected by hormonal activity.

Acnegenic Pertaining to substances thought to be responsible for causing acne vulgaris.

Acnemia 1. Atrophy of the calf muscles. 2. Congenital absence of legs.

Acognosia, acognosy A knowledge of remedies.

Acology Therapeutics.

Acomania Servile submission to those in authority while being over-domineering at home.

Acomia Alopecia, baldness.

Aconative Without the desire or wish to act.

Aconite The dried root of Aconitum napellus, Antipyretic, diuretic, diaphoretic anodyne, cardiac and respiratory depressant, externally analgesic.

Acoprosis Absence or great scanti-ness of fecal matter in the intestines.

Acorea Congenital absence of the pupil of the eye.

Acoria Absence of the feeling of satiety after eating.

Acousma An auditory hallucination in which indefinite sounds such as ringing or hissing are heard.

Acoustic Relating to hearing or the perception of sound.

Acousticophobia Fear of sounds.

Acoustics The science of sounds and their perception.

Acquired Denoting a disease predisposition, that is not congenital but has developed after birth.

Acrania Lack of a cranium.

Acremoniosis A condition marked by fever and the occurrence of gumma like swellings caused by a fungus Acremonium potronii.

Acriflavine An acridine dye, a mixture of 2:8 diamino-10-methyl-acaridinium chloride and 2,8 diaminacridine. A brownish red odorless powder soluble in water. A powerful antiseptic.

a. hydrochloride Acid acriflavine, acid trypaflavine, used as a wound antiseptic. It has been administered intravenously in brucellosis, tularemia, blastomycosis, and trypanosomiasis.

Acrimony The quality of being intensely irritant; biting or pungent.

Acrisorcin Antifungal agent available as 0.2% cream.

Acritochromacy Color blindness.

Acroagnosis Absence of limb sen-sibility.

Acrobrachycephaly Condition in which the anteroposterior diameter of the skull is abnormally short.

Acrocephaly Malformation of the head consisting in a high or pointed cranial vault due to premature closure of the sagittal, coronal and lamboid sutures.

Acrocyanosis A circulatory disorder in which the hands and less commonly the feet are persistently cold, blue, and sweaty. Milder forms are closely allied to chillblains.

Acrodolichomelia Large size and disproportionate growth of the hands and feet.

Acrodynia 1. Peripheral neuritis of the fingers or toes 2. A condition caused in rats by a deficiency of pyridoxine (B6) characterized by redness and swelling of the tips of the ears and nose leading to necrosis of these parts.

Acroesthesia 1. Extreme degree of hyperesthesia 2. Hyperesthesia of one or more extremities.

Acrogeria Premature aging of the skin of the hands and feet.

Acromegaly Acromegalia; Marie disease, a trophic disorder marked by progressive enlargement of the head and face, hands and feet and thorax due to excessive secretion of growth hormone by the anterior lobe of the pituitary gland.

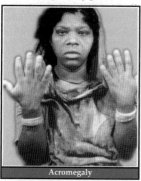
Acromegaly

Acromelagia A vasomotor neurosis marked by redness, pain and swelling of the fingers and toes, headache and vomiting, probably the same as erythromelalgia.

Acromion Acromial process, the outer end of the spine of the scapula which projects as a broad flattened process overhanging the glenoid fosssa; it articulates with the clavicle and gives attachment to the deltoid and some fibers of the trapezius muscles.

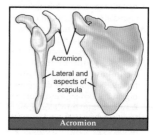
Acromion

Acropachy Hypertrophic pulmonary osteoarthropathy.

Acropathy Simple hereditary clubbing of the digits without associated pulmonary or other progressive disease; often more severe in males, autosomal dominant inheritance.

Acrophobia A morbid dread of elevated places.

Acrose A sugar obtained by the action of a weak alkaline solution on formaldehyde.

Acrosome The juxtanuclear body at the anterior extermity of a spermatid derived from the Golgi apparatus.

Acrotism Absence or imperceptibility of the pulse; pulselessness.

Actin One of the protein components into which actomyosin can be split. Can exist in a fibrous form (f-actin) or a globular form (G-actin).

Actinobacillus A genus of the family Bricellacea, Gram negative non-motile small rods or coccoid forms characterized by the tendency to form aggregates in tissues or culture which resemble the sulfur granules of actinomycosis. Pathogenic for animals, some species attack man.

Actinomyces Ray fungus so called because it occurs in the form of aggregation of radiating clubshaped rods; a genus of the family Actinomycetaceae, containing nonmotile branching filamentous organisms forming a mycelium and fragmenting into elements of irregular sizes. They are mostly anaerobic but some are microaerophilic. A few of the species are pathogenic for man; several cause scab and other potato diseases but the greater number of them are nonpathogenic soil organisms.

Actinomycin An antibacterial crystalline substance isolated from Actinomyces (streptomyces) antiboiticus. Active against Gram positive bacteria, e.g. *Bacillus subtilis;* slightly active against Gram negative bacteria. It is also fungicidal and toxic to animal tissues. There are three close similar compounds termed A, B and C.

Actinomycosis A disease of cattle and swine, sometimes communicated to man, caused by the ray fungus Actinomyces (Nocardia). It affects the jaw most commonly (lumpy jaw) but it may invade the brain, lungs or gastroenteric tract. It is characterized by the formation of granulomas of sluggish growth which eventually breakdown and discharge a viscid pus containing minute yellowish granules; the constitutional symptoms are of a septic character.

Actiophage A virus destructive to actinomycetes.

Actinophore A mixture of three parts cercum dioxide and one part thorium dioxide used in roentgen ray diagnosis.

Activation 1. The act of rendering active 2. An increase in the energy content of an atom or molecule through the raising of temperature absorption or light photons, etc. which renders that atom or molecule more reactive. 3. Techniques of altering the physiologic environment of the brain by stimulating it by light sound or electricity in order to produce hidden or latent abnormal activity in the electroencephalogram. 4. Stimulation of cell division in an ovum by fertilization or by artificial means.

Activator 1. A substance that renders another substance such as an enzyme active. 2. Internal secretion of the pancreas. 3. An apparatus for impregnating water with radium emanation. 4. A catalyst or accelerator for the polymerization of resins.

Active 1. Production effect; not passive. 2. More than usually likely to undergo some chemical– reaction.

a. **transport** The name given to the passage of ions or molecules across a cell membrane not by passive diffusion but by an energy consuming process. Active diffusion can take place against a concentration gradient.

Actomysoin A protein complex composed of the globulin mysoin and actin in the micellae of the muscle fiber. It is the essential contractile substance of muscle.

Actonia A Fungus that causes yellowish patches on the pharyngeal mucous membrane which may be mistaken for diphtheria, belongs to order Endomycetales.

Acuity Sharpness, clearness, distinctness.

a. visual Acuteness of vision; it is indicated by a fraction in which numerator is a number expressing the distance in feet at which the patient sees a line or typed on the chart (usually 20 feet) and the denominator a number expressing the distance in feet at which the normal eye would see the smallest letters which the patient sees at the distance at which he is; thus if at 20 feet he sees only the letters which the normal eye would see at 50 feet the formula of his vision will be V = 20/50.

Acupuncture Puncture made with long fine needles for diagnostic or therapeutic purposes.

Acyclovir Antiviral agent used in herpes.

Acyesis 1. Sterility in the woman. 2. The nonpregnant condition.

N-Acylsphingosine N-Acylsphingol, a condensation product of an organic acid with sphingosine at the amino group of the latter compound.

Adamantine Exceedingly hard specifically relating to the enamel of the teeth.

Adamantinoma A tumor of jaw, arising from enamel cells. May be benign or of low grade malignancy. *SYN*—ameloblastoma.

Adams-Stokes syndrome Black out due to sudden fall in cerebral circulation commonly after heartblock.

Addict A person who finds it difficult to stop some practice especially the taking of drugs or excessive use of alcohol.

Addiction Habituation to some practice, withdrawal from which causes symptoms.

Addisin Factor in gastric tissue and gastric mucosa that acts upon the extrinsic factor to produce the hematinic principle of liver.

Additive A substance not essentially part of a material such as food, fuel, etc. but which is deliberately added to fulfill some specific purpose.

Adducent To draw toward the median line.

Adduction 1. Movement of a limb toward the central axis of the body or beyond it. 2. A position resulting from such movement.

Adductor A muscle drawing a part towards the medianline.

Adenase A deaminating enzyme in the liver, pancreas and spleen that converts adenosine into hypoxanthine.

Adenine One of the two purines found in both ribonucleic acid and deoxyribonucleic acid; found also in various nucleotides of importance to the body, e.g. adenylic acid adenosine triphosphate (ATP) coenzymes I and II, Q-nitrogen.

Adenitis Inflammation of a lymph node or of a gland.

Adenoacanthoma A malignant neoplasm consisting chiefly of glandular epithelium (adenocarcinoma) usually well differentiated with foci of metaplasia to squamous (or epedermoid) neoplastic cells.

Adenoblast An embryonic cell destined to proliferate into cells that will enter into the formation of a gland.

Adenocarcinoma A malignant neoplasm of epithelial cells in glandular or glandlike pattern; frequently with infiltration of adjacent tissue, metastases, recurrence after removal, etc. a malignant adenoma.

Adenocyst A cystic tumor developing from glandular epithelium, adenocystoma.

Adenocystoma Adenoma in which the neoplastic glandular epithelium forms cysts or cysts like structures.

Adenohypophysis Anterior lobe, pars anterior or pars glandularis of the pituitary gland.

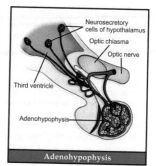

Neurosecretory cells of hypothalamus
Optic chiasma
Optic nerve
Third ventricle
Adenohypophysis

Adenohypophysis

Adenoid Gland like, adeniform, lymphoid; denoting a form of connective tissue found in the lymph nodes, spleen, tonsils, solitary and aggregated nodules of the intestine, red bone marrow and elsewhere; it consists of a connective tissue frame work or reticulum; containing masses of round cells (lymphocytes) in its interestices.

Adenoidism Symptoms and signs associated with enlarged adenoids.

Adenoleiomyofibroma A benign neoplasm of mesodermal origin consisting chiefly of fibroblasts and connective tissue with neoplastic smooth muscle cells, glandular or adenomatous elements.

Adenoma A neoplasm of glandular epithelium.

a. chromophobe A tumor of the chromophobe cells of the anterior pituitary body associated with hypopituitarism, the cells do not stain well with acid or basic dyes.

a. eosinophilic A tumor of the eosinophilic chromophil cells of the anterior pituitary associated with gigantism and acromegaly.

a. getsowa's An adenocarcinoma of the thyroid gland formerly thought to originate in a lateral angle but probably represents a metastasis from a primary neoplasm in the gland per se, termed also struma postbranchiallis.

a. islet cell A benign neoplasm of the pancreas composed of tissue similar in structure to that of the islets of Langerhans. It may contain functioning beta cells and may cause hypoglycemia, sometimes termed insulinoma or Langerhansiana.

a. malignant Sometimes used for adenocarcinoma especially when a portion of an adenoma is thought to be histologically malignant or metastatic neoplasm of similar type is recognised.

a. racemose A benign neoplasm composed of epithelial tissue resembling racemose gland.

a. sebaceum A neoplasm occurring on the face composed of a mass of sebaceous glands and appearing as an aggregation of red yellow and yellow papules; the patients are sometimes mentally retarded with seizure.

Adenomyosis The ectopic occurrence or diffuse implantation of adenomatous tissue in muscle (usually smooth muscle) as in benign invasion of myometrium by endometrial tissue.

Adenomyxoma A benign neoplasm with histologic characteristics of adenoma and myxoma.

Adenosarcoma A malignant neoplasm of mesodermal tissue with adenomatoid element, sometimes applied to sarcoma originating in connective tissue of a gland.

Adenosine A condensation product of adenine and D-ribose a nucleoside which can be found among the hydrolysis products of all nucleic acids and of the various adenine nucleotides.

Adenosine diphosphate A condensation product of adenosine with pyrophosphoric acid, ADP, formed from adenosine triphosphate (ATP) by the hydrolysis of the terminal phosphate group of latter compound.

Adenosis A more or less generalized glandular disease especially one involving the lymphatic nodes.

Adenotome An instrument for the removal of adenoids in the nasopharynx.

Adenylate cyclase An enzyme that synthesizes c-AMP.

Adiaphoresis Absence or deficiency of perspiration.

Adiaphoretic A drug that causes repression of perspiration.

Adipocere A fatty substance of waxy consistency into which dead animal tissues are sometime converted when kept from the air under certain favouring conditions of temperature; it is believed to be produced by the conversion into fat of the proteins of the tissues.

Adipokinn An anterior pituitary factor that brings about mobilization of fat from kidney and liver depots.

Adiposis An excessive local or general accumulation of fat in the body, liposis.

a. dolorosa Dercum's disease, an affection characterized by a deposit of symmetrical nodular or pendulous masses of fat in various regions of the body attended with more or less pain.

a. tuberosa simplex Anders disease, an affection resembling A. dolorsa in which the fat occurs in small more or less circumscribed masses on the abdomen or confined to the extremities; these masses are sensitive to the touch and may be spontaneously painful.

Adipsia Absence of thirst.

Adjuvant That which aids or assists; denoting a remedy that is added to a prescription to assist or increase the action of the main ingredient; synergist.

Adolescence Period of attaining complete growth and maturity

Adolescent Pertaining to the period or state of adolescence.

Adonis The herb Adonis vernalis. It has a digitalis like action and is sometimes used as a cardiac stimulant and diuretic.

Adrenaline Trade name for epinephrine.

Adrenalism A condition resulting from abnormal function of the adrenal (suprarenal) glands, suprarenalism.

Adrenergic Relating to nerve fibers that liberate adrenaline.

Adrenochrome The red oxidation product of epinephrine, was used therapeutically in Germany during the second world war to increase efficiency of diabetic laborers. It is said to produce psychic changes.

Adrenocorticotrophin Adrenocorticotrophic hormone.

Adrenosterone An androgen isolated from the adrenal cortex, also known as andrenosterone and as Reichsteins compound G.

Adriamycin Doxorubicin, an anticancer antibiotic.

Adsorb To attach atoms or molecules to the surface of a substance by means of unsatisfied valence bonds.

Adsorbent A substance which adsorbs, e.g. ADTE, carbon, clay, magnesia, etc.

Adtorsion Internal rotation of both eyes.

Adult Fully grown and mature, a fully grown individual.

Adulterant Impurity, additive that is considered to have an undesirable effect.

Adulteration The alteration of any substance by the deliberate addition of a component not ordinarily part of that substance, usually used to imply that the substance is debased as a result.

Adventitia The outer most covering of any organ or structure which is poorly derived from without and does not form an integral part of such organ or structure specifically the outer coat of an artery; the tunica adventitia.

Adventitious 1. Coming from without; extrinsic. 2. Accidental. 3. Relating to the adventitia of an artery or an organ.

Adynamia Weakness, vital debility, asthenia.

Aerasthenia A psychoneurotic condition marked by worry, lack of self confidence and mild depression occurring in aviators.

Aerobacter A genus of the tribe Escherichia, family Enterobacteriacea, containing rod shaped Gram negative organisms, found chiefly in the intestine.

Aerocystography X-ray of bladder after air has been injected into it.

Aerodynamics The study of air and other gases in motion, the forces that set them in motion, and the result of such motion.

Aerometer An apparatus for determining the density of or for weighing air.

Aerophagia Swallowing of air.

Aeropholia Abnormal and extreme dread of fresh air or of air in motion.

Aeroscope An instrument for the examination of air for visible impurities.

Aetinolol Cardioselective beta-blocker used in hypertension.

Afebrile Nonfebrile, apyretic.

Affect 1. Feeling 2. The sum of an emotion.

Afferent Bringing to or into, denoting certain arteries, veins, lymphatics and nerves.

Affinity 1. Attraction. 2. In chemistry the force that attracts certain atoms to unite with certain others to form compound 3. The selective staining of a tissue by a dye or the uptake of a dye chemical or other substance selectively by a tissue.

Affusion The pouring of water upon the body or any of its parts for therapeutic purposes

Afibrinogenemia The absence of a detectable amount of fibrinogen in the blood, a relatively rare cause of hemorrhages.

Afterbirth The placenta and membranes that are extruded after the birth of the fetus and most other mammals.

Aftercare The care and treatment of a patient after operation, or of one convalescing from an acute or serious illness.

After discharge The prolongation of reflex response after cessation of stimulation.

After image 1. After vision, Spectrum. 2. Ocular spectrum, the image of an object of which the subjective sensation persists after the object has disappeared. It is called positive when its colors are the same as in the original, negative when the complementary colors are perceived

After pains Painful cramplike contractions of the uterus occurring after child birth.

After potential The small changes in electrical potential in a stimulated nerve which follow the main potential change. They follow the "spike" potential of the oscillographic record and consists of an initial negative deflection followed by a positive deflection in the oscillograph record.

Agalactia Absence of milk in the breasts after child birth.

Agammaglobulinemia A condition characterized by 1. A lack or extremely low levels, of gamma globulin in the blood (and lymphoid tissue) 2. Defective formation of antibody and. 3, Frequent occurrence of suppurative and nonsuppurative infectious disease observed in 2 clinical forms, i.e. primary and secondary.

a. acquired A type of primary agammaglobulinemia occurs in both sexes at various ages probably resulting from pathological alteration or destruction of normal lymphoid tissue. Level of gamma globulin likely to be from zero to 100 or 125 mg per 100 ml.

a. congenital A type of primary agammaglobulinemia occurs chiefly in male infants more than 4 to 6 months of age probably resulting from sex linked recessive gene; level of gamma globulin likely to be from zero to 20 or 30 mg per 100 ml.

a. primary As distinguished from hypogammaglobulinemia; includes transient, congenital and acquired forms, probably results from decrease synthesis of gamma globulin with levels usually less than 100 or 125 mg per ml.

a. secondary Probably results from increased rate of catabolism or unusual loss of γ-globulin; levels of gamma globulin usually range from 200 to 400 mg per 100 ml.

a.transient A type of primary agammaglobulinemia occurs in infants of both sexes usually during the second to sixth months of life probably resulting from immaturity of lymphoid tissue, level of gamma globulin likely to be less than 100 to 150 mg per 100 ml.

Agamegenesis Asexual reproduction.

Agamogenetic Indication of a sexual reproduction.

Agamogony Asexual reproduction.

Aganglionosis The state of being without ganglia, absence of ganglion cells from Auerbach plexus in eye, distal colon in congenital hypertrophic dilation of the colon.

Agar A gelatinous substance prepared from seaweed in Japan and India, used in constipation to increase the bulk of the feces and in bacteriology as a base for culture media; when unqualified it is usually called agar-agar.

a. Brodet and Gengou potato blood Glycerine potato agar with 25 percent of blood.

a. Brilliant green bilesalt A culture medium consisting of agar with peptone, lactose, sodium taurocholate, brilliant green and picric acid solution.

a. cholera An alkaline agar medium for cultures of the cholera vibrio.

a. Endo's fuchsin Nutrient agar containing lactose alcoholic solution of fuchsin, sodium sulfite and soda solution; used as a culture medium to differentiate the typhoid bacillus from the colon bacillus and others of that group.

a. eosinmethylene blue EMB Agar lactose medium for isolation of coliform organisms.

a. gelatin Made by dissolving peptone gelatin glucose or mannite sodium chloride and potassium chloride in water and adding agar.

a. lactose litmus Made by adding 2 percent lactose and litmus to acid free nutrient agar. Used in the differentiation of the typhoid bacillus.

a. Mac Conkey's bile salt Made by the addition of 12 to 20 percent of agar to Mac Conkey's bile salt bouillon.

a. Novy and MacNeal's blood A nutrient agar containing 2 volumes of defibrinated rabbits blood suitable for the cultivation of a number of trypanosomes.

Agenosomi Markedly defective formation or absence of the genitalia in a fetus. The condition is usually accompanied by protrusion of the abdominal viscera through an incomplete abdominal wall.

Agent An active force or substance capable of producing an effect.

a. antifoaming Chemicals such as ethylalcohol or 2-ethylhexanol administered with oxygen to patients in pulmonary edema to relieve the respiratory obstruction aggravated by the foam of edema fluid.

a. blocking A drug that blocks transmission at an automatic synapse or myoneural junction.

a. chelating A compound such as calciumdisodium ethylene diamine tetraacetic acid which forms a complex with a metal. The medicinal use of these agents is to render poisonous metal compounds innocuous. The resulting chelate complex is unionizable, stable and nonpoisonous and is excreted in the urine.

a. eaton A living organism of a coccobacillary type 125 to 150 μ that is grown on living cells and on official media and produces a characteristic cold agglutinin.

a. reducing Any substance that has the power of initiating a reaction involving the gain of electrons.

a. sclerosing A compound such as sodium ricinoleate used in the treatment of varicose veins.

Ageusia Loss of the sense of taste.

Agglutinate Pertaining to a specific activity of antibody in an antigen antibody reaction, as a specific hemagglutin as certain red blood cells.

Agglutination Aggregation into clumps or masses of micro-organisms or other cells upon exposure to a specific immune serum or other source of appropriate antibody.

a. cold Agglutination of red blood cells by their own serum or by any other serum when the blood is cooled below body temperature but is most pronounced below 25° C. The phenomenon results from cold agglutinins. Although it is seen occasionally in the blood of apparently normal persons it is more frequent in scarlet fever, staphylococcal infections, pneumonia, certain hemolytic anemias and trypanosomiasis.

Agglutinin Antibody that causes clumping or agglutination of the bacteria or other cells which either stimulate the formation of the agglutinaion or contain immunologically, similar reactive material.

a. cold Agglutinin that agglutinates human group O erythrocytes at zero to 5° C but not at 37° C, found in the serum of less than half of patients with primary atypical pneumonia and also in certain other diseases especially trypanosomiasis, titer is usually at a peak relatively early during recovery.

Agglutinogen An antigenic substance that stimulates the formation of specific agglutinin.

Agglutinoid An agglutinin that has lost its agglutiophore group while retaining its haptophore group, such substances can combine with agglutinogens of bacteria or blood cells but do not produce clumping.

Aggregate 1. To unite or come together in mass or cluster. 2. The total of individual units making up a mass or cluster.

Agitophasia Abnormally rapid speech in which words are imperfectly spoken or dropped out of a sentence.

Aglutition Inability to swallow or great difficulty in swallowing, aphagia, dysphagia.

Agnosia Lack of sensory ability to recognize objects.

a. auditory Central auditory inappreciation of sound, ability to perceive sound at the end organ with inability to interpret it centrally.

a. ideational Loss of the concept due to damage of associate areas.

a. optic Inability to interpret visual images.

a. position Failure to recognize the posture of extremity.

a. tactile Inability to recognize objects by touch.

a. visual spatial Disturbance in spatial orientation and in understanding of spatial relations; apractognosia.

Agonal Relating to the process of dying or the movement of death so called because of the former erroneous notion that dying is a painful process.

Agonist Denoting a muscle in state of contraction with reference to its opposing muscle or antagonist.

Agrammatism Loss, through cerebral disease, of the power to construct a grammatical or intelligible sentence, words are uttered but not in proper sequence, a form of aphasia.

Agranulocytosis Acute condition characterized by pronounced leukopenia with great reduction in the number of polymorphonuclear leucocytes, infected ulcers likely to develop in the throat, intestinal tract and other mucous membranes as well as in the skin.

Termed also sepsis agranulocytica, malignant leukopenia, agranulocytic angina, mucocytis necroticans agranulocytica and Schultz angina.

Agraphia Loss of the power of writing due or to an inability to phrase thought. Acoustic agraphia is acquired inability to write from dictation. In amnemanic agraphia, letters and words can be written but not connected sentences; in verbal agraphia single letters can be written. Musical agraphia is the loss of power to write musical notation.

Albinism Congenital leukoderma or absence of pigment in the skin and its appendages, it may be partial or complete.

Akathisia Motor restlessness.

Albino A person with very little or no pigment in the skin, hair or choroid. A congenital diffuse absence of melanin in the skin and hair.

Albumen 1. White of egg, egg albumin ovalbumin 2. Albumin.

Albumin A simple protein widely distributed throughout the tissues and fluids of plants and animals, it is soluble in pure water, precipitable from a solution by mineral acids and coagulable by heat in acid or neutral solution. Varieties of it are found in blood, milk and muscles.

a. native Protein existing in its natural state in the body, it is soluble in water and not precipitated by diluted acids, the two principal forms are serum albumin and egg albumin.

a. normal human serum A sterile preparation of serum albumin obtained by obtaining blood plasma proteins from healthy persons. Used as a transfusion material and to treat edema due to hypoproteinemia.

Albumin radioiodinatcd serum ^{131}I made by mild iodination of normal human serum albumin; one atom of iodine per 60,000 molecular weight of albumin; ^{131}I emits negative beta particles and gamma radiation, half life of ^{131}I is 8.0 days. Used for the determination of blood and plasma volumes, circulation time and cardiac output and for the detection and localization of brain tumors.

Albuminuria The presence of protein in urine chiefly albumin (but also globulin) usually indicates disease but sometimes results from a temporary or transient dysfunction.

a. adolescent Functional albuminuria occurring at about the time of puberty, it is usually cyclic or orthostatic albuminuria.

a. of athletes A form of functional albuminuria following excessive muscular exertion.

a. bamberagers Hematogenous that is sometimes observed during the later phase of advanced anemia.

a. benign orthostatic Dietetic and similar types of albuminuria that are not the result of pathologic changes in the kidneys.

a. cyclic A functional form sometimes observed intermittently in cycles of 12 to 36 hours duration chiefly in younger persons, the degree of albuminuria is usually slight.

a. dietetic The excretion of protein in the urine following the ingestion of certain foods, also termed digestive albuminuria.

a. essentiala A collective term that includes various forms of functional albuminuria, e.g. of athletes, postural, etc. not associated with recognizable pathologic conditions.

a. functional A collective term designating any albuminuria in which there is no detectable, associated pathologic condition in the kidneys or other tissues; may be observed intermittently during pregnancy or adolescence, in athletes, etc.

a. orthostatic A condition characterized by the appearance of albumin in the urine when the patient is in the erect posture and its disappearance when he is recumbent.

Albuterol A sympathomimetic drug used in bronchial asthma.

Alcaine Proparacaine, a local anaesthetic.

Alcohol 1. One of a series of organic chemical compounds in which the hydrogen (H) in a hydrocarbon is replaced by hydroxyl (OH), the hydroxide of a hydrocarbon radical reacting with acids to form esters as a metallic hydroxide reacts to form salt. 2. Any beverage containing ethyl alcohol. 3. Ethanol a liquid containing 92.3 percent by weight corresponding to 94.9 percent by volume of C_7H_5OH.

a. absolute With a minimum admixture of water at most 1 percent.

a. dehydrogenase A pyridinoen-zyme of the liver catalyzing the dehydrogenation of ethyl alcohol to acetaldehyde.

a. dehydrated Absolute alcohol; ethyl hydroxide C_2H_5-OH. Containing not more than 1 percent by weight of water.

a. denatured Methylated spirit, ethyl alcohol that has been made undrinkable by the addition of one ninth of its volume of methyl alcohol and a small quantity of benzine or the pyridine bases.

a. dilute Eight concentration are official, 90, 80, 70, 50, 45, 25 and 20 percent V/V.

a. diluted Contains 41.5 percent by weight (48.6% by volume) of absolute or ethyl hydroxide.

a. fatty A long chain alcohol, e.g. stearyl alcohol.

a. tertiary An alcohol characterized by the trivalent atom group (CHOH).

a. triatomic or tirhydric One containing three atom Groups (OH), e.g. glycerol.

a. unsaturated Those whose carbon chains contain one or more double or triple bonds.

Alcoholism Poisoning with alcohol.

Alcoholophilia The craving for alcohol.

Alcuronium A neuromuscular blocking agent; non-depolarizing.

Aldolase Zymohexase, an enzyme involved in the glycolytic chain catalyzing the splitting of fructose-1, 6-disphosphate to 3-phosphoglyceraldehyde and phosphodihydroxyacetone.

Aldose A monsaccharide containing the characterizing group of the aldehydes (CHO).

Aldosterone A steroid principle of the adrenal cortex which is more potent than deoxycorticosterone in causing sodium retention and potassium loss. It possesses little or no antirheumatic property. Chemically it differs from corticosterone in having an aldehyde group at C-18.

Aldosterone

Aldosteronism Excessive production or excretion of aldosterone. Two forms are recognized 1. True or Primary, characterized by persistent hypokalemia (with alkalosis), hypertension, polyuria, exacerbation of muscular weakness and normal or elevated serum sodium 2. So-called secondary form that is characterized by conspicuous edema (in contrast to primary) and is associated with congestive cardiac failure, cirrhosis, nephrosis and so on.

Aleukemia 1. Literally a lack of leukocytes in the blood. Term is generally used to indicate varieties of leukemic disease in which the white blood cells count in circulating blood is normal or even less than normal (i.e. no leukocytosis) but a few young leukocytes are observed; sometimes used more restrictedly for unusual instances of leukemia with no leukocytosis and no young forms in the blood 2. Leukopenic myelosis, i.e. leukemic changes in bone marrow associated with a sub-normal number of leukocytes in the blood. See also sub-leukemia.

Aleukia 1. Absence or extremely decreased number of leukocytes in circulating blood, sometimes also termed aleukemic myelosis. 2. Absence or extremely decreased number of blood platelets. See also thrombokopenia.

Aleukocytosis Absence or great reduction (relative or absolute) of the number of white blood cells in circulating blood (i.e. an advanced degree of leukopenia) or the lack of leukocytes in an anatomical lesion.

Alexia Loss of the power to grasp the meaning of written or printed words, sentences, also called optical, sensory or visual alexia in distinction to motor alexia (aphemia or anarthria) in which there is loss of the power to read aloud although the significance of what is written or printed is understood; musical blindness is loss of the power to read musical notation.

Alfentanil Newer more potent opioid analgesic with shorter duration of action.

Algesia State of increased sensitivity, to pain some times provoked by stimuli not normally painful.

Alegesimeter, algesiometer An instrument for measuring the degree of sensitivity to a painful stimulus.

Algesthesia The appreciation of pain especially hypersensitivity to painful stimuli, a form of hyperesthesia.

Algid Chilly cold.

Alimentary Relating to food or nutrition.

Aliphatic 1. Fatty. 2. Denoting the open chain compounds most of which belong to the fatty series.

Alkalies A strongly basic substance alkaline in reaction and capable of saponifying fats, i.e. sodium hydroxide, potassium hydroxide.

Alkaloid A basic substance found in the leaves, barks, seeds and other parts of plants usually constituting the active principle of crude drug. A substance of similar nature is formed in animal tissues. Alkaloids are usually bitter in taste and alkaline in reaction and unite with acids to form salts.

Alkalosis A normally high alkali reserve (biocarbonate) of blood and other body fluids with a tendency for an increase in pH of the blood although it may remain normal. It may result from persistent vomiting, hyperventilation or excessive ingestion of sodium bicarbonate.

a. compensated A rise in the alkali reserve but as a result of compensatory readjustment, e.g. retention of CO_2 or increased excretion of alkali, no rise in pH occurs. Thus compensated alkalosis is usually associated with a subnormal level of bicarbonates.

a. metabolic A condition in which the blood and the other body fluids have pH greater than normal associated with an increased concentration of bicarbonate possibly resulting from an excessive intake of alkaline materials or a great loss of chloride (as in persistent vomiting).

a. uncompensated Usually related to a rise in the alkali reserve of the blood possibly resulting from vomiting (loss of Cl) or intake of bicarbonate and compensatory mechanisms may fail thereby leading to alkalemia.

Alkaptonuria Urinary excretion of alkaptone bodies (e.g. homogentisic acid) which cause a dark color if the urine is permitted to stand or is alkalinized; Represents a defect in the metabolism of tyrosine and phenylalanine; some times associated with ochronosis.

Alkylamine An organic compound containing an NH_2 group, an open chain hydrocarbon.

Alkylation The substitution of an aliphatic hydrocarbon radical for a hydrogen atom in a cyclic or ring compound.

Allantoid 1. Sausage shaped 2. Relating to or resembling the alantois.

Allantoin Ureidohydantoin, glyoxyidiureide, a nitrogeneous crystalline substance present in the allantoic fluid, the urine of the fetus and elsewhere. Used externally to promote wound healing. It is the oxidation product of purine metabolism in animals other than man and other primates.

Allele Any one of a series of two or more different genes that may occupy the same position or locus on a specific chromosome. As autosomal chromosomes are paired each autosomal locus is represented twice in normal somatic cells. If the same allele occupies both loci the individual or cell is homozygous for this allele, if the two loci are different the individual or cell is heterozygous for both.

Allelism State of two or more genes that must occupy the same position or locus on a specific chromosome.

Allergen A substance (usually protein but may be non-protein material) that stimulates an altered cellular response in the animal or human body thereby resulting in

manifestation of allergy as the protein (S) of certain foods, bacteria, pollen and so on.

a. bacterial The specific protein (or other material) in the bacterial cell that may stimulate an allergic response, e.g. tuberculin which is prepared from tubercle bacilli.

a. pollen The material in pollen that may stimulate an allergic response.

Allergic Relating to a recognizable condition of allergy or to any response stimulated by an allergen.

Allergy 1. Any abnormal or altered reaction to an antigen or allergen including greater (hyper) or less sensitivity, the term is now used almost invariably to indicate hypersensitivity of the body cells to a specific substance (antigen, allergen) that results in various types of reaction. The exciting material or antigen may be protein, lipid or carbohydrate in nature. The allergic reaction is basically an antibody reaction and includes anaphylaxis, atopic diseases, serum sickness, contact dermatitis. 2. That branch of medicine which embraces the study diagnosis and treatment of allergic manifestation. 3. An acquired hypersensitivity to certain drugs and biologic preparations.

a. bacterial Increased sensitivity to various substance of certain species of bacteria. Usually result from previous infection with a specific organism but under special condition may occasionally develop after injection of antigenic materials not related to antibody in circulating blood.

a. bronchial Asthma and similar conditions that are allergic in origin.

a. cold Physical allergy produced by exposure to cold.

a. contact Cutaneous reaction caused by direct contact with an allergen to which the person is hypersensitive.

a. delayed Allergic response that is not apparent until several hours or a few days have passed as in hypersensitivity to tuberculin, coccidioidin, and other extracts from microorganism.

a. drug Unusual sensitivity to a drug or other chemical or to combination products of such compounds with various substances in the body.

Alloeroticism Sexual attraction toward another person, as opposed to autoeroticism.

Allogamy The fertilization of the ova of one individual by the spermatozoa of another; the opposite of autogamy.

Allopath One who practises medicine according to the system of allopathy.

Allopathy A therapeutic system in which disease is treated by producing a morbid reaction of another kind or in another part by method of substitution.

Alloploidy The condition of a hybrid individual or cell having two or more sets of chromosomes derived from two different ancestral species.

Allopurinol Xanthine oxidase inhibitor, used in gout and hyperuricemia.

Allosome One of the chromosomes differing in appearance or behaviour from the ordinary chromosomes or autosomes and sometimes unequally distributed among the germ cell, heterotypical chromosome.

Allylestrenol Progestational agent.

Almetrine Respiratory stimulant used in COPD.

Alopecia Acomia, baldness.

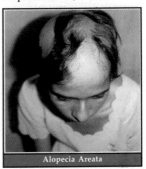
Alopecia Areata

a. areata Condition of unknown etiology producing of circumscribed, noninflamed areas of baldness on the scalp, eyebrows and bearded portion of the face.

Alpha 1 antitrypsin An inhibitor of trypsin deficient in patients of emphysema.

Alpha fetoprotein An antigen present in fetus increased in adults with hepatic cancer.

Alprazolam A benzodiazepine, anxiolytic agent.

a. dynamica Hair loss due to some destructive disease process affecting the hair follicles.

a. follicularis A papular or postular inflammation of the hair follicles of the scalp resulting in scarring and loss of hair in the affected area.

Aluminium A white silvery metal of very light weight. Symbol Al. atomic no 13, atomic weight 26.97 melting point 660°, inhalation of the finely divided dust has been proposed to bind silica, to prevent silicosis.

a. carbonate Aluminium hydroxide carbonate complex; occurs in white lumps, insoluble in water. Used as an aqueous suspension for its powder to bind phosphorus in the intestinal tract; the serum inorganic phosphorus concentration is lowered as a result reabsorption of phosphorus by the renal tubules is increased and its excretion in the urine reduced. Useful in diminishing the tendency towards the formation of phosphatic urinary calculi; also used to reduce gastric acidity especially in the treatment of gastric and duodenal ulcer.

a. chloride White or yellowish white crystalline powder used as an astringent or antiseptic in 10 percent water solution. May be irritating.

a. hydroxide Hydrated alumina a light white powder. Soluble in water, used as an astringent dusting powder. Also used internally as a mild astringent, antacid.

a. oleate A yellow mass insoluble in water. Used locally, on mucous membranes as an astringent antiseptic.

a. phosphate A white infusible powder insoluble in water but soluble in alkali hydroxides. Used for dental cement with calcium sulfate and sodium silicate.

a. subacetate Used in solution as an astringent, and in embleming fluids. Diluted to about 0.5 percent with water it is used as an ingradient in mouth washes.

a. sulfate Cake alum, a white crystaline powder soluble in water, used as an astringent, detergent in skin ulcers.

a. tannate A basic salt of varying composition, a brownish powder insoluble in water. Used as astringent solution for local applications.

a. torotannate A brownish powder. Used as an antiseptic and dusting powder. The tartarte is soluble in water, it is used as a local astringent.

Alveolitis Inflammation of alveoli.

a. allergic Diffuse granulomatous

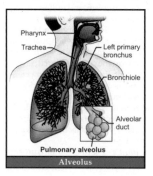

lung disease caused by hypersensitivity to organic dusts.

Alzheimer's disease A disease of unknown etiology causing presenile dementia.

Amalgam A solution of metal in mercury. In dentistry the metal consists mainly of intermetallic compound $Ag_3 Sn$, zinc and copper are useful but not essential. About one part alloy to two parts mercury are mixed and packed, this hardens to almost full strength in 24 hours. Properties of set amalgam depend largely on technique, mixing time, packing, pressure etc. Crushing strengths range from 45,000 to 65,000 pounds per square inch for most.

Amanita A genus of fungi, Agaricus.

a. phallaoides deadly agaric, contains a poisonous principle that causes severe gastrointestinal symptoms and is hemolytic and injurious to the kidneys.

Amantidine An agent used in Parkinsonism, and influenza.

Amaurosis A total loss of vision.

a. fugax Temporary blindness in airoplane pilots when making a circular manoeuvre with head toward the centre of the circle due to centrifugal force causing cerebral ischemia, flight blindness, blackout.

a. partialis fugax Temporary blindness occurring in attacks associated with headache, nausea and scotomas.

a. burn's Postmarital amaurosis; blindness following sexual excess.

a. toxic Blindness due to optic neuritis excited by tobacco, alcohol, wood alcohol, lead, arsenic, quinine or other poisons.

Ambenoniam An anticholinesterase agent.

Amblyoscope An instrument resembling a stereoscope used in training the fusion sense and habituating an amblyopic eye to bear its share of vision.

Amebiasis Infestation with Amoeba histolytica or other pathogenic amebas.

a. hepatic Infection of the liver with entamoeba histolytica, may occur with or without antecedent amebic dysentery.

Amebocyte A cell such as a neutrophil leukocyte having the power of ameboid movements.

Ameboid 1. Resembling an ameba in appearance or characteristic 2. Of irregular outline with peripheral projections.

Ameboma An amebic granuloma, a nodular tumorlike focus of proliferative inflammation sometimes developing in chronic amebiasis especially in the wall of colon; may occur 1. as a fairly well circumscribed solitary lesion or 2. multiple nodular foci or massive lesion comprised of several smaller foci that become coalescent.

Ameiosis A cell division resulting in formation of gametes without reduction in chromosome number.

Amelia Congenital absence of a limb or limbs.

Amelioration Improvement, moderation in the intensity of symptoms.

Amelobastoma A neoplasm originating from epithelial tissue. Related to the enamel organ; consists of rounded cordlike or irregular foci of epithelial cell that frequently surround a stellate reticulum; the basal layers of epithelial cells, resemble amelobasts, but differentiation into keratinizing cells may be observed; enamel is not formed; the stroma is usually loose connective tissue but is sometimes densely fibrous; the stellate reticulum may degenerate there by resulting in one or more cysts, occurs chiefly in the mandible especially in molar region; histologically similar neoplasm rarely occur in the region of the sella turcica and in the tibia. Termed also adamantinoma.

Amenorrhoea Absence or abnormal cessation of the menses.

Amentia 1. Idiocy 2. A form of confusional insanity marked especially by apathy, disorientation and more or less stupor.

Amepthoterin Methotrexata, a cytotoxic drug.

Amiloride A potassium sparing diuretic.

Amikacin An aminoglycoside antibiotic.

Aminacrine Antibacterial, antitrichomonal agent used in vaginal preparations.

Amino caproic acid Antifibrinolytic agent used for vascular plugging in haemorrhage.

Aminopterin 4-Aminopteroyl-glutamic acid, a folic acid antagonist, yellow crystals, soluble in alkali. Used in treatment of acute leukemia and other neoplastic diseases.

Aminopyrine Amidopyrine, pyramidon, dimethylamino antipyrine; odorless white crystals, soluble in 18 parts of water or 1.5 parts of alcohol. Melting point 107° C. Used as an antipyretic and analgesic in rehumatism, neuritis, pulmonary tuberculosis and common colds. May cause leukocytopenia.

Aminosalicylic acid P-Amino-salicylic acid, 4-amino-2-hydroxy-benzoic acid, small crystals slightly soluble in water. Melting point 150°C. A bacteriostatic agent against tubercle bacilli, used as an adjunct to streptomycin. Abbreviated AS or PAS.

Amitriptyline hydrochloride Chemically and pharmacologically related to imipramine hydrochloride. An antidepressant agent with mild tranquilizing properties, used in the treatment of mental depression and maniac depressive states.

Ammonia A volatile alkaline gas, NH_3, very soluble in water combining with acids to form a number of salts.

Ammoniemia The presence of ammonia or some of its compounds in the blood, thought to be formed from the decomposition of urea with weak pulse, gastroenteric symptoms and coma.

Amminoglutethimide Adreno-cortical suppressant used in breast cancer.

Ammonium A group of atoms, NH_4 that behaves as a univalent metal in forming ammonical compound; it has never been obtained in a free state.

a. acetate White, deliquescent, crystals, soluble in water, melting point 112° C. Mild diaphoretic and refrigerant, used in preserving meat.

a. carbonate A mixture of carbon dioxide and carbonate soluble in water, occurs in white masses with ammonical odor. Cardiac and respiratory stimulant and expectorant.

a. chloride White crystalline powder soluble in water. Stimulant-expectorant and cholagogue. Used to relieve alkalosis, also promotes lead excretion.

a. nitrate A white deliquescent crystalline salt, soluble in water. Used in making nitrous oxide gas in freezing mixtures and in fertilizers.

a. salicylate White crystalline powder soluble in water. Used in rheumatism.

Amnesia Loss or impairment of memory, inability to recall past experiences.

a. anterogradea In reference to events occurring after the trauma or disease that cause the condition.

a. retrograde In reference to events that occurred before the trauma or disease that caused the condition.

a. visual Inability to recall to mind the appearance of objects that have been seen or to recognize printed words.

Amnion The innermost or the membranes enveloping the embryo in utero. It consists of a layer of splanchnopleure with its ecto-dermal components toward the embryo and its somatic meso-dermal component external.

Amniorrhea The escape of amniotic fluid or liquor amni.

Amobarbital White crystalline powder of a bitter taste slightly soluble in water, melting point 156° C. A central nervous system depressant, has an intermediate duration of action.

Amodiaquine hydrochloride Camoquine hydrochloride, as the dihydrochloride hemihydrate, yellow crystals soluble in water. A synthetic antimalarial drug, effective against plasmodium vivax in the erythrocytic phase of malaria, less effective against P. vivax falciparum and P. malaria infections. Also used in treatment of amebic hepatitis, rheumatoid arthritis.

Ameba A genus of unicellular protozoan organisms of microscopic size existing in nature in large numbers, many living as parasites, some species pathogenic for man.

Amoxapine Tricyclic antidepressant.

Amoxicillin Ampicillin group of antibiotic with better GI absorption.

Ampere Unit of strength of an electrical current representing a current having a force of one volt and passing through a conductor with a resistance of one ohm.

Amphetamine An acrid liquid racemic synthetic preparation slightly soluble in water, closely related in its structure and action to ephedrine and other sympathomimetic amines. Central nervous system stimulant.

Amphoric Denoting the sound heard in precussion and auscultation resembling the noise made by blowing across the mouth of a bottle.

Amphoteric Having two opposite characteristics especially the capacity of reacting as either acid or base.

Amphotericin B An antibiotic substance derived from strains of streptomyces nodosus, used for the treatment of deep seated myocotic infections.

Ampicillin Semisynthetic broad spectrum penicillin, acid resistant.

Ampoule A hermetically sealed container usually made of glass containing a sterile medicinal solution or powder to be made up in solution, to be used for subcutaneous, intramuscular, or intravenous injection.

Ampulla A sacular dilation of canals, is seen in the semicircular canals of the ear or the lactiferous ducts of the mammary glands.

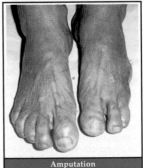
Amputation

Amputation 1. The cutting off of a limb or part of a limb, the breast or other projecting part. 2. In dentistry amputation may be of the root of a tooth or of the pulp or even of a nerve root or ganglion, e.g. the Gasserian ganglion.

Amrinone Bipyocidine derivative with positive inotropic effect, used in heart failure.

Amygdala A nugget like mass of gray matter in the anterior portion of temporal lobe.

Amylase A starch splitting or amyloytic enzyme that causes hydrolytic cleavage of the starch molecule.

Amylnitrate A vasodilator used in angina and cyanide poisoning.

Amylocaine hydrochloride Benzoyl ethyldimethyl — aminopropanyl hydrochloride, a local anaesthetic. Its action is slightly stronger than that of cocaine less toxic but more irritant. It has been used for spinal anesthesia. Side effects and after effects are frequent.

Amyloid A protein (probably combined with chondroitin sulfuric acid) that is microscopically homogeneous hyaline and acidophilic and frequently manifests great affinity for congored; occurs characteristically as pathologic extracellular deposits beneath the endothelium of capillaries or sinusoids in the walls of arterioles and especially in association with reticuloendothelial tissue.

Amyloidosis Deposits of amyloid in various organs tissues. Four types of conditions are recognized, i.e. primary secondary, a localized masses or nodules, and associated with multiple myeloma.

a. primary A form of amyloidosis not associated with other recognized disease, tends to involve diffusely the mesenchymal tissues in the tongue, lungs, intestinal tract, skin, skeletal muscles, and myocardium, the amyloid in this condition frequently does not manifest the usual affinity for congored and sometimes provokes a foreign body type of inflammatory reaction in the adjacent tissue.

a. secondary The most frequent form of amyloidosis occurs in association with another chronic disease, e.g. tuberculosis, osteomyelitis, pyelonephritis and so on; organs chiefly involved are the liver, spleen, and kidneys and the adrenal glands less frequently.

Amylopectin A polysaccharide found in the outer layer of the starch granule, characterized by glucose residues arranged in branched chains.

Amyoplasia Deficient formation of muscle tissue.

Amyotonia Myotonia.

Amyotrophy Muscular wasting or atrophy.

Anabolism The process of assimilation of nutritive matter and its conversion into living substances. This includes synthetic processes and requires energy.

Anabolite Any substance formed as a result of anabolic processes.

Analgesia Loss of sensibility to pain.

Analgia Freedom from pain.

Analogous Resembling functionally but having a different origin or structure.

Analogue 1. One of two organs or parts in different species of animals or plants which differ in structure or development but are similar in function. 2. In chemistry one of two or more compounds with similar structure but different atoms, e.g. nitrogen and carbon monoxide.

Analysis 1. The breaking up of a chemical compound into its simpler elements, a process by which the composition of a substance is determined. 2. The separation of any compound substance into the parts composing it. 3. Applied in electroencephalography to the estimation or recording of the components of a complex wave form in terms of their frequency and amplitude.

a. gastric Analysis of the contents of the stomach after the ingestion of a test meal. The gastric contents are aspirated through a specially designed stomach tube, and the free and total acidities, the pH and the peptic activity are determined. They may also be examined for food residue, bile, blood, mucus etc.

Anamnesis 1. The act of remembering. 2. The medical history of a patient.

Anandria Absence of masculinity.

Anaphase The stage of mitosis or meiosis in which the chromosomes move from the equatorial plate toward the poles of the cell. In mitosis a full set of daughter chromosomes (46 in man) moves towards each pole. In the first division of meiosis one member of each homologous pair (23 in man) now consisting of two chromatids united at the centromere, moves towards each pole. In the second division of meiosis the centromere has divided and the two chromatids separate one moving to each pole.

Anaphoria A tendency of the eyes when in a state of rest to turn upward.

Anaphylactoid Resembling anaphylaxis. A shock may result from intravenous injection of 1. serum that is pretreated with kaolin or starch 2. Trypsin 3. organic colloids. 4. peptone or 5. several other materials. The pathologic changes in a shock are different from those of true anaphylaxis.

Anaphylatoxin According to the humoral hypothesis of the mechanism of anaphylaxis, anaphylaxis results from the in vivo combination of specific antibody (anaphylactin) and the specific. Sensitizing material, when the latter is injected at a shock dose in a sensitized animal.

Anaphylaxis The antithesis of prophylaxis; anaphylaxis is an exaggerated or extreme hypersensitivity that may be induced in various animal species as the result of the injection of even a small dose of foreign material (anaphylactogen) this is usually termed the sensitizing dose. Anaphylaxis develops during an incubation period of 10 to 14 days and then the injection of a second larger dose of the same material (usually termed the shocking dose) promptly results in anaphylatic shock.

Anaplasia 1. A reversion in the case of a cell to a more primitive embryonic type, i.e. to one in which reproductive activity is marked. 2. Loss of structural differentiation.

Anastomosis 1. A natural communication direct or indirect between two blood vessels or tubular structures. 2. An operative union between of two hollow or tubular structures.

a. arteriovenous A situation where blood is shunted from arterioles to venules without passing through capillaries.

a. Braun's After gastroenteros-tomy prevention of reverse peristalsis by anastomosis between loops of jejunum on either side of stomach anastomosis.

a. Clado's Anastomosis between ovarian and appendicular arteries in the broad ligament.

a. Glen's A nerve that connects superior and inferior laryngeal nerves in the larynx and supplies sensory fibres to the latter.

a. isoperistaltic One to allow the contents in the same and natural direction.

a. Schmidel's Abnormal channels of communication between the vena cava and portal system as for example a communication between the coronary veins of the stomach and the azygus vein.

Anatomy 1. The structure of an organism; morpholgy. 2. The science of the morphology or structure of organisms. 3. Dissection. 4. A work describing the form and structure of an organism and its various parts.

a. applied Anatomical knowledge utilized in the diagnosis of disease and in treatment especially surgical treatment.

a. comparative 1. Anatomy of the lower animals 2. The comparative study of the human body with those of other animals and observation of analogous and homologous parts.

a. surface The study of the configuration of the surface of the body especially in its relation to deeper parts.

Ancylostoma A genus of Nematoda, the old word hookworm the members of which are parasitic in the duodenum where they attach themselves to the mucous membrane sucking the blood and causing a state of anemia and mental and physical inertia. The eggs are passed with the feces and the larvae develop in moist soil, they enter the body of man through the skin of the feet and ankles, possibly also in the drinking water and reach maturity in the intestine.

a. caninum A species with three pairs of ventral teeth in the oral cavity infesting dogs, cause of kennel anemia, it occurs also although rarely in man.

a. duodenale A reddish worm with two pairs of hooklike teeth on the ventral surface and one rudimentary minor pair. This species and A. braziliense (with only one pair of ventral teeth) are found in man, the latter in dogs and cats also.

Androlelastoma A relatively infrequent functional neoplasm of the ovary derived from cells of the male anlage and resulting in varying degrees of defeminization and masculinization.

Androgen A generic term for an agent usually a hormone, e.g. testosterone or androsterone that stimulates the activity of the accessory sex organs of the male;

encourages the development of the male sex characteristics.

Androsterone

Androgynoid A man with hermaphroditic sexual characteristics who is mistaken for a woman, a pseudohermaphrodite. Possession of masculine characteristics by a genetically pure female.

Androgynus Female pseudohermaphrodite.

Andropathy Any disease such as prostatitis peculiar to the male sex.

Androstenodione A testosterone precursor.

Anemia (Anaemia) Qualitative or quantitative in reduction in red blood cells.

a. elliptocytic Anemia characterized by elliptical erythrocytes (ovalocytes) resembling those observed normally in camels; 1 to 15 percent of erythrocytes in non-anemic persons may be oval but greater proportions are observed in certain patients with microcytic anemia, latter conditions frequently termed symptomatic ovalocytosis.

a. hyperchromic Characterized by an increase in the ratio of the weight of hemoglobin to the volume of the erythrocyte, i.e. the mean corpuscular hemoglobin concentration is greater than normal with the exception of some instances of hereditary spherocytosis such "supersaturation" does not occur although the weight of hemoglobin per cell may be greater in the macrocytes of pernicious anemia, the increase is proportional to larger volume and such cells are not truly hyperchromic.

a. hypochromic Characterized by a decrease in the ratio of the weight of haemoglobin to the volume of the erythrocyte, i.e. the mean corpuscular hemoglobin concentration (MCHC) is less than normal; the individual cells contains less hemoglobin than they could have under optimal conditions.

a. hypochromic microcytic A type of anaemia caused by a deficiency of iron; the amount of haemoglobin is reduced to a greater degree than the blood red cell count as a result of 1. less than the normal percentage of haemoglobin per cell and 2. the smaller than the normal size of most of the erythrocytes. The mean corpuscular volume (MCV), mean corpuscular haemoglobin (MCH) and mean corpuscular haemoglobin concentration (MCHC) are less than normal.

a. Iron deficiency Any hypochromic microcytic anemia with the exception of that occurring in thalassemia and anemia produced in certain experimental animals that are deficient, in vitamin B_6 or copper.

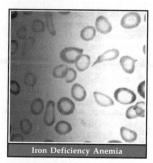
Iron Deficiency Anemia

a. macrocytic Any anaemia in which the average size of circulating erythrocytes is greater than normal, i.e. the mean corpuscular volume (MCV) is 94 cu or more (normal range 82 to 92 cu) includes such syndromes as pernicious anemia, celiac disease, anaemia of pregnancy etc.

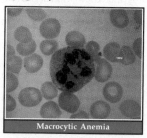
Macrocytic Anemia

a. megaloblastic Any anaemia in which there is a predominant number of megaloblasts and relatively few normalasts among the hyperplastic erythroid cells in the bone marrow (as in pernicious)

a. normochromic Anemia in which the concentration of hemoglobin in the erythrocytes is within the normal range, i.e. the mean corpuscular haemoglobin concentration (MCHC) is around 32 to 36 percent.

Anemic Deficient in hemoglobin.

Anemophobia Morbid fear of wind.

Anencephalus Congenital absence of brain and spinal cord with open cranial cavity and a groove like spinal canal.

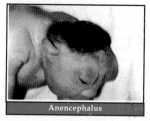
Anencephalus

Anergia Lack of activity

Anergy Impaired ability to react with antigens.

Aneroid Equipment that does not utilize liquid medium for measurement of pressure, e.g. aneroid barometer.

Anesthesia Partial or complete loss of sensation with or without loss of consciousness, (depending upon stage of anaesthesia) induced by administration of an anaesthetic agent.

a. caudal injection of anaesthetic agent into caudal epidural space.

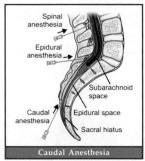

Caudal Anesthesia

a. dissociative A type of anaesthesia characterized by amnesia, analgesia and cataplexy. The patient is dissociated from environment.

a. Gwathmey's Anaesthesia induced by injecting olive oil and either solution into the scrotum.

a. infiltration Local anaesthesia produced by injecting the local anaesthetic solution directly into tissue.

a. inhalational General anesthesia produced by inhalation of vapor or gas anaesthetic like ether, nitrous oxide, halothane, trilene etc.

a. pudendal The pudendal nerve near the spinous process of ischium is blocked; used in perineal and obstetric surgery.

a. sexual Absence of sexual desire.

a. spinal Anaesthesia produced by injection of anaesthetic agent into subarachnoid space.

a. surgical Depth of anaesthesia of which relaxation of muscles and loss of sensation and consciousness are adequate for performance of surgery.

a. twilight State of light anaesthesia.

Anesthesiologist Physician specializing in anaesthesiology.

Anesthetize To induce anesthesia.

Anetoderma Atrophy of skin with soft fibromata forming large pendulous massess.

Aneuploidy Possession of abnormal number of chromosomes.

Aneurysm Localized abnormal dilatation of a blood vessel due to congenital weakness or defect in the wall.

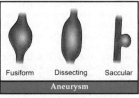

Aneurysm

a. atherosclerotic Aneurysm due to degeneration of arterial wall by atherosclerosis.

a. berry Small saccular congenital aneurysm of cerebral vessel.

a. cirsoid A dilatation of network of vessels, forming a pulsating subcutaneous tumor, usually on the scalp.

a. compound Aneurysm in which some of the layers of vessel wall are ruptured and others dilated.

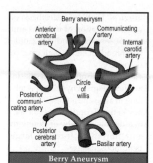

Berry Aneurysm

a. dissecting Aneurysm in which following interruption of wall of a blood vessel, blood enters in between the walls separating them for variable distance and often obstructing the vessel lumen.

a. fusiform Aneurysm in which all the walls of blood vessel dilate more or less equally, forming a tubular swelling.

a. mycotic Aneurysm due to bacterial infection of vessel wall.

a. saccular The dilatation does not involve the entire circumference of vessel.

Aneurysmorrhaphy Surgical closure of sac of an aneurysm.

Angel dust Phencyclidine, a psychodelic.

Angel's trumpet A flowering shrub producing alkaloids like atropine, hyoscyamine and hyoscine.

Angel's wing Posterior projection of scapula caused by paralysis of serratus anterior.

Angelucci's Syndrome Vasomotor disturbances associated with vernal conjunctivitis.

Anger The emotion of extreme displeasure to a person, a situation or an object.

Angiectasia Dilatation of blood and lymph vessel.

Angina Severe pain.

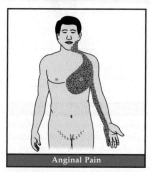

Anginal Pain

a. abdominis Abdominal pain due to ischaemia of gut.

a. agranulocytic Acute sore throat with pain due to agranulocytosis.

a. cruris Leg pain due to vascular obstruction.

a. decubitus Attacks of angina pectoris occurring in recumbent position.

a. Ludwig Deep infection of tissues in the floor of the mouth.

a. pectoris Ischemic pain of cardiac origin manifesting as constriction around heart, faintness; radiation of pain occurring to jaw, neck, left shoulder, upper abdomen and along inner border of left arm.

a. prinzmetal's Angina pectoris with ST elevation due to coronary spasm.

a. unstable Angina of recent onset, abrupt progression; occurring at rest; is due to superadded coronary thrombosis, a fore runner of impending infarction.

a. variant Angina occurring at rest in absence of cardiac acceleration.

Auginous Resembling angina.

Angioblast The mesenchymal cell derivative which ultimately develops into blood vessels.

Angioblastoma Tumor involving blood vessels of brain and meninges.

Angiocardiogram Serial X-rays of heart after intraventricular injection of radio-opaque dye.

Angiocarditis Inflammation of heart and great vessels.

Angioedema An allergic condition characterized by urticaria and edematous areas of skin and mucous membrane or viscera. The reaction is IgE dependent, but is often complement mediated as in hereditary angioedema.

Angioendothelioma A tumor with endothelial cells predominance occurring in bone.

Angiogenesis Development of blood vessels.

Angiogenic factors A group of polypeptides that either stimulate vascular endothelium to proliferate or stimulate macrophages to secrete endothelial growth factors.

Angiography X-ray of blood vessels after injection of radioopaque material.

a. coronary X-ray of coronary circulation to evaluate ischaemic disease.

a. cerebral X-ray picture of cerebral circulation to evaluate stroke, tumor, av malformation, aneurysm or abnormal vascular pattern.

a. digital subtraction A computer aided "subtraction" technique that subtracts images of surrounding tissue from the contrast image to give better resolution and minor details.

Angioid streaks Dark wavy anastomosing striae lying beneath the retinal vessels.

Angiokeratoma Thickening of epidermis of feet with telangictases warty growths.

Angioleukitis Inflammation of lymphatics.

Angiolipoma A mixed tumor containing blood vessels and fatty tissue.

Angiolith Calcareous deposits in walls of blood vessels.

Angiology Science of blood vessels and lymphatics.

Angioma A tumor containing blood vessels (hemangioma) or lymph vessels (lymphangioma), considered to be misplaced fetal tissue undergoing abnormal development.

a. capillary Congenital superficial hemangioma appearing as irregular red discolouration due to overgrowth of capillaries.

a. cavernous Elevated dark red tumor consisting of blood filled vascular spaces; involves sub-mucous and subcutaneous tissue and is pulsatile.

a. senile Hemangioma in elderly due to capillary wall degeneration, producing a compressible mass.

a. serpiginous A Skin disorder characterized by appearance of small, red vascular dots arranged in rings due to proliferation of capillaries.

a. stellate Hemangioma in which telangiectatic blood vessels radiate from a central point *SYN*—spidero nevus.

Angiomalacia Softening of wall of blood vessels.

Angiomatosis Multiple angiomas.

Angiomyolipoma A benign growth containing vascular, muscular and fatty elements.

Angionoma Ulceration of a vessel.

Angiopathy Any disease of blood or lymph vessel.

Angiotensin A vasopressor substance formed by interaction of renin on a serum globulin called angiotensinogen.

a. I Physiologically inactive form of angiotensin.

a. II Physiologically active form of angiotensin; a potent vasopressor and stimulant of aldosterone secretion.

Angiotensinogen A serum globulin fraction formed in the liver; hydrolyzed to angiotensin by renin.

Angle The space outlined by two diverging lines from a common point or by the meeting of two planes.

a. acromial Angle formed by junction of lateral and posterior borders of acromion.

a. alpha Angle formed by intersection of visual line with optic axis.

a. alveolar Angle between the horizontal plane and a line drawn through the base of nasal spine and the midpoint of alveolus of upper jaw.

a. cardiophrenic The angle formed by diaphragm and heart outline.

a. carrying Angle made at the elbow by extending the long axis of forearm and the upper arm. Normally it is around 15° in male and 18° female.

a. costophrenic Angle formed by lateral end of diaphragm with the rib cage.

a. facial Angle made by the lines from the nasal spine and external auditory meatus meeting between upper middle incisor teeth.

a. gamma Angle between line of vision and visual axis.

a. of Treitz Sharp curve at duodeno jejunal junction.

a. sphenoid Angle formed at the top of sella turcica by intersection of lines drawn from nasal point and tip of rostrum of sphenoid bone.

a. visual Angle formed by the line drawn from nodal point of eye to the edges of the object being viewed.

Angor animi The feeling that one is dying as in angina pectoris.

Angstrom unit Unit for measurement of wavelength equal to 10^{-10} meter.

Angular artery Artery at inner canthus of eye.

Anhedonia Lack of pleasure in normally pleasurable acts.

Anhidrosis Absence of sweat secretion.

Anhydrase Enzyme that helps in removal of water from a chemical compound.

Anhydride Compound formed by removal of water from a substance, especially an acid.

Anhydrous Lacking water.

Anicteric Without jaundice.

Aniline The simplest aromatic amine, an oily liquid derived from benzene, used for dyes.

Anilism Chronic aniline poisoning manifesting with vertigo, cardiac conduction defects, muscular weakness.

Anima Soul, individual's innerself.

Animal A living organism.

a. cold blooded An animal whose body temperature changes with that of environment.

a. warmblooded Animals that maintain constant body temperature irrespective of change in environmental temperature.

Animation State of being alive.

a. suspended State of apparent death.

Anion An ion carrying negative charge being attracted to positive pole, anode.

Anion gap It is calculated from subtracting $HCO_3 + Cl^-$ from plasma sodium. Normal value is 8-12 mEq/L.

Aniridia Congenital absence of a part of iris.

Aniseikonia A condition in which the size and shape of ocular image in the both eyes differ from one another.

Anisocoria Inequality in size of pupils.

Anisocytosis Marked inequality in size of cells.

Anisogamy Sexual fusion of two gametes of different form and size.

Anisometropia Condition in which refractive powers of each eye are different.

Anisophoria Muscular imbalance in eye so that horizontal visual plane of one eye is different from other.

Anisotropine A belladona alkaloid derivative, spasmolytic.

Anisindione Anticoagulant agent.

Ankle The hinge joint formed by articulation of tibia, fibula and talus.

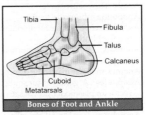

Tibia — Fibula — Talus — Calcaneus — Cuboid — Metatarsals

Bones of Foot and Ankle

a. clonus Repeated contraction and relaxation of leg muscles following mild extension of ankle in patients of corticospinal disease, an evidence of increased muscle tone.

Ankle jerk Plantar flexion of foot due to contraction of calf musculature following a brisk tap to tendo-Achilles tendon.

Ankyloblepharon Adhesion of upper and lower eyelids at lid margin.

Ankylocolpos Imperforated or atretic vaginal canal.

Ankyloglossia Poor tongue protrusion due to abnormally short frenulum.

Ankylosis Immobility of a joint, due to fibrous tissue growth or bony fusion within joint.

a. dental fusion of root cementum with adjacent alveolar bone.

Annular Circular.

Annuloraphy Closure of hernial ring by suture.

Annulus A ring shaped structure.

Anococcygeal body The muscle and fibrous tissue lying in between anus and coccyx; giving attachment to.

Anococcygeal ligament A band of fibrous tissue joining coccyx to external sphincter ani.

Anode The positive pole.

Anodontia Absence of teeth.

Anomaloscope Device for detection of color blindness.

Anomaly Deviation from normal, irregularity.

Anomia Inability in naming objects.

Anopheles A genus of mosquito, vector for plasmodia, the causative agent of malaria.

Anorchism Congenital absence of one or both testes.

Anorexia Loss of appetite.

a. nervosa A psychological malade of young girls who are anorexic for fear of becoming obese.

Anorexigenic Causing loss of apetite

Anoscope Speculum for examining anus and lower rectum.

Anosmia Loss of sense of smell.

Anovulatory Not associated with ovulation.

Anovulatory cycle Menstrual cycle not preceded by ovulation.

Anoxemia Insufficient oxygenation of blood.

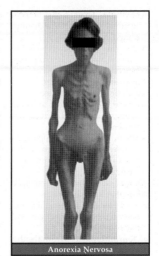

Anorexia Nervosa

Anoxia Reduced oxygenation of tissues from various causes.

a. altitude Insufficient oxygen content of inspired air in high altitude causing anoxia.

a. anemic Anoxia due to decreased oxygen carrying capacity of blood.

a. anoxic Anoxia due to defective pulmonary mechanism of oxygenation, i.e. pulmonary fibrosis, edema, bronchial obstruction, emphysema, etc.

a. stagnant Tissue anoxia due to stagnant peripheral circulation as in cardiac failure, shock.

Ansa Any structure in the form of a loop or arc.

a. cervicalis A nerve loop in the neck formed by fibres from first three cervical nerves.

a. lenticularis Fibre tract from globus pallidus to ventral nucleus of thalamus that winds round in internal capsule.

a. peduncularis Fibre tract from anterior temporal lobe to medio dorsal nucleus of thalamus, extending around internal capsule.

a. sacralis Nerveloop connecting sympathetic trunk with coccygeal ganglion.

Ansamycin A rifamycin derivative, used in tuberculosis.

Ansiform Shaped like a loop.

Antabuse Disulfiram, used to cause aversion in alcoholics by increasing acetaldehyde concentration.

Antacid Agent that neutralizes gastric HCl.

Antagonism Mutual opposite or contradictory action.

Antagonist Agent or any other thing that counteracts the action of something else.

a. narcotic A drug that reverses action of a narcotic hence producing withdrawal symptoms in some.

Antalgesic *SYN*–analgesic, i.e. pain reliever.

Antaphrodisiac Agent that suppresses sexual desire.

Antasthenic Invigorating, strengthening, relieving weakness.

Antazoline An antihistamine used for allergic conjunctivitis.

Ante Prefix meaning before.

Antecedent Some thing coming before; precursor.

Antecibum Before meals.

Antecubital At the bend of elbow.

Antecubital fossa Triangular area lying anterior to and below the elbow, bounded medially by pronator teres and laterally by brachio-radialis.

Anteflexion Abnormal bending forward, e.g. especially of uterine body at its neck.

Antegrade Moving forward or in the direction of flow.

Antemortem Before death.

Antenatal Occurring before birth.

Antenatal diagnosis Diagnostic procedures done to determine the health and genetic status of foetus, e.g. ultrasound, amiocentesis, chorionic villi sampling, biophysical profile, non-stress test.

Antepar Piperazine citrate.

Antepartum Before onset of labor.

Anterior In anatomy refers to ventral portion of body.

Anterior chamber The front chamber of eye bounded infront by cornea, behind by iris and lens; contains aqueous humor.

Anterior horn cell The nerve cells in anterior horn of spinal cord whose axons form the efferent fibres innervating the muscles.

Anterograde Moving frontward.

Anteroinferior Infront and below.

Anterolateral Infront and to one side.

Anteromedian Infront and towards midline.

Anteroposterior Passing from front to rear.

Anterosuperior In front and above.

Anteversion A tipping forward of an organ as a whole, without bending.

Anthelmintic Agents against intestinal worms.

Anthracoid Resembling or pertaining to anthrax.

Anthracometer An instrument for measuring combustion products in the air.

Anthracosis *SYN*–black lung; accumulation of carbon deposits in lungs due to smoking or coal dust.

Anthralin A synthetic hydrocarbon used as ointment to treat fungal infections and eczema.

Anthrax Disease caused by bacillus anthracis, a disease primarily of animals. In man it may occur as cutaneus pustule with black eschar, or a pulmonary form (Wool Sorter's disease) with pulmonary edema, necrotizing mediastinal lymph adenitis, pleural effusion etc.

Anthropogeny Origin and development of man.

Anthropology The study of man; physical, cultural, linguistic and archaeologic.

Anthropometer Device for measuring body parts.

Anthropometry Science of measuring human body, including craniometry, osteometry, skin fold thickness, height and weight measurement.

Anthropomorphism Attributing human qualities to nonhumans.

Anthropophilic Parasites that prefer human host rather than other animals.

Anti Prefix meaning against

Antiadrenergic Counter acting or preventing adrenergic actions.

Antiagglutinin A specific antibody opposing the action of agglutinin.

Antiamebic A medicine used to treat amebiasis.

Antiandrogen Substances antagonizing action of androgen, e.g. ciproterone acetate.

Antibiosis Relationship between two organisms where one is harmful to the other.

Antibiotic Substances that inhibit or destroy micro-organisms; can be bactericidal or bacteriostatic (only inhibit growth).

Antibody A protein substance developed on challenge by an antigen. Antibodies may be present due to previous infection, vaccination, transplacental transfer (IgG only) or unknown idiopathic antigenic stimulation.

a. blocking Antibody that reacts with other antigens and blocks its effects.

a. cross reacting Antibody that reacts with other antigens functionally similar to its specific antigen

a. fluorescent Antigen antibody reaction made visible by incorporating a fluorescent material into the reaction and their examination under fluorescent microscopy.

Antibody coated bacteria Bacteria coated with antibody present in urine. Analysis of antibody pattern can localize the site of invasion of bacteria in urinary tract.

Antibromic Deodorant.

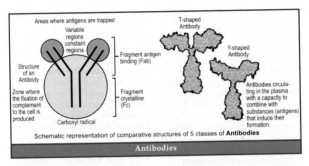

Schematic representation of comparative structures of 5 classes of **Antibodies**

Antibodies

Antiburn scar garment A garment made of stretchable filaments worn to provide uniform pressure over burn graft sites in order to reduce scarring during healing.

Anticholinergic Agents that prevent parasympathetic transmission, e.g. belladona, tricyclic antidepressants, thereby causing dryness of mouth, constipation, urinary retention, blurring of vision and tachycardia.

Anticholinesterase Substance opposing action of choline sterate which causes, breakdown of acetylcholine.

Anticipate To occur before.

Anticoagulant Agents that prevent/ delay clot formation, e.g. sodium citrate; heparin.

Anticodon A triple arrangement of bases in tRNA that complements the triplet on corresponding MRNA.

Anticonvulsant Agents that prevent or control seizure.

Antidepressant Agents that prevent, cure or alleviate mental depression.

Antidiuretic hormone Vasopressin.

Antidote Agents that neutralize poisons or their effects.

a. chemical Antidote that reacts with poison to produce harmless chemical compound, e.g. common salt precipitates silver nitrate to produce silver chloride.

a. mechanical Antidote that prevents absorption of poison, e.g. charcoal, egg albumin, milk casein and fats (fats contraindicated in camphor, phosphorus poisoning).

a. universal Two parts of activated charcoal, one part tannic acid, one part magnesium oxide; given orally mixed with water. Charcoal adsorbs, tannic acid precipitates and magnesium oxide neutralizes poisons. This antidote like chemical antidotes should be removed from stomach after some time.

Antidromic Nerve impulse travelling in opposite direction than normal.

Antiemetic Agent that prevents or relieves vomiting and nausea.

Antiestrogen Substances that block or modify action of estrogen, e.g. clomifene citrate.

Antigen Substance that induces antibody production and interacts with it in a specific way.

Antigen-antibody reaction Combination of antigen with specific antibody that may result in agglutination, precipitation, neutralization, complement fixation or increased susceptibility to phagocytosis.

Antihelix Inner curved ridge of external ear parallel to helix.

Anti-inflammatory Counteracting inflammation.

Antiluetic Agent that cures or relieves syphilis.

Antilymphocytic serum Serum used in certain autoimmune disorders and in transplant patients to reduce chances of rejection.

Antimetabolite 1. A substance structurally similar to metabolite, opposes or replaces a metabolite 2. a class of antineoplastic drugs used to treat cancer.

Antimony A metal whose compounds are used to treat trypanosomiasis.

Antineoplastic Agents that prevent the development growth and proliferation of malignant cells.

Antinuclear antibody A group of antibodies that react against normal components of cell nucleus. They are present in SLE, PSS, scleroderma, polymyositis etc.

Antioxidants Agents that prevent or inhibit oxidation, e.g. vit E.

Antipathy Antagonism, strong aversion.

Antiperistalsis Reverse peristalsis.

Antiplastic Preventing or inhibiting wound healing.

Antiprostaglandins Agents that interfere with prostaglandin activity; used for treatment of arthritis, dysmenorrhoea.

Antiprostate Cowper's gland.

Antipruritic Preventing or relieving itching.

Antipyretic Agent that reduces fever.

Antishock garment Inflatable garment that compresses lower extremity and abdomen to prevent pooling of blood. Useful in aviation and in treating hypotension.

Antiseptic Agent preventing sepsis by inhibiting growth of microorganisms.

Antisudorific Agent that inhibits perspiration.

Antithrombotic Preventing thrombosis or blood coagulation.

Antithrombin III A protein synthesized in liver. Its concentration is lowered in nephrotic syndrome leading to renal veins thrombosis.

Antitoxin Antibody capable of neutralizing a toxin.

Antitrypsin A substance that inhibits action of trypsin.

a. alpha I A low molecular weight glycoprotein whose deficiency is associated with early onset emphysema and neonatal hepatitis.

Antitussive Agent preventing or relieving cough.

Antivenin Serum that contains antibodies against animal or insect venom.

a. black widow spider Horse antivenin against black widow spider.

a. polyvalent Antisnake venom against common snakes.

Antivitamin A vitamin antagonist, agents that oppose action of vitamins.

Antizymotic Agent that prevents or arrests fermentation.

Antrectomy Excision of walls of an antrum.

Antroatticotomy Operation to open the maxillary sinus and the attic of lympanum.

Antrocele Fluid accumulation causing a cystic swelling of antrum.

Antrostomy Opening up of antral wall by surgery.

Antrum Any nearly closed cavity or chamber especially in a bone.

Anulus A ring shaped structure.

a. fibrosus The tough outer portion of intervertebral disk.

Anuresis Absence of urination.

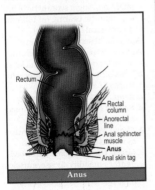

Anus

Anus The lower external opening of GI tract, lying between the folds of buttocks.

Anxiety A feeling of apprehension, worry, uneasiness.

Anxiety neurosis A mental disorder with excessive anxiety not restricted to specific situation or objects and is associated with somatic symptoms like palpitation, tremor, dryness of throat, headache.

Anxiolytic Agents that diminish or counteract anxiety.

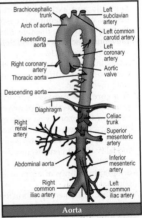

Aorta

Aorta The main arterial trunk arising from left ventricle and lying to the right and anterior to pulmonary artery. The aortic arch ends at level of fourth thoracic vertebra. The branches of aorta are 1. ascending aorta — two coronary arteries, right and left 2. arch of aorta-right innominate, left subclavian 3. thoracic aorta-bronchial arteries, esophageal arteries, intercostal arteries 4. abdominal aorta-celiac artery, renal arteries, mesenteric arteries (superior and inferior).

Aortic regurgitation Leakage of blood from aorta into left ventricle during diastole.

Aortic stenosis Narrowing of aortic valve. Normal valve diameter 2 cm/m^2

Aortic valve The valve between left ventricle and ascending aorta, consists of three semilunar cusps that appose during diastole, thus preventing backflow of blood from aorta to left ventricle.

Aortitis Inflammation of aortic wall, commonly syphilitic or of unknown origin.

Aorto coronary bypass Surgical procedure to direct blood from root of aorta to coronary vessels by putting a saphenous vein graft or internal mammary arteries; a modality of treatment for coronary obstruction.

Aortography X-ray of aorta after contrast injection.

Aortolith Calcareous deposits in the aortic wall.

Apareunia Inability to accomplish sexual intercourse.

Apathetic Indifferent, disinterested.

Apathism Slowness to react to stimuli, (opposite of erethism).

Apatite The deceptive stone, a mineral containing calcium and phosphorus ions.

Apeidosis Slow modification or disappearance of the clinical and histological characteristics of a disease.

Aperient A very mild laxative.

Aperitive Appetite stimulant.

Apert's syndrome Congenital disorder with peaked head, webbed fingers and toes.

Aperture An orifice or opening.

Apex The pointed end of any cone shaped structure.

Apex beat The systolic movement of left ventricular apex against chest wall, felt in 5th intercostal space 1/2" inside midclavicular line.

Apgar score A system of assessing infants' physical condition one minute after birth. The heart rhythm, respiration, muscle tone, response to stimuli and skin colour are assigned a score of 0, 1 or 2. Total score is 10. Those with very low score require immediate attention. Apgar score at birth has a prognostic bearing on ultimate neurological development.

Aphakia Absence of lens of eye.

Aphasia Impairment of speech; may be motor or sensory (Wernicke's).

a. amnestic Loss of memory for words.

a. anomic Forgetful for naming.

a. Broca's Motor aphasia with intact comprehension.

a. global Failure of comprehension as well as speech production.

a. jargon Use of disconnected words.

a. motor Inability to use muscles controlling speech production.

a. semantic Inability to understand meaning of words.

a. syntactic Lack of proper grammatical composition.

Aphemia Motor aphasia.

Aphephobia Morbid fear of being touched.

Apheresis Technique of separating blood into its components.

Aphonia Peripherial failure of speech production; commonly due to a laryngeal lesion.

Aphrasia Inability to speak or understand phrases.

Aphrodisiac Sex stimulant.

Aphthae Small ulcer on mucous membrane.

Aphthous Pertains to aphthae, i.e. recurrent stomatitis.

Apicectomy Excision of apex of petrous part of temporal bone.

Apicitis Inflammation of tooth/lung apex.

Aplanatic lens A lens that corrects spherical aberration.

Aplasia Failure of an organ or tissue to develop normally.

Aplastic Having deficient or arrested development.

Apnea Temporary cessation of breathing.

Apneumatosis Congenital atelectasis.

Apneusis Abnormal respiration with sustained inspiratory effort; caused by pontine lesion.

Apochromatic lens Lens that corrects both spherical and chromatic aberration.

Apocrine Secretory cells that contribute part of their protoplasm to the matter secreted.

Apocrine sweat glands Sweat glands of axilla and pubic region that open into hair follicles rather than directly onto surface.

Apoenzyme The protein portion of an enzyme.

Apoferritin The protein that combine with iron to form ferritin.

Apolipoprotein The nonlipid protein portion of lipoprotein named as B100, AI, AII, B and E.

Apomorphine A grayish white powder; derivative of morphine, used as emetic and cough suppressant.

Aponeurosis A flat fibrous sheet of connective tissue serving to attach muscle to bone.

a. epicranial Fibrous membrane joining occipital and frontal muscles.

a. pharyngeal Fibrous sheet lying between mucosal and muscular layers of the pharyngeal wall.

a. Plantar Connective tissue sheet investing muscles of the sole of the foot fit.

Apophysis An outgrowth from bone without as independent center of ossification.

Apophysitis Inflammation of apophysis.

Apoplexy Bleeding into an organ; sudden loss of consciousness with paralysis due to haemorrhage into brain.

Apoptosis Disintegration of cells into membrane bound particles, that are then phagocytosed by other cells; an important process for limitation of tumor growth.

Apparatus 1. A mechanical device or appliance used in operations or experiments. 2. A group of structures or organs that work together to perform function, e.g. *a auditory, a biliary, a juxtaglomerular, a larcrymal.*

Appendectomy Surgical removal of vermiform appendix.

Appendicitis Inflammation of vermiform appendix. Characterized by pain in right iliac fossa, nausea and vomiting, tenderness and rigidity over right rectus muscle or Mc Burney's point, mild fever, leukocytosis.

a. chronic Follows acute attack with inflammatory adhesions, and formation of a lump.

a. gangrenous Acute appendicitis involving blood vessels with their occlusion and development of gangrene and its vulnerability for rupture.

Appendicolysis Operation to free appendix from adhesions.

Appendicostomy Operation in which opening is made in vermiform appendix to irrigate cecum and colon.

Appendix An appendage.

a. atrial Muscular pouch attached to left and right atria; the sites for atrial thrombi.

a. epiploica Numerous pouches of peritoneum on colon filled with fat.

Appestat Area of brain controlling appetite.

Appetite Strong desire for food in contrast to hunger which is a painful condition due to lack of food.

a. perverted Desire to eat unnatural substances *SYN*— pica.

Appetizer Substance that promotes appetite.

Applanometer Device for measuring intraocular pressure.

Apple Adam's The laryngeal prominence formed by two laminae of thyroid cartilage.

Apple Picker's disease Respiratory involvement due to fungicides used in apple harvesting.

Appliance In dentistry a device used to correct bite such as artificial dentures.

Applicator A rod with cotton swab on end for making local applications.

Apposition Being positioned side by side.

Approach 1. Surgical procedures for exposing any organ or tissue 2. draw near.

Apraxia Inability to perform purposive and learned movements even though there is no motor/ sensory loss.

a. amnestic Patient cannot understand the action asked to perform even though ability to perform the act is intact.

a. constructional Inability to construct two or three dimensional figures due to lack of ability to integrate perception into kinesthetic images.

a. dressing Patient's inability to dress due to lack of knowledge about spatial relations of body.

a. ideational Incorrect use of objects due to inability in perceiving their correct use.

a. motor Inability to perform an action although the components of it are understood.

Apron Outergarment for protection of clothing inside.

Aprosody Absence of normal variations in pitch, rhythm and stress in the speech.

Aprotinin Protease inhibitor used in pancreatitis, carcinoid syndrome and during surgery to reduce blood loss.

Aptitude Inherent ability or skill in learning or performing.

Aptyatism Deficient secretion of saliva.

APUD cells Amine precursor uptake and decarboxylation cells; the class of cell producing hormones like ACTH, insulin, glucagon, thyroxin dopamine, serotonin, histamine, etc.

Aqua Water.

a. aerata Carbonated water.

a. calcariae Lime water.

a. fervens Hot water.

a. fontana Spring water.

Aquanant Persons working under water for carrying research.

Aquaphobia Morbid fear of water.

Aquapuncture Subcutaneous injection of water to produce counter irritation.

Aqueduct Canal or channel.

a. cerebral Canal in midbrain joining third and fourth ventricles.

a. vestibular Passage from vestibule to petrous part of temporal bone.

a. cochleae Canal connecting subarachnoid space and the cochlear perilymphatic space.

Aqueous Watery

Aqueous humor Transparent liquid produced by ciliary processes and filling the posterior and anterior chambers of eye and finally absorbed into venous system by canals of Schlemm.

Arabinose A pentose plant sugar, gum sugar.

Arachidonic acid An essential fatty acid, precursor for prostaglandins, thromboxane and leukotrienes.

Arachnida A class of arthropodes that includes spiders, ticks, mites and scorpions.

Arch Any anatomic structure with a curved or bow like outline, e.g. aortic arch.

a. axillary An anomalous muscular slip across the axilla between pectoralis major and latissimus dorsi.

a. crural The inguinal ligament extending from anterior superior iliac spine to pubic tubercle.

a. longitudinal The antero-posterior arch of the foot; the medial portion is formed by calcaneus, talus, navicular, cuneiform and first three metatarsals and the lateral portion by calcaneus, cuboid and 4th and fifth metatarsals.

a. mandibular The first branchial arch from which upper and lower jawbones and associated structures develop, so also malleus and incus.

a. palmar The superficial arch is formed by termination of ulnar artery and the deep arch by communicating branch of ulnar and the radial artery.

a. plantar Arch formed by external plantar artery and deep branch of dorsalis pedis artery.

a. transverse Transverse arch of foot formed by navicular, cuboid cuneiform and metatarsals.

a. zygomatic Arch formed by malar and temporal bones.

Archenteron The primitive digestive cavity of gastrula.

Archetype Original type from which other types have developed by differentiation.

Archinephron Primordial kidney of embryo.

Archipallium Olfactory cortex.

Architis Inflammation of anus.

Arcuate Shaped like an arc.

Arcus An arch.

a. juvenalis Opaquering at the periphery of cornea in young, may be due to hypercholesterolemia, corneal irritation/inflammation.

a. senilis Opaque white ring at periphery of cornea due to deposit of fat granules or hyaline degeneration.

Ardor A burning sensation during urination.

Area Well defined space with defined boundaries.

a. association Area of cerebral, cortex that is neither sensory nor motor but seat of higher mental processes.

a. Brodman's Division of cerebral cortex into 47 areas in respect to their different functions.

a. Kiesselbach's Area in anterior portion of nasal septum, with rich capillaries, a site of frequent bleed.

a. of Rolando Area infront of fissure of Rolando in anterior central convolution governing motor function of body.

a. silent Any area of brain whose destruction does not produce detectable motor or sensory loss.

Areflexia Absence of reflexes.

Areola 1. A small space or cavity in a tissue. 2. Circular area of different pigmentation, e.g. around nipple.

Areolar glands (Montgomery's glands). Large modified sweat glands beneath the areola secreting a lipoid material that lubricates the nipple.

Areometer Device for measuring specific gravity of fluids.

Argentaffinoma An Argentaffin tumor secreting serotonin that may arise in intestinal tract, bile ducts, pancreas, bronchus or ovary.

Arginine Amino acid obtained from decomposition of vegetable matter, protamines and proteins. On hydrolysis it yields urea and ornithine.

Arginosuccinic acid Formed from citruline and aspartic acid.

Argon An inert gas occupying 1% of atmosphere.

Argyl Robertson pupil Absence of light reflex with preservation of accommodation reflex as in tabes.

Argyria Bluish discolouration of skin and mucous membranes from prolonged administration of silver.

Argyrol Mild silver protein used as an antiseptic for eye, nose, throat and urethral irrigation.

Argyrophil Cells that bind to silver salts producing brown or black stain.

Aristogenics *SYN*-eugenics. The science dealing with genetic and prenatal influences affecting expression of certain characteristics in offspring.

Arithmetic mean In statistics, the number obtained by addition of all the values listed in a group divided by total values.

Armamentarium The total utilities at disposal-like drugs, instruments, books, supplies.

Armature 1. A part of an electric generator consisting of a coil of insulated wire. 2. In biology a structure that serves to protect.

Arm board Board placed under the arm for stabilization during I.V. administration.

Arnold-Chiari deformity A condition in which the inferior poles of cerebellar hemispheres and medulla protrude through foramen magnum causing hydrocephalus. It is commonly associated with spina bifida and meningomyelocele.

Aroma Pleasant odor.

Aromatic 1. Having an aggreable odor. 2. Belonging to a series of compounds in which the carbon atoms form a closed ring (as in benzene) in comparision to aliphatic series where carbon atoms form straight or branched chains.

Aromatic ammonia spirit Solution of ammonium carbonate in diluted ammonia solution, fragrant oils, alcohol and water. It acts as a reflex stimulant on inhalation. Also acts as an antacid and carminative.

Arousal 1. Alertness. 2. Sexual excitement

Arrectores pilorum Involuntary muscle in skin connected to hairfollicle whose contraction due to cold, fright causes erection of hair and goose flesh appearance of skin.

Arrest Cessation of function.

a. cardiac Cessation of heart function.

a. epiphyseal Arrest in growth of long bones.

a. pelvic The foetal presenting part is arrested in its descent in maternal pelvis.

a. respiratory Stoppage of spontaneous respiration.

a. sinus The SA node does not initiate the impulse formation, a feature of sick sinus syndrome.

Arrhenoblastoma An ovarian tumor secreting male sex hormones, causing virilization in females.

Arsenic poisoning Accidental or deliberate ingestion causes acute gastroenteritis with shock, convulsion, paralysis and death.

Arsphenamine 30% arsenic previously used for treatment of syphilis. *SYN*—Salvarsan.

Arterial line A method of haemo-
dynamic monitoring where catheter is put into an artery for recording
blood pressure, arterial gas
analysis.

Arteriogram X-ray of an artery after
injection of radio-opaque material.

Arteriole A minute artery that leads
into capillary.

Arterioplasty Repair or reconstruction of an artery.

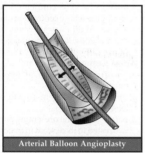
Arterial Balloon Angioplasty

Arteriosclerosis Thickening and
hardening of an artery with loss of
elasticity and contractility. Risk
factors for arteriosclerosis include
ageing, hyperlipidemia, obesity,
diabetes mellitus, smoking etc.

Arteriostenosis Narrowing of the
lumen of an artery.

Arteriostosis Calcification of an
artery.

Arteritis Inflammation of an artery.

a. nodosa Widespread inflammation of
adventia of small and medium sized
arteries with impaired function.

a. temporal Chronic inflammation of
temporal and often occipital and
ophthalmic arteries with presence
of giant cells and occlusion of
vascular lumen.

Artery (from Greek - arteria meaning wind pipe). The ancient Greeks
believed that air travelled through
them. Arteries carry oxygenated
blood from heart to distant body
parts : exceptions are pulmonary
artery and umbilical artery.

a. end Artery whose branches do not
anastomose with those of other

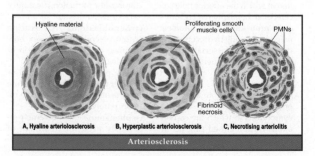

Hyaline material | Proliferating smooth muscle cells | PMNs

Fibrinoid necrosis

A, Hyaline arteriolosclerosis   B, Hyperplastic arteriolosclerosis   C, Necrotising arteriolitis

Arteriosclerosis

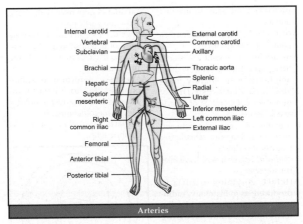

Internal carotid
Vertebral
Subclavian
Brachial
Hepatic
Superior mesenteric
Right common iliac
Femoral
Anterior tibial
Posterior tibial

External carotid
Common carotid
Axillary
Thoracic aorta
Splenic
Radial
Ulnar
Inferior mesenteric
Left common iliac
External iliac

Arteries

arteries, e.g. arteries of brain and spinal cord.

Arthralgia Joint pain.

Arthritide A skin eruption caused by arthritis.

Arthritis Inflammation of a joint usually following trauma, due to degeneration, infection (gonococcal, tubercular, brucella, pneumococcal), rheumatic fever, ulcerative colitis, collagen disorders, SLE, rheumatoid arthritis, gout, synovioma, para or periarticular infections, denervation, e.g. tabes dorsalis.

Arthrocentesis Puncture of a joint to drain joint fluid for analysis.

Arthrodesis The surgical immobilization of joint, ankylosis.

Arthrogram Visualisation of interior of a joint after injection of radio opaque dye into joint space.

Arthrogryposis Fixation of a joint in a flexed position.

Arthrolysis Restoration of mobility of an ankylosed joint.

Arthropathy Any joint disease.

Arthroplasty Reconstruction or reshaping of a diseased joint, even by replacement of joint components.

Arthroscope An endoscope for examination of interior of a joint.

Arthroscopy Visualization of interior of a joint by arthroscope.

Arthrospore A bacterial spore formed by segmentation.

Arthrotome Knife for making incision into joint.

Arthus reaction An immediate hypersensitivity reaction due to preformed antibody to injected antigen.

Articulate 1. To join together as a joint. 2. To speak clearly.

Articulation 1. A joint, classified, being synarthrosis (immovable), amphiarthrosis (slightly movable) and diarthrosis (freely movable) 2. Utterance of words and sentences.

a. apophyseal The joint between superior and inferior articulating process of vertebra.

a. confluent Speech in which syllables run together.

Artefact Anything artificially produced; as in histology/radiology a feature produced by the technique but not occurring naturally.

Artificial Not natural, formed by imitation of nature.

a. insemination donor Artificial insemination of a woman with sperms of anonymous donor.

a. insemination husband Use of husband's sperms for insemination of wife.

a. intelligence Computer performance of congnitive tasks.

a. pneumothorax Introduction of air into pleural cavity to induce collapse of lung as to control haemoptysis in tuberculosis.

Artisan's cramps Muscle cramp involving muscles used in prolonged spells of writting, sewing, telegraphing etc.

Aryepiglottic Pertaining to arytenoid cartilage and epiglottis.

Asafetida A gum resin with strong odor and garlic taste.

Asbestos Fibrous incombustible form of magnesium and calcium silicate used to make insulating material.

Asbestosis A form of pneumoconiosis due to inhalation of asbestos dusts, also responsible for pleural mesothelioma.

Ascariasis Infestation with ascaris lumbricoides.

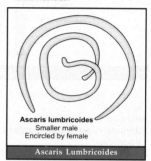

Ascaris lumbricoides
Smaller male
Encircled by female

Ascaris Lumbricoides

Ascaris lumbricoides A species of ascaris inhabiting human intestine, often producing dyspepsia, intestinal obstruction, biliary colic and appendicitis.

Aschheim-Zondek test A pregnancy test where patient's urine is injected into female mice to induce ovulation.

Aschner's phenomenon Slowing of pulse following carotid sinus massage or pressure on eyeball.

Aschoff's cells Large multinucleated cell with vesicular nucleus and basophilic cytoplasm.

Aschoff's nodule Small nodules composed of central fibrinoid necrosis surrounded by giant cells and leukocytes, seen in interstitial tissues of heart in rheumatic myocarditis.

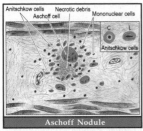

Aschoff Nodule

Ascites Accumulation of fluid in peritoneal cavity.

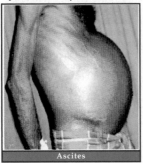

Ascites

a. chylous Milky ascites resulting from rupture of thoracic duct.

Ascorbic acid Vit C.

Aseptic Sterile, free from germs.

Aseptic technique Techniques that prevent contamination of operative wounds.

Asparagine Aminosuccinic acid; a non-essential amino acid.

Aspartame An artificial sweetner, 180 times sweeter than sugar; synthesized from aspartic acid and phenyl alanine. Unsuitable for cooking as the flavor changes on eating.

Aspartic acid A nonessential amino acid, product of pancreatic digestion.

Apergillosis Granulomatous inflammation of skin, lungs, ear canal and mucous membrane by A. fumigatus.

Aspergillin A pigment produced by A. niger which also produces black spores and commonly infects ear canal.

Aspermia Lack of or failure to ejaculate semen.

Aspersion Sprinkling of an affected part with water, a form of hydrotherapy.

Asphyxia Suffocation caused by lack of oxygen due to failure of breathing, tracheobronchial obstruction, drowning, environmental oxygen lack, edema of the lungs.

Asphyxiant An agent, especially gas producing asphyxia.

Asphyxiate To cause asphyxia.

Aspirate To draw in or out by suction.

Aspirator Apparatus for evacuating fluid contents of a cavity.

Aspirin Acetyl salicylic acid.

Assault Violent physical attack on an individual. In legal sense any procedure on an individual without proper permission.

a. sexual Sexual intercourse without consent/against will.

Assay The analysis of a substance or mixture to determine its constituents or the relative proportion of each.

Assimilate To absorb digested food.

Assimilation 1. The processes whereby the products of digestion are absorbed and utilized in the body. 2. In psychology, the absorption of newly perceived information into the existing conscious structure.

Association Relationship; interrelationship of conscious and unconscious; in genetics the occurrence together of two characteristics at a frequency greater than would be predicted by chance.

Association cortex Areas other than motor and sensory cortex which serve to integrate brain functions.

Association test A test in which patient is given a word and he replies with another word to in the first. The time taken in his response is an indicator of his brain function.

Astasia Inability to stand or sit erect due to motor incoordination.

a. abasia A form of hysterical ataxia with inability to stand or walk although all leg movements can be performed while sitting or lying down.

Asteatosis Any diseased condition with scaling of skin due to lack of sebaceous secretion.

Asterognosis Inability to recognize objects or forms by touch.

Astemizole H_1 receptor blocker, antiallergic.

Asterion The junction of lambdoid, occipitomastoid and parietomastoid sutures.

Asterixis Transient lapses of muscle tone with involuntary jerky movements especially of hands as in hepatic failure.

Asteroid Star shaped.

Asthenia Loss of strength, debility.

a. neurocirculatory A psychosomatic disorder characterizes by mental and physical fatigue, dyspnea, giddiness etc.

Asthma Paroxysmal dyspnea and wheezing caused by bronchospasm, bronchial mucosal swelling and retention of viscid sputum.

a. cardiac Asthma secondary to left ventricular failure.

a. extrinsic Asthma due to environmental allergens.

a. intrinsic Asthma where no external cause is identifiable.

Astigmatism A form of ametropia where the curvature of cornea or lens differ in different meridians so that an object is not sharply focussed on retina.

a. compound The horizontal and vertical curvatures are abnormal.

a. simple Only one meridian is defective.

Astragalus Old term for talus.

Astraphobia Fear of thunder and lightening.

Astringent An agent that has constricting or binding effect, i.e. that causes coagulation of proteins and thus contracts organic tissue; thereby checks haemorrhages and secretions. Common examples are salts of lead, iron, zinc, tannic acid.

Astrocyte Star shaped neuroglial cell with many branching processes.

Astrocytoma A tumor of astrocytes; classified in order of increasing malignancy as Grade I—consisting of fibrillary or protoplasmic astrocytes—Grade II composed of astroblasts Grade III-IV—called glioblastoma multiforme composed of spongioblast, astroblast and astrocyte in varying proportion.

Astrophobia Morbid fear of stars and celestial bodies.

Asylum An institution for mentally ill.

Asymmetry Without symmetry.

Asymptomatic Without any symptoms.

Asynclitism An oblique presentation of foetal head during labor.

Asyndesis A form of mental defect in which related thoughts cannot be assembled to form a comprehensive concept.

Asynergia Lack of co-ordination between body parts or muscles that normally act in unison.

Ataraxia A state of complete mental relaxation and tranquility.

Atavism The appearance of characteristics presumed to be present in some ancestors.

Ataxia Defective muscular control and coordination.

a. alcoholic Ataxia due to loss of proprioception in chronic alcoholism.

a. Brun's Ataxia of bilateral frontal lobe lesions with a tendency to stagger and fall backwards.

a. cerebellar Motor ataxia of cerebellar disease. Often with nystagmus, tremor, scanning speech and dysmetria.

a. Friedreich's An inherited disease manifesting in childhood or adolescence. There is degeneration of lateral and dorsal columns of spinal cord. Peripheral neuropathy, high arch palate, kyphoscoliosis are often associated.

a. sensory Ataxia due to loss of proprioceptive impulses.

a. telangiectasia IgA deficiency state of congenital origin manifesting with cerebellar ataxia, telangiectasia and recurrent sinopulmonary infections.

Atelectasis Collapsed or airless condition of lungs; the affected lungs are often unexpanded since birth, can be caused by bronchial obstruction, or compression.

Ateliosis A form of infantilism due to pituitary insufficiency.

Atherogenesis Formation of atheromata in the walls of arteries.

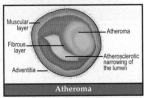

Atheroma

Atheroma Fatty degeneration of arterial wall with cholesterol deposit and smooth muscle hyperplasia.

Atherosclerosis A sclero degenerative disease of arterial wall marked by intimal lipid deposit, fibrous tissue accumulation and smooth muscle cell proliferation.

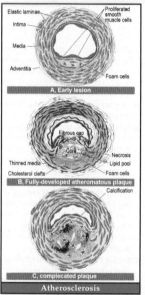

Atherosclerosis

Athetosis Slow irregular twisting involuntary movement of hand and fingers.

Athlete's foot Fungus infection of foot particularly in between toes.

Atlantoaxial Pertaining to first and second curvical vertebrae.

Atlas The first cervical vertebra articulating with occipital bone (Atlas is the Greek God holding the world on his shoulders).

Atom The smallest form of an element consisting of protons, neutrons and electrons.

Atopy An allergy with a genetic predisposition. Principal forms of atopy are bronchial asthma, urticaria, eczema and rhinitis.

Atresia Congenital absence or closure of any tubular structure.

Atrial fibrillation Randomized irregular arrhythmic atrial contractions giving rise to irregularly irregular pulse.

Atrial flutter Rapid regular atrial contraction with a varying but regular ventricular response due to fixed or varying A-V block.

Atrial natriuretic factor A hormone secreted by dilated atria that helps in natriuresis.

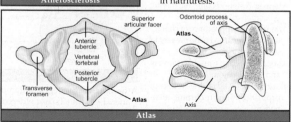

Atlas

Atrichosis Congenital absence of hair.

Atrioventricular bundle The conducting system extending from A-V node till division into left and right bundles.

Atrioventriculares communis Persistence of the common atrioventricular canal manifesting with atrioventricular septal defects and A-V valve incompetence.

Atrium A chamber or cavity in communication with another.

a. of ear Portion of tympanic cavity lying below the malleolus.

Atrophy Decrease in size of tissue or wasting.

a. acute yellow Extensive necrosis of liver cells with jaundice, haemorrhage and mental obtundation.

a. optic Degeneration of optic nerve head, primary or secondary (MS, glaucoma, trauma etc).

a. disuse Atrophy resulting from lack of use of muscle.

a. peroneal muscular A hereditary disease involving peroneal nerves with progressive atrophy of peroneal muscles.

a. sudek's Acute atrophy of bone at the site of injury, possibly due to local vasospasm.

Atropine sulfate A parasympatholytic agent used for preanesthetic medication to decrease bronchial secretions and in organophosphorous poisoning.

Atropinization Administration of atropine till desired effect is obtained.

Attack The sudden onset of an illness, e.g. heart attack.

Attention-deficit-disorder A disease of infancy or childhood, mainly boys characterized by inappropriate attention, hyperactivity and impulsivity.

Attenuate To render thin, weak or less virulent.

Attic The middle ear cavity above the tympanic membrane.

Attitude 1. Behavior towards a person, thing or situation 2. Bodily posture or position assumed, e.g. catatonic posture.

Audible sound Sound with frequency of 15-15000 Hz.

Audiologist A specialist in the evaluation and rehabilitation of persons with hearing disorder.

Audiometry Testing of hearing by audiometer.

Audito-oculogyric reflex Sudden turning of eyes and head towards direction of loud sound.

Auditory bulb The membranous labyrinth and cochlea.

Auditory Evoked Response An objective method of assessing hearing where the hearing stimulus as traverses along its path to auditory cortex produces characteristic electric potentials recorded across the cortex. It is useful in children, in malingerers, and in psychiatric patients. It can pin point as to the site of lesion along the auditory pathway.

Auditory reflex Any reflex produced by stimulation of auditory nerve like blinking of eyes in response to sudden sound.

Auerbach's plexus A plexus formed by sympathetic nerve fibers in muscular coats of GI. tract.

Auer bodies Rod shaped in-tracytoplasmic structure present in myeloblasts in acute myeloblastic leukemia.

Augmentin Amoxycillin-clavulanic acid.

Aura A subjective sensation preceding an attack of epileptic seizure or migraine; epileptic aura may be psychic in nature or sensory in the form of auditory, visual, olfactory or taste hallucinations.

Auranofin Gold preparation for rheumatoid arthritis.

Aureomycin Chlortetracycline hydrochloride.

Auricle 1. Left and right atria 2. Pinna of the ear.

Auriculopalpebral reflex Closure of eye resulting from tactile or thermal stimulation of external auditory meatus. Synonym: Kisch's reflex.

Auriscope Instrument for examination of ear.

Aurotherapy Treatment with gold salts, e.g. rheumatoid arthritis.

Auscultation The technique of listening to sounds produced within body, e.g. passage of air in bronchi, blood in occluded vessels, and A-V malformation, bowel movement, beating of heart, murmurs and adventitious heart sounds, etc.

Austin Flint murmur Diastolic mitral regurgitation in a aortic insufficiency mimicking mitral stenosis but without the opening snap or pre-systolic accentuation.

Australia antigen Hepatitis B surface antigen, existing in serum as part of Dane particle (40-400 nm) or as free particles and rods (22 nm).

Autacoids Generic name for histamine and antihistamine like agents in body.

Autism Mental introversion with attention centered around own ego.

a. infantile A syndrome appearing in childhood with self absorption, aloneness, inaccessibility, rage reactions and behavioral-language problems; a form of childhood psychosis.

Autoagglutinin Agglutinins that agglutinate individuals own red blood cells.

Autoanalyzer Device that analyzes multiple samples automatically.

Autoantibody Antibody acting against the host antigens.

Autocatharsis A form of psychotherapy in which patient gets an insight into his problems by a frank discussion.

Autoclave A device used for sterilization by steam pressure.

Autocrine factor A growth factor probably produced by cells in response to virus infection and playing some role in genesis of malignancies.

Autodigestion Digestion of a tissue by tissue's own products, e.g. pancreatic digestion in acute pancreatitis.

Autoerotism Sexual arousal or gratification by using one's own body as in masturbation.

Autograft A graft transferred from one part of body to another.

Autohemolysis Hemolysis of ones blood by person's own serum.

Autohemotherapy Injection of patient's own blood.

Autoimmunity Condition in which antibodies are produced against body's own tissues.

Autoimmune disease Diseases in which antibodies are produced against body's own tissues to cause organ damage, e.g. rheumatoid arthritis, SLE, glomerulonephritis, rheumatic carditis, myasthenia gravis.

Autoinfection Infection produced by an agent already present within the body.

Autoinfusion Forcing blood from extremities to body core by applying tight bandages.

Autoinoculation Inoculation of a person by organisms obtained from the same individual.

Autologous blood transfusion Use of patient's own blood for transfusion, the blood being collected prior to operation or during operation from wound site; thus avoiding dangers of mismatch and transfusion associated infections like; HBV, AIDS.

Automatism Behavior without conscious volition or knowledge, the individual appearing normal but amnesic for the events.

Autonomic nervous system The part of nervous system controlling involuntary functions like heart beat, glandular secretions, bowel and bladder contraction and other smooth muscle function. It is divided into parasympathetic or craniosacral system and sympathetic or thoracolumbar system.

Autopsy Postmortem examination to ascertain cause of death.

Autoregulation A phenomena where the involved tissue regulates events like blood flow into/through it according to its requirement, e.g. as in brain.

Autosomes Any of the chromosomes other than sex chromosomes.

Autosplenectomy Multiple infarcts of spleen that cause it to shrink as in sickle cell anaemia.

Autotrophic Self nourishing, e.g. green plants and bacteria forming protein and carbohydrate from inorganic salts and bicarbonates.

A-V block A block in atrioventricular node whereby impulses arising from atria cannot reach ventricles or are delayed; divided into first degree (prolonged PR), second degree (mobitz type I and II) and third degree A-V block.

Avascular Having poor blood supply.

Avalanche theory Theory that nervous impulses are reinforced and thereby become more intense as they travel peripherally.

Aversion therapy A form of behavior therapy where unpleasant and undesired (e.g. alcohol) stimuli are presented to patient simultaneously so that patient associates the undesired stimulus with the unpleasant one and thus discontinues the undesired stimulus.

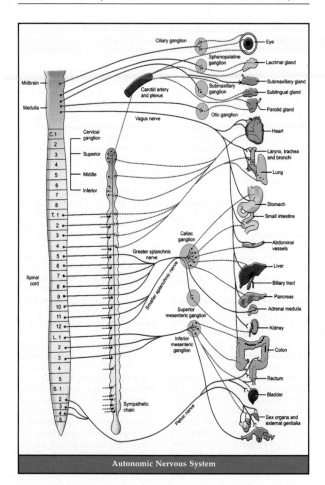

Autonomic Nervous System

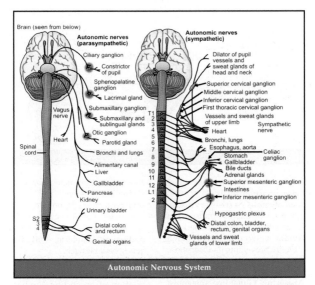

Autonomic Nervous System

Avidin A protein of egg white inhibiting biotin.

Avulsion A tearing away forcibly of a part or structure.

Axilla Armpit.

Axanthopsia Yellow blindness.

Axial line A line running in the main axis of body. The axial line of hand runs through second digit.

Axis 1. A line running through the center of the body. 2. The second cervical vertebra bearing the odontoid process about which atlas rotates.

a. cardiac A graphic representation of the main conduction vector of the heart. Normal axis is 0 to + 90°.

a. visual The line passing from object through center of cornea and lens to the fovea.

Axis deviation Deviation of cardiac axis, like left axis deviation −10° to −90°, right axis deviation + 91 to −90°.

Axis traction Traction made on the fetus in the direction of long axis of birth canal.

Axon A process of nerve cell conducting impulse away from the cell body.

Axoneme Axial thread of a chromosome.

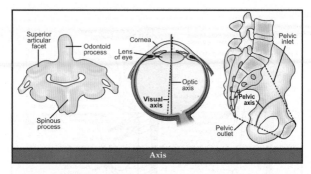

Axis

Axonometer Device for determining axis of astigmatism.

Axonotemesis Nerve injury disrupting nerve impulse transmission but without severing the nerve.

Avidin A glycoprotein that binds to biotin, preventing its absorption.

Azapropazone A pyrazolon, aspirin like agent, potent uricosuric.

Azaserine Glutamine antagonist, potent inhibitor of purine nucleotide biosynthesis.

Azathioprine An immunosuppressant.

Azauridine A pyrimidine analog.

Azoospermia Complete absence of sperms in the semen.

Azotemia Increased blood urea.

Azotobacter Gram negative rod-shaped gram negative non-pathogenic bacteria that fix atmospheric nitrogen.

Azygos Occurring singly, not in pairs.

Azygos vein The thoracic continuation of ascending lumbar vein through aortic hiatus in diaphragm entering superior vena cava at the level of D_4 vertebra.

B

Babesia A genus of the order Haemosporidia found in the cattle, sheep, horse, dogs and other vertebrate animals, transmitted by tick.

Babesiosis A disease caused by intraerythrocytic protozoan parasite.

Babesia microti Principally manifesting with fever, chills and hemoglobinuria.

Babinski's reflex Dorsiflexion of great toe and fanning out of other toes on stimulation of lateral part of sole of foot is called positive Babinski's reflex; commonly results from pyramidal tract interruption; also positive in infants below 6 months (before myelination).

Bacampicillin A long acting ampicillin given in twice daily dose.

Bacillemia Presence of bacilli in blood.

Bacillus Any rod shaped microorganism.

b. abortus (undulant fever in man).

b. cereus anaerobic spore bearing opportunistic invader in immunocompromised.

b. Doderleins (identical with lactobacillus acidophilus).

b Dcrey (causes soft sore).

b. Friedlander's (Klebsiella pneumoniae).

b. Koch-Weeks (*Haemophilus aegyptius* causing conjunctivitis).

b. melaninogenicus (gram negative bacillus causing vincents angina).

b. morax Axenfeld. (causes angular conjunctivitis).

Bacitracin Topically used antibacterial agent.

Backache Any pain in back; due to muscle spasm, disease of disk, ligaments, vertebral body, nerve roots, and meninges.

Baclofen GABA inhibitor used to reduce muscle spasticity.

Bacteria Any micro-organism, of the class Schizomycetes; can be spherical or ovoid (cocci); rod shaped (bacilli) or spiral.

Bacteriocin Protein produced by certain bacteria which is lethal to other bacteria.

Bacteriocinogen A plasmid that produces bacteriocin.

Bacterioclasis Fragmentation of bacteria.

Bacteriophage A virus that infects bacteria.

Bacteriuria Presence of bacteria in urine, significant if concentration exceeds 10^5/ml.

Bacteroides A genus of non-spore forming, gram negative, anaerobic bacteria frequently found in necrotic tissue.

Bagasosis Hypersensitive pneumonitis due to inhalation of bagasse dust, the moldy fibrous waste of sugarcane.

Baker's cyst Synovial cyst in popliteal fossa.

Balanitis Inflammation of the glans penis and mucous membrane beneath it.

Balantidiasis Infestation with *B. coli*.

Balanoposthitis Inflammation of glans and prepuce.

Ballottement Palpatory technique for examining floating objects, e.g. foetus in uterus, hydronephrotic kidney.

Balneology Science of baths and bathing.

Balser's fatty necrosis Gangrenous pancreatitis with fatty necrosis of pancreas and often of bone marrow.

Bandage A piece of gauze to be wrapped around a body part as dressing.

b. barton Double figure of eight bandage for the lower jaw.

b. butterfly Adhesive bandage used to hold wound edges together.

b. buttocks T or double T bandage or open triangle bandage for buttocks.

b. cravat Triangular bandage folded to form a band around any injured bony part, e.g. knee elbow, hand, wrist, head, clavicle.

b. figure of eight Bandage in which turns cross each other like the figure 8. Used to fix and elevate the shoulders in fracture clavicle, to fix splints for the foot or hand.

b. spica Bandage in which a number of figure of 8 turns are applied, each a little higher or lower with some overlapping. Used for breasts, shoulders, great toe etc.

b. suspensory used for support of breast and scrotum.

Banti's syndrome A combination of anaemia, cirrhosis and splenic enlargement.

Bandl's ring Ring like thickening at the junction of upper and lower uterine segments.

Barber's itch Folliculitis of face mostly by Staph. aureus.

Barbotage Repeated injection and withdrawal as in withdrawal of CSF and injection of drugs into SA space.

Baresthesia Pressure sense.

Barium An alkaline metallic compound used as barium sulphate for upper GI studies, colon and GI tract

Baritosis Barium dust induced pneumoconiosis.

Barlow's disease Vit. C deficiency state.

Barognosis The ability to estimate weight.

Baroreflex Reflex mediated by pressure changes within great vessels through stimulation of mechanoreceptors.

Barotrauma Trauma due to changes in atmospheric pressure.

Barr body Sex chromatin mass seen within the nuclei of normal female somatic cells, representing inactivated X-chromosome.

Barrel chest Rounded chest due to air trapping as in emphysema. In normal chest, AP diameter is more than transverse, hence elliptical shape.

Bartholin's gland A compound mucus gland lying in lateral wall of vestibule of vagina, at the junction upper and middle one third.

Bartholin's duct Duct of sublingual salivary gland that runs parallel with Wharton's duct and opens with it.

Bartonellosis Infection due to bartonella bacilliformis (oroya fever) characterised by fever and haemolysis; transmitted by female sandflies and treated with chloramphenicol.

Bartter's syndrome Hyperplasia of Juxtaglomerular cells with hypokalemia, hyperaldosteronism but without a rise in blood pressure.

Basal ganglia Four masses of gray matter (caudate, lentiform, amygdaloid and claustrum) lying deep in cerebral hemispheres.

Basal metabolic rate (BMR) Normal value is 40 kcal/m^2/hour, a test of thyroid function.

Base Any substance that accepts hydrogen ion; strong bases feel slippery and are corrosives.

Base pair In double stranded helical DNA the connecting chemicals, i.e. base pairs adenine-thymine, guanine-cytosine bind the strands.

Basion Mid point of anterior border of foramen magnum.

Basiphobia Fear of walking.

Basisphenoid An embryonic bone that becomes the lower portion of sphenoid.

Bassini's operation Surgical repair of inguinal hernia.

Battered child syndrome Physical injuries inflicted upon children.

Battery Assault.

Bazin's disease Erythema induratum.

B cells Bone marrow derived lymphocytes, which when stimulated by antigen, transform to antibody producing plasma cells.

BCG vaccine Bacilli-Calmette-Guerin, indicated for vaccination of tuberculin negative children.

Beaker Wide mouthed glass vessel.

Beau's line White lines on finger nails.

Beclomethasone Synthetic corticosteroid.

Becquerel (BQ) A measure of radioactivity of radionuclides equal to 3.7×10^{10} curies.

Bedlam Asylum for insane.

Bedsore Pressure Sore, i.e. ischaemic necrosis of tissue esp. over bony prominences.

Behcet's syndrome A symptoms complex of recurrent orogenital ulceration, uveitis and joint pains, 5 times more frequent in males.

Belching Expulsion of stomach gas through mouth and nose.

Bell's palsy Sudden unilateral lower motor facial palsy due to swelling/ischemia of the nerve in bony canal.

Bellini's tubule The straight connecting tubule of the kidney.

Bence Jones protein A low molecular weight protein that disappears when urine is boiled to above 60°C but reappears once urine is cooled, commonly seen in multiple myeloma.

Benedict's sol A solution of copper sulfate, sodium citrate and sodium carbonate, used for testing presence of reducing sugars in urine.

Benedict's test 8 drops of urine is added to 5 ml. of Benedicts Sol. and boiled to see for green, yellow, red precipitate.

Benign Not recurrent, nor progressive.

Benign Prostatic Hypertrophy (BPH) Prostatic enlargement in elderly due to hyperplasia causing obstruction of prostatic urethra.

Benoxynate HCL Topically used ophthalmic local anaesthetic.

Benserazide Inhibitor of amino acid decarboxylase, used in parkinsonism.

Bentonite Hydrated alumino - silicate, used as a suspending agent.

Benzalkonium chloride An antimicrobial preservative, used as detergent and germicide.

Benzafibrate Lipid lowering agent

Benzene A volatile liquid used in synthesis of dyes and drugs.

Benzidine Used for test of occult blood in stool, (to a solution of benzidine in glacial acetic acid is added 3% H_2O_2 and the stool sample. Appearance of blue colour indicates presence of blood.

Benznidazole A nitroimidazole for Chaga's disease.

Benzobromarone Uricosuric agent used in gout.

Benzocaine Topical anaesthetic.

Benzodiazepine Psychotropic agents with potent hypnotic and antianxiety effects.

Benzoic A plant resin used as inhalant, or protective coating for ulcers.

Benzoic acid Antifungal agent.

Benzoyl peroxide Keratolytic agent (for acne).

Benzthiazide Diuretic of thiazide group.

Benztropine mesylate Antiparasympathomimetic agent for treatment of parkinsonism.

Benzyl benzoate Scabicide.

Bephenium hydroxynaphthoate Anthelmintic for hookworm and mixed infestation.

Beraud's valve A fold of mucous membrane at the mouth of lacrymal duct in the lid.

Beri beri A disease due to thiamine deficiency characterized by cardiac failure (wet type) or fatigue, neuritis, poor memory, anorexia (dry type).

Benzoic acid   **Benzoic alcohol**   **Benzocaine**

Benzoic Acid

Berylliosis Beryllium induced pulmonary fibrosis.

Bestiality Sexual intercourse with animals.

Beta adrenergic receptors Specific receptors in blood vessels, heart, bronchi intestine, etc. for action of adrenaline and noradrenaline.

Beta adrenergic receptor blockers Drugs that block both Beta$_1$ and Beta$_2$ receptors.

Betahistine Drug used for vertigo.

Betaine An alkaloid from beet, used orally as a source of HCl.

Betadine Povidone-iodine.

Betalactamase An enzyme produced by certain bacteria that inactivates antibiotics.

Beta methasone Synthetic glucocorticoid.

Betatron Electron accelerator that produces high energy electrons or X-rays.

Bethanicol Choline ester used for relief of urinary retention.

Betz cells Giant pyramidal cells in the motor cortex whose axons form pyramidal tract.

Bezoar A hardmass of entangled material found in stomach or intestine, hair ball (trichobezoar) hair and vegetable fiber (trichophyto bezoar).

Biblio mania Obsession with collection of books.

Biceps A muscle with two heads.

b. brachii flexor of elbow and supinater.

b. femoris muscle on posterior lateral side of thigh, flexor of knee and rotates it outwards.

BCNU Carmustine, an antineoplastic agent.

Biconcave Concave on each side.

Biconvex Convex on both sides.

Bicornis Uterus with two horns due to incomplete union of müllerian ducts.

Bicuspid Having two cusps or leaflets. mitral, often aortic.

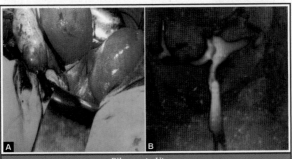

Bikornuate Uterus

Bicuspid tooth Permanent premolars are bicuspid.

Bicycle ergometer Stationary bicycle used for cardiac exercise, i.e. MUGA testing/intraoperative exercise test.

Bifid Cleft or split into two parts.

Bifocal Eye glasses with lenses for distant and near vision.

Bifonazole An imidazole with antifungal activity.

Bigemini Group of two beats separated by a long pause. Commonly due to regular extrasystoles, (e.g. digitalis toxicity).

Bile A thick viscid fluid with bitter taste secreted by liver. The bile when secreted in liver is straw coloured but down below is yellow-brown or green in colour.

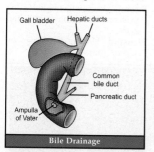

Bile Drainage

Bile acids Cholic, taurocholic and glycocholic acids that exist as salts in bile and are helpful for intestinal fat absorption (micelle formation).

Bile pigment Bilirubin and biliverdin, imparting brown colour to urine and faeces and give positive reaction in Vandenberg's test.

Biticyanin A blue or purple pigment, an oxidation product of biliverdin.

Biligenesis Formation of bile.

Bilirubin Bile pigment; yellow to orange coloured, can be direct acting when conjugated to glucuronic acid or indirect acting when unconjugated.

Biliverdin Greenish pigment, formed by oxidation of bilirubin.

Billroth's operation BI: Excision of pylorus and gastroduodenal anastomosis BII: Partial gastrectomy followed by side to side gastrojejunal anastomosis.

Bimanual Examination by both hands.

Bimodal Means a graphic presentation with two peaks.

Bioassay Determination of strength of a drug in live animal/humans.

Bioavailability The rate and extent to which an active drug or metabolite enters the general circulation to be available at the acting site.

Biochemistry Chemistry of living things.

Biodynamics The science of force or energy of living matter.

Biofeedback A training programme aimed at controlling in function of autonomic nervous system.

Biogenic amines Chemical compounds important in neuro transmission, e.g. dopamine, norepinephrine, serotonin and histamine.

Biokinetics Study of growth changes and movements in developing organisms.

Biometry Computation of life expectancy, application of statistics to biological science.

Biophysics Application of physical laws to biological processes and function.

Biostatistics Application of statistical processes and methods to the analysis of biological data, e.g. morbidity rate, mortality rate etc.

Biot's breathing Short breaths in succession followed by long apnea as seen in raised intracranial pressure.

Biotin Otherwise known vit. H; deficiency manifests with poor mental and physical development, alopecia, impaired immunity, etc.

Biparietal Distance between both parietal eminences important for foetal descent and delivery.

Bipolar In bipolar disease patient has alternating mania and depression.

Birth mark Nevus, pigmentation or vascular tumor.

Bisacromial Pertains to two acromial processes.

Bismuth Silvery metallic element whose salts are astringent, protective, soothing and antidiarrhoeal.

Bite In dentistry denotes the angle and manner at which upper and lower teeth meet when jaw is closed.

b. closed lower incisors lie behind upper incisors.

b. open gap existing between upper and lower incisors.

b. over upper incisors overlap lower ones.

b. under lower incisors pass in front of upper ones.

Bite wing radiograph X-ray showing crown and upper third of root of upper and lower teeth.

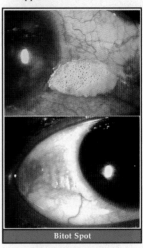

Bitot Spot

Bitot's spots Triangular, shinny, gray spots on conjunctiva seen in vit A deficiency.

Bjerrum's screen Used for mapping the field of visions esp. central and paracentral scotomas.

Blackhead A plug of dried sebum in a sebaceous gland (Acne).

Black eye Bruising, discoloration and swelling of eyelids following trauma.

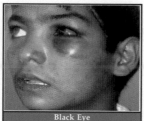
Black Eye

Black measles Also called haemorrhagic measles implying a severe
hemorrhagic measle eruption.

Blackout Sudden loss of consciousness.

Black water fever Haemoglobinuria
following P. falciparum induced
hemolysis.

Black widow A species of poisonous
spider: Latrodectus mactans,
whose bite causes severe
abdominal cramps.

Bladder Receptacle to hold secretions,
(urinary bladder, gallbladder).

b. autonomous Bladder with loss of
both efferent and afferent limbs of
reflex arc, constant dribbling with
large amount of residual urine.

b. exstrophy Congenital eversion of
bladder.

b. neurogenic Any bladder dysfunction due to interruption of its
innervation.

b. worm Larval form of tapeworm
with a rounded cyst or bladder into
which scolex is invaginated.

Blanch To lose colour. In blanching
test, the nail is pressed quickly and
then released. When circulation is
good, colour returns within 5
seconds.

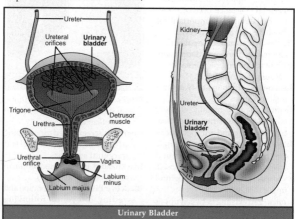
Urinary Bladder

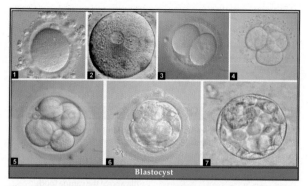

Blastocyst

Bland diet Diet without irritant foods, e.g. milk, cream, prepared cereals, eggs, lean meat, fish, cheese, custard, cookie etc.

Blandin's glands Glands on each side of frenulum of tongue.

Blastocyst A stage of mammalian embryo next to morula and consists of outer trophoblast to which is attached an inner cell mass. The enclosed cavity is blastocele.

Blastoma Neoplasm composed of immature undifferentiated cells.

Blastomere One of the cells resulting from cleavage of a fertilized ovum.

Blastomyces A genus of yeast like budding fungi pathogenic to man.

Bleaching powder Calcium hypochlorite or chlorinated lime.

Bleeding time Time required for blood to stop flowing from a pin prick. Normal range 1-3 minutes (Dukes) or 1-9 minutes (Ivy).

Blennorrhagia A discharge from mucous membranes.

Bleomycin Anti-tumor agent used for carcinoma of skin, lungs, head and neck.

Blepharitis Inflammation of lid margins including hair follicles and the glands.

Blepharodiastasis Excessive separation of eyelids.

Blepharospasm Twitching or spasm of orbiculares oculi muscle.

Blindness Amauresis.

Blindspot Physiological scotoma situated 15° to outside of visual fixation point, corresponding to optic disc.

Blister Collection of fluid within epidermis.

Blood brain barrier A barrier membrane, i.e. endothelium and basement membrane, that prevent entry of damaging substances into CNS.

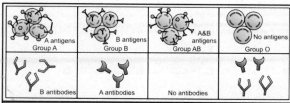

Blood Groups

Blood group A genetically determined system of antigens located on surface of RBC. AB, and O system is the commonly accepted one. There are 30 Rh antigens too.

Blood pressure Pressure exerted by moving blood on the vessel wall. A value beyond 140/90 mm Hg in those below 50 years and 160/95 mm Hg in those above 60 years is abnormal.

BP diastolic BP in between heart beats; depends upon elasticity of arteries and peripheral vascular resistance.

Blumenbach's sign Sign indicative of peritonitis, pain is experienced while pressure is relieved, on the abdomen by examining hand.

Boa's point A tender spot left of 12th dorsal vertebra, in patients with gastric ulcer.

Bochdalek's ganglion Ganglion of plexuses of dental nerve in the maxilla above the canine tooth.

Body

b. ketone They are acetone, acetoacitic acid and betahydroxy butyric acid.

b. amygdaloid Almond shaped gray matter in the lateral wall and roof of third ventricle of brain concerned with memory.

b. Aschoff Microscopic areas of central fibrinoid degeneration with sorrounding chronic inflammatory cell infiltration seen in rheumatic fever.

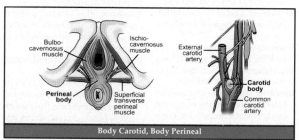

Body Carotid, Body Perineal

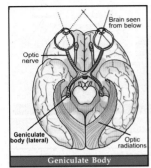

Geniculate Body

b. carotid Flat structure at bifurcation of common carotid, containing baroreceptors.

b. chromaffin Also known as paraganglia, ectodermal in origin, lie along both sides of dorsal aorta.

b. donovan Chlamydia granulomatis, causative organism of granuloma inguinale.

b. medial geniculate Lie in posterior dorsal thalamus and receive acoustic fibers from medullary centers passing to it via inferior colliculus.

b. lateral geniculate Receives afferent fibers from retina through optic tracts.

b. Leishman-Donovan Leishman donovan parasite seen both extra- and intracellularly in kala-azar (Dum-Dum fever).

b. malpighian Renal corpuscle consisting of glomerulus and the Bowman's capsule.

b. mammilary It is a rounded eminence projecting into inter peduncular fossa. It acts as a relay station for olfactory impulses.

b. Negri Inclusion bodies in nerve cells of CNS in patients of rabies.

b. Nissl Large inclusion bodies in nerve cells.

b. pacchionian Arachnoid granulation.

b. pineal Located near splenium of corpus callosum secreting melatonin.

b. psammoma Laminated calcareous body seen in certain tumors (meningioma).

b. restiform Inferior cerebellar peduncle.

Body mass index Body weight in kg divided by height in meters squared (W/H^2), an index for estimating obesity.

Body rocking Rhythmic purposeless body movements.

Boeck's sarcoid Older name for sarcoidosis.

Boil A furuncle, acute inflammation of subcutaneous tissue including glands and hair follicles.

Bombesin A neuropeptide present in gut and brain.

Bone

b. alveolar bone of maxilla and mandible supporting the teeth.

b. sesamoid bone found embeded in tendons and joint capsule.

Bone age Estimation of biological age based on development of ossification centers of wrist and long bones.

Borborygmus A gurgling, splashing sound heard in abdomen caused by passage of gas.

Boric acid An odourless white crystaline powder used as a mild antiseptic solution especially for eyes, mouth and bladder.

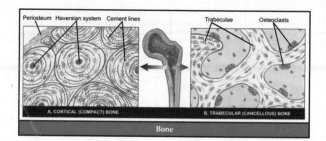

Bone

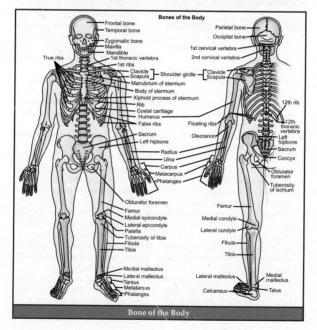

Bone of the Body

Bornholm disease Pleurodynia caused by coxackie B. virus.

Botulin The neurotoxin responsible for botulism.

Botulism A severe form of food poisoning due to botulinous toxins A,B,C,D,E,F and G.

Bougie A slender flexible instrument for dilating tubular organs, e.g. urethra.

Boutonniere deformity Proximal IP joint flexion and DIP hyper-extension, characteristic of rheumatoid deformity.

Bowleg Outward bending of lower limbs (genu varum, due to rickets).

Bowman's capsule A bilayered membrane closely applied to glomerulus. functioning as a filter for formation of urine.

Bowman's membrane Thin homogeneous membrane separating corneal epithelium from corneal substance.

Boyle's law The law states that at a constant temperature, the volume of gas varies inversely with pressure.

Brachium pontis Middle cerebellar peduncle.

Brachycheilia Abnormally short lips.

Brachydactylia Abnormally short fingers and toes.

Brachytherapy Radioactive material implant (radium, cesium, indium or gold) at the malignancy site.

Bradycardia Sinus rhythm, < 60/minute in adult, 100/minute in a child and 120/minute in fetus.

Bradyarrhythmia Slow and irregular heart rate.

Bradykinesia Slowness of movement (parkinsonism).

Bradyphrasia Slowness of speech.

Braille Raised dots system for education of blind.

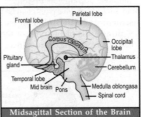
Midsagittal Section of the Brain

Brain Composed of neurones and neuroglia, average weight 1350-

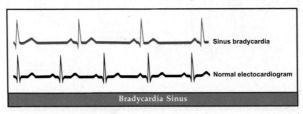
Bradycardia Sinus

1400 g in of which 2% in spinal cord and 85% is cerebrum, divided into 1. diencephalon (thalamus, hypothalamus, epithalamus) 2. mesencephalon (tegmentum, crura cerebri, medulla) 3. metencephalon (cerebellum, pons) and 4. telencephalon (cerebral cortex).

Brain death Isoelectric EEG for at least 30 minutes with no change in response to sound and pain stimuli; absent respiration and all reflexes, (barbiturate, diazepam, methaqualone can produce short periods of isoelectric EEG).

Bran Outer layer or husk of grains/ cereals composed of undigestible cellulose, adding bulk to stool.

Branchial arches Five pairs of arched structure that form lateral and ventral walls of pharynx of the embryo from which structures of face and neck are formed.

Branchial clefts Openings between branchial arches.

Brandt-Andrews maneuver Expression of placenta from uterus during third stage of labour by gentle traction on cord by one hand, the other hand pressing uterus backwards and upwards.

Braxton-Hicks sign Painless intermittent uterine contractions occurring after 3rd month of pregnancy.

Break bone fever Dengue fever (group B arbovirus).

Breathing Act of inhaling and exhaling air.

b. bronchial Prolonged high pitched expiration with often a tubular quality.

Breech presentation Foetal buttocks present at pelvic inlet.

Bregma That point on skull where coronal and sagittal sutures join.

Breisky's disease Kraurosis vulvae.

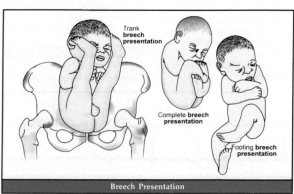

Trank breech presentation

Complete **breech presentation**

Footing **breech presentation**

Breech Presentation

Brenner's tumor Benign fibro-epithelioma of ovary.

Bretylium Antiarrhythmic agent.

Briquets syndrome A personality disorder with alcoholism and somatization disorder.

Brittle diabetes Changing and unpredictable response to insulin leading to ketosis, particularly in childhood diabetes.

Broca's area Posterior end of left inferior frontal gyrus which contains motor speech area controlling movements of lips, tongue and vocal cord.

Brodies's abscess Subacute osteomyelitis usually due to tuberculosis or Staph. aureus infection.

Bromocryptine mesylate A dopaminergic ergot derivative that is used in hyperprolactinemia.

Bronchiectasis Chronic irreversible and permanent dilatation of bronchi, may be congenital or acquired.

Bronchiocele Circumscribed dilatation of bronchus.

Bronchiole Respiratory bronchiole is the last division of bronchial tree and continues as alveolar duct into alveolus. Terminal bronchiole is next to last subdivision of a bronchiole.

Bronchiolitis Inflammation of bronchioles, commonly in small children.

Bronchitis Inflammation of mucous membrane of bronchi.

Bronchogram Radioopaque material opacification of bronchi.

Broncholith A calculus in the bronchus.

Bronchophony The voice as heard over normal bronchus by use of stethoscope.

Bronchopneumonia Inflammation of terminal bronchioles and alveoli.

Bronchoscope An endoscope for visualization of tracheobronchial tree, biopsy and foreign body removal.

Bronchoscopy Examination of bronchial tree by a bronchoscope.

Broncho vesicular Sounds intermediate between bronchial and alveolar sounds.

Bronchus The hollow tubes formed by division of trachea at the level of D_4.

Brown Sequard's syndrome Hemisection of spinal cord with loss of pain and temperature on opposite side, motor paralysis on the same side with loss of position and vibratory sense.

Brucellosis Infection caused by Brucella organism (B. abortus, suis and mellitensis),

Bruch's membrane The membrane lying between choroid membrane and the pigmented epithelium of retina.

Bruck's disease A combination of muscle atrophy and skeletal disorder like multiple fracture, ankylosis.

Bruise Injury with effusion of blood into subcutaneous tissue and skin discolouration with intact skin.

Bruit An adventitious sound of arterial or venous obstruction narrowing.

Brunner's glands Compound glands of duodenum and upper jejunum secreting mucus.

Brush border Hollow microvilli in the renal tubules and intestinal epithelium.

Brushfield spots Gray or pale yellow spots present at the periphery of iris in Down's syndrome.

Bruxism Grinding of teeth particularly during sleep.

Bryant's traction Traction applied to lower leg vertically in treating femur fracture in children.

Buck's traction Traction of lower extremity applied in line with long axis of the leg.

Buclizine Antihistamine used for motion sickness.

Buerger's disease Thromboangitis obliterans, a vasospastic disease, often nicotine induced, responding to sympathectomy, revascularization and vasodilators.

Buffalo hump Excess fat deposition in cervical and upper thoracic region due to cortisone excess.

Buffer A substance that maintains hydrogen ion concentration in blood. Principal blood buffers are: bicarbonates, carbonates, carbonic acid, dibasic phosphates, Hb and plasma proteins.

Bufotenine A hallucinogen from plant, N-methylation product of - 5HT.

Bulb Any rounded or globular structure; *bulbar paralysis*-paralysis due to disease of medula oblongata.

Buffy coat A light coloured layer containing white cells that forms

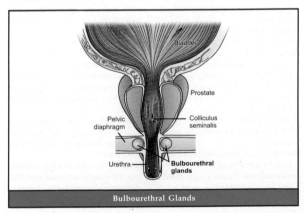

Bulbourethral Glands

when blood is centrifused or is allowed to stand in a test tube.

Bulbitis Inflammation of urethra in its bulbous portion, e.g. posterior portion of corpus spongiosum found between the two crura of penis.

Bulbocavernosus reflex Contraction of bulbocavernosus muscle on percussing of dorsum of penis.

Bulbomimic reflex Contraction of facial muscles following pressure on eye ball.

Bulbourethral glands Cowper's glands: Two small glands about the size of a pea, one on each side of prostate gland secreting a viscid fluid adding to semen.

Bulimia Excessive and insatiable appetite. Bouts of over eating followed by vomiting in young girls.

Bulla A large blister or skin vesicle filled with fluid.

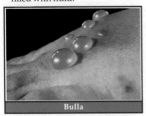
Bulla

Bumetanide A diuretic.

Bunion Inflammation and thickening of the bursa of the joint of great toe often with lateral displacement of the toe.

Buphthalmos Infantile glaucoma with uniform enlargement of eye esp. cornea.

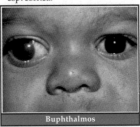
Buphthalmos

Buprenorphine Semisynthetic morphine analog, very potent analgesic.

Burr A device that rotates at high speed, used by dentist or surgeon to make holes in cranium.

Burkitt's lymphoma Undifferentiated lymphoblastic lymphoma involving sites other than lymph nodes and RE system, with strong association with EB virus infection.

Burnett's syndrome Milk-alkali syndrome.

Burning foot syndrome Burning in the sole of feet due to vitamin deficiency and chronic renal failure.

Bursa A pad like cavity in the vicinity of joint lined with synovial membrane, acting to reduce friction between tendon and bone.

Bursitis Inflammation of a bursa.

Bursolith Calculus formed in bursa.

Burton's line A blue line along the margin of the gum visible in chronic lead poisoning.

Buspiron Antianxiety agent.

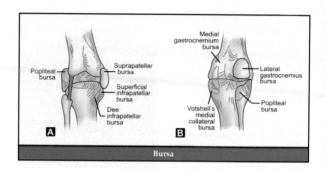

Bursa

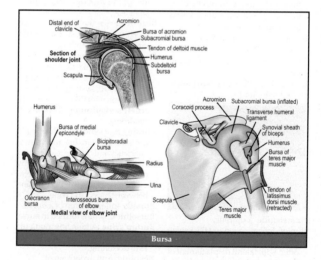

Bursa

Butterfly rash Skin rash on both cheeks joined by an extension across the bridge of nose.

Butorphanol Morphine conzener, acts like pentazocine.

Butoxamine Beta$_2$ adrenergic antagonist.

Butyric acid A fatty acid used in disinfectants, emulsifying agent.

Butyrophenone A class of chemicals of which haloperidol is a member, antipsychotic agents.

Byssinosis Pneumoconiosis of cotton and textile workers.

C

Cabot's Ring Blue stained thread like inclusions in red blood cells in severe anaemia.

Cachectin Tumor necrosis factor alfa.

Cachet Used for administering medicines with a bitter taste.

Cachexia A state of ill health, malnutrition, wasting.

Cacogenesis Abnormal development or growth.

Cacogeusia Unpleasant taste in the mouth.

Cacosmia Unpleasant odor (olfactory hallucination).

Cadaver Dead body, corpse cadaverine-malodorous substance, cadaverous; resembling corpse.

Cadence Rythmic movements.

Cafe-au-lait spots Spots of patchy pigmentation of skin, usually light brown in color-characteristic of neurofibromatosis.

Caffein An alkaloid of tea, coffee. CNS stimulant, analgesic.

Caissons disease A condition that develops in divers when air pressure is rapidly reduced while ascent to the surface. Symptoms are due to bubbling out of dissolved nitrogen.

Calamine A pink powder containing zinc oxide and little ferric oxide, used as protective, astringent.

Calcaneus The heel bone articulating with talus and cuboid.

Calcareous Having the nature of lime, chalky.

Calcicosis Pneumoconiosis caused by inhalation of lime stone dusts.

Calciphylaxis Calcification of tissue due to induced tissue sensitivity

Calcitonin Calcium lowering hormone, used in hypercalcemia, Paget's disease secreted by D cells thyroid.

Calcium A silvere white metallic element, calcium phosphate constitutes 85% of mineral matters of bone; calcium is essential for blood coagulation, enzyme activation and acid base balance, muscle and myocardial contraction and maintenance of membrane permeability.

c. carbonate is used as antacid, Cachloride is given IV for ionic balance.

c. cyclomate is an artificial sweetner.

c. disodium edetate binds metallic ions;

c. gluconate is used orally and IV.

c. hydroxide is used in dentistry as cavity liner or pulp capping material under a layer of zinc phosphate.

c. lactate/levulinate used IV.

c. oxalate a constituent of renal stone; Caoxide used as disinfectant and geremicide;

C. phosphate used as antacid.

Calcium Channel blockers A group of drugs that act by slowing the influx of calcium ions into muscle cells resulting in decreased arterial resistance and decreased myocardial O_2 demand.

Calciferol Vit D_2, ergocalciferol.

Calcitrol A sterol of vit D activity, very potent.

Calculus Any abnormal concretion in the body.

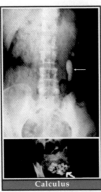

Calculus

Calf Fleshy muscular back part of leg formed by gastrocnemius and soleus.

Calefacient Agent that gives sense of warmth when applied to the body.

Calcivirus Cause epidemics of viral gastroenteritis in adult and children

Calisthenics An exercise programme to bring suppleness and gracefulness of body combined with music.

Calomel Mercurous chloride

Calyx Any cuplike organ or cavity.

Callosity Localized hypertrophy/ thickening of skin at friction/ pressure points.

Callus See callosity.

Calmodulin Intracellular proteins that combine with calcium and activate a variety of cellular responses.

Calvaria The dome like superior portion of cranium.

Calve-Perthe's disease Aseptic necrosis of femoral head epiphysis.

Campylobacter A gram negative rod shaped spirally coiled bacteria, flagellated and mobile causing diarrhoea

C of Lambert Broncho alveolar communication channels that prevent hatelectasis

C pterygoid A canal in sphenoid bone transmitting Pterygoid vessels and nerves.

C of Sclemm Spaces at sclero corneal junction draining aqueous humor.

C Volkman's canals on periosteum through which blood vessels pass to connect to those in haversian canals

Canal Channel, passage way.

c. adductor: triangular space lying beneath the sartorius muscle and between the adductor longus and vastus medialis muscles; transmits femoral vessels and saphenous nerve; also called **Hunter's canal.**

c. Alcock's Canal on the pelvic surface of abturator internus formed by obturator fascia, transmits pudendal vessels and nerve.

c. femoral the medial division of femoral sheath, containing some lymphatic vessel and a lymph node.

c. inguinal 1½" long oblique passage extending from internal inguinal ring to external inguinal ring transmitting spermatic cord, ilioinguinal nerve in male and round ligament of uterus and ilioinguinal nerve in female.

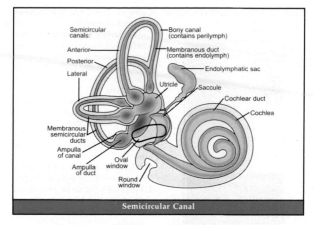

Semicircular Canal

c. semicircules Three half circular, interconnected tubes present in the inner ear.

Canaliculus Small channel or canal.

Cancer Malignant tumor which is invasive and metastasizes to new sites by lymph/blood.

Cancrum A rapidly spreading ulcer.

Candida A genus of yeast like fungi that develop a pseudomycelium and reproduce by budding.

Candidiasis Infection of skin and mucous membrane by candida.

Cane Sugar Sucrose.

Canker Ulceration of mouth and lips.

Cannabis Dried flowering tops of the cannabis saliva.

Cannibalism Eating of human flesh (kuru)

Canthridin Keratolytic for removal of warts.

Canthoplasty Enlargement of palpebral fissure by division of external canthus.

Capitellum The round eminence at lower end of humerus articulating with the radius

Capitulum A small rounded articular end of a bone.

Caplan's syndrome Rheumatoid arthritis with progressive massive lung fibrosis in pneumoconiosis.

Capreomycin A second line tuberculostatic drug.

Capsid Protein covering around the central core of virus particle protecting the virus particle from destructive enzymes.

Capsule Gelatin enclosure for drug delivery.

c. articular A two layered covering for sinovial joints. The inner layer is sinovial and outer layer is fibrous.

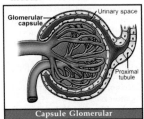

Capsule Glomerular

c. Glisson: outer fibrous capsule covering liver and portal vessels.

c. Tenon: the thin fibrous sac enveloping the eyeball.

c. glomarculus fibrous capsule covering the glameruli.

Captopril AC enzyme inhibitor, blocking conversion of angiotensin I to angiotensin II. A vasodilator useful for hypertension and congestive failure.

Caput succedaneum Swelling on presenting part of foetal head during labour.

Caramel Flavoring and colouring agent made by heating sugar or glucose, destroying the sweet taste in the process.

Carbachol Cholinergic drug for producing miosis, also used for emptying bladder.

Carbamazepine Antiepilepsy drug used for temporal lobe epilepsy and trigeminal neuralgia.

Carbenoxolone Oleandane derivative used in peptic ulcer.

Carbasone Contains 28% arsenic antiamoebic agent.

Carbenicillin Broad spectrum antibiotic, penicillin derivative.

Carbidopa Dopa decarboxylase inhibitor, used in combination with levodopa for parkinsonism.

Carbimazole Antithyroid drug.

Carbohydrate Chemical substances containing carbon, oxygen and hydrogen, e.g. sugar, glycogen, starches, dextrin and celluloses. Sucrose is glucose + fructose; maltose is 2 D glucose; lactose is glucose + galactose.

Carbon ^{14}C is radioactive isotope of carbon with halflife of 5600 years. Used in archeology dating and as tracer element in metabolic studies.

Carbon dioxide Final metabolic product of carbon compounds present in food. CO_2 combining power is a test of buffer capacity of blood. Solid CO_2 (-80°C) used for removal of naevi, telangiectasis, warts, haemorrhoids etc.

Carbon monoxide Present in automobile exhaust fumes, displaces O_2 from haemoglobin, hence diminishing O_2 transport.

Carbon tetrachloride A colourless toxic anesthetic liquid, previously used for ankylostomiasis but toxic to liver and kidney.

Carboxyhemoglobin Compound formed by CO and Hb.

Carboxylase An enzyme that catalyzes the removal of carboxyl group (COOH) from amino acids in the presence of Vit. B_1 acting as an coenzyme.

Carboxylation Replacement of hydrogen by a carboxyl (COOH) molecule.

Carboxylic acid Organic acid with COOH group.

Carbuncle Spreading inflammation of deeper skin.

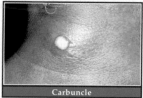
Carbuncle

Carbutamide An oral hypoglycemic agent.

Carcino embryonic antigen A class of antigen in fetus and expressed by colonic tumors. CEA level returns to normal after complete removal of colonic tumor.

Carcinogen Carcinoma inducing chemicals, e.g. benzpyrines.

Carcinoid Tumor of Argentaffin cells in the GI tract, bronchi, ovary, secreting serotonin.

Carcinoid syndrome Syndrome due to metastatic carcinoid tumors secreting serotonin, bradykinin, histamine and prostaglandin. Symptoms are diarrhoea, flushing, hypotension and heart valve lesions.

Carcinoma Malignant growth of epithelial tissue; *basal cell carcinoma* is from basal layer of skin, rarely metastasizes (rodent ulcer) *epidermoid carcinoma:* tumor on the surface either wartlike or infiltrating. *Medullary carcinoma:* Carcinoma that is soft because of predominance of cells and paucity of fibrosis. *Squamous cell cancer:* Cancer from squamous epithelium with rolled out everted edges. *Scirrhous carcinoma:* A form of cylindrical carcinoma with a firm, hard structure.

c. cylindrical Carcinoma of glands usually entodermal origin.

Carcinophilia Having affinity for cancer cells.

Cardarelli's sign Pulsating movement of trachea with aortic aneurysm.

Cardiac cycle The period from beginning of one heart beat to beginning of next beat It comprises atrial systole 0.1 second, ventricular systole 0.3 second and ventricular relaxation of 0.5 seconds.

Cardiac failure Condition resulting from inability of heart to pump sufficient blood to meet the body needs.

Cardiac output Blood ejected from left/right ventricle per minute, usually 3 lit/m².

Cardiac plexus Branches of vagus and sympathetic trunk encircling base of heart.

Cardiac reflex Slowing of heart rate from stimulation of sensory nerve endings in the walls of carotid sinus from a rise in arterial blood pressure. (Marey's law).

Cardiac reserve The capacity of heart to increase cardiac output and raise blood pressure to meet body requirements.

Cardiectasis Dilatation of heart.

Cardinal Important or of primary importance.

Cardiocele Herniation of heart through an opening in diaphragm or chest wall.

Cardiocentesis Puncture of heart.

Cardiac cirrhosis Cirrhosis of liver secondary to a cardiac cause. Commonly constructive pericarditis.

Cardiodynia Pain in the region of heart.

Cardioesophageal reflux Reflux of gastric contents into esophagus.

Cardiogenesis Formation and growth of embryonic heart.

Cardiogenic In relation to heart itself.

Cardiogram Recording of electrical activity of heart.

Cardiograph Machine that picks up electrical activity of heart.

Cardiolipin An extract of beef heart used for test of syphilis.

Cardiomegaly Enlargement of heart

Cardiomyopathy Primary disease of heart muscle.

Cardiomyopexy Stitching of pectoral muscle to cardiac muscle in order to augment vascular supply to heart muscle.

Cardiomyoplasty Reinforcement of cardiac muscle contractility by transfer of latissimus dorsi to surround the heart and to contract synchronously with cardiac muscle.

Cardiomyotomy Surgical therapy of achalasia in which the muscle surrounding cardioesophageal junction is cut but the mucous membrane is left intact.

Cardioplegia Deliberate arrest of cardiac function by use of hypothermia, potassium, etc.

Cardiopulmonary resuscitation Emergency medical care to a person whose heart and lung function is going to stop or has recently stopped. Artificial respiration and cardiac massage are the two principal components of CPR.

Cardiorrhexis Rupture of heart.

Cardioverter Defibrillator that delivers electric shockwaves for treating cardiac arrhythmia/ventricular standstill.

Caries Tooth decay with loss of enamel and dentin G.V. Black's classification of dental caries: class I-occlusal, class II-interproximal of bicuspids and molars; class III-interproximal surfaces involving incisal surfaces; class IV-interproximal but not involving incisal surface. Root of tooth in more susceptible to decay due to lack of enamel covering.

Cariogenic Conducive to dental caries formation.

Carisoprodol A muscle relaxant, acting through CNS.

Carminative Agent that helps to get rid of gas in intestine.

Carmustine Antineoplastic agent.

Carnal Related to desires or appetite of flesh.

Carnitine A chemical important in metabolism of palmitic and stearic

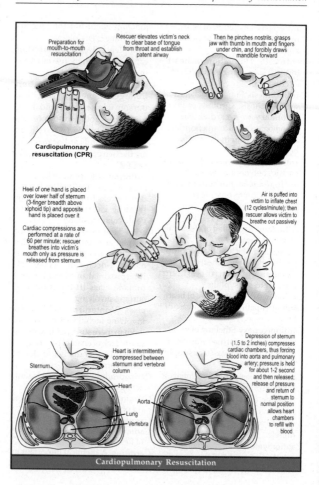

Preparation for mouth-to-mouth resuscitation

Rescuer elevates victim's neck to clear base of tongue from throat and establish patent airway

Then he pinches nostrils, grasps jaw with thumb in mouth and fingers under chin, and forcibly draws mandible forward

Cardiopulmonary resuscitation (CPR)

Heel of one hand is placed over lower half of sternum (3-finger breadth above xiphoid tip) and opposite hand is placed over it

Cardiac compressions are performed at a rate of 60 per minute; rescuer breathes into victim's mouth only as pressure is released from sternum

Air is puffed into victim to inflate chest (12 cycles/minute); then rescuer allows victim to breathe out passively

Depression of sternum (1.5 to 2 inches) compresses cardiac chambers, thus forcing blood into aorta and pulmonary artery; pressure is held for about 1-2 second and then released; release of pressure and return of sternum to normal position allows heart chambers to refill with blood

Heart is intermittently compressed between sternum and vertebral column

Sternum

Heart

Aorta

Lung

Vertebra

Cardiopulmonary Resuscitation

acid. Used therapeutically in treatment of myopathy due to carnitine deficiency.

Carnivorous Flesh eating.

Carotinase Enzyme that converts carotine into Vit A.

Carotene Yellow cristalline pigments of plant and animal tissue, converted to Vit A in liver.

Carotenemia A benign condition with high blood caroten level causing yellow colouration of skin but not of conjunctiva.

Carotid body A pressure and hypoxia sensitive flat structure present at carotid bifurcation.

Carotid sinus A dilated area at the bifurcation of common carotid, richly supplied with sensory nerve endings, responding to changes in concentration of O_2 and blood pressure.

Carotid siphon The S shaped terminal portion of internal carotid artery.

Carotidynia Pain elicited by pressures on common carotid artery.

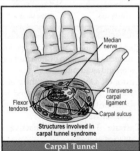

Median nerve

Flexor tendons

Transverse carpal ligament

Carpal sulcus

Structures involved in carpal tunnel syndrome

Carpal Tunnel

Carpal tunnel The canal beneath flexor retinaculum of wrist in which flexor tendons and median nerve pass.

Carpal tunnel syndrome Pain, tenderness and weakness of muscles of thumb caused by pressure on median nerve in carpal tunnel.

Carphology Involuntary picking at bed clothes, muttering etc. the signs of impending end.

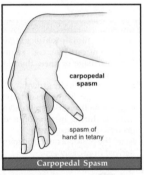

carpopedal spasm

spasm of hand in tetany

Carpopedal Spasm

Carpopedal spasm Spasms of hand and feet seen in tetany and hyperventilation.

Carrier A person who harbors a pathogenic organism without any sign or symptom of disease but is capable of spreading the organism to others.

Cartilage A type of dense connective tissue capable of withstanding high pressure and tension. Cartilage is avascular and is without nerve supply.

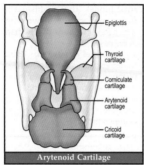

Arytenoid Cartilage

c. hyaline Bluish-white glassy translucent cartilage, e.g. semilunar cartilage of knee, thyroid cartilage.

Caruncle Small fleshy growth.

Carvallo's sign Murmurs of heart originating from tricuspid valve increase during inspiration and decrease during expiration.

Casein The principal protein in milk derived from casinogen.

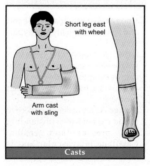

Casts

Casoni's test Appearance of wheal surrounded by erythematous zone following intradermal injection of sterile hydatid fluid. The test is false positive in 40% cases in diagnosis of Echinococcus granulosus.

Cast 1. A solid mold of a part, usually applied for immobilization of fracture, dislocation and severe injuries. 2. In dentistry a positive copy of tissues of jaw over which denture base is to be made. 3. Pliable or fibrous matter which mould to the shape of the part in which they accumulate. According to source they can be classified as bronchial, intestinal, nasal, esophageal, renal, vaginal etc. According to constituents casts can be bloody, fatty, hyaline, granular, waxy etc.

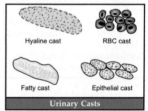

Urinary Casts

Castellani's paint Composed of phenol, resorcinol, used as a disinfectant for skin and as an antifungal.

Castor oil Obtained from the plant *Ricinus communis*, hydrolyzed in intestine to ricinoleic acid that acts as laxative.

Castrate To remove or inactivate ovaries or testes.

Casuality Accident/injury/death.

Catabolism Breakdown of complex substances into simpler substances with consumption of energy; opposite of anabolism.

Catagen Intermediate phase of hair growth lying between anagen (growing) and telogen (Resting phase).

Catalase An enzyme that helps in breakdown of hydrogen peroxide into water and oxygen.

Catalepsy A trance like state with diminished responsiveness but often intact perception.

Catalysis Enhancement of a chemical reaction by a catalyst.

Catalyst A substance that speeds up chemical reaction without itself being permanently altered, e.g. HCl catalyzes hydrolysis of sucrose.

Catamenia Menstruation.

Cataphasia Involuntary repitition of same word.

Cataphoria Tendency of visual axes to incline below the horizontal plane.

Cataphylaxis The process of carrying antibodies and leukocytes to the site of an infection.

Cataplexy The brief sudden loss of muscle control brought on by strong emotion, i.e. excitement, anger.

Catapres Clonidine, an antihypertensive agent.

Cataract Opacity of lens nucleus, capsule or both. Immature stage: lens swollen, anterior chamber shallow mature stage: lens shrinks, no iris shadow on transillumination cataract can be polar, lamellar, nuclear, cortical, congenital, traumatic, diabetic but senility is the single most common cause.

Catarrh Inflammation of mucous membranes esp. of head and throat.

Catatonia A phase of schizophrenia in which patient is unresponsive and tends to assume fixed posture.

Catecholamine Biologically active amines like epinephrine and nor epinephrine derived from amino acid tyrosine.

Catgut Suture made up of ship's intestine. Chromium trioxide treatment enhances strength of the suture.

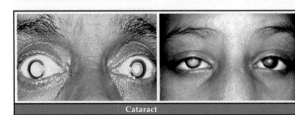

Cataract

Catharsis Purgation.

Cathartic Agent causing purgation.

Cathepsin D An estrogen induced lysosomal protease, a predictor of breast cancer recurrence

Cathepsis Synthesis of proteins in living animals or autolysis in dead.

Catheter A hollow tube for evacuation and injection of fluids. Arterial and venous catheters for recording of pressure, pacing catheter for a trial/ventricular pacing; self retaining bladder catheter; Tenckoff peritoneal catheter for peritoneal dialysis.

Cathexis The emotional or mental energy used in concentrating on an object or idea.

Cathode Negative electrode, opposite of anode.

Cation An ion with positive charge that travels onto cathode.

CAT scan Computerized axial tomography: computerized X-ray picture of any body part.

Cat scratch fever Febrile disease with lymphadenopathy transmitted by cats.

Cauda Tail or tail like structure. Terminal portion of spinal cord — cauda equina. Inferior portion of epididymis—cauda epididymidis.

Caudate Possessing a tail.

Causalgia Intense burning pain accompanied by trophic skin changes, due to injury to sympathetic innervation.

Caustic An agent particularly an alkali that destroys living tissue.

Cauterization Destruction of tissue by caustic, electric current, freezing, etc.

Cautery The means of destroying tissue.

Cavalry bone Sesamoid bone in adductor longus of thigh in riders.

Cavernitis Inflammation of corpus cavernousum of penis.

Cavernoma Cavernous haemangioma.

Cavernous Containing a hollow space.

Cavitis Inflammation of vena cava.

Cavity A hollow space in a viscus or tooth.

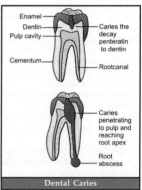

Enamel — Dentin — Pulp cavity — Cementum — Caries the decay penteratin to dentin — Rootcanal — Caries penetrating to pulp and reaching root apex — Root abscess

Dental Caries

Cavity preparation Artificial cavity prepared in teeth for tooth restoration, e.g. root canal treatment.

CD4 A cluster differentiation protein receptor specific to mature T lymphocytes; through it HIV binds to T lymphocytes.

c. clue Vaginal epithelial cell coated with cocobacillary organisms, a clue to bacterial vaginosis.

Cecectomy Surgical removal of caecum.

Cecopexy Surgical fixation of ceeum to abdominal wall.

Cecum The first portion of large intestine, 6 cm in length, 7.5 cm in width, with appendix arising at its lower end.

Cefadroxyl Long-acting oral cephalosporin.

Celiac disease Intestinal malabsorption syndrome mostly gluten induced.

Celiac plexus Sympathetic plexus near origin of celiac artery.

Cell The basis structural unit of all plants and animals containing protoplasm and nucleus.

c. argentaffin Epithelium of digestive tract containing grannules that stain with silver.

c. basket 1. branching basal cell of salivary gland 2. Certain cells of cerebellar cortex.

c. Betz Large pyramidal cells of motor cortex.

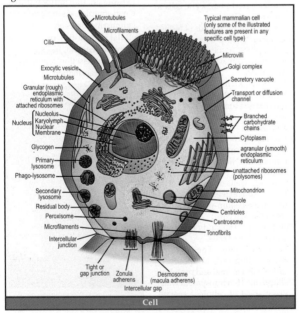

Cell

c. beta Insulin secreting cells of pancreas (islets of Langerhans).

c. chief Parathormone secreting cells, pepsin secreting gastric cells, chromophobe cells of pituitary.

c. columar Cells with height breadth.

c. cuboid Cell with height equal to width and depth.

c. endothelial Flat cells outlining blood vessels, peritoneum and pleura-pericardium.

c. Hela Cells cultured from patients of carcinoma of cervix.

c. Kuffer Fixed phagocytic cells in sinusoids of liver.

c. Leydig Interstitial cells of testes.

c. Littoral Macrophages in sinuses of lymphatic tissue.

c. mast Cells containing heparin and histamine.

c. natural killer A line of B lymphocytes that kill the virus infected and tumor cells.

c. neuroglia Supporting cells in CNS and retina.

c. Niemann-Pick At foamy lipid filled cell present in spleen and bone marrow in Niemann and Pick's disease.

c. Purkinje Cells of cerebral cortex whose axon extend to brain stem nuclei, cerebellum or anterior horn cells of spinal cord.

Cell kinetics The study of growth and division of cells.

Cell membrane The envelop surrounding cell, composed of carbohydrate, lipid and protein.

Cellophane Thin transparent water proof sheet of cellulose acetate, used as dialysis membrane.

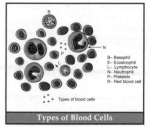

B– Basophil
E– Eosinophil
L– Lymphocyte
N– Neutrophil
P– Platelets
R– Red blood cell

⁖ Types of blood cells

Types of Blood Cells

Cell organelle Structures in the cytoplasm like mitochondria, Golgi complex, endoplasmic reticulum, ribosomes etc.

Cellular immunity T-cell mediated immune reaction, basis of organ transplant rejection, lepromin test and BCG vaccination.

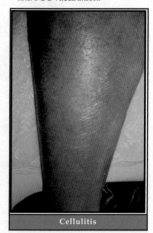

Cellulitis

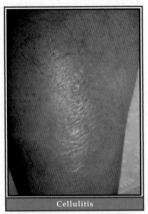
Cellulitis

Cellulitis Inflammation of cellular or connective tissue.

Cellulose A plant polysaccharide, the supporting framework of most plants. It is undigestible and adds to bulk of stool.

Celsius scale Temperature scale where boiling point of water is 100 and melting point is of ice is 0°.

Cement Material that makes one substance bind to another.

Cementitis Inflammation of dental cementum.

Cementoblast Cells lining the developing tooth depositing cementum.

Cementoclast Multinucleated large cells that remove cementum (i.e. odontoclasts).

Cementoma A benign fibrous connective tissue growth usually at root of tooth containing small masses of cementum.

Cementum Thin layer of calcified tissue formed by cementoblast covering the root of tooth.

Center A group of nerve cells in CNS subserving special function.

c. apneustic Center in brainstem regulating breathing.

c. auditory Center for hearing in the anterior part of transverse temporal gyri.

c. autonomic Center controlling autonomic functions located in hypothalamus, brainstem and spinal cord.

c. cardioaceleator and c. cardioinhibitory Both present in medulla oblongata, innervating the heart through sympathetic and para-sympathetic fibers.

c. Broca's Center in inferior frontal gyrus (area) controlling speech.

c. ciliospinal Center in spinal cord giving rise to sympathetic fibers dilating the pupil.

c. defecation Two centers located in medulla oblongata and in S_2-S_4 segments of spinal cord.

c. deglutition Center in medulla oblongata on the floor of fourth ventricle that controls swallowing.

c. heat regulating A heat loss and a heat production center located in medulla.

c. micturition Located in S_2-S_4, medulla and hypothalamus controlling micturition.

c. pneumotaxic Center in pons that rythmically inhibits inspiration.

c. respiratory The inspiratory, expiratory and pneumotaxic centers in medula oblongata controlling the respiratory movements.

c. satiety An area in ventromedial thalamus that modulates eating behavior.

Centigram Hundredth of gram, 10 mg.

Centiliter Hundredth of liter, 10 ml.

Centimeter Hundredth of meter, 10 mm.

Centepede Arthropod with long flat segmented body each with a pair of legs.

Central core disease A form of benign familial polymyopathy characterized by hypotonia, and nonprogressive muscle weakness.

Central venous pressure The pressure within superior vana cavs; normally 5-10 mm Hg.

Centrifugal Force directed outwards from center of rotation.

Centrifuge A machine that spins test tubes at high speed, causing heavy particles to settle down to the bottom. RBCs settle down at bottom, and WBCs form a thin layer between RBC and plasma.

Centrilobular Concerning the center of a lobule.

Centriole A minute organelle consisting of a hollowed cylinder closed at one end and open at the other. During mitosis the centrioles migrate to opposite poles of the cell to which spindle fibers are attached.

Centripetal Directed towards the axis, i.e. center.

Centromere The constricted central portion of chromosome that divides chromosome into two.

Cephalgia Headache, pain in the body.

Cephalexin Analog of antibiotic cephalosporin.

Cephalhematoma Subcutaneous swelling containing blood found on the head of a newborn baby disappearing within 2-3 months.

Cephalic Index Maximal length of head divided by maximal breadth × 100.

Cephalometry Measurement of the head using various bony points used to assess growth and in determining orthodontic or prosthetic treatment

Cephaloridine An analogue of the antibiotic cephalosporin.

Cephalotomy Perforating the foetal head to facilitate delivery.

Cercaria A free swimming stage in the development of fluke or trematode.

Cerebellum Largest portion of rhombencephalon lying dorsal to pons and medulla oblongata; involved in coordination of fine movements, maintenance of posture, equilibrium, muscle tone, etc.

Cerebral palsy A nonprogressive neurological impairment occurring in early childhood due to cerebral insult or congenital anomalies.

Cerebromalacia Softening of cerebrum.

Cerebroside A lipid constituent of nerve tissue.

Cerebrospinal fever Inflammation of brain and meninges.

Cerebrospinal fluid The cushioning fluid formed in the choroid plexuses of the lateral and third ventricle. Normal amount 100-140 ml, specific gravity 1003-1008.

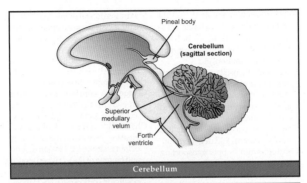

Cerebellum

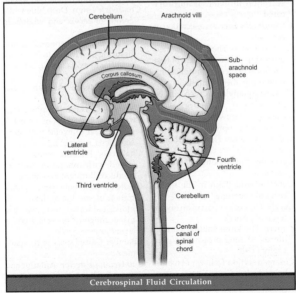

Cerebrospinal Fluid Circulation

Cerebrovascular accident (CVA) Ischemic or haemorrhagic cerebral events due to embolism, thrombosis, vasculitis, aneurysm, A.V. malformation, etc.

Cerebrum Consists of two hemispheres united by two commissures; corpus callosum, anterior and posterior hippocampal commissures.

Ceroma A waxy tumor that has undergone amyloid degeneration.

Ceruloplasmin Copper transporting glycoprotein in blood,

Cerumen The wax like, soft brown secretion in external auditory canal.

Ceruminosis Excessive secretion of cerumen.

Cervical plexus The plexus formed by joining of anterior rami of first 4 cervical nerves, communicating with sympathetic ganglia.

Cervical spondylosis Osteoarthritis of cervical vertebra with osteophytic growths often causing nerve root compression.

Cervical vertebra First seven bones of spinal column.

Cervicitis Inflammation of uterine cervix.

Cervicodynia Pain in the neck, cervical neuralgia.

Cervix The neck or part of an organ resembling neck.

c. uteri The lower tubular part of uterus, 1" long protruding into vaginal valt.

Cesarean section Delivery of foetus by giving incision on uterus, either extraperitoneal or intraperitoneal. Commonly done in cephalo-pelvic disproportion, breech presentation and foetal distress.

Cesium ^{137}Cs an radioactive isotope of metal cesium is used for radiation of cancer tissue.

Cestoda A subclass that includes tapeworms that have a scolex and a chain of segments (proglottids).

Chaddock's reflex 1. Extension of great toe when outer edge of dorsum of foot is stroked. 2. Flexion of wrist and fanning of fingers when tendon of palmaris longus is pressed; positive in corticospinal tract lesions.

Chadwick's sign Deep blue violet colour of cervix and vagina, in early pregnancy

Chafing Erythema, maceration and fissuring of skin due to friction of clothing in axilla, groin, between digits.

Chaga's disease African trypanosomiasis.

Chalasia Relaxation of sphincters.

Chalazion Distention of a meobomian gland of eyelid with hard secretions, resembling tumor.

Chalicosis Pneumoconiosis associated with inhalation of dust produced during stone cutting.

Challenge In immunology, administration of specific antigen to an individual known to be sensitive to that antigen in order to produce an immune response.

Chamber Closed space or compartment.

c. anterior, posterior Anterior and posterior chambers of eye contain-

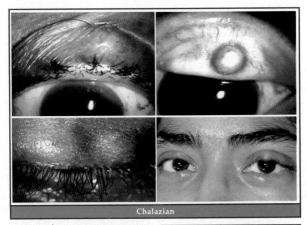

Chalazian

ing aqueous humor, lying between cornea and iris, iris and lens respectively.

c. Boyden Chamber used to measure chemotaxis.

c. hyperbolic Closed chamber with high internal air pressure, e.g. hyperbaric oxygen chambers for treatment of frost bite, gangrene decompression sickness.

c. pulp The chamber within crown of tooth containing nerve endings and blood vessels.

Chancre Hard painless syphilitic primary ulcer on exposed part with, slough leather base.

Chancroid Non-syphilitic venereal ulcer due to haemophilus ducrey.

Charcoal Activated charcoal used for adsorption of gas and poisonous alkaloids in GI tract.

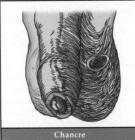

Chancre

Charcot Bouchard aneurysm Micro aneurysms in cerebral small vessels due to weakening of media in hypertension.

Charcot's joint Denervated degenerating joint in syrin-gomyelia, tabes dorsalis or spinal cord injury with hypermobility.

Charcot-Leyden Crystal Colourless, hexagonal, double pointed and often needle like crystals found in sputum of asthmatic patients and in faeces of patients of intestinal amoebiasis.

Charcot-Marie-Tooth Disease A form of hereditary progressive neuro-muscular atrophy usually developing in childhood, commonly males. (SYN-peroneal muscular atrophy).

Charcot's triad Combination of nystagmus, intention tremor, and scanning speech; frequently associated with multiple sclerosis.

Charle's law At constant pressure, a given amount of gas will expand in direct proportion to absolute temperature.

Charting The process of making a tabulated record of the progress of patient during hospital stay in relation to temperature, blood pressure, intake, etc.

Chediak-Higashi syndrome AR disease in which neutrophils contain peroxidase positive inclusion bodies. Partial albinism, photophobia and pale optic fundi are the clinical features. Children usually die between 5-10 years of age due to lymphoma like disease.

Cheilitis Inflammation of lips.

Cheilosis Red lips, with fissured angles of mouth commonly due to riboflavin deficiency.

Chelation The process of chelating; meaning to hold ionic metallic compounds preventing their absorption or action at target sites, e.g. calcium disodium edetate.

Chemabrasion Use of chemicals to destroy superficial dayers of skin to treat scars, tatoos, abnormal pigmentation.

Chemical warfare Warfare with toxic-chemical/biological agents. The chemicals used are nerve gases/disease producing organisms.

Chemiluminscence Light produced by chemical reactions without production of heat, e.g. light production during bacterial killing by neutrophils, fire flies.

Chemodectoma Tumor of chemoreceptor system, e.g. para ganglioma.

Chemoprophylaxis Use of drugs to prevent occurrence of disease.

Chemoreceptor A sense organ or sensory nerve ending that is stimulated by and reacts to certain chemical stimuli; usually located outside CNS, e.g. carotid and aortic bodies, taste buds olfactory cells of nose.

Chemosis Edema of conjunctiva.

Chemotaxis Movement of cells in response to a chemical stimulus or message, e.g. movement of neutrophils to site of injury.

Chemotherapeutic index The ratio of the toxicity of the drug, expressed as maximum tolerated dose/kg body weight to the minimal curative dose/kg of body weight.

Chemotropism Ability of impulse to progress or turn in certain direction in response to certain stimuli.

Chenodeoxy cholic acid Used for dissolution of gallstones.

Cherry red spots Red spot in retina of Tay-Sachs disease.

Chest The body part accommodating heart and lungs.

c. emphysematous Short and round thorax with AP diameter equal to transverse diameter, horizontal ribs (barrel chest).

c. flail Paradoxical chest movement due to multiple rib fracture.

c. flat Chest deformity with short AP diameter, long thorax, oblique ribs and prominent scapula.

c. pigeon Prominent sternum with prominent sternal ends of the ribs.

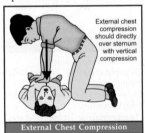

External chest compression should directly over sternum with vertical compression

External Chest Compression

Chest thump A sharp blow to chest in precordial area in order to revert a VT or restore normal rhythm in cardiac arrest.

Cheyne-Stokes respiration Breathing pattern in which period of apnea is followed by gradually increasing depth and frequency of respiration.

Common in diencephalic and frontal lobe dysfunction.

Chiari-Frommel syndrome Persistent amenorrhoea and lactation following child birth due to hyperprolactinemia.

Chiasm A crossing or decussation.

c. optic An incomplete crossing of the optic fiber.

Chilblain A form of cold injury characterized by local erythema, itching and often blistering.

Child abuse Emotional, physical and sexual injury to a child.

Chill Shivering with sensation of coldness and pallor of skin.

Chimpanzee An intelligent ape native to parts of Africa.

Chinese Restaurant Syndrome Headache, perspiration and chest pain after eating monosodium glutamate.

Chiropodist Podiatrist

Chiropractic A system of health care which emphasizes on good relatioship between organs for proper functioning.

Chi-square (x^2) A statistical test to determine the similarity of the number of occurrences being investigated to the expected occurrences.

Chlamydia A genus of micro organisms causing ornithosis, lymphogranuloma venereum, trachoma and genital infection.

Chloasma Skin pigmentation (localized) following trauma, idiopathic or pregnancy.

Chloral hydrate Colourless, caustic, hypnotic agent

Chlorambucil Cytotoxic agent used to treat CLL, Hodgkin's disease, etc.

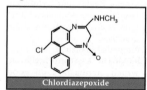
Chloramphenicol

Chloramphenicol Antibiotic isolated from *Streptomyces venzualae*, specific for treatment of enteric fever.

Chlordane An insecticide.

Chlordantoin Topical antifungal agent.

Chlordiazepoxide

Chlordiazepoxide A benzodiazepine, used to treat anxiety, alcohol withdrawal syndrome etc.

Chloremia Increased chloride concentration in blood.

Chlorhexidine Topical anti-infective agent.

Chlorinated lime Calcium hypochlorite and calcium chloride, used as bleaching agents and antiseptic.

Chlorite A salt of chlorous acid, used as disinfectant and bleaching agent.

Chlorbutanol Antiseptic and local anaesthetic used in dentistry and as a preservative.

Chlormezanone Antianxiety sedative agent.

Chloroguanide Antimalarial agent.

Chloroma Sarcoma of periosteum of cranial bones (green cancer).

Chlorophane Green yellow pigment in retina.

Chloroquine An antimalarial; also used in amoebiasis, SLE arthropathy.

Chlorphenothane An insecticide known as DDT.

Chlorophyll The green pigment in plants.

Chlorothiazide

Chlorothiazide A diuretic.

Chlorpheniramine An antihistamine agent.

Chlorphenoxamine Drug for parkinsonism.

Chlorpromazine Tranquilliser used in psychosis.

Chlorpropamide Oral hypoglycemic agent of sulfonyl urea group.

Chlorprothixene Antidepressant.

Chlortetracycline Bacteriostatic antibiotic of tetracycline group.

Chlorthalidone Diuretic.

Chloroxazone Muscle relaxant

Choana Funnel shaped opening esp. on the posterior nares.

Choking Obstruction within respiratory passage or constriction in the neck obstructing breathing and circulation to brain.

Cholangiectasis Dilatation of bile ducts.

Cholangiography Radiography of biliary system.

Cholangioma Tumor of bile ducts.

Cholangitis Inflammation of the bile ducts.

Cholecystectomy Excision of gallbladder.

Cholecystitis Inflammation of gall bladder manifesting with fever, chills, upper abdominal pain and mild jaundice; nearly always caused by gall stones.

Cholecystokinin Hormone secreted by duodenum that stimulates gall bladder contraction and pancreatic secretion.

Cholelithiasis Stone formation within gall bladder.

Cholemia Hyperbilirubinemia.

Cholera Profuse watery diarrhoea and vomiting with dehydration caused by vibrio cholerae.

Choleriform Resembling cholera.

Cholesteatoma An epithelial pocket filled with keratin debris.

Cholesterol A monohydric alcohol, principal constituent of gall stones and constituent of cell membrane, percursor of hormones.

Cholesterosis Cholesterol deposition in tissues.

Cholestyramine An ion exchange resin to treat itching of hyperbilirubinemia.

Cholic acid A bite acid.

Choline An amine, constituent of lecithin and other phospholipids; involved in protein metabolism.

Cholinergic Nerve endings that liberate acetyl choline.

Cholinergic fibers They include all preganglionic fibers, all postganglionic parasympathetic fibers, postganglionic sympathetic fibers to sweat glands and, efferent fibers to skeletal muscle.

Cholinesterase Enzyme that catalyzes the hydrolysis of choline esters, i.e. acetyl cholinesterase breaks down acetylcholine into acetic acid and choline.

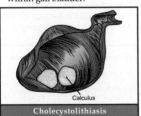

Calculus

Cholecystolithiasis

Cholesterol

Chondrin Gelatin like material obtained by boiling of cartilage, (the basic substance of cartilage).

Chondritis Inflammation of cartilage.

Condrodysplasia Multiple exostoses of epiphysis esp. of long bones, metacarpals and phalanges.

Chondrogen Basal substance of cartilage and corneal tissue, which changes to chondrin on boiling.

Chondroitin Substance present in connective tissue, including cornea and cartilage.

Chondroma A painless, slow growing tumor of cartilage.

Chondromalacia Softening of articular cartilage, usually involving patella.

Chondrosarcoma Cartilaginous sarcoma.

Chorda A cord or tendon.

c. tympni branch of facial nerve whose efferent fibers innervate submandibular and sublingual glands and affarent fibers convey taste sensation from anterior two thirds of tongue.

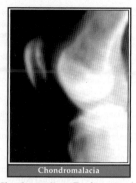
Chondromalacia

Chordae tendinae Tendinous cords connecting free edges of A-V valves to papillary muscles.

Chorditis Inflammation of vocal/spermatic cord.

Chordoma A tumor along vertebral column composed of embryonic nerve tissue.

Chorea A movement disorder due to extrapyramidal damage characterized by quasipurposive,

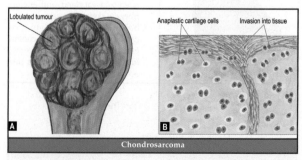
Chondrosarcoma

involuntory, non-repetitive limb movements, e.g. Sydenham's (rheumatic) chorea, chorea gravidarum, Huntington's chorea.

Choreoathetosis Jerky bizarre involuntary muscle contraction, usually more proximal than distal.

Chorioadenoma Adenoma of chorion, the outer membrane enclosing the foetus.

Chorioamnionitis Inflammation of membranes covering foetus, i.e. amnion and chorion.

Choriocarcinoma Malignant neoplasm of chorion usually following hydatid mole, abortion or often normal pregnancy.

Choriomeningitis Inflammation of meninges.

c. lymphocytic is of viral origin.

Chorion An extraembryonic membrane that covers outerwall of blastocyst from which develop chorionic villi.

Chorionic Villi Sampling The procedure of obtaining samples of chorionic villi for prenatal evaluation of foetus.

Chorioretinitis Inflammation of choroid and retina.

Choristoma A neoplasm of embryonic rudiments at sites where the tissue is usually not found.

Choroid Dark brown vascular layer of eye in between sclera and retina.

Choroideremia X-linked choroid degeneration manifesting as night blindness progressing to absolute blindness.

Choroiditis Inflammation of the choroid.

Christion-Weber disease Nodular, nonsuppurating panniculitis with fever.

Christmas factor A thromboplastin activator present in plasma.

Chromaffin cells Pigment cells of adrenal medulla and paraganglia

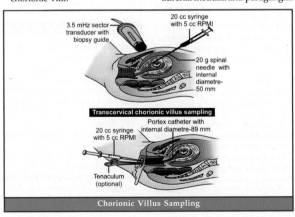

Chorionic Villus Sampling

containing granules that stain with chromium salts.

Chromatid Replication of chromosome into two before mitosis joined at centromere.

Chromatin It is a DNA structure present in the cell nucleus. Males are chromatin negative and females are chromatin positive (inactivated X-chromosome).

Chromatography A method of separating two or more chemical compounds in solution by passing across the surface of an absorbent paper.

Chromatophore A pigment bearing cell.

Chromatoptometry Measurement of color perception.

Chromoblasts An embryonic cell that becomes a pigment cell.

Chromolysis Dissolution of chromophil substance (Nissle bodies) in neurons in certain pathological conditions.

Chromomycosis Fungal infection of skin marked by warty plaques.

Chromophil Easily staining cell of anterior pituitary which is usually secretory.

Chromosome The structures containing DNA that store genetic information. There are 22 pairs of autosomes and one pair of sex chromosome in every cell.

Chronic fatigue syndrome A disease of unknown cause probably caused by EB virus with excessive fatigue, mild fever and myalgia

Chronic granulomatous disease A disease of children characterized by inability of neutrophils to kill ingested organisms.

Chronic obstructive lung disease (COLD) Included in this group an chronic asthma and bronchitis witt dyspnoea, poor FEV$_1$, and maximum breathing capacity.

Chronological Description of an event in natural sequence according to time.

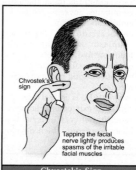

Chvostek's sign

Tapping the facial nerve lightly produces spasms of the irritable facial muscles

Chvostek's Sign

Chvostek's sign Spasm of facial muscle by tapping over area of facial nerve, a sign of tetany.

Chyle The protein and fat rich fluid of lymphatic channels drained to left subclavian vein via thoracic duct

Chylemia Chyle in peripheral circulation.

Chylomicron Small particles of fat rich in triglycerides.

Chyluria Presence of chyle or fat globules in urine.

Chymopapain An enzyme related to papain.

Chymotrypsin A proteolytic enzyme present in the intestine that hydrolyses proteins to peptones.

Cicatrix Scar left by a healed wound.

Cicatrization Healing by scar formation.

Ciclopirox Locally applied antifungal agent.

Cilia Hair like processes projecting from epithelial cells of bronchi propelling up mucus and foreign particles.

c. immotile syndrome A group of inherited conditions characterized by immotility of cilia of respiratory mucosa and sperms. *SYN–* Kartagener's syndrome.

Ciliary ganglion The ganglion in orbital fossa receiving preganglionic fibers from Edinger-Westphal nucleus and giving rise to 6 short ciliary nerves that innervate ciliary muscles, sphincters of iris and smooth muscles of blood vessels.

Ciliary muscles Smooth muscles of ciliary body, by contraction loosen suspensory ligament of lens allowing lens to become more spherical for accomplishing near vision.

Ciliary process About 70 folds arranged meridionally so as to form a circle, secrete nourishing fluid for cornea, lens and vitreous.

Ciliary reflex Normal contraction of pupil during process of accommodation.

Ciliospinal reflex Dilatation of pupil following stimulation of the skin of the neck.

Ciliospinal center Center in spinal cord that controls dilatation of pupil.

Cimetidine H_2 receptor antagonist inhibiting gastric acid secretion.

Cinnarazine Drug used for vertigo.

Cinchona Dried bark of cinchona tree containing quinine, cinchonine.

Cinchophen Old agent for gout frequently producing fatal hepatitis.

Cineangiocardiography Graphic record of heart and blood flow dynamics after constrast injection.

Cingulotomy Excision of anterior half of cingulate gyrus for control of intractable pain.

Cingulum A band of association fibers in the cingulate gyrus extending from anterior perforated substance to hippocampal gyrus.

Cinoxacin A quinolone, antibacterial agent.

Ciprofloxacin A quinolone with broad spectrum antibacterial activity.

Circadian Pertains to events that occur approximately at 24 hours interval.

Circle of Willis The anastomosis at base of brain where posterior cerebral and middle cerebral vessels meet.

Circulation fetal Oxygenated blood from placenta is carried to fetal heart by umbilical vein and ductus venosus. The blood enters aorta via ductus arteriosus bypassing fetal lung.

Circulation time the time required for a drop of blood to complete systemic and pulmonary circulation normal circulation time from arm vein to tongue is 10-16 seconds. It is prolonged in heart failure and shortened in anaemia and hyperthyroidism.

Circulatory failure Inadequate cardiac pump action to meet oxygen demand of body tissues. Peripheral circulatory failure means pooling of blood in expanded vascular space consequent to vasodilatation resulting in decreased venous return to heart.

Circumcision Removal of extra prepucal skin covering glans penis.

Circumduction Circular movement performed by the limb, the joint performing the movement is at the apex of the cone.

Circumflex Winding around.

Circumvalate papillae V-shaped row of papillae at base of tongue.

Cirrhosis Chronic liver disease characterized by bridging fibrosis, hepatic cell degeneration and regeneration and evidence of portal hypertension.

c. alcoholic 20% of chronic alcoholics develop cirrhosis.

c. biliary Cirrhosis following chronic bile stasis.

c. cardiac Chronic heart failure leading to passive congestion of liver ending in cirrhosis.

c. infantile Childhood cirrhosis due to protein malnutrition.

c. macronodular Cirrhosis characterized by broad bands of fibrous tissue and large irregular regene-

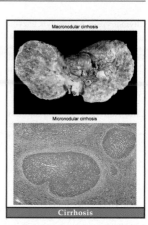

Macronodular cirrhosis

Micronodular cirrhosis

Cirrhosis

rating nodules, e.g. post necrotic/ post hepatic cirrhosis.

Cisplatin Antineoplastic agent for treatment of ovarian and testicular tumors.

Cisterna A reservoir or cavity.

Cisvestitism Wearing of clothes contrary to ones profession.

Citric acid A tribasic acid present in juice of citrous fruits.

Citrovorum factor Folinic acid used with dihydrofolate reductase inhibitors.

Citruline Amino acid formed from ornithine, present in water melons.

Citric acid cycle (Kreb's cycle) The cycle involving oxidative metabolism of pyruvic acid to CO_2, and H_2O, releasing energy (36 ATP).

Clark's rule A formula for calculating pediatric dose, i.e. weight of the child in lb. × adult dose/150.

Clasmatocyte A large wandering uninucleated cell with many branches, a fixed macrophage of loose connective tissue.

Claude's Syndrome Third cranial nerve palsy, contralateral ataxia and tremor, caused by lesion around red nucleus.

Claudication Pain in calf muscle during walking due to inadequate Wood supply.

Claustrophilia Dread of being in an open space, a morbid desire to remain within with windows shut.

Claustrophobia Fear of closed space.

Claspknife rigidity Passive flexion of the joint causes increased resistance of the extensors. This gives way abruptly if flexon is continued, a sign of pyramidal tract lesion.

Clavulanic acid Beta lactamase inhibitor.

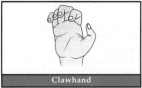
Clawhand

Clawhand A hand characterized by hyperextension of proximal phallanges and extreme flexion of middle and distal phallanges.

Clawfoot Excessively high longitudinal arch of foot with dorsal contracture of toes.

Clean catch method Contamination free urine specimen collection.

Cleavage Splitting a complex molecule into two or more simple ones.

Cleft A fissure or elongated opening.

c. alveolar An anomaly resulting from lack of fusion between median nasal process and the maxillary process, commonly

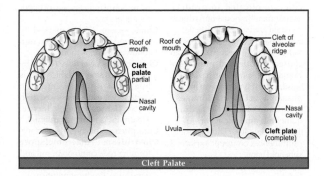
Cleft Palate

associated with cleft lip and cleft palate.

c. bronchial An opening between branchial arches of an embryo.

Cleft foot A bipartite foot resulting from failure of a digit and its corresponding metatarsal to develop.

Clenching With the teeth in contact, forcible repeated contraction of jaw muscles.

Cleptomania Impulsive stealing in which motive is not related to value of stolen object.

Clidinium bromide Parasympathetic inhibitor used for treatment of peptic ulcer.

Climacteric Menopause or end of woman's reproductive ability. Male climacteric points to lessening male sexual activity.

Climax Sexual orgasm, period of greatest intensity.

Clindamycin hydrochloride An antibiotic against gram-positive cocci, implicated to produce pseudomembranous colitis due to resistant claustridium dificile.

Clinocephaly Congenital flatness or saddle-shape of the top of the head caused by bilateral premature closure of the sphenoparietal sutures.

Clinodactyly Hypoplasia of middle phalanx as in Down syndrome.

Clinoquinol Iodochlor hydroxy quine, anti-amoebic agent.

Clinoid processes Three pairs of prominences on upper surface of sphenoid bone.

Clithrophobia Morbid fear of being locked in.

Clitoris Small erectile body beneath anterior labial commissure of female, homologous to penis of male.

Clitorism Recurring painful erection of clitoris, akin to priapism in male.

Clitoris Crises Involuntary orgasm in female in tabes dorsalis.

Clivulus A surface that slopes as in sphenoid bone.

Clofazimine Antileprotic agent that stains skin.

Clofibrate Lipid lowering agent, may be carcinogenic and causes gall stones.

Clomid Clomiphene citrate, a nonsteroidal agent to stimulate ovulation in females and spermatogenesis in males.

Clonazepam Anticonvulsant for myoclonic seizure.

Clonidine Antihypertensive agent, also used for migraine prophylaxis.

Clonus Alternate contraction and relaxation of muscles, sign of upper motor lesion.

Clonic spasm Spasm marked by repeated muscular contraction followed by relaxation.

Clonorchiasis Liver fluke caused by chlonorchis sinensis which infects bile duct of man. Infection contacted by eating uncooked fresh water fish containing larvae. Treatment is with praziquantel.

Chlorphene A phenol, disinfectant

Clostridium Anaerobic spore forming rods common in soil and GI tract of animal and man.

c. botulinum Produces botulism.

c. difficile Causes pseudomembranous colitis.

c. histolytium Proteolytic, isolated from gas gangrene.

c. perfringens Causes gas gangrene (C. welchii)

c. tetani Produces tetanus.

Clotrimazole Antifungal agent for treatment of vulvovaginal candidiasis.

Cloxacillin Betalactamase resistant penicillin.

Clozapine Diabenzodiazepine group of antipsychotic agent.

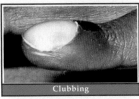

Clubbing

Clubbing Bulbous enlargement of finger and toes tips with exasserated lateral and longitudinal curvatures. Most commonly found in infective endocarditis, suppurative lung disease, cyanotic heart disease and often congenital.

Clumping Thick grouping of microorganisms in a culture when specific immune serum is added.

Cluster headache Nocturnal headache, 2-3 hours after falling asleep, continuing for months associated with watering from eyes.

Clutton's joint Hydroarthrosis of knee joint often associated with interstitial keratitis, seen in congenital syphilis.

Cluquet's canal The hyaloid canal through vitreous in fetus.

Coagulation The process of clotting, dependent upon availability of prothrombin, calcium, fibrinogen and thromboplastin. Prothrombin is converted to thrombin by the

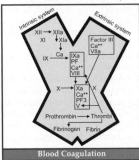

Blood Coagulation

action of thromboplastin in the presence of calcium ions. Thrombin then converts soluble fibrinogen to insoluble fibrin mesh work on which RBCs are entangled. Thromboplastin is produced from injured vessel wall or by activated platelets.

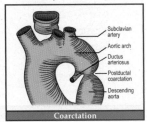

Coarctation

Coarctation A stricture, compression of walls.

Coat's disease Development of large white masses in blood vessels of retina.

Cobalt 60 Radioactive isotope for treating malignancies.

Cocaine CNS stimulant, in toxic doses causes CNS depression, cardiac arrhythmia, and respiratory depression.

Coccidioidomycosis A coccidioidal granuloma.

Coccygeal body Small arteriovenous anastomosis at the level of coccyx.

Cochlea A winding cone-shaped tube resembling a snail shell, winding two and three quarter turns about a central bony axis, organ responsible for hearing.

Cochlear implant An electronic device that receives sounds and transmits the resulting electric signals to implanted electrodes in cochlea so that the sound is perceived. *SYN*–Cochlear prosthesis.

Cochlear nerve 8th cranial nerve supplying cochlea with nucleus at pons and medulla.

Cochleo-palpebral reflex Contraction of orbicularis oculi from sudden noise near the ear.

Cocktail Any beverage or product containing several ingredients.

Cock-up splint a static aplint designed to keep the wrist either in extension or dorsal flexion.

Codeine Derivative of opium used as analgesic-hypnotic.

Cod liver oil Oil extracted from liver of fish rich in vitamin A and D.

Coenzyme A diffusible heatstable of enzyme which when combines with apoenzyme forms active complete enzyme, e.g. riboflavin, coenzyme I and II.

Coenzyme A precursor for biosynthesis of fatty acids and sterols.

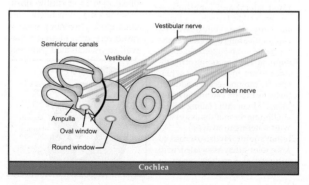

Cochlea

Cogan's syndrome Interstitial keratitis associated with tinnitus, vertigo and usually deafness.

Cognition Awareness with perception, reasoning, judgement, memory, etc.

Cogwheel Combination of tremor and rigidity as in extrapyramidal disease, i.e. Parkinson's disease.

Coherent Sticking together, adhesiveness.

Cohort The component of population born during a period and traced through life.

Cohort Study In epidemiology, a method of investigation is a cohort, q.v.; is followed prospectively or retrospectively.

Coilonychia Dystrophy of fingernails with spoon shaped surface, feature of iron deficiency anaemia.

Coin test A test for pneumothorax, a coin placed on chest is struck with another coin. A metallic ringing sound is heard at a distant site of the chest in pneumothorax.

Coitus Sexual intercourse between male and female.

Colchicine Antigout medicine, may produce GI side effects.

Cold agglutinin The agglutinin agglutinating RBCs at 4°C, commonly seen in viral and mycoplasma infections.

Cold common *SYN*–nasal catarrh, acute catarrhal inflammation of mucous membrane of nasal cavity, sinuses and pharynx caused by rhinovirus.

Cold pack Wrapping patient in cold water soaked clothing to reduce fever, for relief of pain and diminution of swelling in bruise.

Colestipol Ion exchange resin akin to cholestyramine.

Colic Spasmodic pain originating from any hollow viscus.

c. biliary Gall stone in bile duct/cystic duct causing pain.

c. intestinal Abdominal pain due to worms, infection, spasm of intestines.

c. renal Passage of stone, clot along ureters with pain in loin radiating to groin, genitalia and inner aspect of thigh.

c. uterine Dysmenorrhoeic pain due to retained clots.

Colistin Potymyxin, an antibiotic effective against many organisms including pseudomonas.

Colitis Inflammation of colon.

c. ulcerative Inflammation involving rectum with skip lesions, cobble stone appearance, friable mucosa and bloody offensive diarrhea.

Collagen Fibrous insoluble protein of skin, bone, ligaments and cartilages.

Collagenase Enzyme responsible for breakdown of collagen.

Collagen vascular diseases A group of diseases of blood vessels of unknown etiology manifesting with joint pain, skin rash, muscle ache and bleeding manifestations. Included in this group are SLE, rheumatoid arthritis, systemic sclerosis etc.

Collapse 1. An abnormal retraction of the walls of an organ 2. A sudden exhaustion, prostration or weakness due to poor circulation.

Collapsing pulse Pulse of aortic regurgitation.

Collapse therapy Unilateral pneumothorax induced to promote healing/stop bleeding of Koch's lesion.

Collecting tubule Small ducts in renal medulla that receive urine from several renal tubules. These ducts form papillary ducts of Bellini that open into renal papillae.

Colle's fascia Inner layer of superficial fascia of perineum.

Colle's fracture Transverse fracture of distal end of radius with displacement of lower fragment backwards, upwards and laterally.

Coloboma a fissure or cleft in iris/ciliary body/choriod

Colon irritable Motility disorder of colon manifesting with abdominal pain, frequent small ribbon like stools, usually triggered by anxiety.

Colonic irrigation Flushing out of colon prior to surgery of colon, colonoscopy.

Coloproctectomy Surgical removal of colon and rectum.

Colour blindness Defective perception of colour; colour blindness in which all colours are perceived as gray is called monochromasia.

Colorimeter Instrument for measuring intensity of colour.

Colostomy Opening up of colon to exterior through abdominal wall.

Colostrum Breast fluid secreted during first 2-3 days after delivery, rich in protein, calories and antibodies.

Colpectomy Surgical removal of vagina.

Colpostenosis Narrowing of vagina.

Colposcopy Examination of vagina and vaginal portion of cervix by colposcope, usually to select sites of abnormal epithelium for biopsy in patient with abnormal papsmear.

Column A cylindrical supporting structure.

c. clarkis A group of large cells in the medial portion of the base of the posterior gray column of spinal cord.

c. anterior The anterior portion of the gray-matter on each side of the spinal cord.

c. lateral A column in the lateral portion of gray matter of spinal cord containing preganglionic nurones of sympathetic nervous system.

c. of Morgagni One of the several vertical ridges in the mucous membrane at the junction of anus and rectum.

c. posterior Posterior horn of gray matter in spinal cord.

c. vertebral The axial skeleton containing vertebrae (7 cervical, 12 thoracic, 5 lumbar, sacrum and the coccyx) and encasing the spinal cord.

Coma A state from which patient cannot be aroused by painful stimuli and he does not respond to inner needs.

Comedo Blackhead, discoloured dried sebum plugging an excretory duct of the skin, e.g. acne involving face, back and neck in adolescents.

Comma bacillus Vibrio comma, organism of cholera.

Comma tract of Schultze The fasciculus interfascicularis, a tract of descending fibers located between the fasciculus cuneatus and fasciculus gracilis in the posterior funiculus of spinal cord.

Commensal Organisms that live in an intimate non-parasitic relationship.

Comminuted fracture A fracture where the bone is splintered or crushed.

Comminution Reducing a solid body to varying sizes by grating, pulverizing, slicing etc.

Commissure A transverse band of nerve fibers passing over the midline in the CNS.

c. anterior cerebral Band of white fibers that passes across lamina terminalis connecting the two cerebral hemispheres.

c. posterior Commissure just above the midbrain containing fibers that connect the superior colliculi.

Commissurotomy Surgical incision of any commissure. Commonly refers to mitral commissurotomy in mitral stenosis.

Communicable disease A disease that may be transmitted directly or indirectly from one person to another.

Compartment syndrome Compression of nerve and vessels within a tight musculofascial compartment e.g. of leg in burn or infection.

Compatibility Ability of two individuals or groups to live together without strife or tension.

Complement A series of enzymatic proteins in normal serum that once activated augment immune mechanisms by leukocyte chemotaxis, and bacterial opsonization.

Complement fixation Some antigen antibody reactions fix complement for completion of reaction. This process is the basis of Wasserman reaction for syphilis.

Compliance The property of altering size and shape in response to application of force, weight or release from such force, e.g. pulmonary compliance a measure of the force required to expand the lungs. Children have higher pulmonary compliance in comparision to adults.

Compound fracture Fracture with communication to exterior by breach in the skin.

Compound astigmatism Myopia/hypermetropia of differing diopters in both longitudinal and vertical axes.

Compulsion Repetitive stereotyped act performed to relieve fear connected with obsession; dictated by patient's subconscious mind against his wishes and if not performed causes uneasiness.

Compulsion neurosis Obsession that compels one to perform an absurd act.

Compulsive ideas An idea that continues to haunt against one's will.

Computer An electronic device for storing and retrieving numerical or textural information.

Computer assisted design Computer use to assist in designing objects, e.g. reshape body parts in plastic surgery, artificial hip implant, crown preparation.

Concanavalin A A lectin that stimulates proliferation of T lymphocyte but not B lymphocytes.

Conceive To become pregnant, to form an idea, to form a mental image.

Concentration Strength of a substance in solution; fixation of mind on one subject with exclusion of all other thoughts.

Conception Union of male spermatozoa with ovum.

Concha The outer ear or pinna; the turbinate inside nasal cavity.

Conchotomy Surgical incision of nasal concha.

Concoction Mixture of two medicinal substance aided by heating.

Concomitant Occurring at the same time.

Concussion cerebral Transient loss of consciousness from external cranial trauma.

Conditioning Improving physical capability by an exercise programme.

c. operant Learning of a particular action or type of behavior that is followed by reward.

Condom A latex sheath used for contraception, can be used by male or female (polyurethane) and can often be costume made.

Conduction The transfer of electron, heat, ions or sound wave through a conducting medium or the process whereby a state of excitation is transmitted.

Condyle A rounded protruberance at the end of a bone forming an articulation.

Condyloma A wart like growth in the skin around anus/external genitalia.

c. acuminata Usually venereal, caused by virus.

c. latum A mucous patch on the vulva or anus characteristic of syphilis.

Confabulation A form of memory loss in which the patient fills his memory gaps with inappropriate words.

Confluent Running together, merging together.

Confusion Disorientation in respect to time, place or person.

Congener Two or more muscles with same function, or two substances with similar origin, function or line structure.

Congestion The presence of excessive amount of blood or tissue fluid in an organ or tissue.

c. active Congestion arising out of increased blood flow or vasodilatation.

c. passive Vascular congestion due to impaired pumping action by heart.

c. pulmonary Pulmonary vascular congestion due to increased LA pressure (MS) or LVF.

Coniology The study of dust and its effects.

Coniotomy Cricothyrotomy.

Conization Excision of a cone of tissue as in chronic cervicitis.

Conjugate Paired or joined.

c. deviation Deviation of both eyes to either side.

c. diagonal Distance measured from center of sacral promontory to the back of symphysis pubis. True conjugate is 1.5 to 2 cm less than diagonal conjugate.

c. true It is anterior-posterior diameter of pelvic inlet; the distance between the midline superior point of the sacrum and the upper margin of symphysis pubis.

Conjugation A coupling together. In biology, the union of two unicellular organisms accompanied by an interchange of nuclear material.

Conjunctiva Mucous membrane that lines eyelids and is reflected onto eyeball.

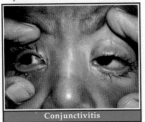
Conjunctivitis

Conjunctivitis Inflammation of conjunctiva.

c. actinic Conjunctivitis from exposure to actinic (ultraviolet rays).

c. angular Conjunctivitis involving angles of eyes, due to Morax Axenfield bacillus.

c. catarrhal Conjunctivitis with mucoid discharge due to foreign body, allergy, heat, cold, etc.

c. epidemic haemorrhagic Viral infection of eye with swollen eyelids, and subconjunctival haemorrhage.

c. inclusion Purulent inflammation of conjunctiva due to chlamydia trachomatis.

c. phlyctenular Nodules around limbus, particularly in allergy to Koch's bacillus.

c. vernal Allergic sping conjunctivitis.

Conjunctivoma A tumor of conjunctiva.

Conn's syndrome Primary hyperaldosteronism with muscle weakness, polyuria, hypertension, hypokalemia and alkalosis.

Consanguinity Blood relationship, i.e. being descended from a common ancestor.

Consciousness A state of awareness, i.e. orientation in time, place and person. Stupor is a state from which only intense stimulus can arouse the patient. Normal motor reflex. In coma patient does not perceive the environment and intense stimuli produce only rudimentary response if any at all.

Consensual Reflex stimulation of another or opposite part.

Consensual light reflex Contraction of opposite pupil from focussing of light on one side.

Consent Granting permission by patient for a procedure.

c. implied Consent presumed in certain circumstances, i.e. when patient sits on a dental chair thereby implying examination.

c. informed The understanding between the person and institution conducting an experimental medical investigation involving human subjects.

Consolidation The act of becoming solid, especially solidification of lung due to pathological engorgement of the tissue as occurring in pneumonia.

Constipation Infrequent defecation with passage of unduly hard and dry fecal material, sluggish action of bowels.

c. obstructive Obstructive colonic/ intestinal lesion causing constipation.

c. atonic Constipation due to weakness of muscles of colon and rectum.

c. spastic Constipation due to excessive tonicity of intestinal wall.

Consummation The completion of marriage by the first act of sexual intercourse.

Contact Mutual touching or apposition of two persons/objects or one who has recently been exposed to contagious disease.

Contact dermatitis Dermatitis due to an irritating or sensitizing chemical.

Contact lens Device, either rigid or flexible that rests on cornea to improve refractive error.

Contagious Communicable; transmitted readily from one person to another either directly or indirectly.

Contagium The agent causing infection or contagion.

Contamination 1. Introduction of disease germs, or infectious materials into normally sterile objects. 2. Radiation in or on a place where it is not wanted.

Continent Capable of controlling urination and defecation or sexual indulgence.

Contortion A twisting into an unusual shape.

Contour Surface configuration of a part.

Contraception Prevention of conception.

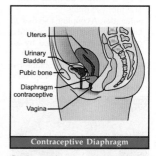

Contraceptive Diaphragm

Contraceptive Any process, device or method that prevents contraception. They include spermicides, estrogen-progesterone pills, and physical barriers like IUD.

Contract To contract a disease/ infection, to shorten or reduce in size.

Contraction isotonic Muscular contraction in which the muscle maintains constant tension by changing its length during contraction.

Contraction isometric Muscular exercise where muscle does not change its length.

Contracture Permanent contraction of a muscle due to paralysis/spasm/ischaemia.

c. Dupuytrens Contraction of palmar fascia leading to deformity of fingers.

c. Volkman's Atrophy of forearm muscles with pronation and flexion of the hand resulting from constricting cast/bandage on brachial artery.

Contraindication Inadvisable form of therapy.

Contralateral Opposite side of body.

Contrast In radiology, radiopaque material to provide a contrast in density between tissue or organ being X-rayed.

Contrecoup injury Injury to one part of brain with lesion on opposite side, e.g. blow to the back of head causing injury to frontal lobes as they are forced against anterior portion of cranial valt.

Contusion A bruise, injury with subcutaneous hemorrhage but intact skin.

Conus Shaped like a cone.

c. arteriosus The portion of right ventricle giving rise to pulmonary arteries.

c. medullaris Lower conical portion of spinal cord.

Convalescence The period of recovery after an illness/operation.

Convection Heat transfer through liquids or gases.

Convergence The moving of two or more objects at same point.

Conversion reaction Hysterical neuroses denoting a psychological conflict translated into physical ailment.

Convolution A turn, fold or coil of anything that is convoluted. In anatomy, a gyrus, one of the many folds on the surface of cerebral hemispheres that are separated by grooves, sulci or fissures.

Convulsion Paroxysms of involuntary muscle contraction and relaxation.

Cooley's anemia Thalassemia major, an inherited disorder of hemoglobin synthesis.

Coombs' test A test for detection of antiglobulins in blood, helpful in diagnosis of autoimmune hemolytic anemia.

Cooper's ligament Supporting fibrous bands in female breast.

Co-ordination Working together of various muscles for performing certain movements.

Copolymer A polymer composed of two different kinds of monomers.

Copper sulfate Deep blue crystals/granules, used as algicide/astringent.

Coprolalia The use of vulgar, obscene language as in schizophrenia and Gilles dela Tourette syndrome.

Coprolith Hard feces.

Coprophilia Unusual preoccupation with feces, a perversion in adults.

Coproporphyria Excessive copro-porphyrin excretion in feces, as in inherited porphyrias.

Coproporphyrin A porphyrin present in urine and feces.

Copula Any connecting part.

Copulation Sexual intercourse.

Coracoid Resembling in shape acrow's beak.

Coracoid process Process on anterior upper surface of scapula.

Cord A string like structure.

c. spermatic The channel for sperms to pass from testes to seminal vesicle.

c. spinal Extension of CNS into the spinal canal upto upper border of first lumbar vertebra.

c. umbilical Cord that connects fetal circulatory system to the placenta, consists of two umbilical arteries and one umbilical vein.

Cordotomy Resectional of lateral spinothalamic tracts in the cord to relieve intractable pain.

Cori cycle In carbohydrate metabolism, the breakdown of muscle glycogen with formation of lactic acid which is converted to glycogen in liver. Liver glycogen is released as glucose which is taken up by muscles being then reconverted to muscle glycogen.

Corn Hardening or thickening of skin that has a conical shape extending into dermis causing pain.

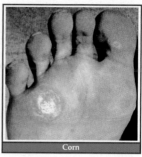
Corn

Cornea The clear, transparent anterior portion of eye covering 1/6 the surface of globe functioning as an important refractive medium. It is composed of 5 layers: epithelium, Browman's membrane, substantia propria, Descemet's membrane and layer of endothelium.

Cornea reflex Closure of eyelid on touching the cornea: Afferent limb by trigeminal and efferent by facial nerves.

Corneal transplant Either partial thickness or full thickness transfer of cornea from a healthy cadaver, donor to treat corneal opacity obstructing vision.

Corneoblepharon Adhesion of eyelid to cornea.

Cornification The process by which squamous epithelial cells are converted into hard horny material, e.g. horns, hairs, nails, feathers etc.

Cornu Any projection like a horn.

Corona Any structure resembling a crown.

Coronal plane Plane dividing into front and back portions.

Corona radiata Ascending and descending fibers of internal capsule that above corpus collosum extend in all directions to reach cerebral cortex.

Coronary arteries A pair of arteries, left and right arising from left and right coronary sinuses supplying blood to myocardium. The left artery is usually dominant.

Coronary angiography Opacification of coronary arteries by injection of iohexol or urograffin or any such contrast agent.

Coronary bypass Surgically established shunt between root of aorta and involved coronary distal to block or diverting internal mammary to augment myocardial blood flow.

Coronary care unit A specially, equipped unit in a hospital providing intensive care to patients of coronary artery disease, i.e. myocardial infarction, unstable angina etc.

Coronary plexus A plexus of autonomic nerve fibers supplying the heart.

Coronary sinus The channel carrying venous drainage of heart into right atrium.

Corona virus The virus particle surrounded by a crown, e.g. common cold virus.

Coronoid fossa An oval depression on anterior surface of distal end of burner us articulating with coronoid process of ulna.

Cor pulmonale Right heart failure secondary to pulmonary pathology.

Corpus The principal part of any organ or body.

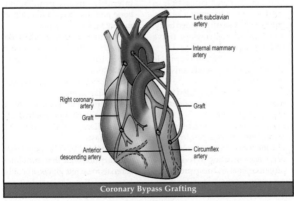

Coronary Bypass Grafting

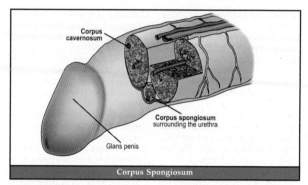

Corpus cavernosum
Corpus spongiosum
surrounding the urethra
Glans penis

Corpus Spongiosum

c. callosum The commissure joining two cerebral hemispheres.

c. cavernosum Erectile tissue of penis, clitoris, bulb of vestibule etc.

c. spongiosum Mass of spongy tissue within the penis surrounding the male urethra

c. striatum The structures in cerebral hemispheres consisting of caudate and lentiform nuclei.

Corpuscle Any small rounded body, an encapsulated sensory nerve ending, blood cell.

c. malphigian A renal corpuscle consisting of a glomerulous and Bowman's capsule.

c. Meissner's An encapsulated touch receptor in the epidermis of skin esp of palm, hand and feet.

c. Pacinian A large ovoid sensory end organ consisting of concentric layers of connective tissue surrounding nerve ending acting as receptor of proprioception and deep pressure.

Corrigan's pulse A full bounding pulse of aortic insufficiency.

Corrosive poisoning Poisoning by strong alkalies, acid, antiseptics, e.g. hydroxides of sodium, ammonium, potassium.

Corrugator The muscle of eye drawing eyebrow medially and interiorly, arising from frontal bone and inserted on the skin of medial half of eyebrows.

Cortex Outer layer of an organ like kidney, adrenal, ovary, lymph node, thymus, cerebrum and cerebellum.

Corticoid Steroid hormone secreted by adrenal cortex.

Corticosterone Hormone of adrenal cortex influencing carbohydrate metabolism, Na^+ and K^+ homeostasis.

Corticotrophin (ACTH) The anterior pituitary hormone that stimulates adrenals to secrete glucocorticoids.

Corticotrophin releasing factor The hypothalamic factor regulating secretion of corticotrophin.

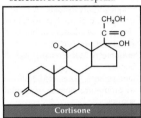

Cortisone

Cortisone Adrenal hormone, largely inactive till converted to active cortisol. Influences metabolism of fat, carbohydrate, protein, N^+ and K^+

Corynebacterium Gram positive nonmotile drum stick shaped rod, causing diphtheria.

Coryza Acute nasal catarrh with profuse watery secretion.

Cosmetic Agents or methods of improving physical appearance, (appearance promoters)

Cosmetic surgery Commonly known as plastic surgery done to improve appearance, i.e. correction of ugly burns and scars, elephantiasis, localized obesity, pendulous breast, facial wrinkles.

Cosmic Universe.

Costens syndrome Temperomandibular arthritis.

Cosyntropin Synthetic corticotropin used to test adrenal insufficiency.

Continine Principal metabolite of nicotine excreted in urine.

Cotton wool spots Soft wooly exudates in retina in hypertension and uremia, probably superficial infarcts.

Couching Forcible downward displacement of lens caused to improve vision in cataract patients.

Cough Forceful expiratory effort with closed glottis, to expectorate mucous and foreign body.

Counselling Providing of advice and guideline to a patient by health professional.

Counter Geiger Device for detection and counting of ionizing radiation.

Counter current exchanger The exchange of chemicals between two counter current streams separated by a membrane.

Counter immunoelectrophoresis A process in which antigen and antibodies are placed in separate wells and an electric current is passed through diffusion medium. Antigens migrate to anode and antibodies to cathode. If the antigen and antibody correspond to each other, they upon meeting in the diffusion medium will precipitate and will form a precipitin band or line.

Counter incision A second incision made to facilitate drainage or to reduce tension on the stitches.

Counterirritant An agent applied locally to produce mild inflammatory reaction to relieve pain of adjacent or deeper structure.

Counter shock An electric shock applied to heart to correct arrhythmia.

Countertraction Application of a force in a direction opposite to the force of traction, usually in fracture reduction.

Couple To join together, to have sexual union.

Courvoisier's law Sudden obstruction of bile duct by gallstone does not cause enlargement of gall bladder as opposed to gradual obstruction as in malignancy of pancreas/ampulla of Vater which consistently causes marked enlargement of gall bladder.

Covalent Sharing of electrons between two atoms.

Cowden's disease Multiple hamartomas.

Cowling's rule Age of child on next birth day divided by 24 to give pediatric dose.

Cowper's gland A pair of compound tubular mucous glands beneath the bulb of male urethra, akin to Bartholin glands in female.

Coxalgia Pain in the hip.

Coxiella burnetti Causative organism of Q fever.

Coxsackie virus A member of picorna virus causing herpangina, aseptic meningitis, pleurodynia, epidemic conjunctivitis, myocarditis.

Crab louse Louse infecting pubic regions (phthirus pubis)

Cracked pot sound Percussion note resembling cracked pot as in pulmonary cavity, hydrocephalus.

Cramp Spasmodic painful contraction of a muscle.

Cranioclast Instrument for crushing foetal skull to facilitate delivery of large dead foetus.

Craniocleidodysostosis A congenital condition that involves defective ossification of bones of face, head, and clavicle.

Craniometry Measurement of skull bones.

Craniostenosis Contracted skull due to premature closure of cranial sutures.

Cranio ostosis Congenital ossification of cranial sutures.

Craniotabes Abnormal softening of skull bones.

Cravat bandage Triangular bandage folded to form a band around the injured part.

Crazybone Name for medial epicondyle of humerus, as slight trauma to it causes pain and tingling in fingers due to stimulation of ulnar nerve.

c. reactive protein Acute phase reactant, aserum globulin whose concentrations is increased in acute infections like rheumatic fever.

Creatine Methylglycocyamine, a colourless substance excreted in urine. Combines with phosphate to form creatine phosphate.

Creatine kinase Enzyme present in skeletal and cardiac muscles that acts in breakdown of ATP to ADP. Serum level is increased in myocardial infarction, skeletal muscle injury, and muscle dystrophy.

Creatinine Formed from creatine.

Crede's method Expulsion of placenta by putting downward pressure on the uterus through anterior abdominal wall and squeezing uterus but inversion is a danger.

Cremaster A fascia like muscle suspending and enveloping testicles and spermatic cord.

Cremasteric reflex Retraction of testes on stimulation of innerside of thigh, a superficial reflex mediated via L_1, L_2 segment.

Crepitation Crackling sound heard 1. in lungs in pneumonia, 2. movement of fractured bones, 3. in soft tissues in anaerobic gasforming infections and in 4. subcutaneous emphysema.

Crescent Shaped like sickle, e.g. menisci of knee joint, choroid atrophy in myopics (myopic crescent).

Cresol Coal tar derivative disinfectant containing 5% phenol.

Cresomania Hallucination of possession of great wealth.

Crest Ridge or elongated prominence, e.g. alveolar crest that surrounds teeth whose resorption can be delayed by flurbiprofen.

Crest Syndrome Calcinosis, Raynaud's phenomenon, esophageal dismotility, sclerodactyly and telangiectasia, a variant of systemic sclerosis.

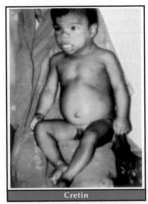
Cretin

Cretin Hypothyroidism in babies manifesting as rough skin, mental subnormality, potbelly, coarse features, hypoactivity and delayed dentition.

Crevice A small fissure or crack, e.g. gingival crevice: a fissure produced by the marginal gingiva with tooth surface.

Crib A small bed with high legs and sides for infants and babies.

Cribiform Sieve like, e.g. 1. Cribiform plate, the thin perforated medial portion of ethmoid bone perforated by olfactory nerve fibers. 2. Cribiform fascia, the part of deep fascia of thigh covering fossa ovalis.

Cricoid Shaped like a signet ring, e.g. cricoid cartilage; the lower most cartilage of larynx, the broad portion being posterior and anterior portion forming the arch.

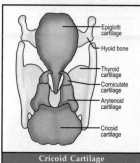

Epiglotti cartilage
Hyoid bone
Thyroid cartilage
Corniculate cartilage
Arytenoid cartilage
Cricoid cartilage

Cricoid Cartilage

Cri-du-chat syndrome A chromosomal deletion disorder characterized by cry like a cat, microcephaly, mental retardation, dwarfism and laryngeal defect.

Crisis Critical period, e.g. 1. Addisonian crisis., (acute adrenal failure) 2. Sickle cell crisis (acute bone/abdominal pain of sickle cell anemia due to thrombotic infarcts) 3. Thyroid crisis: Fever, delirium and extreme tachycardia of sudden deterioration of hyperthyroidism. 4. Sudden fall in temperature in pneumonia.

Crista A crest or ridge, e.g. 1. Crysta ampularis, the localized thickening of membrane lining the ampulla of semicircular canals. 2. Crista supraventricularis of heart.

Crocodile tear Production of tear during mastication in patients with facial palsy due to abnormal regeneration, so named because crocodiles are believed to weep after eating their victims.

Crohn's disease Regional enteritis, a granulomatous inflammation involving all the three coats of small intestine and often colon.

Cromolyn sodium Disodium chromoglycate, useful in bronchial asthma, mast cell stabilizer.

Cross fertilization Fusion of male and female gametes from different persons.

Crossmatching A test for compatibility in blood transfusion A where donor red cells are matched with recipient plasma and vice versa.

Cross over Reciprocal exchange of genetic material between chromosomes.

Crotamiton Ascabicide used as 2% ointment

Croup Laryngitis marked by barking cough, stridor, and respiratory difficulty usually due to formation of diphtheritic membrane.

Crouzon's disease Congenital disease characterised by hypertelorism (wide spaced eyes) craniofacial dysostosis. exophthalmos, optic atrophy and divergent squint.

Crowning Showing of fetal head in vulva during parturition.

Cruciate Cross shaped as in cruciate ligament of knee.

Crura Divergent bands resembling legs, e.g. crura of diaphragm, connecting to spinal column; crura cerebri; cerebral peduncles.

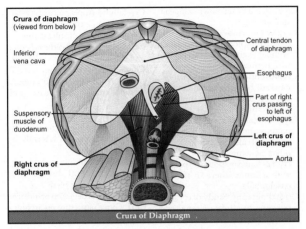

Crura of diaphragm
(viewed from below)

Inferior vena cava

Suspensory muscle of duodenum

Right crus of diaphragm

Central tendon of diaphragm

Esophagus

Part of right crus passing to left of esophagus

Left crus of diaphragm

Aorta

Crura of Diaphragm

Crush syndrome Renal failure following crush injury with myoglobinuria.

Crutch paralysis Crutch induced paralysis of brachial plexus/ radial nerve.

Cryocautery Cold application for therapeutic objective.

Cryoextraction Use of liquid nitrogen/carbon dioxide probe to anterior lens aiding in its extraction.

Cryoglobulin An abnormal globulin that precipitates when cooled but dissolves on heating, found in multiple myeloma, leukemia and mycoplasma pneumonia.

Cryoprecipitate Precipitation of immunecomplexes in patients with autoimmune diseases when their serum is stored in cold.

Cryopreservation Preservation of biological material, e.g. sperm, organs, tissue, plasma in subzero temperature.

Cryosurgery Tissue destruction by application of cold probe (-20 C or below) as to control pain, bleeding, e.g., haemorrhoidectomy, tonsillectomy, conization of cervix, thalamotomy.

Crypt Small cavity, i.e. anal crypts, lying behind junction of anal skin and rectal mucosa, tonsillar crypts on tonsils surrounded by lymphnodules.

Cryptitis Inflammation of anal crypts.

Cryptococcosis *SYN*–torulosis: Systemic fungal infection involving skin, brain, lungs caused by cryptococcus neoformans.

Cryptogenic Of unknown or indeterminate origin.

Cryptomenorrhoea Monthly subjective symptoms of menstruation without vaginal bleed usually due to unperforated hymen.

Cryptosporidiasis Acute diarrhoea caused by protozoa cryptosporidium usually in immunocompromised.

Crystal Small particles with definite pattern and angles, e.g. apatite crystals of calcium phosphate with other elements; Charcot-Leyden crystals found in sputum of patients with asthma where in there is eosinophilia.

Crystallography Study of crystals, pertains to study of renal and biliary calculi.

Crystalluria Appearance of crystals, in urine, commonly after administration of sulfa drugs.

c. terminal The alpha carboxyl group of last amino acid.

Chemoreceptor trigger zone (CTZ) The area of medulla oblongata whose stimulation causes vomiting.

Cubital fossa The hollow anterior to elbow bounded medially by pronater teres and laterally by brachioradialis.

Cubitus Forearm

c. valgus lateral deviation of forearms beyond 16-18°.

c. varus medial deviation of forearm.

Cuff Glove, structure encircling a part.

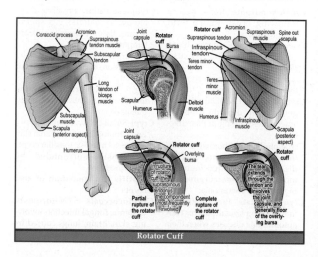

Rotator Cuff

Cul-de-sac A blind pouch or cavity.

Culdocentesis Perforation of posterior upper vaginal wall for draining rectouterine pouch for diagnostic/therapeutic purposes.

Culdoscopy Examination of pelvic cavity by passing endoscope into posterior vaginal fornix.

Culex Mosquito responsibe for filariasis.

Culicide Agents that destroy gnats and mosquitoes.

Cullen's sign Bluish discoloration of periumbilical skin due to intraperitoneal hemorrhage, usually following pancreatitis, tubal pregnancy rupture.

Culmen Top or submit of a thing.

Cult People following an ideal or principle.

Culture Propagation of micro-organisms or living tissue in special media.

Cumulus Small elevation.

Cupid's bow The normal bow shape of upper lip.

Cupola The dome at the apex of cochlea; the dome of pleura covering apex of lung.

Cuprous Monovalent copper Cu^+; Cupric is Cu^{++}.

Curarization Anticonvulsant medication, by administration of agents negating effects of acetylcholine, i.e., suxamethonium.

Currett A spoon shaped scrapping instrument used in dentistry, gynaecology and orthopedics.

Curie Unit of radiation equivalent to $10^{10} \times 3.7$ disintegration per second.

Curling ulcer Peptic ulcer following severe stress, i.e. burn injury.

Current A flow, usually of electrical impulse.

c. *alternating* Current that periodically flows in opposite directions.

c. *direct* Unidirectionally flow of current.

Curriculum Course of study.

Crushmann's spirals Coiled spirals in sputum of asthmatic patients.

Curvilinear Concerning or pertaining to a curved line.

Cushing's disease Hypersecretion of ACTH with hypercortisolism manifesting with trunkal obesity, hyperglycemia, hypokalemia purplish striae and osteoporosis.

Cushing's syndrome Symptoms arising out of hypercortisolism.

Cusp Points on crown of tooth, leaf like portions constituting heart valves.

Cutis The skin.

Cyanemia Blue colour of blood.

Cyanhemoglobin Cyanide haemoglobin compound where blood appears cherry red as in cyanide poisoning.

Cyanocobalamin Vit B_{12}

Cyanosis Bluish discolouration of skin due to raised (≥ 4 gm%) of reduced hemoglobin in blood.

c. *central* Occurring by admixture of venous and arterial blood in heart/lungs, e.g. pulmonary a-v fistula, Fallot tetralogy and TGV

c. *peripheral* Local cyanosis over cold parts due to increased oxygen extraction, e.g. CHF *c. differential* Cyanosis of feet but not arms in Eisenmenger syndrome in patent ductus arteriosus.

Cyclamate Artificial sweetner 30 times more sweet than sugar.

Cyclandelate Vasodilator.

Cyclazocin Used in opioid addiction.

```
Cyclic AMP          NH₂
                     |
                     C
Adenine       N   ⁄     ⁀   N
               ‖  C              ⁀ CH
              HC    ⁀ N    C   N⁄
Phosphate        Ribose
            O ⁀ CH₂
            |           O
O= P ⁀ O  C        C
            | H   H |
            H    C ⁀ C  H
             |    |
             HO   OH
```
Cyclic AMP

Cyclic AMP Adenosine 3'5' cyclic monophosphate, an intracellular messenger of end organ stimulation.

Cyclitis Inflammation of ciliary body.

Cyclodialysis Drainage operation for treatment of glaucoma in which communication is established between supra arachnoid space and angle of anterior chamber.

Cyclizine Antihistamine for motion sickness.

Cyclooxygenase Enzyme converting arachidonic acid to prostaglandin.

Cyclophosphamide Antineoplastic and immunosuppressant.

Cycloplegia Paralysis of ciliary muscles leading to dilatation of pupils.

Cyclopropane Gaseous anaesthetic agent.

Cycloserine Broad spectrum antibiotic used in tuberculosis.

Cyclosporine Immune suppressant used in transplant patients.

Cyclotron A particle accelerator in which the particle is rotated between the ends of a magnet, gaining speed with each rotation.

Cylindroma Malignant tumor containing a collection of cells forming cylinders.

Cyproheptadine Antiserotonin drug used in allergy and dumping syndrome.

Cyst A closed sac or pouch with a definite wall containing fluid, semi-solid material.

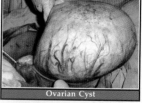
Ovarian Cyst

c. alveolar Cyst at tooth apex, air containing cyst in lungs due to ruptured alveoli.

c. colloid Cyst with gelatinous contents.

c. dentigerous A fluid filled cyst around crown of an unerupted tooth.

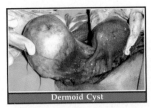

Dermoid Cyst

c. dermoid Cyst containing epidermal elements like hair, nail, teeth.

c. Gartner Cyst developing from a vestigeal mesonephric duct (Gartner's duct) in female.

c. meibomian Cyst of meibomian gland of eyelid, usually post inflammatory.

c. nabothian Retention cyst of nabothian glands of cervix.

c. pilonidal Midline cyst over sacrum lined with stratified squamous epithelium.

c. porencephalic Anomalous cystic cavity in cortex communicating with ventricular system.

Cystadenoma An adenoma containing cyst, may be serous when filled with clear fluid or pseudomucinous when contains thick viscid fluid.

Cystathionine An intermediate compound in the metabolism of methionine to cystine.

Cysticercosis Formation of cysts by encapsulation of larvae of tapeworm (T. solium).

Cystic fibrosis Inherited disease of exocrine gland affecting respiratory tract, pancreas and intestine characterized by dry viscid mucus, respiratory infection, pancreatic insufficiency, increased sodium content of sweat SYN– mucoviscidosis.

Cystitis Inflammation of urinary bladder; usually bacterial/viral/ chemical.

c. interstitial a disease of young females with chronic bladder irritation of unknown etiology but marked voiding symptoms.

Cytarabine Compound of cytosine and D ribose.

Cytochrome A pigment important for cellular respiration.

Cytochrome oxidase Enzyme responsible for electron transfer from cytochromes to oxygen thus activating oxygen to combine with hydrogen to form water.

Cytochrome P450 A protein similar to Hb in the microsomes of liver cells, catalyzing metabolism of steroid hormones and detoxification of many chemicals.

Cytogenesis Origin and developments of cell.

Cytokine More than 100 distinctive protein secreted by white blood cells regulating inflammation, immunity and tissue repair e.g. interleukins, interferon's, tumor necrosis factor, erythropoietin and colony stimulating factors.

Cytomegalic inclusion disease A viral disease that often affects fetus in utero and immunocompromised (AIDS victims) with hepatosplenomegaly, microcephaly, mental retardation.

Cytoskeleton Internal supporting framework of a cell consisting of microfilaments, intermediate filaments and microtubules.

Cytotrophoblast The thin inner layer of trophoblast with cueboidal cells secreting hormones.

Czemak's spaces Spaces in dentin caused by failure of calcification.

D

Dacarbazine An alkylating agent used in treatment of malignant melanoma, Hodgkin's disease.

Dacryo cystitis Inflammation of lacrimal gland.

Dacryostenosis Narrowing of lacrimal duct.

Dactinomycin Antitumor antibiotic.

Dactylitis Chronic inflammation of phalanges and metatarsals.

Dalton's law In a mixture of gases total pressure is equal to sum of partial pressure of each gas.

Danazol A progesterone used in endometriosis and fibroadenosis of breast.

Dance saint vitus *SYN*–chorea, i.e. involuntary quasipurposive non-repetitive jerky movements.

Dandruff Seborrhoea, exfoliation of epidermis of scalp with white greasy, dry scales.

Dandy-Walker syndrome Congenital hydrocephalus due to blockage of foramen of Luschka and Magendie.

Dane particle 42 nm sphere of hepatitis B virus.

Dantrolene A muscle relaxant.

Dapsone Diamino diphenyl sulphone, a bacteriostatic antileprotic agent.

Daraprim Pyrimethamine, used in malaria.

Darier's disease (Keratosis follicularis) a congenital disorder characterized by verrucous papular growths that colaesce into plaques of various sizes on scalp, face, neck and trunk.

Dark room Light tight room for processing X-ray films.

Dartos The subcutaneous muscle of scrotum.

Datura The plant, source of scopalamine and hyosciamine, the anticholinergic agents.

Daunorubicin Anthracycline antineoplastic antibiotic used for leukemia and malignancies.

Davidson's sign Decreased or absent pupillary light reflex when electric light is held in closed mouth as in tumor or fluid in maxillary sinus.

Dawn phenomenon A phenomena in diabetes mellitus with morning hyperglycemia due to growth hormone release.

DDT Dichlordiphenyl trichlorethane (chlorphenothane) an insecticide used in mosquito control.

Dead space The portion of tidal volume not participating in gas exchange

d. alveolar volume of alveolar gas not perfused with capillary blood

d. anatomical the air from nose to bronchial tree, not participating in gas exchange.

Deafness Complete or partial loss of ability to hear

d. conduction resulting from obstruction to sound waves reaching the normal cochlea, e.g. otosclerosis, wax, eustachian catarrh.

d. perceptive deafness due to lesions of cochlea or cochlear nerve/nucleus.

Deamination Removal of NH_2 radicals from amino compounds.

The process being oxidative or hydrolytic.

Death Permanent cessation of all vital functions including that of brain, heart, lung.

Death rate Number of deaths per 1000 population in a given time.

Death rattle Rattle sound produced by passage of air through accumulated mucous in the bronchi in terminal patients due to want of cough reflex.

Debridement Removal of foreign material along with devitalized tissue.

Debrisoquin Antihypertensive agent.

Decadron Dexamethasone, a long acting corticosteroid.

Decadurabolin Nandrolone decanoate, an anabolic steroid.

Decameter A measure of 10 meters.

Decapitation Beheading.

Decarboxylase Enzyme catalyzing release of carbon dioxide from compounds like amino acids.

Deceleration Decrease in velocity.

Decibel The unit expressing degree of intensity or loudness of sound.

Decidua Endometrium of uterus during pregnancy with outer compact layer and inner spongy layer.

d. basalis That unites with chorion to form placenta.

d. capsularis That surrounds chorionic sac.

Deciduoma Uterine tumor containing decidual tissue, when malignant termed choriocarcinoma.

Deciduous teeth Primary dentition of 20 teeth that erupt between 6 months and 3 years.

Deciliter 100 ml or 10 centi liter.

Decimeter 10 cm or 1/10 of meter.

Decision analysis A logically consistent approach to the common clinical problem of needing to make a decision when its consequences cannot be foretold with certainty. The biological variation, inconsistent drug response and poor clinical outcome data on many drug/therapeutic procedures make decision analysis a charter so that patient can be foretold in advance all about the possible outcome of treatment and he can choose the one he thinks best.

Decision making The process of using all the informations available about a patient and arriving at a decision concerning therapeutic plan.

Declaration of Geneva The declaration adopted in 1948 by World Medical Association at Geneva which reads as "At the time of being admitted as a member of medical profession I solemnly pledge my life to the service of humanity cond..

Declaration of Hawaii The guidelines laid down by General Assembly of world psychiatric association for psychiatrists in 1976 at Hawaii.

Decline Progressively decrease.

Decoction A liquid medicinal preparation made by boiling vegetable substances with water.

Decompensation Failure of heart to maintain adequate circulation to meet oxygen demand of tissues.

Decomposition Decay, putrefaction.

Decompression illness Illness arising from rapid reduction of surrounding pressure as in sea divers suddenly coming to surface. Symptoms are due to release of dissolved nitrogen.

Decongestant Reducing congestion or swelling.

Decortication Removal of surface layer of an organ, e.g. removal of pleura, renal capsule.

Decorticate posture The typical posture like flexed arms, clenched fists and extended legs in a comatose patient with lesion above upper brainstem.

Decrudescence Decrease in the severity of symptoms of a disease.

Decubitus ulcer Skin ulceration due to prolonged pressure, commonly over bony prominences.

Decussation A crossing of structures in the form of X.

De differentiation 1. The return of parts to a homogeneous state, 2. process by which mature differentiated cells or tissues at sites of origin of immature elements of the same type, as in some cancers.

Deduction Reasoning from general to particular.

Deep reflex Reflexes influenced by higher cortical centers, e.g. ankle, knee, supination, biceps jerks.

Defecation Bowel evacuation.

Defecation syncope Syncope occurring during or immediately after defecation.

Defecography Imaging of anorectal region after instilling barium into rectum – a procedure to know puborectalis function during defecation

Defeminization Loss of female sexual characteristics.

Defense Resistance to disease.

Defensins Antimicrobial peptide secreted by leukocytes.

d. silver fork forearm deformity following Colle's fracture

d. sealfin lateral deviation of fingers in rheumatoid arthritis

d. Sprengel's congenital upward displacement of scapula

Deferens Carrying away.

Deferoxamine Iron chelating agent used in thalassaemia major, haemosiderosis.

Defibrillation Stoppage of fibrillation of heart by drugs or electrical current.

Definition The precise.

Definitive Clear and final without ambiguity.

Deformity An alteration in the natural form or alignment of an organ.

Degeneration Deterioration in organ structure or function.

d. fatty deposition of abnormal amounts of fat replacing normal cells.

d. calcareous Deposition of calcium salts.

d. cystic Degeneration with cyst formation.

d. hyaline The degenerated tissues assume a homogeneous and glossy appearance.

d. hydropic Appearance of water droplets in cytoplasm.

d. pigmentary Degenerated cells change their colour.

d. spongy familial demyelination of deep cerebral cortex.

d. subacute combined Degeneration of lateral and posterior columns of spinal cord as in Vit. B$_{12}$ deficiency.

Dehydration Excessive fluid loss or inadequate fluid intake resulting in haemoconcentration and renal failure.

Dehydrocholic acid A bile salt that stimulates production of bile from the liver.

Dehydrocholesterol Precursor of vit. D.

Dehydrocorticosterone Adrenal corticosteroid.

Dehydroepiandrosterone A 17 ketosteroid with androgenic activity.

Deiter's cells Supporting cells in organ of corti.

Deiter's nucleus Cell collection behind auditory nerve nucleus.

Deja entendu The illusion or experience of hearing a thing which he has previously heard.

Deja vu The illusion or experience of seeing some thing which as if has seen/experienced previously, (unreasonable familiarity with person/surrounding).

Deladelaphus Twins fused above thorax, but separated below.

Deleterious Harmful.

Deletion The loss of genetic material from one chromosome.

Delinquent One with antisocial/ criminal behavior.

Delirium A state of mental confusion in which patient is disoriented for time and place with illusions and hallucinations. This may occur during fever, after head injury, drug intoxication, etc.

d. of persecution Delirium in which patient feels persecuted by others.

d. tremens Delirium in patients of chronic alcoholism following abstinence or illness. Usually benign but convulsion is a danger.

Delivery Child birth.

Deltoid ligament Internal lateral ligament of knee joint.

Deltoid muscle The prominent muscle covering shoulder — attached to deltoid ridge of humerus.

Delusion A false belief inconsistent to ones knowledge and experience, and with evidence to contrary.

d. nihilistic Victim believes that everything has ceased to exist.

d. grandeur Victim feels himself wealthy, rich and extraordinary and behaves so.

d. persecution Patient feels that every body around him are against him and may persecute him.

d. reference Delusion that causes the victim to read a meaning not intended in the acts or words of others.

d. systematized Logical correlation with false reasoning and deduction.

d. unsystematized Delusion without any correlation between ideas and surroundings.

Demeclocycline An antibiotic of tetracycline group.

Dementia Global impairment of intellectual function (cognition) interfering with social and occupational activities.

Demerol Meperidine hydrochloride, opium derivative.

Demilune A crescent shaped group of serous cells forming a caplike structure over a mucous alveolus, commonly present in submandibular gland.

Demineralization Loss of minerals: calcium and phosphorus from bone.

Demography Statistical and quantitative study of characteristics of human population like size, growth, density, sex, age, etc.

Demorphinization Gradual decrease in the dose of morphine in morphine addicts.

Demulcent Soothening agent acting on mucous membrane like honey, glycerin, olive oil.

de. mussets sign Head nodding with each cardiac contraction in severe aortic incompetence.

Demutization Overcoming mutism by teaching the patient to speak or use sign language.

Demyelination Destruction of myelin sheath.

Denaturation Addition of substances to ethyl alcohol to make it toxic and unfit for human consumption.

Denatured protein A protein that has lost some of its physical and chemical properties by treatment.

Dendrite A branched protoplasmic process of a neurone that conducts impulses to cell body.

Denervation Depriving a structure or organ from its nerve supply.

Dengue A group B arbovirus disease caused by bite of *Aedis egypti* mosquitoes, characterized by fever, myalgia, lymphadenopathy and often purpuric spots.

Densimeter An instrument for measuring optical density of a radiograph.

Densitometry Determining the amount of ionizing radiation to which a patient is being exposed.

Dental arch The arch formed by cutting and chewing surfaces of teeth.

Dental consonant A consonant pronounced with the tongue at or near the front upper teeth.

Dental disk The disk with abrasive powder for cutting or polishing teeth.

Dental formula A brief method of expressing the dentition of mammals.

Dental plaque A gummy mass of micro organisms and minerals that grows on the crown and causes dissolution of enamel and tooth substance.

Dental pulp The embryonic connective tissue rich in vessels and nerves occupying the central space within the tooth and its roots.

Denticle A small tooth like projection, A calcified structure within pulp of tooth.

Dental scalants Application of plastic films to the chewing surfaces of teeth to seal the pits and grooves where food and bacteria can be trapped.

Dentifrice A powder or other substance used for cleaning the teeth.

Dentin The calcified hard part of tooth surrounding the pulp chamber, covered by enamel in the crown and by cementum in the root area.

Dentinogenesis Formation of dentin in development of a tooth.

Dentition The type, number and arrangement of teeth in the dental arch.

Dentulous Having one's natural teeth.

Denture Artificial teeth substituting natural teeth.

Deodorant An agent that masks or absorbs fowl odour.

Deontology Study of professional obligations and commitments.

Deoxycorticosterone A renal hormone with mineral corticoid activity.

Deoxycholic acid $C_{24}H_{40}O_4$, a bile acid.

Deoxycoformycin Anti leukemic agent.

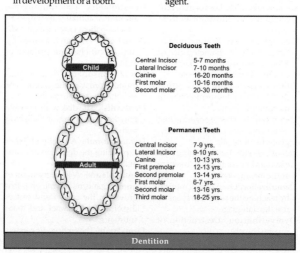

Deciduous Teeth

Central Incisor	5-7 months
Lateral Incisor	7-10 months
Canine	16-20 months
First molar	10-16 months
Second molar	20-30 months

Permanent Teeth

Central Incisor	7-9 yrs.
Lateral Incisor	9-10 yrs.
Canine	10-13 yrs.
First premolar	12-13 yrs.
Second premolar	13-14 yrs.
First molar	6-7 yrs.
Second molar	13-16 yrs.
Third molar	18-25 yrs.

Dentition

Deoxyribonuclease Enzyme causing hydrolysis of DNA.

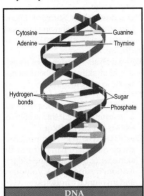

DNA

Deoxyribonucleic acid A protein consisting of deoxyribose, phosphoric acid, two purine bases (adenine and guanine) and two pyrimidines (thymine and cytosine), principally present in cell nucleus; principal protein of genes and chromosomes.

Deoxyribose A phosphoric ester of a pentose sugar.

Dependence Psychic craving for a drug that may or may not be accompanied by physiological dependence.

Depersonalization disorder The belief that ones own reality is lost or altered.

Depilation The process of hair removal.

Depletion Removal of substances like water, electrolyte, blood from the body.

Depolarization Reversal of electrical changes on cell membrane.

d. secretory diarrhea due to excess pouring of fluid and electrolytes into intestine as in carcinoid syndrome, Z.E. syndrome, mudullary carcinoma thyorid, VIPOMA and some pancreatic adenomas.

Depolymerization The breakdown of polymers into monomers.

Depomedrol Methyl prednisone acetate.

Depot Storage, e.g. fat depot.

Depressant Agent that depresses body function or nerve cell activity.

Depression 1. Altered mood with loss of interest in pleasurable activities, feeling of worthless, excessive guilt, self reproach, suicidal ideation. 2. lowering of a part, 3. Decrease in the activity of a vital organ.

d. bipolar depression with alternating periods of elation and grief.

d. endogenous depression without apparent cause.

d. reactive depression following adverse life situations.

de. Quervain's disease Tenosynovitis involving tendon sheaths of abductor pollicis longus and extensor pollicis brevis.

Dercum's disease *SYN*–adiposis dolorosa. Painful areas of fat accumulation in menopausal women.

Dereism In psychiatry, activity and thought based on fantasy and wishes rather than logic or reason.

Derivative Derived from another.

Dermalaxia Morbid relaxation or softness of skin.

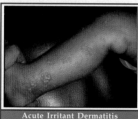
Acute Irritant Dermatitis

Dermatitis Inflammation of skin, may be allergic, actinic, infective, exfoliative, etc. characterized by redness, itching, etc.

d. atopic Dermatitis of unknown etiology, usually familial mostly self limited in children, often with lichenification.

d. contact Secondary to contact with such agents like deodorants and perfumes, usually in hypersensitive skin.

d. exfoliative Constitutional symptoms, desquamation and extensive involvement. Pigmentation is frequent.

d. herpetiformis Chronic inflammatory disease with vesicular, bulbous or pustular eruptions with linkage to HLA-B_8 and gluten. Responds to oral dapsone.

d. seborrheic Rounded irregular or circinate lesions on scalp, eye brows, nasolabial folds with greasy, shinny yellow or yellow gray scales.

Dermatoglyphics Study of lines of hand and feet for drawing inference about one's susceptibility to disease.

Dermatolysis Tendency of hypertrophied skin and subcutaneous tissue to hang in folds.

Dermatome 1. Area of skin innervated by one segment of spinal cord 2. Instrument to cut thin section of skin as in skin grafting.

Dermatomyositis A connective tissue disorder characterized by skin edema, dermatitis and inflammation/dysfunction of voluntary and involuntary muscles.

Dermatophobia Excessive fear about skin disease.

Dermatophyte A fungus that grows in skin or its appendage, e.g. epidermophyton, trichophyton and microsporum.

Dermatophytosis Fungus infection of skin of hand and feet.

Dermatosis Any disease of skin; inflammation may not be there.

Dermis The true skin below epidermis, containing nerve fibers and blood vessels.

Dermoid Resembling the skin.

Dermoid cyst A non malignant cystic tumor containing ectodermal elements like skin, hair and teeth.

Dermonosology The science of classification of skin disease.

Dermotropic Acting especially on the skin.

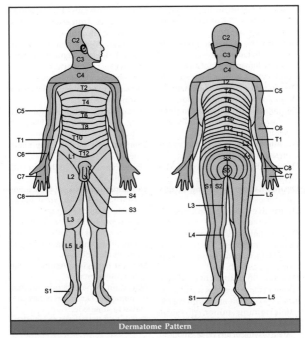

Dermatome Pattern

Dermodidymus A malformed foetus with two heads and neck but a single body and normal limbs.

Desalination Removal of salt, e.g. removal of salt from sea water to make the water drinkable.

Desaturation A process where by a saturated organic compound is converted into an unsaturated one.

Descemet's membrane Membrane between endothelial layer of cornea and substantia propria.

Desensitization Prevention of anaphylaxis usually by administering repeated small doses of the agent causing anaphylaxis/allergy.

Desert fever Coccidioidomycosis.

Desferrioxamine Iron chelating agent.

Desiccant Agent causing dryness.

Desipramine Antidepressant (tricyclic group).

Deslanoside Cardiac glycoside similar to lanatoside - C

Desmitis Inflammation of a ligament.

Desmocyte A supporting tissue cell.

Desmodynia Pain in a ligament.

Desmoid Resembling a tendon.

Desmoplasia An abnormal tendency to form fibrous tissue or adhesive bands.

Desmopressin Synthetic vasopressin analogue.

Desmorrhexis Rupture of the epidermis.

Desquamation Shedding of the, epidermis.

Destructive Causing ruin, opposite to constructive.

Detachment Becoming separate.

Detail In radiology, the sharpness with which an image is presented on a radiograph.

Detector An instrument for determining the presence of something.

d. lie A polygraph, an instrument for determining minor physical changes assumed to occur under stress of lying or any other emotion.

Detergent Cleansing agents, either anionic or cationic.

Deterioration Retrogression.

Determinant That which determines the character of any thing.

Determination Establishing the nature or precise identity of a substance, organism or event.

Detonation A violent noise caused by an explosive.

Detoxify To remove toxic quality of a substance. To treat toxic overdose of a drug/alcohol.

Detrition Wearing away of a part usually due to friction as that of teeth.

Detritus Degenerative matter produced by disintegration.

Detrusor External muscular coat of urinary bladder.

Detumescence Subsidence of swelling, esp. of erectile tissue like penis and clitoris.

Deuteranopia Green colour blindness.

Deuterium Heavy hydrogen with two atoms.

Developer In radiology, the solution used to make the latent image visible on the radiograph.

Developmental milestones Development of skills like crawling, fitting, laughing, walking in infants and children.

Deviant behavior Actions considered abnormal.

Deviation Departure from normal.

d. conjugate Deviation of face and eyes to same side.

d. standard In statistics, the measure of variability from the central tendency of any frequency curve. It is the square root of variance.

Device intrauterine contraceptive Devices placed in uterus to prevent contraception, e.g. copper T.

Devitalization Loss of vitality; esp. anesthetizing the pulp of a tooth.

Devolution Degradation, or destructive process.

Dexamethasone Synthetic glucocorticoid.

Dex chlorpheniramine Antihistaminic (polaramine).

Dexterity Motor skill.

Dextrality Right handedness.

Dextran A plasma volume expander, a polysaccharide fermented from sucrose.

Dextrase Enzyme splitting dextrose into lactic acid.

Dextrin $(C_6H_{10}O_5)_{11}$, a carbohydrate produced during digestion of starch.

Dextriferron Ferric hydroxide used in treating iron deficiency.

Dextroamphetamine An isomer of amphetamine, a CNS stimulant.

Dextrocardia Heart positioned in right side of thoracic cavity.

Dextrocardiogram Electrocardiogram representing right ventricular forces.

Dextroduction Movement of visual axis to right.

Dextromethorphan A cough suppressant.

Dextrophobia Abnormal aversion to objects on right side of body.

Dextropropoxy phene Analgesic with high addiction potency.

Dextroposition Displaced to right.

Dextrose $C_6H_{12}O_6$ (SYN-glucose), a simple monosaccharose sugar.

Dextrothyroxine A thyroxine like drug used to treat type II hyperlipoproteinemia.

Diabetes A general term for diseases causing excessive urination.

d. brittle Patient's glucose tolerance variable especially, in type I diabetes mellitus.

d. bronze (hemochromatosis) iron storage disease with hepatomegaly, darkening of skin, pancreatic endocrine deficiency often with cardiac dysfunction.

d. insipidus Polyuria and polydipsia due to inadequate antidiuretic hormone secretion by posterior pituitary.

d. mellitus A disorder of carbohydrate metabolism due to either insulin deficiency, insulin resistance or insulin antibodies characterized by hyperglycemia and glycosuria.

Diabetic tabes Diabetic neuropathy with neuritic leg pain and loss of knee jerk.

Diabenese Chlorpropamide, an oral sulphonyl urea.

Diacele Third ventricle of brain.

Diacetic acid Acetoacetic acid, a ketone found in urine in diabetic ketoacidosis.

Diacetyl morphine Heroin, strong addictive potential.

Diadochokinesia Ability to make antagonistic movements like pronation and supination in quick succession.

Diagnosis The term used to denote the name of disease or diseased process using scientific and skillful methods.

d. antenatal Diagnostic procedures to determine the health of the foetus, e.g. amniocentesis, biochemical profile (L.: S ratio, estriol assay), amnioscopy, non-stress test, ultrasound, chorionic villous biopsy.

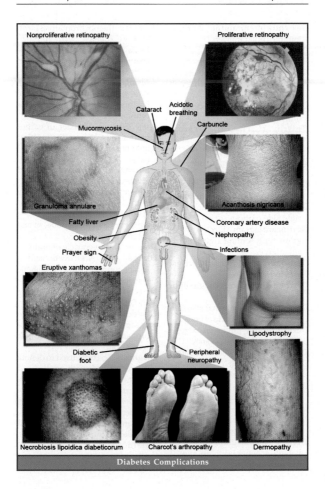

Diabetes Complications

d. differential Comparison of diseases having some what similar presentation.

Dialysate The dialysis fluid used to remove or deliver compounds or electrolytes that the failing kidney cannot excrete or retain in proper concentration.

Dialysis The process of diffusing blood across a semipermeable membrane to remove toxic materials.

d. continuous ambulatory peritoneal Patient is put on continuous peritoneal dialysis by an implanted peritoneal catheter and attached disposable dialysate bags; a substitute to chronic haemodialysis.

d. dementia Neurologic disturbances like speech difficulties, dementia, seizure, myoclonus, etc. after chronic dialysis, probably related to increased aluminium concentration in brain.

d. disequilibrium The symptoms of nausea, vomiting, drowsiness, headache and seizures that appear shortly after starting hemo/peritoneal dialysis. The cause is brain edema as urea in brain remains relatively higher in comparison to serum.

d. haemo The patient's blood and dialysate are passed in opposite directions across a semipermeable membrane (a coil, plate) in a dialysis machine. More effective than peritoneal dialysis.

d. peritoneal Dialysis in which the lining endothelium of peritoneal cavity is used as dialysis membrane. 2 liters of dialysis fluid are introduced into peritoneal sac in 20 minutes, is retained for 20 minutes and is then drained off in 20 minutes (one cycle), 8 cycles in a day.

Diameter Distance from one point to another diagonally opposite point on the perimeter of a sphere.

d. antero-posterior of pelvic inlet Distance between posterior surface of symphysis pubis to sacral promontory usually 11 cm in adult female.

d. antero-posterior of pelvic outlet Distance between tip of coccyx and lower edge of symphysis pubis.

d. biparietal Transverse diameter between parietal eminences of both sides (about 9.25 cm).

d. bitemporal Distance between two temporal bones (about 8 cm)

d. bitrochanteric Distance between highest point of two trochanters (useful for breech delivery).

d. bizygomatic Distance between most prominent points of zygomatic arches.

d. cervico bregmatic Distance between anterior frontal and junction of neck with floor of mouth.

d. diagonal conjugate Distance from the upper part of symphysis pubis to the most distant part of brim of pelvis.

d. external conjugate Antero posterior diameter of pelvic inlet measured externally, i.e. distance from the skin over the upper part of symphysis pubis to the skin over a

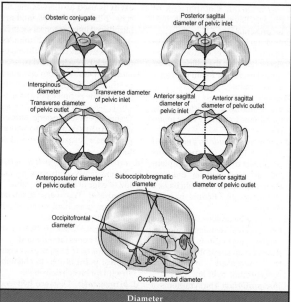

Obsteric conjugate

Posterior sagittal diameter of pelvic inlet

Interspinous diameter

Transverse diameter of pelvic inlet

Transverse diameter of pelvic outlet

Anterior sagittal diameter of pelvic inlet

Anterior sagittal diameter of pelvic outlet

Anteroposterior diameter of pelvic outlet

Suboccipitobregmatic diameter

Posterior sagittal diameter of pelvic outlet

Occipitofrontal diameter

Occipitomental diameter

Diameter

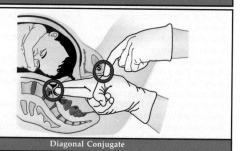

Diagonal Conjugate

point corresponding to the sacral promontory.

d. mento bregmatic Distance from chin to the middle of anterior fontanel.

d. occipito frontal Distance from posterior fontanel to the root of nose.

d. occipito mental Greatest distance between the most prominent portion of the occiput and point of chin (13.5 cm).

d. of fetal skull In full term fetus, the various diameters are: sub-occipitobregmatic: 9.5 cm, cervicobregmatic 9.5 cm, frontomental: 8.1 cm, occipitomental: 12.7 cm. Occipitofrontal: 11.4 cm, biparietal: 9.5 cm. bitemporal: 8.1 cm.

Diamox Acetazolamide, a carbonic anhydrase inhibitor.

Diapedesis Passage of blood cells esp. leukocytes by amoeboid movement through the intact wall of capillary.

Diaphane A very small electric light utilized in transillumination.

Diaphanometer A device for estimation of the amount of solids in a fluid by its transparency.

Diaphanography Transillumination of breast.

Diaphanoscope Device for transillumination of body cavities.

Diaphoresis Profuse sweating.

Diaphoretic Agents that increase sweating/perspiration.

Diaphragm The musculo membranous wall separating abdomen from thoracic cavity. It contracts with each inspiration permitting descent of base of lung. The attachment is to 6th rib anteriorly and 11-12th ribs posteriorly. Diaphragmatic contraction aids in defaecation, parturition and urination by increasing intra-abdominal pressure. It becomes spasmodic in hiccough and sneezing. Contribution of both diaphragms to respiratory inflow is 40% and nerve supply is by phrenic nerves.

d. pelvic Formed by levator ani and coccygeus muscles pierced in midline by vagina, urethra and rectum.

d. urogenital Urogenital trigone or triangular ligament that lies between ischiopubic rami. It lies superficial to the pelvic diaphragm and in the male surrounds the membranous urethra; in females it surrounds vagina.

d. contraceptive A rubber or plastic cup that fits on to the cervix to prevent entry of sperms into uterus.

d. of microscope The apparatus controlling illumination in the instrument

Diaphysis The middle part of long bone.

Diapophysis An upper articular surface of transverse process of vertebra.

Diarrhoea Frequent passage of unformed watery stool due to inflammation, irritation, retention, emotion, etc.

d. traveler's Diarrhoea in travellers due to *E. coli*

Diascope A glass plate held against the skin for examining superficial lesions. Erythematous lesions blanch but not haemorrhagic lesions.

Diastage The enzyme converting starch to sugar.

Diastasis The last part of diastole, of 0.2 second duration and is immediately followed by atrial contraction.

Diastematomyelia A congenital fissure of spinal cord, often associated with spina bifida cystica.

Diastole That period of cardiac cycle (usually of 0.5 sec) during which the heart dilates, ventricles fill with blood.

Diastolic pressure The period of least pressure in the arterial vascular system.

Diathermy The therapeutic use of a high frequency current to generate heat within some part of body.

d. short wave Employs wavelengths of 3-30 meters.

d. surgical Diathermy of high frequency for electrocoagulation or cauterization.

Diathrosis A hinge joint.

Diatom One group of unicellular microscopic algae seen in lungs of patients with antemortem drowning.

Diatrizoate meglumine Radioopaque dye for arterial use (gastrograffin).

Diatrizoate sodium Radiopaque dye for visualisation of bladder, urinary tract, reproductive system.

Diaxon A neurone having two axons.

Diazepam Antianxiety benzodiazepine useful in treatment of cocaine poisoning, status epilepticus, convulsion and a variety of anxiety disorders valium.

Diazo reaction A deep red colour in urine produced by action of ammonia and p-diazobenzene sulfuric acid on aromatic substances of urine.

Diazoxide Drug used IV to treat hypertensive crisis and hypoglycemia.

Dibasic Substance with two atoms of hydrogen in each molecule replaceable by a base.

Dibenzyline Trade name for phenoxybenzamine.

Dibucaine hydrochloride Local anaesthetic similar to cocaine.

Dicalcium phosphate Dibasic calcium phosphate, used for calcium supplement.

Dichloramine A germicide, disinfectant containing chlorine.

Dichlorphenamide Carbonic anhydrase inhibitor used for glaucoma.

Dichotomy Dividing into two parts.

Dichromation Ability to distinguish only two primary colours, i.e. red and green.

Dick test A skin test for susceptibility to scarlet fever similar to shick test for diphtheria.

Dicloxacillin sodium A semisynthetic penicillin for treatment of penicillinase resistant staphylococci.

Dicophane DDT.

Dicrotic Relates to a double pulse.

Dicrotic notch The notch on descending limb of pulse wave.

Dicrotic wave The positive wave following dicrotic notch.

Dictyoma A tumor of capillary epithelium.

Dicumarol An anticoagulant that increases prothrombin time.

Dicyclomine An anticholinergic agent.

Didactic Pertains to teaching by lectures or texts as opposed to clinical or bedside teaching.

Didelphic Pertains to double uterus.

Didymodynia Pain in the testicle.

Didymitis Inflammation of testicle.

Diechoscope A stethoscope for simultaneous auscultation from two different sites.

Dieldrin A chlorinated hydrocarbon used as insecticide.

Diencephalon The portion of brain encompassing epithalamus, thalamus, metathalamus and hypothalamus.

Dienestrol Synthetic estrogen.

Dientameba fragilis Parasitic ameba inhabiting small instestine and causing diarrhoea.

Diet Food substances normally consumed in the course of living.

d. balanced diet adequate in energy providing all tissue building materials, vitamins and proteins.

Diethazine hydrochloride Anticholinergic used in treatment of Parkinsonism.

Diethylcarbamazine Antifilarial agent.

Diethylpropion An adrenergic drug with actions similar to amphetamine.

Diethyl stilbestrol Synthetic estrogen.

Diethyl toluamide Insect repellent.

Diethyl tryptamine Hallucinogenic agent.

Dietitian A person experienced in field of nutrition and dietetic advice.

Dietl's crisis Renal colic from partial obstruction of ureter.

Dieulafoy's triad Tenderness, muscular rigidity and skin hyperesthesia at McBurney's point in acute appendicitis.

Differential blood count Determination of number of each variety of leukocytes in one micro litre of blood.

Diffraction The deflection that occurs when light rays are passed through crystals, prisms or other deflecting media.

Diffusion A process by which various gases intermingle as a result of incessant motion of their molecule, i.e. there is always a tendency of molecule or substances (gas, liquid, solid) to move from a region of high concentration to a low concentration.

Digestion The process by which food is broken down by enzymatic action into absorbable forms.

Digital radiography Radiography using computerized imaging instead of conventional film or screen imaging.

Digitalis Cardiotonic glycoside that increases myocardial contraction and refractory period of AV node.

Digital reflex Sudden flexion of terminal phalanx when nail is suddenly tapped.

Digitoxin Cardiotonic glycoside.

Dihydroergotamine Vasoconstrictor used in migraine.

Dihydrosphingosine An amino alcohol present in sphingo lipids.

Dihydrotachysterol A sterol obtained by irradiation of ergosterol and functions as Vit D.

Dihydroaluminium aminoacetate An antacid.

Dihydroxycholecalciferol Sterols with hormonal properties akin to vit. D, e.g. calcitrol.

Diiodohydroxyquin Iodoquinol.

Diktyoma Tumor of ciliary epithelium.

Dilantin A derivative of glyceryl urea, (diphenyl hydantoin sodium) used as antiepileptic, best for clonic/toxic clonic seizure.

Dilatation Expansion of a vessel or an orifice.

Dilation and curettage Cervical canal dilatation and scraping of uterine cavity.

Dilation and evacuation Cervical canal dilatation and evacuation of product of conception by suction/forcep.

Dilators Instruments used to dilate canals, cavities or openings.

Diltiazem Calcium channel blocker, useful for ischaemic heart disease.

Dimenhydrinate A drug for control of dizziness, vomiting and nausea.

Dimercaprol Used as an antidote for gold, arsenic, mercury, etc. injected IM mixed with benzyl benzoate and alcohol.

Dimethicone A silicone oil used to protect the skin against water soluble irritants.

Dimethindene maleate Antihistamine.

Dimethisterone Progesterone compound.

Dimethylphthalate An insect repellant.

Dimethyl sulfoxide A solvent used to facilitate absorption of medicines through the skin.

Dimethyl tryptamine An agent with properties similar to hallucinogens like LSD.

Dimple sign A sign used to differentiate dermatofibroma from malignant nodular melanoma. Upon application of lateral pressure, the dermatofibroma will dimple or become indented, but melanoma protrudes above plane of skin.

Dinoprost tromethamine A drug causing uterine contraction hence used to induce abortion.

Dioctyl calcium, sodium/potassium/sulfosuccinate A stool softner.

Diopter Refractory power of lens with focal length at 1 meter.

Dioxybenzone Chemical for protecting skin from sun.

Dipeptidase An enzyme that catalyzes the hydrolysis of dipeptides to amino acids.

Diphemanil methyl sulfate An anticholinergic agent used for treatment of peptic ulcer.

Diphenhydramine hydrochloride Antihistamine, (Benadryl).

Diphenoxylate Antidiarrheal agent smooth muscle relaxant (Lomotil).

Diphenyl hydantoin sodium Anti convulsant.

Diphenyl pyraline An antihistamine.

Diphonia Simultaneous production of two voice tones.

2-3 *diphosphoglycerate* An organic phosphate that effects affinity of haemoglobin for RBC and is depleted in stored blood.

Diphtheria Acute infectious disease, characterized by fever, sore throat, cervical lymphadenopathy and formation of gray pseudomembrane at the site of infection, i.e. tonsil, pharynx larynx nose, etc. Causative agent is club shaped bacillus, coryne bacterium diphtheriae.

Diphtheroid Resembling diphtheria or diphtheria bacillus.

Diphyllo bothrium Genus of tape worm, D-latum is fish tapeworm infesting humans, causing B_{12} deficiency.

Diplegia Paralysis of legs and hands of one side.

Diplomyelia Doubling of spinal cord due to a length wise fissure, often seen in patients of spina bifida.

Diploë Spongy tissue between the two layers of compact bone.

Diploid Having two sets of chromosomes.

Diplopia Double vision.

d. binocular Double vision occurring when both eyes are used due to diseases of cranial nerves, cerebrum.

d. monocular Double vision with one eye open (hysterics).

d. uncrossed SYN — homonymous diplopia; each image appears on the same side as the eye that sees the image.

d. crossed Images are on the side opposite to the eye that sees the image.

d. vertical Diplopia with one of the two images higher than other.

Dipole Two equal and opposite charges separated by a distance.

Dipsesis Extreme thirst or craving for abnormal fluids.

Dipsomania A morbid craving for alcohol.

Dipstic A chemical impregnated paper strip used for analysis of chemical constituents in urine.

Direct current An electric current flowing continuously in one direction only.

Direct light reflex Contraction of pupil on focussing a light beam on it.

Dirofilaria A genus of micro filaria.

Disaccharidase Carbohydrate composed of two monosaccharides, e.g. sucrose.

Discitis Inflammation of inter vertebral disk.

Disconnection syndrome Disturbances of visual and language functions due to section of corpus callosum or occlusion of anterior cerebral artery, manifesting as inability to match an object held in one hand with that in the other when eyes are closed.

Discordance In genetics, the expression of a trait in only one of the twin pair.

Discrete Separate, distinct.

Discrimination The process of distinguishing or differentiating.

d. tonal ability to distinguish one tone from the other, a function dependent upon integrity of transverse fibers of the basilar membrane in organ of corti.

d. two point ability to localize two points of pressure when applied to skin as separate sensations.

Disdiadochokinesia Inability to make quick alternating movements like pronation and supination common to cerebellar disease.

Disease Literally the lack of ease, or illness/suffering.

d. autoimmune A state of immune aberration where body produces antibodies against healthy host tissues as in some cases of glomerulonephritis, haemolytic anaemia, rheumatoid arthritis, myasthenia gravis, thyrotoxicosis, SLE, scleroderma, etc.

d. heavy chain Diseases in which heavy chain production of immunoglobulins is in excess. IgA chain excess manifests with abdominal lymphoma and malabsorption, IgM with repeated bacterial infections, lymphadenopathy and Ig D chain with picture similar to multiple myeloma.

d. hereditary Where disease is transmitted from parent to offspring.

d. motor neurone There is degeneration of anterior horn cells of spinal cord, cranial nerve nuclei in the brainstem, and pyramidal tracts, e.g. progressive muscular atrophy, amyotropic lateral sclerosis.

d. psychosomatic Psychological factors contribute to initiation or exacerbation of the disease, e.g. asthma, tension headache, neurodermatitis, peptic ulcer, etc.

Disengagement The emergence of foetal head from within the maternal pelvis.

Disinfectant A substance that prevents infection by killing pathogenic organisms.

Disinfection The process of making rooms/linens/organs germ free. The common methods of disinfection are by autoclaving, boiling in water, ethylene oxide/formal dehyde gas, alcohol, iodine, phenols, etc.

Disinfestation The process of killing infesting insects/parasites.

Disintegration The falling apart of constituents of a substance.

Dislocation Displacement of any part.

d. monteggia Dislocation of the hip in which the head of femur lies near anterosuperior spine of ileum.

d. Nelaton's Dislocation of ankle in which talus is forced up between the end of the tibia and fibula.

Dismutase superoxide An enzyme that destroys superoxide (O_2^-) formed by flavo enzymes. The enzyme protects aerobic bacteria from superoxide being present in them. Now being used for myocardial protection soon after infarction.

Disodium edetate A chelating agent used to treat hypercalcemia.

Disopyramide phosphate Antiarrhythmic agent of class II.

Disorientation Inability to be aware of time, place and person.

Dispensary Place for dispensation of drugs.

Disperate Suspension of finely divided particles in liquid.

Dispersion Dissipation or disappearance of colloid in a fluid.

Dispersonalization Mental state in which individual denies presence of some of his body parts or personality.

Displacement Removal from normal place. In psychiatry, transference of emotion from the original idea with which it was associated to a different idea.

Disposition Individuals aptitude, behavior as sum total of such evident characteristics.

Disproportion A part being different in size from that considered to be normal.

Dissect To split, to go into detail, to separate various parts of cadaver.

Dissection The cutting of parts for purpose of separation and study.

Disseminated Scattered or widely distributed.

Disseminated intravascular coagulation A coagulation disorder with bleeding tendency due to

consumption of clotting factors and platelets due to thrombin generation in bloodstream.

Dissipation Dispersion of matter.

Dissociation Separation of complex compounds into simpler ones.

Dissociation AV Atria and ventricles beat independently as sinus node impulse does not reach the ventricle.

d. of personality Split in consciousness resulting in two different phases of personality, neither being aware of words, acts or feelings of others.

Dissolution Breaking up the integrity of anatomical entity.

Dissolve Dispersion of a solid within a liquid.

Dissonance Disagreement.

Distal Farthest from the center, from a medial line.

Distance Space between two objects.

d. focal Distance from the optical center of lens to focal point.

Distend To stretch; to inflate.

Distensibility The property of being stretchable.

Distichiasis Maldirection of eye lashes, commonly directed inwards.

Distillation Condensation of vapor that has been obtained from a liquid heated to volatilization point.

Distillate Substance obtained by distillation.

Distome A fluke with two suckers.

Distomiasis Infestation with flukes.

Distortion Change from regular to irregular/altered shape.

Distractibility Inability to focus ones attention) or mental wandering.

Distraction State of mental confusion.

Distraught The mental state of being deeply troubled, having conflicting thoughts.

Distress Physical or mental agony.

Distribution The lay out pattern, or spreading/supply of nerve, blood vessels, etc.

Districhiasis Two hairs growing from the same hair follicle.

Disulfiram Drug used to create aversion from alcohol.

Diuresis Passage of large amounts of urine.

Diuretic An agent that increases formation of urine.

Diurnal Daily.

Divalent A molece with two electric charges.

Divergence Separation from a common center.

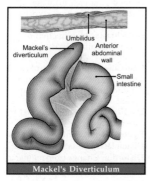

Mackel's Diverticulum

Diverticulum A pouch or sac in the wall of a hollow organ.

d. false Diverticulum without muscular coats in the wall of the pouch.

d. Meckle's Diverticulum due to persistence of omphalomesenteric duct.

d. of colon Most are asymptomatic and cause symptom when inflamed.

d. of jejunum and duodenum Diverticulum commonly located near entrance of common bileduct and pancreatic duct into duodenum. Jejunal diverticula are usually symptomatic and cause severe bleeding.

d. Zenker: See: Zanker's diverticulum.

Diving reflex Emersion in cold water or sprinkling of cold water on body causes parasympathetic stimulation with reduced cardiac output and increasing AV block. Hence used to treat paroxysmal supraventricular tachycardia.

Division Separation into parts.

Divulsion Forcibly pulling apart.

Dizygotic twins Twins who are roducts of two ova.

Dizziness A sensation of unsteadiness or whirling.

DNA finger printing DNA analysis to settle paternity, and in criminal investigations.

DNA probe A method of identifying defective genes and genetic constitution of a cell through employment of recombinant DNA technology.

Doctor To teach, A person qualified to practice medicine.

d. bare foot A practitioner of traditional or native medicine in China who have not attended any medical school.

Dobutamine A beta-adrenergic agonist, used in hypotension.

Doctrine The system of principles taught or advocated.

Docusate sodium A stool softner.

Dohle bodies Inclusions in neutrophils as seen in burn, trauma, infection and neoplastic diseases.

Dolicocephalic Having a skull with long antero posterior diameter.

Dolicomorphic A long and slender body (ectomorph).

Dolophine hydrochloride Methadone.

Dolorimeter Device for measurement of degree of pain.

Domiciliary Carried on in a house.

Dominance 1. Genetic quality through which one gene of pair of allele expresses, while the other is suppressed. 2. Preferred hand or side of body. 3. In psychiatry the tendency to control others.

Domperidone Antiemetic increases gastric motility, useful in dyspepsia.

Donath-Landsteiner phenomenon A test for paroxysmal cold haemoglobinuria where cold haemolysin combines to RBCs at 5°C and upon warming these red cells haemolyze.

Donan's equilibrium A equilibrium is established between two solutions separated by a semipermeable membrane so that the sum of anions and cations on one side is equal to that on other side.

Donor One who donates blood, tissue or an organ for use in another person.

d. universal One with blood group 'O' which is compatible with blood of all other persons, though this is not universally true as there are many other blood antigens besides A, B, and O.

Donovan body Organism of granuloma inguinale, i.e. chlamydia trachomatis.

Dopa 3:4 dihydroxy phenylalanine, produced by oxidation of tyrosine by tyrosinase.

Dopamine hydrochloride A vasopressor catecholamine and neurotransmitter, also implicated in some forms of psychosis and abnormal movement disorder. Doping In sports medicine, use of drugs to improve sports performance; commonly androgenic anabolic steroids.

Doppler A method to measure blood flow in arteries and veins.

Doraphobia Aversion to touching the hair or fur of animals.

Dorllo's canal A bony canal in the tip of temporal bone enclosing abducens nerve.

Dorsal Pertains to back, opposite of ventral.

Dorsal nerves Branches of spinal nerves that pass dorsally to innervate structures near to vertebral column.

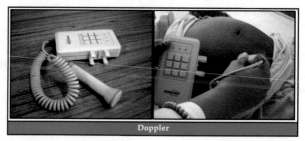

Doppler

Dorsal slit A surgical method of making the foreskin of penis easily retractable. The foreskin is cut in dorsal midline but not far enough to extend to mucous membrane next to glans.

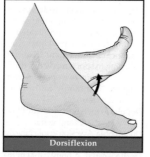

Dorsiflexion

Dorsiflexion Bending a part towards posterior aspect of body.

Dosage Pertains to quantity, frequency and number of doses of a drug/radiation.

Dose calculation for children Young's formula

$$= \frac{\text{Age in years}}{\text{Age} + 12} \times \text{Adultdose}$$
or
Body surface, area of child/1.7 × adult dose.

Dose Amount of medicine/radiation to be given at one time.

d. absorbed Dose of ionizing radiation imparted to a tissue or target.

d. cumulative Total dose of radiation resulting from repeated exposures.

d. maximum permissible The maximum amount of radiation exposure permitted to person whose occupation requires working with radioactive agents.

d. therapeutic Dose required to produce therapeutic effect.

Dose response curve A graph showing the degree of effect of a drug in relation to its doses.

Dosimeter Device for measuring radiation.

Double blind technique A method of scientific investigation in which neither the subject nor the investigator knows what treatment the subject is receiving. The code is only broken at the end of completion of treatment.

Double contrast examination Radiographic examination in which both a radiopaque and a radioluscent contrast medium are used simultaneously to visualize internal anatomy.

Double personality Dual personality seen in hysteria and schizophrenia.

Douche A current of vapour or stream of hot/cold water directed against a part.

d. vaginal Douche of vagina is used for deodorant, antiseptic, stimulating or haemostatic purposes. Douching in healthy women is not warranted as it may alter vaginal pH and flora predisposing to vaginitis.

Douglas pouch Peritoneal space lying between uterus and front of rectum.

Douglas fold The arcuate line of the sheath of rectus muscle.

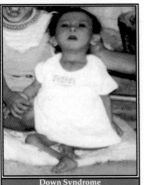
Down Syndrome

Down syndrome Congenital anomaly due to trisomy 21 manifesting with mental retardation, skeletal anomalies and light yellow spots at periphery of iris.

Doxapram Respiratory stimulant.

Doxepin Tricyclic - antidepressant.

Doxorubicin Anthracycline antitumor antibiotic.

Doxycycline Broad spectrum tetracycline used in b.i.d dose.

Doxylamine A sedative.

Dracontiasis *SYN*–Dracunculiasis, i.e. infestation with d. medinesis.

Drain To draw off a fluid, exit or tube for discharge of body fluid.

Drainage The free flow of fluid from a wound/cavity.

d. closed Drainage without access of air into drained site via the tube.

d. negative pressure Drainage where negative pressure is maintained within the tube, e.g. pneumothorax drainage.

d. open Drainage without exclusion of air.

d. postural Drainage of sinuses and bronchi by gravity.

Dramamine Diphenhydramine, an agent for vertigo.

Dramatism Dramatic behavior and lofty speech as in lunatics.

Drastic Acting strongly.

Draught A liquid medicinal dose to be gulped at once; drink.

Drawer sign Sign of cruciate ligament rupture of knee.

Draw sheet The rubber cloth spread on the bed to protect the mattress and linen from drainage and soilage.

Drepanocyte Resembling sickle cell.

Dressing Protective or supportive covering for injured part.

d. occlusive Dressing that seals the wound completely thus preventing infection and also preventing moisture from the wound escaping through the dressing.

d. pressure Dressing that applies pressure on the wound, e.g. following skin grafting.

Drift Movement due to an external force, in an aim less fashion.

Drill (*SYN*-burr) Device for rotating sharp cutting instrument, e.g. cavity preparation in dentistry.

Drip Infusion of a liquid drop by drop.

d. post nasal Post nasal discharge as in chronic sinusitis.

Dromostanolone An antineoplastic agent.

Dromotropic Fibers in cardiac nerves influencing conduction.

Dronabinol Synthetic tetrahydro canabinol, a psychoactive substance.

Droperidol A neuroleptic, sedative and tranquilizer.

Droplet infection Infected particles coming as spray from patient's mouth and nose.

Dropsy Generalized edema.

Drowning Asphyxiation due to immersion in liquid.

Drowsiness The state of almost falling asleep.

Drug abuse Self administered drug overuse.

Drug addiction A condition caused by excessive or continued use of habit forming drugs.

Drug dependence A psychic and often physical dependence upon a drug.

Drug fever Fever caused by drugs.

Drug interaction Interaction between drugs taken concurrently.

Drug rash Rash produced in some individuals by intake or application of drugs.

Drug reaction Adverse and undesired reactions to a substance.

Drug receptors The protein molecules on cell surface that bind to a particular drug and then activate a series of reactions through which the drug produces the desired pharmacological effect.

Drunkenness Alcoholic intoxication with blood ethyl alcohol level exceeding 0.3-0.4%.

Drusen Small hyaline, globular pathological growths formed on Descemet's membrane.

Duazomycin Glutamine antagonist, anticancer drug.

Dubin-Jonson syndrome Inherited defect of bile metabolism with conjugated hyperbilirubinemia.

Ducrey's bacillus Small rod shaped organism found in pairs, causative agent of soft sore.

Duct A narrow tubular vessel or channel to convey secretions from gland.

d. alveolar A branch of respiratory bronchiole that leads to alveolar sacs of lungs.

d. commonbile Duct formed by joining of hepatic duct with cystic duct and draining to duodenum at ampulla of vater.

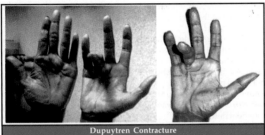

Dupuytren Contracture

d. endolymphaticus Duct connecting endolymphatic sac with the utricle and saccule.

d. Gartner A remnant of wolfian duct extending from parovarium through the broad ligament into vagina.

d. lacrimal Two ducts, superior and inferior draining tear from eye into lacrimal sac.

d. mesonephric Duct in embryo connecting mesonephros with the cloaca. In the male, it develops into reproductive ducts.

d. mullerian Ducts in the embryo that form the uterus, vagina and fallopian tubes.

d. right lymphatic Duct draining lymph from right side of body above diaphragm into right innominate vein.

d's of skene's Two slender ducts of skene's glands that open on either side of female urethral orifice.

d. thoracic The left lymphatic duct that drains the lymph from body below diaphragm and the left thorax into left innominate vein.

Ductus arteriosus The channel communicating ascending aorta to left pulmonary artery in the fetus.

Ductus venosus The duct through which the umbilical vein drains into inferior vena cava in fetus.

Duffy system A blood grouping system.

Dumping syndrome Dumping of stomach contents into the intestine manifesting with weakness and sweating soon after food in patient's of gastrojejunostomy.

Duodenal bulb First part of duodenum beyond pylorus.

Dupuytren Contracture Contracture of palmar fascia causing flexion deformity of ring and fifth fingers.

Dura mater The outer membrane covering the brain and spinal cord.

Duritis *SYN* – pachymeningitis, inflammation of dura.

Duroziez murmur Systolic and diastolic murmur heard over an artery when pressure is applied just distal to stethoscope.

Dust Minute fine particles of earth.

d. ear Fine calcareous bodies found in gelatinous substance of otolith membrane of ear.

d. house Matters included in house dust are mites, hairs, pollen, and smoke particles.

Dwarf An abnormally shorter undersized person.

d. achondroplastic Normal trunk, small extremities, large head and prominent buttocks.

Dyclonine hydrochlorides A topical anaesthetic.

Dye Any coloured or colouring agent, employed for staining slides for histopathological examination or manufacturing test reagents.

Dynamic Pertains to vital force or inherent power; opposite of static.

Dynamograph Device for recording muscular strength.

Dyne Force needed for imparting acceleration of 1 cm per second to a 1 gm mass.

Dynorphins An endogenous opioid peptide.

Dysacusis Difficulty in hearing, dycomfort caused by loud noise.

Dysarthria Difficulty in articulation or speech.

Dysautonomia A hereditary disease involving autonomic nervous system characterized by motor inco-ordination, fluctuating blood pressure, mental retardation, etc.

Dysbasia Difficulty in walking.

Dyscalculia Inability to solve mathematical problems.

Dysdiadochokinesia Inability to perform quick alternating movements.

Dysentery Inflammation of mucosal lining of GI tract with passage of blood, pus and mucus in stool.

Dysesthesia Abnormal sensation on the skin with tingling, numbness, burning, etc.

Dysgammaglobulinemia Disproportion in the concentration of gammaglobulins in blood.

Dysgenesis Defective development.

Dysgerminoma Malignant neoplasm of ovary.

Dysgeusia Impairment or perversion of gustatory sense so that normal taste is interpreted as being unpleasant.

Dysgraphia Difficulty in writting.

Dyshidrosis Disorder of sweating; recurrent vesicular erruption on the limbs with intense itching (pompholyx)

Dyskeratosis Altered keratinization of epithelial cells of epidermis, characteristic of many skin disorders.

Dyskinesia Defect in voluntary movement.

d. tardive Slow rhythmical, involuntary stereotyped movements especially with use of psychotropic drugs.

Dyslexia Inability to interpret written language even though vision is normal.

Dysmaturity *SYN* – small-for-date infants, intrauterine growth retardation; infant's weight is less for his length or age.

Dysmenorrhoea Painful menstruation.

d. congestive Caused by pelvic congestion.

d. membranous Passage of uterine casts causing pain.

d. spasmodic Spasmodic uterine contractions causing pain.

Dysmetria Rapid jerky movement as patient is unable to control range and strength of muscular contraction, as seen in cerebellar disease.

Dysostosis Defect in ossification.

Dysoxia Inability of mitochondria to utilize oxygen properly.

Dyspareunia Painful sexual intercourse.

Dyspepsia Imperfect digestion with abdominal bloating, heart burn, flatulence, anorexia nausea, etc. can be gastric, hepatic, biliary, alcoholic in origin.

Dysphagia Difficulty in deglutition, can be due to spasm of pharyngo esophageal musculature, stricture, neoplasm, paralysis.

Dysphasia Impairment of speech both articulation and comprehension.

Dysphonia Difficulty in speaking but s comprehension is normal; hoarseness.

Dysphoria Excessive depression feeling without apparent cause.

Dysplasia Abnormal tissue growth/differentiation.

d. ectodermal Absence of sweat glands, hair follicles and abnormality of nail, teeth, and mental development

d. monostotic Replacement of bone by fibrous tissue.

d. polystotic fibrous Replacement of bone by vascular fibrous tissue with bone deformity and fracture.

Dyspnea Labored or difficulty in breathing either due to vigorous physical activity, anemia, cardiac or pulmonary disease.

Dyspraxia A disturbance in the programming, control and execution of volitional movements.

Dyssynergia Difficulty in proper muscular co-ordination.

Dysthymia A form of minor depression with low mood more than half the time for 2 years in

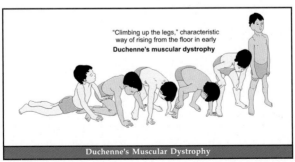

"Climbing up the legs," characteristic way of rising from the floor in early **Duchenne's muscular dystrophy**

Duchenne's Muscular Dystrophy

adult or 1 year in children and adolescents.

Dystocia Difficult labor, can be due to abnormal passage (small out let), passenger (large foetus) or power (uterine inco-ordination)

Dystonia Increased muscle tone.

d. musculum deformans Progressive disorder of childhood with distorted twisting body movements.

Dystopia Displacement of any organ.

Dystrophy Defective muscle power, nutrition and metabolism.

d. Landouzy-Dejerine Childhood progressive muscular dystrophy involving muscles of shoulder girdle, face characterized by myopathic facies, inability to raise arms above head, inability to whistle.

d progressive muscular Familial disease with atrophy of muscles, occurring at early childhood.

d pseudohypertrophic muscular Affected muscles are bulky but weak at the beginning but ultimately become atrophic.

Dysuria Painful micturition either due to concentrated acid urine, urinary crystals/concretions, urinary infections, pelvic pathology and prolapse uterus.

E

Eale's disease Retinal vein thrombophlebitis with recurrent hemorrhages into retina and vitreous.

Ear dust Calcareous concretions in the membranous labyrinth.

Ear plug Device for plugging the external auditory canal, there by preventing access of sound to internal ear.

Ear wax Sticky honey coloured cerumen secreted by glands at outer one-third of ear canal mixed with dust.

Eaton agent Mycoplasma pneumoniae.

Ebanation Removal of bone fragments from wound

Ebola fever A RNA virus form monkeys causing haemorrhagic fever in human with high mortality

Ebstein anomaly Downward displacement of septal leaflet of tricuspid valve with gross tricuspid regurgitation.

Ecchondroma Cartilaginous tumor.

Eccrine sweat glands Sweat glands of skin with density of over 400 per sq. cm. on the palms and about 80 per sq. cm. on thigh.

Eccyclomastopathy Lesion of breast made up of connective tissue and epithelial cells.

Echeosis Mental disturbance caused by noise.

Echinococcosis Infestation with T, echinococcus.

Echinococcus A genus of tape worm. Consisting of scolex and three or four proglottids.

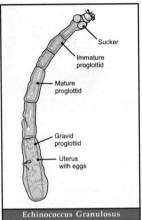

Echinococcus Granulosus

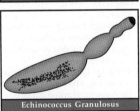

Echinococcus Granulosus

e. granulosus A species of tape worms infesting carnivores causing hydatid cyst in liver or lungs.

Echinocyte Abnormal erythrocyte with multiple spiny projections from surface.

Echinostoma A genus of fluke found in aquatic birds.

Echo A reverberating sound produced when sound waves are reflected back to their source.

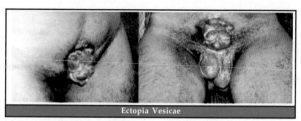
Ectopia Vesicae

Echocardiography The technique of imaging the cardiac structures non-invasively through passage of ultrasound.

Echoencephalogram Recording of midline shift of brain structures by ultrasound waves.

Echokinesia Involuntary repetition of another's gestures.

Echopraxia Imitation of actions of others.

ECHO virus Enterocytopathogenic human orphan virus causing viral meningitis, enteritis, pleurodynia, myocarditis, etc.

Eclampsia Coma and convulsion occurring after 28th week of pregnancy and in immediate post-partum.

Eclecticism An old system of medicine where treatment is dependent upon individual signs and symptoms rather than the disease as a whole.

Econazole A topical antifungal agent.

Economo's disease Encephalitis lethargica.

Ecstasy An exhilarated trance like state; a designer drug- MDMA (3-4 methylene dioxymethamphetamine.

Ectasia Dilatation of any tubular structure.

Ecthyma A shallow skin lesion with crusting, often followed by pigmentation and scarring.

Ectocervix The portion of cervical canal outlined by squamous epithelium.

Ectoderm The outer layer of cells in developing embryo giving rise to skin, teeth, nervous system, organs of special sense, pituitary, pineal and suprarenal glands.

Ectomorph Linear slender body build with poor musculature.

Ectoparasite Parasite living on outer surface of body, e.g. lice, fleas, ticks.

Ectopia Malposition or displacement.

e. cordis Malposition of heart with the organ lying outside the thorax.

e. lentis Displacement of lens in the eye.

e. vesicae Displacement of bladder, e.g. extrophy.

Ectopic In an abnormal position, e.g. ectopic heart beat.

Ectopic pregnancy Implantation of fertilized ovum outside the uterine cavity; can be abdominal, tubal, or ovarian with liability for rupture and hemorrhage.

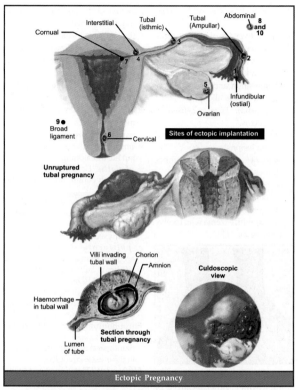

Sites of ectopic implantation

Unruptured tubal pregnancy

Villi invading tubal wall — Chorion — Amnion

Haemorrhage in tubal wall

Culdoscopic view

Lumen of tube

Section through tubal pregnancy

Ectopic Pregnancy

Ectopic rhythm Any abnormal or irregular cardiac rhythm.

Ectoplasm The outer most layer of cell protoplasm.

Ectostosis Formation of bone beneath periosteum.

Ectothrix Fungus growing on hair shafts.

Ectotrichophyton Fungi causing hair and skin infection.

Ectozoon Parasite living on another animal.

Ectromelia Hypoplasia of long bones of limbs.

Ectropion Eversion of eyelid margin.

Eczema Acute or chronic cutaneous lesion with erythema, papule, vesicles, and crusts leading to itching, lichenification and pigmentation; mostly atopic or allergic.

e. marginatum Eczema caused by ringworms.

e. nummular Coin or oval shaped eczema lesions!

e. pustular Follicular or impetiginous form of eczema.

e. seborrheic Eczema with seborrhea.

e. vaccinatum Generalized vaccinial lesion or local lesions elsewhere in persons with eczema who receive vaccination.

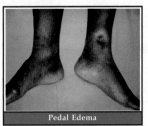

Pedal Edema

Edema Excessive tissue accumulation water, either localized or generalized, can be due to poor venous drainage, lymphatic obstruction, increased venous pressure (CHF), hypoalbuminemia, or increased water retention.

e. angioneurotic Local edema due to hypersensitivity to drugs food, physical agents (cold) or idiopathic.

e. brain Brain swelling due to water accumulation as following injury, toxemia or infection.

e. cardiac Dependent edema of congestive heart failure.

e. high altitude Pulmonary edema of mountaineers related to low partial pressure of oxygen.

e. larynx Usually of allergic origin but life threatening.

e. of glottis Usually follows infection with cough, hoarseness and dyspnea.

e. nonpitting Myxomatous tissue accumulation appearing as edema without any dimple on pressure, e.g. myxedema.

e. pulmonary Increased fluid accumulation in lungs following left heart failure, toxic gas inhalation, or ARDS.

Edge A margin or border.

Edrophonium chloride A cholinergic drug (anticholinesterage).

Edrophonium test A test for myasthenia gravis. A positive test demonstrates brief improvement in the muscle strength.

Effacement Dilatation of cervix and stretching of birth passage.

Effect Result of an action or force.

e. cumulative Drug effect on repeated administration of a drug.

Effector One of the nerve endings having the efferent process and in a gland or muscle cell. Also applied for effector organs (muscle and glands).

Effeminate A male having physical characteristic or mannerism of a female.

Efferent Carrying away from a central organ.

Efferent nerve Nerves that carry impulses away from the nerve cell, (motor nerve).

Effervescence Formation of bubbles of gas rising to surface of fluids.

Effluent Fluid discharged from sewage treatment or industrial plant.

Effusion Escape of fluid/air into a cavity, e.g. hydropneumothorax, chylothorax, pleural effusion.

Eflornithine An antineoplastic and antiprotozoal agent

Ego 1. In psychoanalysis, the three divisions are id, ego and superego. The ego possesses consciousness and memory and serves to mediate between the primitive instinctual or animal drives (the id), internal social prohibitions (super ego) and reality. 2. Selfishness or self love.

Egoism An inflated estimate of one's value or effectiveness.

Egophony A nasal sound like bleating of a goat, present on lung tissue above effusion.

Ehlers-Danlos syndrome An inherited disorder of elastic connective tissue characterized by fragile hyperelastic skin, hyper mobile joints.

Eiconasoids Metabolites of arachidonic acid metabolism like prostaglandins, thromboxane and leukotrienes.

Eisenmenger's complex In a case of congenital heart disease with left to right shunt (ASD, VSD, PDA, etc.) when the pulmonary vascular resistance equals or exceeds systemic resistance it is called Eisenmenger complex.

Ejaculation Ejection of seminal fluid from male urethra.

e. retrograde Lax internal sphincter due to autonomic dysfunction in diabetics or following prostatectomy, the ejaculation occurs retrogradely to bladder.

Ejaculatory duct The terminal portion of seminal duct formed by the union of the ductus deferens and excretory duct of the seminal vesicle.

Ejection fraction The percentage of blood ejected from LV into aorta with each cardiac contraction.

Elastase Proteolytic pancreatic enzyme.

Elastic Stretchable.

Elastic bandage Bandage that can be stretched to exert continuous pressure.

Elastic cartilage Yellow cartilage of epiglottis, pharynx, external ear, auditory tubes.

Elastic stocking Stocking applied to aid in return of blood from the extremity to heart (e.g. in varicosity).

Elastic tissue Connective tissue supplied with elastic fibers as in tunica media of vessels.

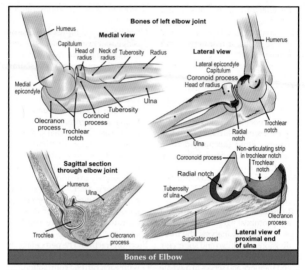

Bones of Elbow

Elastin The protein of elastic tissue.

Elastometry The measurement of elasticity of tissues.

Elbow Joint between arm and forearm, consisting of humeroulnar, humeroradial and proximal radioulnar articulations.

e. tennis Tendinitis of lateral forearm muscles near their origin from lateral epicondyle of humerus (lateral epicondylitis).

Elective therapy A planned convenient therapy/operation.

Electra complex In psychoanalysis, a group of symptoms due to suppressed sexual love of daughter for father.

Electricity A form of kinetic energy having magnetic, chemical, mechanical and thermal effects; formed from interaction of positive and negative charges.

Electric shock Tissue injury from passage of electricity.

Electroanalgesia Pain relief by use of low intensity electric currents.

Electrocardiogram Record of electric activity of heart.

Electrocardiograph The machine used to record electrocardiogram.

Electrocautery Cauterization by an arc heated by electric current.

Electrocoagulation Coagulation of tissue by means of a high-frequency current.

Electroconvulsive therapy The used of shock to produce convulsion,

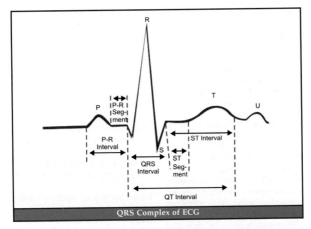

QRS Complex of ECG

indicated for acute psychosis and depression with suicidal tendency.

Electrocution Death by electric current.

Electrode A medium intervening between an electric conductor and the object to which the current is to be applied.

Electrodesiccation Drying of cells or tissues by means of high frequency electric spark used for achieving hemostasis following bleeding from small capillaries and veins during surgery.

Electrodialysis A method of separating electrolytes from colloids by passing current through the solution.

Electrodynamometer Instrument used to measure strength of current.

Electroejaculation Production of ejaculation by electrical stimulation from a probe placed in rectum, e.g. in paraplegics for artificial insemination.

Electroencephalogram (EEG) Recording of electrical activity of brain through surface electrodes.

Electroencephalograph The machine recording EEG.

Electrogoniometer Electrical device for measuring angles of joints and their range of motion.

Electrology The branch of science dealing with properties of electricity.

Electrolysis Dissolution of tissue by electric current, e.g. destruction of hair follicle.

Electrolyte 1. A solution which conducts electricity. 2. Ionised salts in blood, tissue fluids and cells.

Electrometer An instrument for measuring differences in electric potential.

Electromotive force (EMF) The difference in potential that causes the flow of electricity. It is measured in volts.

Electromyography Preparation, study and interpretation of electromyograms.

Electromyogram A graphic record of the contraction of muscle on electric stimulation,

Electron The negatively charged particle of an atom.

Electronics The science of all systems involving use of electric devices, e.g. communication, data control and processing.

Electro-oculogram Recording of electric currents produced by eye movements.

Electronystagmography A method of recording nystagmus from electrical activity of extraocular muscles.

Electrophoresis The movement of charged colloidal particles as a result of changes in electric potential.

Electrophysiology Branch of physiology dealing with relationships of body functions to electrical phenomena.

Electroretinogram (ERG) A record of action currents of retina produced by visual or light stimuli.

Element A substance that cannot be further broken down to substances different from it, e.g. carbon, sodium, calcium, etc.

Elephantiasis Hypertrophy of skin and subcutaneous tissue due to lymphatic stasis, e.g. in filariasis that involves scrotum, penis, legs, breasts and hands.

Elevator Surgical instruments used to raise depressed fractures (e.g. skull), extracting teeth.

Eliminate To expel, to get rid of body waste product.

Elimination diet A diet regime used to determine which foods cause allergic response. Offending food then is discovered when one by one food is gradually introduced into diet.

Elixir Sweetened hydro-alcoholic liquid.

Ellipsoid Spindle shaped.

Elliptocyte Oval shaped red blood cell. Normally 15% of human RBC are oval and bird and reptiles have normally all RBC in eliptocytic form.

Elliptocytosis Benign hereditary disease, causing haemolytic anaemia.

Ellis-van Creveld syndrome Congenital syndrome consisting of polydactyly, chondrodysplasia and congenital heart defect (ASD).

Emaciation To become excessively lean.

Emasculation Castration; excision of entire male genitalia.

Embalming Use of antiseptics and preservatives to prevent premature biodegradation of dead body.

Embarrass To interfere with or compromise function.

Embden-Meyerhof pathway Anaerobic metabolism of glucose to lactic acid in humans.

Embolectomy Removal of embolus from a vessel, e.g. in stroke, pulmonary embolism.

Embolism Obstruction to blood flow by mass of red blood cells and fibrin mesh. Atrial fibrillation and pelvic-leg vein thrombosis predispose to embolism.

Embolotherapy Use of embolic materials for therapeutic obliteration of vessels e.g. aneurysms, bleeding vessel, or malformation.

Embolus A mass of undissolved matter in blood vessel, may be clot, fat, air bubble, clumps of bacteria, amniotic fluid.

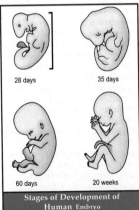

28 days 35 days

60 days 20 weeks

Stages of Development of Human Embryo

Embryo 2nd through 8 weeks of fetal development.

Embryoscopy Visualization of embryo by inserting an endoscope trans abdominally or through vagina into chorionic space for correction of congenital defects, and collection of amniotic fluid for analysis.

Embryogeny The growth and development of an embryo.

Embryology The science that deals with origin and development of an organism.

Emergency cardiac care (ECC) Care necessary to deal with an acute cardiopulmonary event like infarction, arrhythmia, pulmonary embolism.

Emesis Vomiting, due to gastric, CNS, systemic or metabolic factors.

Emetic Agent producing vomiting, e.g. apomorphine.

Emetine Ipecac derivative, used for extraintestinal amebiasis.

Emigration Passage of WBC through walls of capillaries.

Eminence Prominence or projection esp. on a bone.

Emissary An outlet.

Emission Discharge.

e. nocturnal Involuntary discharge of semen during sleep.

Emmetropia When the eyes are at rest parallel rays are focussed exactly on retina, i.e. normal refraction.

Emmetropic Normal vision.

Emolient An agent that smoothens and softens the skin when applied.

Emotion A mental state or feeling such as fear, hate, grief, joy with some change in cardiorespiratory function.

Empathy Objective awareness of and insight into the feelings, emotions and behavior of another person and their meaning and significance.

Emphysema 1. Pathological distension of tissues by air/gas. 2. Chronic pulmonary disease with dilatation of airspaces beyond terminal bronchioles.

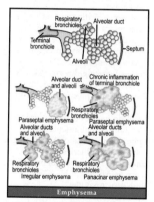

Emphysema

Empirical Based on experience rather than scientific principle.

Emprosthotonus A form of spasm in which body is flexed forward opposite to opisthotonus.

Empyesis Any pustular skin lesion.

Empyocele Suppurating hydrocele.

Emulsification Breaking down of large fat globules into smaller ones by bile acid that lower surface tension.

Emulsion A mixture of two liquids not mutually soluble.

Enalapril Converting enzyme inhibitor, used in heart failure, hypertension.

Enamel Hard dense glistening white substance forming a covering on crown of teeth.

Enamel organ A cup shaped structure that forms on the dental lamina of an embryo.

Enathem Eruption on mucous membrane.

Enantiopathy Treatment of one disease by using another disease that produces symptoms antagonistic to former.

Encapsulation The process of formation of a capsule around a structure.

Encephalalgia Deep seated headache.

Encephalitis Inflammation of brain parenchyma, manifesting with changes in level of consciousness, increased intracranial pressure, sensory motor dysfunction.

Encephalocele Protrusion of brain substance through a cranial defect.

Encephalogram (air) X-ray of brain with air injected into ventricular system.

Encephalomeningocele Softening of brain.

Encephalomeningocele Protrusion of membrane and brain parenchyma through cranial defect.

Encephalomyelitis Inflammation of brain and spinal cord.

e. acute disseminated that following acute exanthema but fewer symptoms.

Encephalopathy Any dysfunction of brain.

Enchondroma A benign cartilaginous tumor occurring within a bone and expanding the diaphysis.

Encopresis Condition associated with constipation and passage of watery colonic content across the hard fecal mass, mimicking diarrhoea.

Endarterectomy Surgical removal of lining endothelium of an artery.

Endarteritis Inflammation of intima of an artery resulting from syphilis, trauma, infective thrombi.

Endemic A disease occurring repeatedly in a particular population confering some immunity and hence low mortality.

Endocarditis Inflammation of endothelial lining of heart chambers and heart valves; may be due to invasion of microorganisms or abnormal immunologic response.

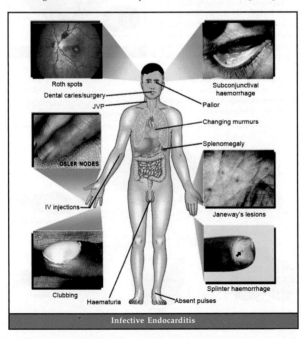

Roth spots
Dental caries/surgery
JVP
OSLER NODES
IV injections
Clubbing
Haematuria
Subconjunctival haemorrhage
Pallor
Changing murmurs
Splenomegaly
Janeway's lesions
Splinter haemorrhage
Absent pulses

Infective Endocarditis

e. verrucous Nonbacterial endocarditis associated with wasting diseases, e.g. SLE, *SYN* — Libman–Sack.

e. subacute bacterial Caused by streptococcus viridans group.

e. ulcerative Rapidly destructive acute bacterial endocarditis.

Endocervicitis Inflammation of mucus lining of endocervix.

Endocrine glands Glands secreting directly into bloodstream.

Endocytosis A method of ingestion of a foreign substance by a cell.

Endodontics A branch of dentistry concerned with diagnosis, treatment and prevention of diseases of dental pulp and its surrounding tissue.

Endogenous Produced or arising from within a cell or organism.

Endolymax nana A nonpathogenic parasite in human gut.

Endolymph Pale transparent fluid within the labyrinth of ear.

Endometer Electronic device used to determine the length of tooth root canal.

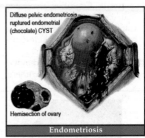

Diffuse pelvic endometriosis ruptured endometrial (chocolate) CYST

Hemisection of ovary

Endometriosis

Endometriosis Proliferation of endometrium at ecopic sites, i.e. sites other than ulterine cavity.

Endometritis Inflammation of endometrium.

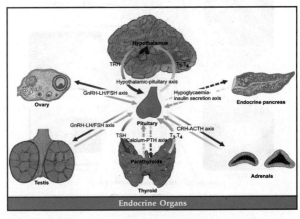

Endocrine Organs

e. dissecans Endometritis accompanied by development of ulcers and shedding of mucous membrane.

Endomorph Body build characterized by predominance of tissues derived from endoderm.

Endomysium A thin layer of connective that tissue surrounds each striated muscle fiber.

Endoneurium A delicate connective tissue sheath that surrounds nerve fibers.

Endonuclease Enzyme that clears ends of poly nucleotides.

Endopelvic fascia The downward continuation of the parietal peritoneum of abdomen that supports pelvic viscera.

Endopeptidase Proteolytic enzyme that cleaves peptides.

Endophthalmitis Inflammation within substance of eye.

Endorgan The expanded end of a nerve fiber in a peripheral tissue.

Endorphins Polypeptides produced in the brain tissue that bind to opioid receptors and block them, there by producing analgesia. The most important is beta endorphin.

Endosalpingitis Inflammation of lining of fallopian tubes.

Endoscope A device containing optical system for observing or conducting surgery in hollow structures like abdomen, pelvis.

Endosome The vacuole formed when material is absorbed in the cell by process of endocytosis. The vacuole fuses with lysosome.

Endosteitis Inflammation of the endosteum of medullary cavity.

Endothelioma Malignant tumor of endothelial cells lining any cavity, blood vessel lumen.

Endotheliosis Increased growth of endothelial cells.

Endothrix Fungus growth within hair.

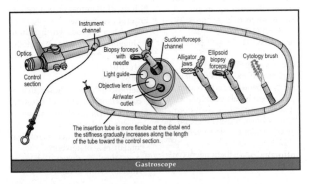

Gastroscope

Endotoxemia Toxemia due to presence of endotoxin in blood.

Endotoxin Bacterial toxin released after death of bacteria.

Endotracheal tube Tube that provides an airway through trachea while preventing aspiration by its inflated cuff.

Endplate The terminal end of nerve fibre to a muscle.

End product The final product of a chemical/metabolic process.

Enema Stimulation of bowel activity by introduction of soothning, cleansing and chemical agents into rectum. Drugs can be given as enema, e.g. steroids in ulcerative colitis, paraldehyde.

e. double contrast Enema of barium and air for colonography.

e. retention e.g. saline or steroids for purpose of nutrition/medication.

Energy The capacity of a system in doing work.

Energy expenditure basal (BEE) Harris Benedict equation.

For women 6.55 + (9.6 × W) + (1.8×H)-(4.7×A)

For men 66 + (13.7 × w) + (5 × H)-(6.8 × A).

Where A = Age in years H = Height in cm and W = Weight in kg. Energy expenditure is increased by 13% over basal needs for each C° rise in temperature than normal. Stress, burn, trauma increase the need of calories to the extent of 40-100%.

Enflurane Anaesthetic agent (volatile)

Engagement In obstetric descent of presenting part into true pelvic cavity, i.e. the part is immobile.

Engorgement Vascular congestion.

Enkephalins Polypeptides produced in brain that bind to opioid receptors to produce analgesia.

Enolase An enzyme present in muscle tissue that converts phosphoglyceric acid to phosphopyruvic acid.

Enophthalmos Recession of eyeball into orbit.

Enriched Addition of something extra.

Entameba A genus of parasitic ameba found in human digestive tract, e.g. E. coli, E gingivalis, E histolytica E. undulans.

Enteral tube feeding Feeding patient with a tube passed into stomach.

Enteric coated Tablet or capsule coated with special coating that only dissolves in intestine.

Enteritis Inflammation of intestine.

Enterobacteriaceae Gm -ve non-spore bearing rods which include Shigella, Salmonella, Klebsiella, Yersinia, Proteus, Escherichia.

Enterobiasis Infestation with pinworms.

Enterococcus Any species of streptococcus inhabiting human intestine.

Enterocolitis Inflammation of intestine and colon.

e. necrotizing Unknown necrotizing fatal disease of newborn.

Enterocolostomy Surgical joining of small intestine to colon.

Enterocystoplasty Use of a portion of small intestine to enlarge the bladder.

Enteroenterostomy Establishing communication between two intestinal segments that are not continuous.

Enterogastrone A hormone secreted by intestinal mucosa that decreases gastric emptying. Fat stimulates its secretion.

Enterolith Concretions in intestine.

Enteromyiasis Disease caused by maggots (larva of flies) in the intestine.

Enteron The elementary canal.

Enteropathogen Microorganism that causes intestinal infection.

Enteropeptidase Enzyme of duodenal mucosa that helps conversion of trypsinogen to trypsin.

Enteropexy Fixation of intestine to abdominal wall.

Enterovirus A class of picornavirus, that includes polio, coxsackie and ECHO viruses.

Enterozoon Any intestinal parasite.

Enthesis The use of metallic or other inert substances to substitute or replace lost tissue.

Enthesitis Inflammation at site of tendon insertion to bone

Enthiasis A depressed fracture of skull

Entoderm Innermost primary germ layer giving rise to epithelium of digestive tract, and associated glands, the respiratory tract, bladder, vagina and urethra.

Entome A knife for division of urethral stricture.

Entomology Study of insects and their relationship to disease.

Entoptic phenomena Visual phenomena like seeing floating bodies, circles of light, black spots, transient flashes of light.

Entropion Inward turning of an edge, e.g. margin of eyelid.

e. cicatricial Inversion resulting from scar tissue (e.g. trachoma)

e. spastic Inversion resulting from spasm of orbicularis oculi.

Enucleate To remove eyeball, to remove a part of mass or entire mass.

Enuresis Involuntary passage of urine in bed after the age of 5 years, often a familial tendency.

Envenomation Introduction of poisonous venum into body by bite or sting.

Enzootic Endemic disease confined to animals.

Enzyme Complex proteins catabolizing reactions but without being changed themselves; can be synthesizing, coagulating, branching, debranching, digestive, fermenting, glycolytic, lipolytic, mucolytic.

e. mucolytic Enzyme that depolymerizes mucus by splitting mucoproteins, e.g. mucinase, hyaluronidase.

e. respiratory Enzymes acting within cells catalyze oxidative reactions with release of energy (ATP), e.g. cytochromes, flavoproteins.

Enzyme induction Increase in enzyme level due to its increased production or decrease degradation. Drugs commonly causing hepatic enzyme induction are barbiturates.

Enzyme linked immunosorbent assay (ELISA) A test to detect antigen or antibody, hormones.

Eosin Synthetic rose colored dye used for staining tissues/body fluids for microscopic examination.

Eosinophil Granular leukocyte staining with acid stain eosin.

Eosinophilia Increased blood eosinophil count beyond 6-8% or 300/cmm.

Ependyma Membrane lining the cerebral ventricles and central canal of spinal cord.

Ependymitis Inflammation of ependyma.

Ependymoma A tumor of ependymal elements.

Ephebiatrics Adolescent medicine.

Ephebology Study of puberty and its changes.

Ephedrine Sympathomimetic agent used locally as decongestant and systemically for bronchodilation and raising blood pressure.

Epiandrosterone Androgenic hormone normally present in urine.

Epiblast *SYN* — ectoderm; outer layer of cells of blastoderm.

Epiblepharon A fold of skin passing across either lids so that eye lashes are pressed against eye.

Epicanthus A vertical fold of skin extending from root of nose to the median end of eye brow covering inner canthus and caruncle.

Epichordal Dorsal to notochord.

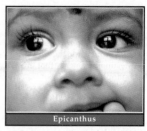
Epicanthus

Epichorion The portion of decidua of placenta that covers the ovum.

Epicondyle Bone element above the condyle, i.e. articular surface of bone.

Epidemic Appearance of a disease in a high proportion not expected for a community in a geographical area.

Epidemiology Science concerned with study and analysis of inter-relationship of factors that determine disease frequency.

Epidermis Outer layer of skin, avascular, consists of 4 layers from inwards to outwards, i.e. stratum germinatum, stratum granulosum, stratum luciderm and stratum corneum.

Epidermization Conversion of deeper germinative layers of cells into outer layers of epidermis.

Epicyte An epithelial cell.

Epidermoid A tumor arising from aberrant epidermal cells.

Epididymis A small long convoluted organ lying behind testes and containing the ducts of testes. It ends in spermatic duct.

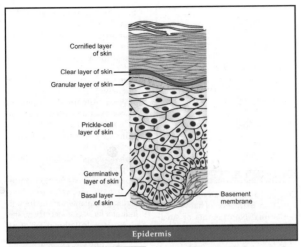

Epidermis

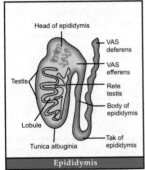

Epididymis

Epididymitis Inflammation of epididymis, usually as a complication of gonorrhoea, syphilis, tuberculosis, mumps, filariasis, etc.

Epididymography Radiographic examination of epididymis after introduction of contrast.

Epididymo orchitis Inflammation of epididymis and testes.

Epidural Outside dura.

Epigastric reflex Contraction of upper portion of rectus abdominis when skin of epigastric region is scratched.

Epigastrium Region over pit of the stomach.

Epiglottis Leaf shaped flat membrane covering entrance of larynx during swallowing.

Epiglottitis Inflammation of epiglottis, usually bacterial, often threatens airway obstruction if treatment is delayed.

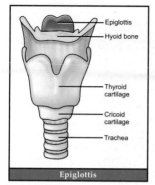

Epiglottis

Epilate To extract hair by the roots.

Epilation Extraction of hair.

Epilemma Neurilemma of small branches of nerve filament.

Epilepsy Recurrent, paroxysmal electrical dysfunction of brain characterized by altered consciousness and motor/sensory phenomena.

Epileptic Concerning epilepsy.

Epileptiform Mimicking epilepsy.

Epiloia A syndrome of mental retardation, convulsion, hypertrophic sclerosis of brain, adenoma sebaceum, tumors of kidneys.

Epimorphosis Regeneration of a part of organism by growth from cut surface.

Epimysium Outermost sheath of connective tissue surrounding a skeletal muscle.

Epinephrine Hormone of adrenal medulla, synthesized from phenylalanine having ionotropic, bronchodilator and sympathomimetic effects.

Epinephritis Inflammation of adrenal gland.

Epinephroma Lipomatoid tumor of kidney.

Epineurium Connective tissue sheath of a nerve.

Epiphora Abnormal overflow of tears either due to excess secretion or blockage of lacrimal duct.

Epiphylaxis Increase in defensive power of body.

Epiphysiolysis Separation of an epiphysis.

Epiphysis An ossification center separated from parent bone by a cartilage in infants and children; an indicator for assessment of bone age.

Epiphysitis Inflammation of an epiphysis especially that of knee, hip shoulder in infants.

Epiplocele Hernia containing omentum.

Epiploic Pertains to omentum.

Epipygus A developmental anomaly where accessory limb is attached to the buttocks.

Epirubicin Antitumor antibiotic.

Episcleral Overlying sclera of eye.

Episiotomy Incision of perineum to facilitate delivery and avoid laceration.

Epispadius Congenital opening of urethra on dorsal aspect of penis, or clitoris.

Episplenitis Inflammation of splenic capsule.

Epistasis Suppression of any discharge.

Epistaxis Bleeding from Kiesselbach's area of nose.

Epitendon The connective tissue holding a tendon within its sheath.

Epithelial cells Cells irregular in shape, having a single nucleus.

Epithelial tissue Those tissues covering outer surface of body and lining the internal passages or cavities. The cells lie in close proximity of each other with little intercellular substance.

Epithelioid Resembling epithelium.

Epithelioma Malignant tumor arising from epithelium, e.g. skin or mucous membrane.

e. adamantinum Tumor of jaw arising from enamel organ usually of low grade malignancy, may be cystic.

Epoprostinol PGI_2.

Epsom salt = $MgSO_4$ a, cathartic.

Epsilon-aminocaproic acid Synthetic substance, antifibrinolytic, used to check bleeding.

Epstein Barr virus A member of herpes virus family causing mononucleosis, nosopharyngeal cancer.

Epstein's pearls Whitish yellow accumulation of epithelial cells or retention cyst on hard palate in newborn.

Epulis A fibrous sarcomatous tumor of lower jaw.

Equivalent to weight The weight of an element that is equivalent to and will replace in chemical reaction a hydrogen atom.

Eradication Complete elimination of disease.

Erben's reflex Slowing of pulse when head and trunk are forcibly bent forward.

Erb's paralysis Paralysis of muscles supplied by C_5 and C_6.

Erectile tissue Spongy vascular tissue which when filled with blood becomes erect and rigid, e.g. penis, clitoris, nipple.

Erection Swelling, hardness and stiffness of penis on sexual arousal/physical handling.

Erector spinae reflex Irrigation of skin of back causes hardening due to contraction of erectorspinae.

Erethism Excessive excitation or irritation.

Erg In physics, the amount of work done when a force of 1 dyne acts through a distance 1 cm.

Ergasthenia Weakness due to overwork.

Ergocalciferol Vit D_2.

Ergocristine An ergot alkaloid.

Ergograph An apparatus for recording contractions of muscles and measuring the amount of work done.

Ergometer An apparatus for measuring amount of work performed.

Ergonomics The science concerned with how to fit a job to man's anatomical, physiological and psychological characteristics in a way that will enhance human efficiency and well-being.

Ergonovine maleate An ergot derivative used in treatment of migraine. It also stimulates contraction of uterus.

Ergosterol The sterol of plant and animal tissue that can be converted to vitamin D_2 on irradiation.

Ergotamine tartarate Ergot alkaloid used to treat migraine or to enhance uterine contraction.

Ergotism Ergot poisoning.

Erode To wear away.

Erosion Destruction of surface layer.

e. dental Enamel loss.

e. cervix Alteration of the epithelium, squamous cells replacing columnar cells following low grade infection.

Erotism Sexual desire.

e. auto Self gratification of sexual instincts by manual stimulation of erogenous areas like penis, clitoris.

Erotology The study of love and its manifestations.

Erotomania Pathological exaggeration of sexual behavior.

Erotophobia Aversion to sexual love or its manifestations.

Erratic Floctuating, unpredictable.

Error Mistake, miscalculation.

Eructation Belching, bringing out gas from stomach.

Eruption Appearance of a lesion such as redness or spotting on the skin or mucous membrane.

e. creeping A skin lesion characterized by a tortuous, elevated red line that progresses at the other usually caused by migration of larva of Ankylostomas.

e. drug Drug ingestion causing skin eruption.

Erysipelas Spreading inflammation of skin and subcutaneous tissue accompanied by systemic disturbance.

Erysipeloid An infective dermatitis resembling erysipelas.

Erythema Diffuse macular redness of skin.

e. induratum Chronic vasculitis of skin occurring in young adult females; often breaking down with formation of atrophic scar.

e. multiforme A macular erruption with dark red papules or tubercles that appear as rings, disc shaped patches, figured arrangements.

e. marginatum A form of erythema multiforme with central fading area but elevated edges.

e. nodosum Red and painful nodules on legs, often caused by drugs, toxins.

Erythrasma Red brown eruption in patches in axillae and groin caused by *Corynebacterium* minutissimum.

Erythredema An infantile disease characterized by itchy lesions of hands and feet, and polyarthritis.

Erythrityl tetranitrate Anti anginal agent.

Erythroblast Nucleated red blood cell, may be pronormoblast, basophilic normoblast, polychromatic normoblast, orthochromatic normoblast.

Erythroblastosis fetalis Hemolytic disease of newborn usually due to Rh incompatibity or ABO mismatching.

Erythrocyanosis Red or bluish discolouration of skin with swelling, burning and itching.

Erythrocyte The non nucleated biconcave disc of 7.7 micron matured red blood cell containing hemoglobin, involved in oxygen transport

e. crenated RBC with serrated or crenated edge.

Erythrocythemia Increased red cell mass.

Erythrocytopenia Decrease in number of red cells.

Erythrocytorrhexis Breaking down of RBC, with some amount escaping to plasma.

Erythrocytosis Increase in red cell mass.

Erythroderma Abnormal redness of skin.

Erythrodontia Reddish brown staining of teeth.

Erythroid Concerning red blood cells.

Erythroleukemia A variant of acute myeloid leukemia with anaemia, bizarre red cell morphology, erythroid hyperplasia in bone marrow.

Erythromania Uncontrolled blushing.

Erythromelia Painless erythema of extensor surface of arm.

Erythromelalgia Burning and throbbing in feet that come and go.

Erythromycin Antibiotic from *Streptomyces erythreus* effective for many gm + ve and few gram -ve organisms.

Erythropoitin An alfaglobulin secreted by kidney that stimulates erythropoisis.

Erythropsin Pigment in external portion of rods of retina.

Erythrosine Sodium A dye (2%) used as dental disclosing agent.

Esculent Suitable for use as food.

Esophagoenterostomy Making communication between esophagus and intestine following resection of stomach as in gastric malignancy.

Esophagomyotomy Incision of muscular coat of esophagus as in achalasia cardia.

Esophagoplication Reduction of dilatation of esophagus by taking tucks in its walls.

Esophagotomy Surgical incision into the esophagus as in achalasia cardia.

Esophoria Amount of inward turning of eye, *SYN*-esotropia.

ESR Electron spin resonance, a newer medical technique for imaging, e.g. NMR studies.

ESP Extrasensory perception.

Essence Alcoholic solution of volatile oil.

Essential Indispensable.

ESRD End stage renal disease with GFR below 10 ml/minute.

EST Electroshock therapy.

Ester Compound formed by organic acid with alcohol.

Ester Enzyme catalyzing hydrolysis of esters.

Esthesia Perception, feeling, sensation.

Esthesiometer Device for measuring tactile sensibility.

Estradiol $C_{18}H_{24}O_2$. Steroid hormone of ovary with estrogenic properties.

Estriol $C_{18}H_{24}O_3$ Metabolic product of estrone and estradiol.

Estrone

Estriol

Estradiol

Estrogen

Estrogen Substance having estro-genic activity, i.e. development of female sex characteristics, cyclic changes in endometrium and vaginal epithelium, breast changes.

Estrone $C_{18}H_{22}O_2$. Natural estro-genic hormone less active than estradiol but more active than estriol.

Estrus The cyclic period of sexual activity in mammals; during estrus animal is said to be 'in heat'.

Etching Application of corrosives material to a glass/metal to create a pattern or design.

Ethambutol Antitubercular bacteriostatic agent.

Ethanol Ethyl alcohol.

Ethaverine hydrochloride Mild coronary artery dilator.

Ethchlorvynol Hypnotic agent.

Ether diethyl $C_4H_{10}O$ inflammable anaesthetic agent.

Ethics Moral principles or standards governing conduct.

Ethinamate Mild sedative-hypnotic agent.

Ethinyl estradiol An estrogenic hormone.

Ethionamide Bacteriostatic second line antitubercular drug.

Ethionine Progestational agent used in contraceptive.

Ethomoid bone Sieve like spongy bone forming roof of nasal fossa and partly floor of anterior cranial fossa containing ethmoidal air cells.

Ethmoiditis Inflammation of ethmoidal air cells causing pain in between eyes, headache and nasal discharge.

Ethnic Groups of people with one cultural system.

Ethnology Comparative study of cultures using ethnographic data.

Ethopropazine Anticholinergic used in parkinsonism.

Ethosuximide Anticonvulsant, principally used for absence seizure.

Ethotoin Sparingly used anti-convulsant.

Ethyl chloride C_2H_5Cl. Volatile liquid used for topical anaesthesia.

Ethyl cellulose Ether of cellulose, used for drug preparation.

Ethylene glycol Antifreeze, poisnous.

Ethylene oxide C_2H_4O a fumigant. Also used for sterilizing articles that cannot withstand heat.

Ethylenediamine Solvent for theophyline.

Ethylenediaminetetraacetic acid (EDTA) A chelating agent.

Ethyl morphine Used as cough suppressant.

Ethylnorepinephrine Adrenergic drug used in asthma.

Etidronate Drug used in Paget's disease.

Etofamide An intraluminal amoebicide.

Etoposide Podophylotoxin for malignant diseases.

Etretinate Retinoid used for acne.

Eucalyptus oil Oil distilled from eucalyptus leaves, used as an expectorant.

Eucapnia Normal CO_2 concentration in blood.

Eudiometer Instrument for testing purity of air and making analysis of gases.

Eugenics The science dealing with genetic and prenatal influences that affect the expression of certain characteristic in offsprings.

Eugenol A topical analgesic used in dentistry. Used with zinc oxide to make temporary filling.

Eunuch Castrated male; male without secondary sexual characteristics.

Eunuchoidism Deficient male sexual characteristics.

Euphoria Exaggerated feeling of well-being.

Euploidy In genetics, a state of having complete sets of chromosomes.

Eustachian tube 4 cm long mucus lined tube extending from middle ear to pharynx.

Eustachian valve Valve at the entrance of inferior vena cava.

Euthanasia Mercy killing; dying easily, quietly and painlessly; ending ones life with an incurable disease.

Euthenics The science of improvement of population through modification of environment.

Euthyroid Normal thyroid function.

Evacuate To discharge especially. bladder and bowel; to transfer patient from one site to another.

Evaluation Assessment.

Evanescent Not permanent, brief duration.

Evans blue A dye used IV as diagnostic agent.

Evaporation Change from liquid to gaseous state.

Evenomation Removal of venom from biting site.

Eventration Removal of contents of abdominal cavity, partial protrusion of abdominal contents through an opening in the abdominal wall.

Eversion Turning outwards.

Evisceration Removal of viscera.

Evoked response Study of function of sense organs even though patient is unconscious by giving sensory stimuli and recording the electric

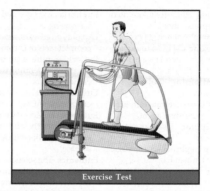
Exercise Test

response along the propagation pathway to brain.

Ewing's tumor Diffuse endothelioma causing a fusiform swelling of long bone.

Exacerbation Aggravation of symptoms.

Exanthem Eruption of skin rash.

Exchange transfusion Transfusion and withdrawal of small amounts of blood until blood volume is entirely replaced; used in auto-immune haemolytic anaemia, hyperbilirubinemia.

Excipient The vehicle for the drug.

Excise Removal by surgery.

Excitability Property of muscle or nerve fiber to contract or produce action potential on stimulation respectively.

Excitation wave The wave of irritability originating in sino-atrial node and moving across atria and conduction system to ventricular muscles.

Excoriation Abrasion of epidermis by chemicals, burns, irritation.

Exenteration Evisceration.

Exercise Performed activity of muscles.

e. isometric Active contraction of muscle without shortening of muscle length.

e. isotonic Active muscle contraction where muscle length is decreased.

e. static Alternate contraction and relaxation of muscle without movement of joint.

Exercise electrocardiogram *SYN* – stress test.

Exercise tolerance test A test to determine the efficiency of cardio-respiratory system, e.g. treadmill testing.

Exflagellation The formation of microgametes (flagellated bodies) from microgametocytes. Occurs in plasmodia in the stomach of mosquito.

Exfoliation The shedding of cells.

Exhalation The process of breathing out.

Exhaustion Fatigue

e. heat A state of salt and water deficit on constant exposure to high temperature.

Exhibitionism Tendency to attract attention to oneself by any means.

Exhumation Removal of a dead body from grave.

Exner's nerve Nerve from pharyngeal plexus to cricothyroid membrane.

Exocrine Secretion of a gland to exterior lumen.

Exodontology Branch of dentistry dealing with dental extraction.

Exoerythrocytic Occurring outside RBC.

Exomphalos Umbilical hernia.

Exophoria Tendency of visual axes to diverge outwards.

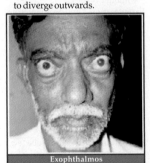
Exophthalmos

Exophthalmos Abnormal excessive protrusion of eyeballs due to thyrotoxicosis, retro orbital tumors, aneurysm, secondary to leukemic deposit.

Exoplasm Outer protoplasm of a cell.

Exostosis Outgrowth from bone surface.

Exotic Not native.

Exotoxin Toxins produced by microorganism to surrounding medium.

Exotropia Divergent squint.

Expectoration The act of expulsing sputum.

Expiration Breathing out of inhaled air. It may be active or passive.

Explode To burst.

Exponent The mathematical method of indicating the power.

Exposure The amount of radiation delivered/received.

Exsanguination Excessive blood loss to the point of death.

Extrophy Congenital turning inside out of an organ.

Extension Movement by which both ends of a part are pulled apart.

Extinction The process of extinguishing or putting out.

Extirpation Excision of a part.

Extorsion Rotation of a part outward.

Extracorporeal Outside the body.

Extracapsular Outside the joint capsule.

Extracorporeal membrane oxygenator (ECMO) A device for oxygenation of blood used for patients of acute respiratory failure.

Extracorporeal shock wave lithotripsy: (ECSWL) shock wave dissolution of renal and gallstones.

Extract To pull out forcibly, e.g. teeth; Active principle of a drug obtained by distillation or chemical process. It can be alcoholic, aqueous.

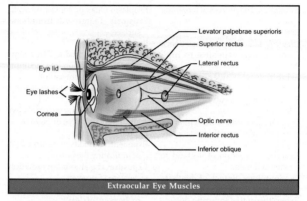

Labels: Levator palpebrae superioris, Superior rectus, Lateral rectus, Eye lid, Eye lashes, Cornea, Optic nerve, Interior rectus, Inferior oblique

Extraocular Eye Muscles

Extradural Outside dura mater.

Extramural Outside the wall of an organ or vessel.

Extraocular eye muscles Muscles attached to the capsule of eye controlling its movements.

Extrapyramidal Outside the pyramidal tracts of CNS.

Extrapyramidal syndrome Syndrome arising out of disease or degeneration of basal ganglia and their connections manifesting with tremor, rigidity, in coordination.

Extrasensory perception Perception of external events by other than the five senses.

Extrasystole Premature contraction of heart muscle by a stimulus originating in the conduction system or musculature. It can be atrial, junctional, nodal or ventricular.

e. atrial Normal QRS complex with altered P. waves.

e. ventricular Wide bizarre QRS without P waves.

Extravasation Fluid escaping from vessel.

Extremity The terminal part of any thing, an arm or leg.

Extroversion Eversion, turning inside out.

Extrovert Opposite of introvert. One who is interested mainly in external objects and actions.

Extrusion In dentistry, position of a tooth when pushed forward from line of occlusion.

Extubation Removal of tube, e.g. laryngeal.

Exuberant Excessive growth of tissue, joyful, happy.

Exudate A protein rich fluid, high in cell count can be pus, catarrhal, haemorrhagic, fibrinous.

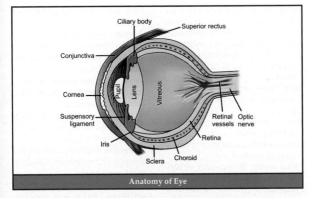

Anatomy of Eye

Exude To pass out slowly through the tissues.

Eye Organ of vision consisting of outer layer (cornea and sclera), middle layer (choroid, ciliary body and iris) and inner retina.

e. aphakic Eye without lens.

e. black Ecchymosis of tissue surrounding eye.

e. dominant Eye which one preferentially uses as in seing through mono-ocular microscope, while using a gun.

Eye bank An organization that collects corneas and stores them for transplantation.

Eyelids Movable protective folds closing the anterior surface of eye ball; the upper is the larger and more movable, raised by contraction of levator palpebrae superioris.

Eye muscle imbalance Incoordinate action of extraocular muscles causing esophoria or exophoria.

Eye strain Tiredness of eye due to errors of refraction, overuse, debility, anaemia.

F

Fabrication Deliberately false statement told as if it were true, present in Korsakoff's syndrome.

Fabry's disease An inherited disorder of metabolism with accumulations of glycolipid in tissues.

Face Anterior part of head from forehead to chin, composed of 14 bones.

Facet A small smooth area on a bone or hard surface.

Facetectomy Excision of articular facet of vertebra.

Facial center Brain center responsible for facial movements.

Facial nerve Seventh cranial nerve supplying facial muscles, platysma, submandibular and sublingual glands, and carrying taste sensations from anterior two thirds of tongue.

Facial reflex Contraction of facial muscles following pressure on eye ball.

Facial spasm Involuntary contraction of muscles supplied by facial nerve.

Facies The expression or appearance of face.

f. adenoid Dull lethargic appearance with open mouth due to chronic mouth breathing.

f. aortica Seen in aortic insufficiency; with bluish sclera, sunken cheeks and sallow face.

f. hepatica Shunken eyes, yellow conjunctiva.

f. hippocratic Face of long continued illness with hollow cheeks, sunken eyes, lead complexion and relaxed lips.

f. leonine Lion like face of lepromatous leprosy with thick inelastic skin, depressed bridge of nose and leprosy nodules.

f. masklike Expressionless face with little or no animation/blinking as seen in parkinsonism.

f. mitralis Face of mitral insufficiency with dilated capillaries, pink and often cyanotic cheeks.

f. myopathic Fades due to muscular atrophy and relaxation, lids drop and lips protrude.

Facilitation Hastening of an action.

Factitious False, not natural, artificial.

Factitious disorder Disease not genuine, produced voluntarily for gain, etc. Munchausen syndrome.

Factor An essential element

f eosinophilic chemotatic a substance released from mast cells;

f. epidermal growth: a macrophage produced cytokine that stimulates growth of smooth muscle cells and fibroblasts;

f. hepatocyte growth formed by platelets, fibroblasts, macrophages, endothelial and smooth muscle cells stimulating growth of hepatocytes;

f. intringic secreted by parietal cells of gastric mucosa essential for vit B_{12} absorption.

Facultative In biology and bacteriology, having the ability to live under certain conditions. Thus a bacteria can be facultative with respect to O_2 and be able to live with or without O_2.

Faculty A normal mental attribute or sense; teaching staff.

Faget's sign a pulse slower than corresponding body temperature

f. brown fat around major blood vessels in newborn, burnt for thermogenesis as shivering mechanism is lacking

Fahrenheit A temperature scale with freezing point of water at 32° and boiling point at 212° point.

Failure Loss of function of an organ.

f. heart Poor pump function secondary to myocardial anoxia, necrosis, abnormal pre/after load or electrical disturbance.

f. renal Loss of kidney function with uremia due to infection, diabetes, hypertension, glomerulonephritis, etc.

f. respiratory Inability of lungs to oxygenate the blood and expel carbon dioxide, occurring due to disease of diaphragms/intercostal muscles or lung parenchyma, (ARDS,COPD).

f. hepatic Liver failure with cholemia due to cirrhosis, acute hepatic necrosis, etc.

Faint syncope About to lose consciousness.

Faith healing Healing through divine power, without medical aid.

Falciform Sickle shaped.

Falciform ligament Triangular ligament attached to sides of sacrum and coccyx by its base.

Falciform ligament of liver Sickle shaped reflection of peritoneum attaching liver to diaphragm and separating right lobe from left lobe.

Falciform process That portion of falciform ligament along the inner margin of ramus of ischium.

Fallopian tube The 4½" long tube joining peritoneal cavity near the ovary to lateral side of fundus of uterus. It serves to convey ovum from ovary to uterus. It has three parts: the infundibulum, isthmus and ampulla.

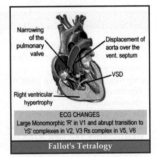

Fallot's Tetralogy

Fallot tetralogy Congenital cyanotic heart disease characterized by overriding of aorta, infundibular stenosis, right ventricular hypertrophy and a ventricular septal defect.

Fall out Settling of radioactive fission products from atmosphere after nuclear explosion.

False positive A test indicating that the disease is present when in fact it is not

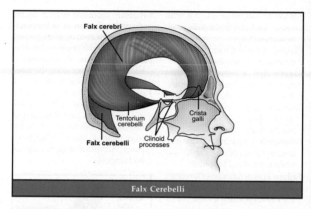

Falx Cerebelli

False negative A test indicating that the disease is not present when actually it is present.

False ribs The lower five pairs of ribs that do not unite directly with the sternum.

Falx Any sickle shaped structure.

f. cerebelli A vertical fold of dura partitioning the two halfs of cerebellum.

f. cerebri A fold of dura mater lying in longitudinal fissure, separating the two cerebral hemispheres.

f. inguinalis The conjoint tendon that forms the origin of transverse abdominis and internal oblique muscles.

Familial Disease occurring more frequently in a family than would be expected by chance.

Familial Mediterranean fever Inherited autosomal recessive disorder in persons of Irish or Italian descent manifesting with periodic fever, chest/abdominal pain and a propensity for amyloidosis.

Familial periodic paralysis Paralysis occurring at awakening with hypokalemia or even normokalemia.

Family 1. A group of individuals descending from a common ancestor. 2. A group of people living in a household who share common attachments, such as mutual caring, emotional bonds, common goal, etc. 3. In biology the division between an order and genus.

Family planning Planning and spacing of child birth according to wishes of the couple rather than to chance.

Famotidine H2 receptor blocker, used for peptic ulcer disease.

Fanconi's syndrome Rickets with aminoaciduria, hypoplastic anaemia, growth failure.

Fang A sharp pointed tooth.

Fantasy The mechanism of creating in one's mind.

Farad A unit of electrical capacity. The capacity of a condenser that charged with 1 coulomb, gives a difference of potential of 1 volt.

Faradism Therapeutic use of an interrupted current to stimulate muscles and nerves.

Farmer's lung Hypersensitive alveolitis on exposure to moldy hay.

Farsightedness An error of refraction in which parallel rays are focussed at a point behind retina, so that near objects are not seen clearly.

Fascia Fibrous membrane covering, supporting or separating muscles, uniting skin with underlying tissue.

f. Buck's Facial covering of penis derived from Colle's fascia.

f. Cloquet's Femoral fascia.

f. cribiform Fascia of thigh covering saphenous opening.

f. pelvic It maintains strength of pelvic floor.

f. Scarpa's The deep layer of superficial fascia of abdomen.

f. transversalis Fascia located between the perineum and transversalis muscle.

Fascicle A fasciculus.

Fasciculation Involuntary contraction or twitching of muscle fibers.

Fasciculus A small bundle especially of muscle or nerve fibers.

f. cuneatus Triangular shaped bundle of nerve fibers in the dorsal column carrying sense of proprioception and deep touch. *Syn* — column of Burdach.

f. gracilis It lies medial to f. cuneatus *SYN* — Column of Goll.

Fasciectomy Excision of a portion of fascia.

Fasciolopsis buski A fluke infesting intestinal tract of certain mammals including man.

Fasciorrhaphy Repair of fascia.

Fascitis Inflammation of fascia.

Fastidium Aversion to eating.

Fastigium The highest point; The most posterior portion of fourth ventricle in brain.

Fasting Accepting no food.

Fat Adipose tissue of body serving as energy reserve, providing fat soluble vitamins.

Fatigue Feeling of tiredness resulting from continuing activity.

Fatty acids Omega-3 Unsaturated fatty acids present in fish and certain vegetables, not synthesized in body. They reduce platelet adhesiveness and. lower serum triglyceride; hence used in coronary artery disease prevention.

Fatty change Abnormal accumulation of fat within the cell.

Fauces The constricted opening leading from mouth to the pharynx bounded by soft palate, base of the tongue and palatine arches.

Faucial reflex Sensation of vomiting resulting from irritation of fauces.

Favism Hereditary hypersensitivity to a kind of bean, vicia faba characterized by fever, hemolytic anemia, vomiting; common to patients of G_6-PD deficiency.

Favus Fungal infection of skin characterized by yellowish crusts over hair follicle with itching and musty odor.

Fazadinium Neuromuscular blocking agent.

Fc fragment A part of immunoglobulin for antigen recognition and processing by macrophages.

Fc receptor Present in neutrophils, monocytes and macrophages that binds to Fc fragment of immunoglobulin.

Fear Emotional reaction to external or internal threat, a feature of depression.

Febrile convulsion Convulsion precipitated by fever.

Feces Excreta, stool.

Fechner's law A theory stating that the magnitudes of sensations produced by given stimuli form an arithmetical progression; 1 the stimuli forming a geometrical progression.

Feculent Having sediment.

Fecundation Fertilization, impregnation.

Fecundity Fertility, ability to produce children.

Feedback Return to original place, can be positive or negative.

Feeder A device permitting independent eating by severe neurologically disabled person.

f. artificial Tube feeding, the tube passed through esophagus or rectum.

Feeling The conscious phase of nervous activity. Emotions are centrally stimulated feelings.

Fehling's solution A solution for testing urine sugar; prepared by dissolving 34.66 gm of copper sulfate in 500 ml of water to make solution A and 173 gm potassium iodide and 50 gm of sodium hydroxide in 500 ml of water to make (solution B). When urine containing sugar is boiled after addition of both the solutions, a red precipitate of cuprous oxide is formed.

Felon Abscess of soft tissue in terminal portion of finger.

Felty's syndrome Rheumatoid arthritis associated with splenomegaly, neutropenia, anemia and often thrombocytopenia.

Female Woman, sex that produces ova.

Feminism Male developing secondary sexual characteristic of female.

Feminization testicular An apparent female with genetic characteristic of male due to tissue resistance to androgenic hormones secreted by testes.

Femoral artery A branch of external iliac artery.

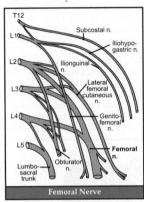

Femoral Nerve

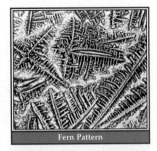

Fern Pattern

slide; dependent on salt concentration in mucus which is further dependent upon amount of estrogen in the mucus. This test is only positive in mid cycle. If positive in late cycle, indicates lack of progesterone.

Femoral nerve Largest branch of lumbar plexus supplying the skin in front of thigh and muscles involved in straightening the leg.

Fenestra An aperture frequently closed by membrane.

Fenfluramine An adrenergic agent.

Fenofibrate Lipid lowering agent.

Fenoprofen calcium Non steroidal anti inflammatory agent.

Fenoterol Beta adrenergic agonist used in bronchial asthma.

Fentanyl citrate Synthetic potent analgesic.

Ferment To decompose.

Fern A flowerless plant, whose extracts are used as anthelmintic.

Fern pattern Palm leaf (arborization) pattern of cervical mucus when allowed to dry on a glass

Ferritin Iron-phosphorus protein complex containing about 23% iron, the principal tissue storage form of iron.

Ferrokinetics Study of absorption, utilization, storage and excretion of iron.

Ferroprotein Important oxygen transferring enzyme.

Ferrous Bivalent iron.

Ferric Trivalent iron, oxidized form.

Ferule A bond or ring of metal applied to the end of the root or crown of tooth in order to strengthen it.

Fertilization Union of ovum with spermatozoa or union of male and female gametes in plants.

Fervescence Increase of fever.

Festinant Increase in speed, accelerating.

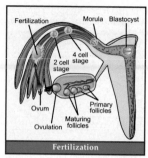

Fertilization

Festish An object thought to have magical supernatural power.

Fetal alcohol syndrome Birth defects and mental retardation in babies born to alcoholic mothers who continued alcohol ingestion during first trimester.

Fetal circulation Oxygenated blood from placenta passes via umbilical vein and ductus venosus to inferior vena cava bypassing liver and thence to right atrium and then via foramen ovale to left atrium, left ventricle and aorta.

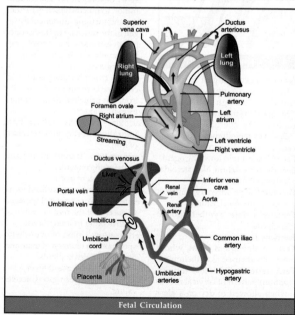

Fetal Circulation

Some blood from right atrium also enters right ventricle and pulmonary artery to be shunted to aorta via ductus arteriosus. Blood to placental villi are returned via the two umbilical arteries which are continuation of hypogastric arteries.

Feticide Killing of the fetus.

Fetoprotein A fetal antigen often present in adults. Amniotic fluid fetoprotein level can indicate about fetal well being and maturity. Level is increased in defects of neuroaxis. Increased level in adults indicates hepatoma.

Fetoscope An flexible optical device of fiberoptic material used for direct visualization of fetus *in utero*.

Fetotoxic Materials toxic to developing fetus, e.g. alcohol sedatives, tetracycline, tobacco.

Fetus Child *in utero* from third month to birth.

f. amorphus Shapeless fetus, barely recognizable as fetus.

f. calcified Fetus dyeing *in utero* with calcification.

f. in fetu A small imperfect fetus is contained within body of another fetus (e.g. desmoid).

f. mummified A dead fetus that has assumed mummified form.

f. papyraceus In twin pregnancy, the dead fetus is pressed flat by living fetus.

FEV1 Forced expiratory volume in 1 second. After full inspiration patient exhales as hard and as fast

as possible into spirometer and the amount of air exhaled in 1 second is recorded. FEV_1 is reduced in obstructive lung disease.

Fever Elevation of body temperature above 37°C (98.6°F). Rectal temperature is 0.5-1°F higher than oral temperature. Body calorie expenditure is increased by 12% for each 0°C of fever.

f. continuous Fever with diurnal variation of below 2°F as in enteric, typhus.

f. drug Almost any drug can cause fever as a side effect.

f. of unknown origin (FUO) Fever above 38°C on several occasions continuing for more than 3 weeks but without a diagnosis even with 1 week of hospital investigation. Common causes are neoplasms, collagen vascular diseases, pulmonary embolism, drug fever.

f. periodic Inherited disease of unknown etiology manifesting with joint pain, abdominal pain, pleurisy, etc.

f. blister Herpes simplex (type I) eruption of lips.

Fiber Thread like element, can be nerve fiber, muscle fiber or a cellular product like collagen fiber, elastic fiber, reticulin fiber.

f. afferent Fiber carrying impulses towards nerve cell.

f. dietary Undigestible elements of food, i.e. cellulose, hemicellulose, lignin, pectin that add bulk to stool. Foods rich in fiber include whole grain, fruits, leafy vegetables, and their skin. High fiber intake prevents constipation, prevents diverticulosis, lowers cholesterol and sugar and possibly prevents colon cancer.

f. efferent Nerve fiber carrying information away from nerve cell.

f. medullated Nerve fiber whose axis cylinder is covered by myelin sheath.

Fibril A small fiber, often the component of a cell or a fiber; can be myofibril or neurofibril.

Fibrillation Spontaneous contraction of individual muscle fibers.

f. atrial Rapid, irregular and incomplete contraction of atria.

f. ventricular Similar to above, with ineffectual contraction of ventricles. May result from mechanical injury to heart, coronary artery disease, drugs, electrocution, electrolyte imbalance, etc. Life threatening unless immediately treated.

Fibrin Whitish filamentous protein formed by action of thrombin on fibrinogen. Fibrin entangles RBC and platelets to produce the clotting.

f. foam A sponge like substance prepared from human fibrin used as hemostatic in surgery.

Fibrinogen A coagulation protein of plasma that is precursor of fibrin.

Fibrinogenolysis Dissolution of fibrin.

Fibrinogenopenia Reduction in blood fibrinogen.

Fibrinoid Resembling fibrin.

Fibrinoid change Change in connective tissue with immunologic injury, the tissue becoming homogeneous, swollen and band like.

Fibrinokinase Enzyme of animal tissue that activates plasminogen.

Fibrinolysin *SYN*— plasmin that dissolves fibrin.

Fibrinolysis The process of dissolution of fibrin by plasmin.

Fibrinopeptide The substance removed from fibrinogen during blood coagulation; fibrin degradation product.

Fibrinosis Excess fibrin in blood.

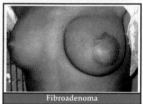
Fibroadenoma

Fibroadenoma Adenoma with fibrous tissue stroma.

Fibre angioma A fibrous tissue angioma.

Fibrocartilage A type of cartilage in which the matrix contains thick bundles of white or cartilaginous fibers. Found in the intervertebral disks.

Fibrocyst A fibrous tumor having undergone cystic degeneration.

Fibrocystic disease of breast Painful lump in breast, the pain and size fluctuating with menstrual cycle; 50% of women in reproductive age have this problem and carry a

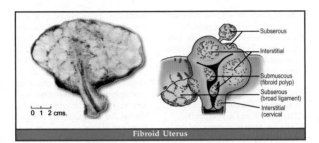

Fibroid Uterus

2-5% greater risk of developing breast cancer.

Fibrocystic disease of pancreas Cystic fibrosis.

Fibroid Fibromyoma of uterus which may grow inwards or outwards to become subperitoneal.

Fibroma Encapsulated, irregular, firm slow growing connective tissue tumor. Can arise within muscle, breast, uterus, (causes menorrhagia).

Fibromatosis Simultaneous development of multiple fibromas.

f. gingivae An inherited condition in which there is hypertrophy of gums prior to eruption of teeth.

Fibromyositis Inflammation of muscle and surrounding connective tissue, a nonspecific illness characterized by pain, tenderness, stiffness of joint capsule.

Fibromyxoma A fibroma that has undergone partial myxomatous degeneration.

Fibromyxosarcoma A sarcoma containing fibrous and myxoid tissue or sarcoma that has undergone mucoid degeneration.

Fibropapilloma Mixed fibroma and papilloma seen in bladder.

Fibrosarcoma A spindle celled sarcoma containing abundant connective tissue.

Fibrosis Abnormal fibrous tissue formation.

f. diffuse interstitial pulmonary SYN — Hamman rich syndrome, causing respiratory distress of newborn.

f. of lungs Formation of scar tissue in lungs following pneumonia, lung abscess, tuberculosis.

f. retroperitoneal Of unknown etiology, causes obstruction of ureter and great vessels.

Fibula The outer and smaller bone of leg, often sacrificed in bone grafting.

Pick method A method to determine cardiac output.

Field A specific area in relation to an object.

Fifth cranial nerve Trigeminal nerve, a mixed nerve with its sensory-motor nuclei in Pons-medulla.

Fifth disease Parvovirus infection with rash mimicking rubella.

FIGLU excretion test Test for folic acid deficiency. When histidine is administered to a patient with folic acid deficiency formimino-glutamic acid excretion in urine is increased.

Filament Thread like coil of Tungsten found in X-ray tube.

Filaria A long filiform nematode found in lymphatics, serous cavities and connective tissue, e.g. f. bancrofti.

Filariasis A chronic disease due to filaria species.

Filiform Hair like, filamentous.

Film A thin membrane/covering; photographic film usually cellulose coated with a light sensitive emulsion.

f. bitewing Technique used for taking film of several teeth at the same time.

f. badge A badge containing a film to calculate the total exposure of an individual to X-rays.

Filter Device for filtering light, liquid, radiation, etc.

f. Berkefeld A diatomaceous earth filter designed to remove bacteria from solutions passed through it. (excepting viruses).

f. infrared Filter that permits only passage of infrared waves of certain wave lengths.

f. optical Device that only permits a portion of the visible light spectrum. The filter absorbs the unwanted wave length.

f. umbrella Filter placed in blood vessels in order to prevent passage of emboli, e.g. inferior vena cava umbrella filter placement to reduce pulmonary embolism in patients of pelvic or deep leg vein thrombosis.

f. wood's A glass screen allowing passage of ultraviolet rays and absorbing rays of visual light, useful for diagnosis of fungus infection of hair.

Filtrate The fluid that has been passed through a filter.

f. glomerular The protein free plasma filtered while passage of blood through glomeruli.

Filum A thread like structure.

f coronaria A fibrous band extending from the base of the median cusp of tricuspid valve to the aortic annulus.

f. terminate A long slender filament at the terminal end of cord terminating in coccyx.

Fimbriate Having finger like projections.

Fine motor skills Skills pertaining to synergy of small muscles of hand.

Finger One of the five digits of hand.

f. clubbed Enlarged terminal phalanx of the finger. Present in cyanotic heart disease, pulmonary suppuration and malignancy, bacterial endocarditis.

f. hammer Permanent flexion of terminal phalanx due to damage of extensor tendons.

Finger print An imprint made by the cutaneous ridges of fingers, used for the purpose of identification.

First aid Emergency assistance to injured sick individuals prior to physician's care or transportation to hospital. Common situations necessitating first aid are: foreign body, coma, convulsion, burn, poisoning, etc.

First cranial nerve Nerve carrying smell sensation from olfactory mucosa,

First degree AV block Partial block of conduction in AV node characterized by prolonged PR interval. When occurring independently does not need treatment but if with anterior myocardial infarction or bundle branch block, it may progress to complete heart block and hence needs permanent pace maker.

Fish skin disease A disease of skin characterized by increase of the horny layer and deficiency of the skin secretion.

Fission Splitting into two or more parts, method of asexual reproduction in bacteria, protozoa and other lower forms of life.

Fissiparous Reproducing by fission.

Fissure A groove or natural division, cleft or slit, break in enamel of tooth, crack like sore, deep furrow in an organ like brain, lung, liver, spinal cord.

f. anal Linear painful ulcer at anal margin.

f. auricular Fissure of petrous part of temporal bone.

f. Broca Fissure encircling the third left frontal convolution of the brain.

f. inferior orbital Fissure at the apex of orbit, through which pass the infraorbital blood vessels and maxillary branch of trigeminal nerve.

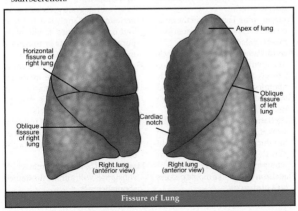

Fissure of Lung

f. of Rolando Fissure separating frontal and parietal lobes.

f. of Sylvius Fissure separating frontal and parietal lobes from temporal lobe.

f. transverse 1. Fissure between cerebrum and cerebellum of brain. 2. Fissure on the lower surface of liver serving as the hilum for entrance of hepatic vessels and exit of ducts.

Fistula An abnormal free passage from cavity/or inner organ to exterior/another organ.

f. arteriovenous Direct communication between artery and vein.

f. horseshoe Perianal fistula in which the tract goes round the rectum and communicates with skin at one or more point.

f. thyroglossal A midline fistula about thyroid that connects the persistent embryonic thyroglossal duct to exterior.

Fixation point The fovea or the point on the retina where the visual axes meet for clearest vision.

Flaccid Paralysis with loss of muscle tone, reduction or loss of tendon reflexes, atrophy of muscles, usually due to lesion of lower motor neurone.

Flagellate A protozoon with one or more flagella.

Flagellation Whipping, massage by strokes, a form of sexual aberration in which sexual urge is brought about by being whipped or whipping the partner.

Flagellum A hair like motile process on a protozoon.

Flagyl Metronidazole.

Flail chest A condition arising from fracture of a number of ribs, or ribs at many points, resulting in the flail rib segment moving in paradoxically with inspiration and out with expiration.

Flail joint Joint with excessive mobility due to paralysis of acting, muscles.

Flange In dentistry, the part of an artificial denture that extends from embedded teeth to the border of denture.

Flank The part of body between ribs and upper border of ilium.

Flap A mass of partially detached tissue used in plastic surgery.

f. pedicle Flap made by suturing the edges to form a tube. Then one end of the tube is severed and sutured to another site. By use of this jump flap technique, such a flap may be moved in several stages, a great distance.

f. periodontal Gingival flap removed or repositioned to eliminate periodontal pockets or to correct mucogingival defects.

Flare A spreading area of redness that surrounds a line made by drawing a pointed instrument across the skin. It is due to dilatation of blood vessels.

Flashbacks The return of imagery and hallucinations after the immediate effect of hallucinogens is worn off.

Flash point The temperature at which substance will burst into flames spontaneously.

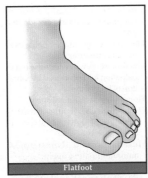
Flatfoot

Flatfoot Abnormal flatness of sole and loss of arch on innerside of foot.

Flatness Resonance heard on percussion over solid organs or when there is fluid in the thoracic cavity.

Flatulence Excessive formation or passage of gas from GI tract.

Flatus Expulsion of gas from anus. Average person excretes 400-1200 cc of gas everyday, containing hydrogen, methane, skatoles, indoles, carbon dioxide, small amounts of oxygen and nitrogen. Flatulogenic foods are milk, legumes, fried items.

Flatus tube A rectal tube which is pushed to facilitate expulsion of gas.

Flavin One of a group of natural water soluble pigments occurring in milk, yeast, bacteria and some plants.

Flavism Having a yellow tinge.

Flavi virus Previously called group B arbo virus responsible for yellow fever, dengue fever and encephalitis.

Flavobacterium A group of bacteria producing orange-yellow pigments in culture. Flavobacterium meningosepticum causes virulent meningitis in prematures.

Flavoprotein A group of conjugated proteins that constitute yellow enzyme for cellular respiration.

Flavour The quality that affects the sense of taste.

Flaxedil Gallamine triethiodide.

Flea Wingless blood sucking insects that have legs adapted for jumping. Xenopsella species transmit plague from rats to humans. Fleas may transmit tularemia, endemic typhus and brucellosis.

f. chigger Sand flea.

Fleccainide acetate Antiarrhythmic agent.

Fleece of Stilling Meshwork of white fibers that surrounds the dentate nucleus of cerebellum.

Fleming Alexander Scottish physician who in 1945 was awarded Nobel prize for discovering penicillin.

Flesh Soft tissues of animal body, esp. the muscles.

Fletcher factor A blood clotting factor, prekallikrein.

Flexibility Adaptibility, quality of being bent without breaking.

Flexion The act of bending forward.

Flexor Muscle that bends a part in proximal direction.

f. left colic Bend in colon where transverse colon continues as descending colon *SYN* — splenic flexure.

f. right colic Bend in colon where ascending colon becomes the transverse colon *SYN* — hepatic flexure.

Flexure A bend

Flicker The visual sensation of alternating intervals of brightness caused by rhythmically interrupting light stimuli.

Flight of ideas Continuous but fragmentary stream of talk may be seen in acute mania.

Floaters Translucent specks of various sizes and shapes that float across the visual field; usually small bits of protein or cells.

Flocculation The gathering together of fine dispersed particles in a solution into larger visible particles.

Flocculus 1. A small tuft of wool like fibers. 2. lobes of cerebellum behind the middle cerebral peduncle.

Floppy - valve syndrome Mitral valve prolapse.

Floss To use dental floss or tape to remove plaque or calculus.

Flour Ground wheat powder.

Flowmeter Device for measuring flow of gas or liquid, i.e. flow of anesthetic gases.

Flow state An altered state of consciousness in which the mind functions at its peak, time may seem to be distorted and a sense of happiness seems to pervade that period.

Floxuridine An antimetabolite used in cancer treatment.

Fluctuation A wavy impulse felt in palpation and produced by vibration of body fluid.

Flucytosine Antifungal agent.

Fludrocortisone Synthetic corticosteroid with high mineral retaining property.

Flufenamic acid Nonsteroidal antiinflammatory agent.

Flufenazine enathate A phenothiazine type antipsychotic drug.

Fluid amniotic Clear yellowish fluid of specific gravity 1.006 composed of albumin, urea, water mixed with lanugo, epidermal cells, vernix caseosa, and meconium.

Fluid cerebrospinal Fluid found in central canal of spinal cord, in the ventricles of brain and in the subarachnoid space.

Fluid synovial Fluid contained within synovial cavities, bursae and tendon sheaths.

Fluid balance Regulation of water homeostasis in body.

Fluke A parasite belonging to class trematoda.

f. blood Schistostoma hematobium, *S. mansoni, S. japonicum,* belong to this group inhabiting mesenteric and pelvic veins.

f. hepatica Fasciola hepatica, chlorosis sinensis.

f. intestinal Fasciolopsis buski.

f. lung Paragonimus westermani.

Flumethasone Synthetic cortico-steroid.

Flunarizine Calcium channel blocker for migraine.

Fluocinolone acetonide Synthetic corticosteroid.

Fluorescein sodium A red crystal-line powder, used to for corneal staining and angiography.

Fluorescence Property of certain substances to emit light when exposed to ultraviolet radiation.

Fluorescent Luminous when ex-posed to other light rays.

Fluorescent antibody A body tagged with fluorescent material, for diagnosis of various kinds of infections.

Fluorescent treponemal antibody absorption test (FTA-ABS) Test for syphilis using fluorescent antibody.

Fluoridation Addition of fluorides to water to prevent dental caries in the concentration of 1 mg/1000 ml of water drinking to assure daily fluoride intake of 0.25 to 0.5 mg.

Fluorometer Device for determining amount of radiation produced by X-rays.

Fluoroscope A radiological tool consisting of a fluorescent screen by means of which the shadows of objects interposed between the tube and screen are made visible.

Fluoroscopy Patient examination by fluoroscope.

Fluorosis Chronic flourine poisoning causing mottling of tooth enamel, and hyperlucency of bone.

Fluorouracil Antimetabolite, anti-cancer agent.

Fluoxetine 5HT antagonist, anti-depressant.

Fluoxymesterone An anabolic and androgenic hormone.

Flupenthixol Antipsychotic agent.

Flurandrenolide A corticosteroid.

Flurbiprofen Propionic acid deri-vative NSAID.

Flurazepam Sedative-hypnotic agent.

Fluoroapatite A compound formed when the enamel of teeth is treated with appropriate concentration of fluoride to form hydroxyapatite which is less acid soluble, hence resistant to caries.

Flurogestone A progestational drug.

Fluroxene An anesthetic agent administered by inhalation.

Flush 1. Sudden redness of skin. 2. Irrigation of cavity with water.

f. hot Flush accompanied with sensations of heat, common in menopausal syndrome and neu-roses.

Flutter A tremulous movement.

f. atrial Rapid atrial contraction (200-400/min) but with a regular heart beat due to 1:2/1:3 AV block.

f. diaphragmatic Rapid diaphrag-matic contraction.

f. mediastinum Abnormal side to side motion of diaphragm.

Flux An excessive flow or discharge from an organ or cavity of body.

Foam Production of gas bubble interspersed with fluid.

Foam solubility test Procedure for determining the presence or absence of surfactant active material in amniotic fluid. Surfactant deficit is diagnostic of respiratory distress syndrome.

Focus The point of convergence of light rays or waves of sounds.

Fog Water droplets in air.

Fogging 1. A method of testing vision used particularly in testing astigmatism and in post cycloplegic examination. 2. Unwanted density on the radiographic film resulting from exposure to secondary radiation, light, chemicals, heat, etc.

Foil A thin pliable sheet of metal. Gold foils are used in dental restoration work.

Fold A doubling back.

f. aryepiglottic The ridge like lateral walls of the entrance to larynx.

f. gastric Gastric mucosal folds; mostly longitudinal.

f. rectum Transverse mucosal folds of rectum, *SYN* – valves of Houston.

Foliaceous Resembling leaf.

Folic acid $C_{19}H_{19}N_7O_6$, chemically pteroyl glutamic acid, found in green plant tissue, liver and yeast. Deficiency causes megaloblastic anaemia.

Folinic acid The active form of folic acid.

Follicle A small secretory sac or cavity.

f. aggregated *SYN* – Peyer's patch. An aggregation of solitary nodules or group of lymph nodules at the junction of ileum with colon at the anti mesentric border.

f. graffian Developing primary oocyte in the cortex of ovary.

f. hair An invagination of the epidermis from which hair develops.

f. lymphatic The densely packed collection of lymphocytes and lymphoblasts that make up cortex of a lymph node.

f. nabothian Dilated cyst of glands of uterine cervix.

f. ovarian A spherical structure in the cortex of ovary consisting of an oocyte and surrounding follicular cells.

f. primordial Follicle of ovary with ovum enclosed in a single layer of cells.

f. of thyroid Spherical structure lined with a single layer of cuboidal epithelium secreting thyroid hormones.

Follicle-stimulating hormone (FSH) Hormone of anterior pituitary stimulating spermatogenesis in male and maturation of graffian follicle in female.

Follicular tonsillitis Inflammation of follicles on surface of tonsils which become filled with pus.

Foliculitis barbae Ringworm of heard.

Folliculoma A tumor of ovary originating in graffian follicle in which cells resemble the cells of stratum granulosum.

Folliculosis Presence of an abnormal quantity of lymph follicles.

Follow-up The continued care or monitoring of a patient after the initial visit or examination.

Fomentation A hot, wet application for the relief of pain or inflammation.

Fomes (fomite) Any substance that adheres to and transmits infectious material.

Fontana's spaces Spaces between the processes of ligamentum pectinatum of iris, conveying aqueous humor.

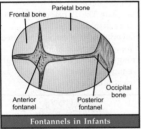

Parietal bone
Frontal bone
Occipital bone
Anterior fontanel
Posterior fontanel

Fontannels in Infants

Fontanel Unossified space lying between cranial bones of the skull.

f. anterior Lying at the junction of coronal, frontal and sagittal sutures.

f. posterior Lying at the junction of sagittal and lambdoid sutures.

Food additives Substances other than basic food stuffs that are present in food during production, processing, storage or packaging.

Food adulterants Substances making food impure or toxic like toxic organisms, pesticide residues, poisonous substance or substances added to increase weight or bulk of food.

Food allergies Allergic reaction resulting from ingestion of food to which one has become sensitized. Common offenders are: milk, egg, shellfish, chocolate, oranges.

Food and drug administration (FDA) In USA, an official regulatory body for food, drugs, cosmetics, and medical devices, a part of Department of health and human services.

Food ball Gastric stone made up of fruit and vegetable skins, seeds and fibers. *SYN* — phytobezoar.

Food chain Sequential transfer of food energy from green plants to herbivorous animals and then to man through animal flesh. Interruption of this chain can result in ecological disaster.

Food poisoning Illness resulting from ingestion of foods containing poisonous substances, e.g. mushroom poisoning, insecticides contaminating food, milk from cows that have eaten some poisonous plants, ingestion of putrefied or decomposed food.

Food requirement Requirement of calorie and protein depending upon age, muscular work and environment. Average active healthy (70 kg) man requires 2700 cal/day and average healthy woman 2000 cal/day. Persons in sedentary work require less calories. Protein requirement of adult is 1 gm/kg of their ideal weight. Pregnancy and lactation demand 15-25% extra calories. In growing children protein requirement is 2-3 gm/kg/day.

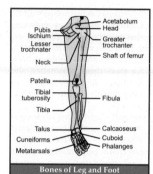

Bones of Leg and Foot

Foot Terminal portion of lower extremity.

f. arches Four arches: internal longitudinal, outer longitudinal, and two transverse arches.

f. athlete's Fungus infection of interdigital spaces.

f. cleft A condition where cleft extends between the digits to the metatarsal region, usually due to a missing digit.

f. flat The inner longitudinal and anterior transverse metatarsal arches are depressed and flat; very often asymptomatic.

f. immersion Resulting from prolonged immersion of foot in cold water or exposure of foot to extreme cold swampy atmosphere resulting in impaired circulation and anesthesia.

f. madura Bone hypertrophy and degeneration, frequently followed by suppuration and gangrene, causative agents are - mycetomas.

f. splay Flat wide foot.

Foot and mouth disease A viral disease of cattle and horses.

Foot board A device that helps to prevent foot drop.

Foot candle An amount of light equivalent to one lumen per square foot.

Foot drop Plantar flexion of foot due to paralysis of muscles in anterior compartment of leg. (lateral popliteal palsy).

Foot plate The flat part of stapes, the bone of middle ear.

Foot print An impression of foot used for identification of infants.

Forage Creating a channel through enlarged prostate by use of an electric cautery.

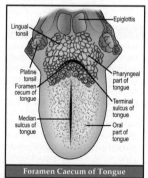

Foramen Caecum of Tongue

Foramen A passage; opening; an orifice; a communication between two cavities.

f. apical Opening at the end of root canal transmitting blood, lymph and nerve supply to dental pulp.

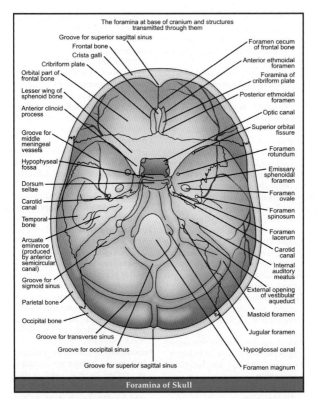

The foramina at base of cranium and structures transmitted through them

Groove for superior sagittal sinus
Frontal bone
Crista galli
Cribriform plate
Orbital part of frontal bone
Lesser wing of sphenoid bone
Anterior clinoid process
Groove for middle meningeal vessels
Hypophyseal fossa
Dorsum sellae
Carotid canal
Temporal bone
Arcuate eminence (produced by anterior semicircular canal)
Groove for sigmoid sinus
Parietal bone
Occipital bone
Groove for transverse sinus
Groove for occipital sinus
Groove for superior sagittal sinus

Foramen cecum of frontal bone
Anterior ethmoidal foramen
Foramina of cribriform plate
Posterior ethmoidal foramen
Optic canal
Superior orbital fissure
Foramen rotundum
Emissary sphenoidal foramen
Foramen ovale
Foramen spinosum
Foramen lacerum
Carotid canal
Internal auditory meatus
External opening of vestibular aqueduct
Mastoid foramen
Jugular foramen
Hypoglossal canal
Foramen magnum

Foramina of Skull

f. Caecum of tongue a median opening on the dorsum of the posterior part of tongue.

f. condyloid Opening above the condyle of occipital bone for passage of hypoglossal nerve.

f. epiploic Opening connecting the peritoneal cavity to lesser sac *SYN*— foramen of Winslow.

f. internal auditory The opening in the petrous portion of sphenoid bone through which 7th and 8th cranial nerves pass.

f. intervertebral Opening between adjacent articulated vertebrae for passage of nerves.

f. jugular Opening at base of skull permitting passage of sigmoid and inferior petrosal sinus and 9th, 10th, and 11th cranial nerves.

f. magnum Opening in the occipital bone through which passes the spinal cord.

f. of Monro Communication between third and lateral ventricles of brain.

f. optic Opening in the lesser wing of sphenoid bone permitting passage of optic nerve and ophthalmic artery.

f. ovale Opening between the two atria in fetal heart which often continues into adulthood.

f. rotundum Opening in greater wing of sphenoid in which maxillary branch of trigeminal nerve passes.

Forbe's disease Type III glycogen storage disease.

Force A push or pull exerted upon an object, measured in Newtons. 1 Newton is equivalent to 0.225 pound force.

f. electromotive Energy that causes flow of electricity in a conductor.

Forceps Pincers for holding/ extracting.

f. alligator Toothed forceps with a double clamp.

f. artery Forceps for holding ends of an artery in order to perform ligation.

f. clamp Any forcep with automatic lock.

f. dental Forceps of varying shapes for grasping teeth during extraction.

f. obstetrics Forceps used to extract the fetal head from pelvis.

f. towel/tissue Forceps for clipping towels to operation site or grasping delicate tissue.

Fordyce's disease Enlarged ectopic, sebaceous glands in mucosa of mouth and genitals.

Fordyce-Fox disease A disease similar to prickly heat in which itchy follicular papules are present in axilla, areola of breast, labia, etc.

Forensic Pertains to legal.

Forensic dentistry Application of science of dentistry for the purposes of law, e.g. establishing identity.

Forensic medicine Medicine in relation to law, legal aspects of medical ethics and standards.

Foreskin Prepuce; loose skin covering end of penis/clitoris.

Fore waters Mucus discharge from vagina during pregnancy.

Fork turning An elongated instrument that bifurcates at one end, used for testing hearing, bone conduction and vibration.

Formaldehyde A colorless pungent irritant gas formed by oxidation of methyl alcohol, used as disinfectant, preservative in histology and for sterilizing feces, urine, sputum.

Formalin Aqueous solution of 37% formaldehyde.

Formation A structure, shape or figure.

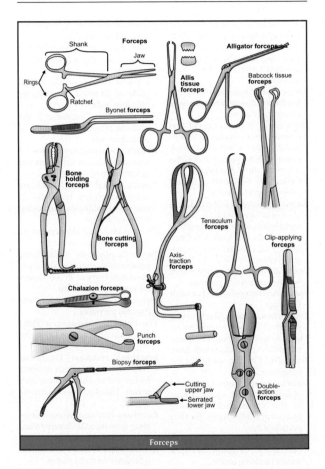

Forceps

f. reticular Found in medulla oblongata between the pyramids and floor of the fourth ventricle, supposed to be the activating or arousal system for consciousness.

Forme fruste An aborted or incomplete form of disease arrested before running its course.

Formic acid A clear pungent acid obtained from oxidation of formaldehyde or wood alcohol, responsible for pain and swelling following stings and bites.

Formication Sensation of insects creeping upon the body.

Formiminoglutamic acid (FIGLU) A chemical intermediate in the metabolism of histidine to glutamic acid. In folic acid deficiency states FIGLU excretion is increased in urine.

Fornication Sexual intercourse between unmarried partners.

Fornix Anything of arched or vault like shape.

f. conjuctivae Loose fold connecting palpebral and bulbar conjuctivae.

f. uteri Anterior and posterior spaces into which upper vagina is divided.

Forskolin Cardiac stimulant for congestive failure.

Fortification spectrum Appearance of dark patch with zigzag outline in the visual field causing temporary blindness in that portion of eye.

Fossa A shallow depression.

f. claudius Triangular area accommodating ovary.

f. condylar Depression behind the occipital epicondyle.

f. coronoid Depression on the anterior surface of lower end of humerus.

f. ethmoid The groove in cribiform plate of ethmoid occupied by olfactory bulb.

f. Rosenmüller Depression in the pharynx posterior to opening of eustachian tube.

Fourchette Transverse band of mucous membrane at the posterior commissure of vagina.

Fourth cranial nerve Trochlear nerve emerging from dorsal surface of midbrain, supplying superior oblique.

Fovea A pit or cup like depression, e.g. fovea centralis of eye.

Fowler's position Semisitting position with angulation of upper portion of body at 45°-60°; knees may or may not be bent.

Foxglove Common name for plant digitalis purpurea.

Fraction of inspired oxygen (FiO$_2$) The concentration of O$_2$ in the inspired air.

Fractional testmeal Fractional examination of stomach contents for free and total hydrochloric acid.

Fracture Dissolution in continuity of bone.

f. avulsion Tearing of a piece of bone away from the main bone by force of muscular contraction.

f. comminuted Fracture where bone is broken into many pieces.

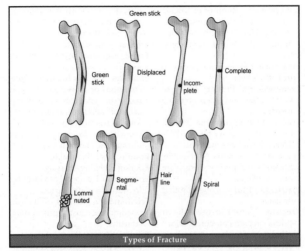

Green stick

Green stick Dislpaced Incom-plete Complete

Lommi nuted Segme-ntal Hair line Spiral

Types of Fracture

f. compound Fracture where bone fragment protrudes through skin or there is communication between fracture site and exterior.

f. compression Fracture of vertebra by pressure along long axis of the vertebral column.

f. epiphyseal Separation of epiphysis from bone, occurs only in young patients.

f. fissured A narrow split in the bone, the split not extending to other side of bone.

f. greenstick Fracture when one cortex fractures, the other being intact.

f. hair line A. Thin narrow incomplete fracture line not extending through the entire bone.

f. impacted Fracture where one end is wedged into the interior of other.

f. pathologic Fracture of a weakened bone produced by a force, that would not have fractured a healthy bone.

f. pingpong Depressed fracture of skull resembling indentation made on pingpong ball by compression.

f. Pott's Fracture of lower end of fibula with outward displacement of the ankle and foot.

Fragile-x-syndrome Mutation in x-chromosome manifesting with mental retardation and greatly enlarged testicles after puberty.

Fragilitas Brittleness as of the hair.

Fragility State of brittleness.

f. erythrocyte Rupture of RBC in various strengths of salt solution. Normal blood starts hemolyzing at about 0.44% and complete at 0.35%.

Frambesia Infectious disease caused by a spirochete.

Frambesioma Primary lesion of yaws in the form of a protruding nodule.

Franceschetti's syndrome Mandibulo facial dysostosis *SYN*– Treacher-Collins syndrome.

Francisella tularensis Non motile, encapsulated, gram -ve organism causing plague.

Fratricide Murder of one's brother or sister.

Freckle Small brownish or yellowish pigmentation of skin.

Freiberg's infarction Osteochondritis of head of second metatarsal bone.

Fremitus Vibrating tremors esp. those felt through the chest wall by palpation or auscultation.

French scale A system indicating outer catheter diameters. Each unit of scale is equivalent to 1/3 mm.

Frenotomy Cutting of the frenum esp. of tongue.

Frenulum linguae A fold of mucous membrane that extends from floor of mouth to the inferior surface of tongue along midline.

Frenzy A state of violent mental agitation or excitement.

f. response In electrodiagnostic study of spinal reflexes, the time required for a stimulus applied to a motor nerve to travel in the opposite direction up the nerve to the spinal cord and return.

Fretum A constriction.

Freud, Sigmund Austrian neurologist and psychoanalyst.

Freudian Freud's theories of unconscious or repressed libido on past experiences or desires as the cause of various neuroses, and cure for which is the restoration of such conditions to consciousness through psychoanalysis.

Friable Easily breakable.

Friction Rubbing, massage.

Friction rub The sound produced by friction of two dry surfaces.

Friedländer's bacillus Klebsiella pneumoniae causing pneumonia, sinusitis.

Friedrich's ataxia An inherited disease involving degeneration of dorso-lateral columns of spinal cord, kyphoscoliosis and muscular weakness of lower limbs.

Fright Extreme sudden fear.

Frigid Cold, irresponsive to emotions or lack of sexual desire in women.

Frigidity Partial or complete inhibition of sexual excitement.

Frogbelly Flaccid atonic abdomen of children with rickets.

Frog face Facies of chronic sinusitis.

Fröhlich's syndrome Obesity, hypogonadism, due to hypothalamic disturbance.

Froin's syndrome High CSF protein content that rapidly coagulates and is yellow caused by spinal canal obstruction.

Fromet's sign Flexion of distal phalanx of thumb when a sheet of paper is held between thumb and index finger, a feature of ulnar nerve palsy.

Frontal lobe 4 main convolutions infront of central sulcus of cerebrum.

Frontal plane Plane parallel with the long axis of body and at right angles to the median sagittal plane.

Frontal sinus A pair of hollow asymmetrical spaces in the frontal bone above the orbits, filled with air and lined by mucous membrane.

Front tap reflex Contraction of gastrocnemius muscles when stretched muscles of extended leg are percussed.

Frost uremic Deposit of urea crystals on skin in uremia patient.

Frostbite Freezing and death of a body part due to cold exposure.

Frottage Orgasm produced by pressing against some body, massage technique using rubbing.

Frozen section A technique of examining and reporting on pathological tissue cut from a patient while on surgical table, thus deciding future course of action in the theatre itself.

Frozen shoulder restricted shoulder mobility due to adhesive capsulitis

Fructose $C_6H_{12}O_6$, fruit sugar, monosaccharide akin to glucose.

Fructose intolerance Inability to metabolize fructose in absence of enzyme aldolase thus producing nausea, vomiting, sweating, tremor, hypoglycemia on fructose consumption.

Fructokinase Enzyme that transfers high energy phosphate from a donor to fructose.

Frustration Disappointment.

Fucose A mucopolysaccharide present in blood group substances and in human milk.

Fucosidosis Hereditary disease with thick skin, heart disease, hyperhydrosis and poor neural growth resulting from improper metabolism of fucose.

Fugitive Inconstant symptoms, transient, wandering.

Fugue A dissociative disorder in which a person acts in normal manner but has complete amnesia for that period of action.

Fulguration Destruction of tissue by high frequency electric sparks.

Full term In obstetric child born between 38-41 weeks of gestation.

Fulminant Coming like flashes of pain, as in tabes dorsalis. Synofulgurant.

Fumaric acid One of the organic acids in the citric acid cycle.

Fumigation Use of poisonous gases for destroying living organisms like insects, rats, mice, etc. root disinfection.

Functional disease Emotional response to physical disease, taking the form of conversion or hysterical response.

Fundoplication Surgical reduction in size of opening into fundus of stomach, used in treating reflux esophagitis.

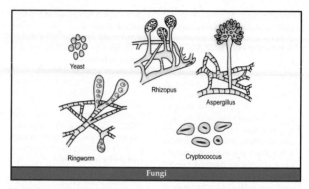

Fungi

Funduscopy Visual examination of fundus of eye.

Fundus The portion of an organ most remote from its opening.

Fungus Plant like organism including yeasts and molds but without chlorophil, hence of having parasitic or saprophytic existence.

Fungiform papillae Small rounded eminences on the tongue.

Funicular process That part of tunica vaginalis covering spermatic cord.

Funiculitis Inflammation of spermatic cord.

Funiculopexy Suturing the spermatic cord to tissues in cases of undescended testes.

Funiculus Any small structure resembling cord.

Funnel Conical wide mouthed device for pouring through it with a tubular end.

Funnel chest Sternal depression resembling funnel.

Funny bone Medial epicondyle of humerus.

Fur fur Dandruff scales.

Furgemia Presence of fungi in blood.

Furor Extreme violent outbursts of anger.

Furosemide Loop diuretic, kaliuretic.

Furrow A groove.

Furuncle A boil.

Furunculoid Resembling boil.

Furunculosis Condition resulting from boil.

Fuscin A dark brown pigment present in pigment epithelium of retina.

Fusiform Spindle shaped, i.e. tapering at both ends.

Fusion Meeting and joining together.

Fusobacterium A genus of nonspore forming, non-motile-non encapsulated gram -ve rods causing gingivitis, and seen in necrotic lesions.

f. waves Flutter waves in atrial fibrillation.

G

Gadfly A kind of fly that lay eggs under the skin of victim causing swelling simulating a boil.

Gadolinium A rare element used as NMR contrast agent.

Gag reflex Gagging and vomiting resulting from irritation of fauces.

Gaisbock's syndrome synonymspurious erythrocytosis or pseudopolycythemia vera .

Gait Manner of walking.

g. ataxic Staggering unsteady gait, e.g. alcoholics.

g. cerebellar Staggering broad based gait.

g. double step Gait in which alternate steps are of a different length or at a different rate.

g. equine High stepping gait of peroneal nerve palsy.

g. festinating Walking on toes as if pushed from behind. Starts slowly and then accelerates till he holds on to something that stops him, e.g. parkinsonism.

g. hemiplegic The paralyzed limb abducts and makes a circle to come to front to touch the ground.

g. scissor Gait in which legs cross while walking, e.g. cerebral palsy.

g. slapping High stepping ataxic gait due to loss of proprioception as in tabes dorsalis.

g. Waddling Walk resembling that of a duck as in muscular dystrophy.

Galactogogue Agent promoting secretion of milk.

Galactan A complex carbohydrate that forms galactose on hydrolysis.

Galactase A proteolytic ferment of milk.

Galactemia Milky condition of blood.

Galactocele A tumor caused by occlusion of a milk duct; hydrocele containing milk like fluid.

Galactokinase Enzyme transferring high energy phosphate groups from a donor to D-Galactose.

Galactometer Device for measuring specific gravity of milk.

Galactoplania Secretion of milk in any other part of body other than breast.

Galactopoitic Substance promoting secretion of milk.

Galactorrhoea Excessive flow of milk, continuation of lactation even without childbirth.

Galactose $C_6H_{12}O_6$ a monosaccharide, isomer of glucose converted to glycogen in liver.

Galactosemia An autosomal recessive inborn error of metabolism characterized by inability to convert galactose to glucose due to absence of enzyme galactose-1 phosphate uridyl transferase. Symptoms are diarrhoea and vomiting with failure to thrive after birth. Infants urine contains high galactose. Intrauterine diagnosis possible from amniocentesis.

Galactosuria Excretion of galactose in urine.

Galeazzi's sign A clinical test for determining presence of congenital hip dislocation in infants and toddlers; with the child lying supine, knees and hips flexed to 90°; dislocation is evidenced if one knee is higher than other.

Galen's veins These veins run through the tela chorodiae formed by the joining of the terminal and choroid veins. They form venacerebra magna, that empties into straight sinus.

Gallamine triethiodide A drug that inhibits transmission of nerve impulses across myoneural junction of voluntary muscles. Trade name flaxedil.

Gallbladder Pear shaped sac on under surface of right lobe of liver holding bile and discharging it into common bile duct through cystic duct during digestion.

Gallium Radio nucleide of gallium used in bone scan.

Gallon Measure of liquid equivalent to 4.55 liters.

Gallstone Concretion formed in the gallbladder or common bile duct,

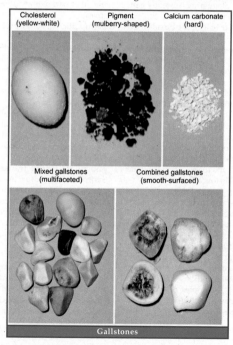

Cholesterol (yellow-white)
Pigment (mulberry-shaped)
Calcium carbonate (hard)

Mixed gallstones (multifaceted)
Combined gallstones (smooth-surfaced)

Gallstones

commonest being cholesterol stone. Excess of cholesterol or decreased bile acid concentration in bile help to precipitate cholesterol leading to stone formation.

Galvanic current Direct electric current from battery.

Galvanometer An instrument for measurement of current.

Galvanoscope An instrument that shows presence and direction of galvanic current.

Gamete A mature male or female reproductive cell.

Gamete intrafallopian transfer (GIFT) The process involves obtaining ova through laparoscope and mating it with sperms and then placing in fallopian tube for completion of fertilization and transfer to uterus.

Gametocide Agents that destroy malaria gametocytes.

Gametes The sexually differentiated form of protozoa that when enters mosquito reproduces into sporozoites.

Gametogenesis Development of gametes.

Gamma benzene hexachloride Scabicidal agent and insecticide.

Gamma globulin Immunoglobulin fraction in plasma containing IgG, IgA, IgD and IgE.

Gamma rays Electromagnetic waves of extremely short wave length emitted by radioactive substances having high tissue penetration.

Gammopathy Diseases with high gammaglobulin, e.g. multiple myeloma.

Gamophobia Neurotic fear of marriage.

Gancyclovir An antiviral used IV in CMV infection

Gangliocyte A ganglion cell.

Ganglioma Tumor of lymphatic gland.

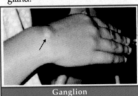
Ganglion

Ganglion 1. A mass of nervous tissue composed principally of nerve cell bodies lying outside brain and spinal cord. 2. Cystic tumor developing in a tendon or aponeuroses.

g. cardiac Tiny ganglion towards which converge the fibers of superficial cardiac plexus, lying on the right side of the ligamentum arteriosum.

g. carotid Ganglion formed by filamentous threads from the carotid plexus beneath the carotid artery.

g. celiac One pair of paravertebral or collateral ganglia located near the origin of celiac artery.

g. dorsal root Ganglia located in dorsal nerve root containing cell bodies of sensory nerves.

g. geniculate Ganglion on the pars intermedia, the sensory root of facial nerve.

g. jugular Ganglion located on the root of vagus nerve lying in upper portion of jugular foramen.

g. otic A small ganglion located in zygomatic fossa below the foramen ovale.

g. sphenopalatine Ganglion associated with the great superficial petrosal nerve and maxillary nerve, transmitting both sympathetic and parasympathetic fibers to nasal mucosa, palate, pharynx and orbit.

g. spiral A long coiled ganglion in the cochlea of ear containing bipolar cells whose peripheral processes terminate in organ of corti. The central processes form the cochlear nerve to terminate in medulla.

g. vestibular A bipolar ganglion located in the vestibular branch of 8th cranial nerve at the base of internal acoustic meatus. Its incoming fibers arise from macules of utricles and saccules and cristae of ampullae of semicircular canals.

Ganglioneuroma A nerve cell tumor containing ganglion cells.

Ganglion blockade Blockage of neurotransmission in autonomic ganglia by drugs that occupy receptor sites for acetylcholine or stabilize postsynaptic membrane against action of acetylcholine liberated in presynaptic nerve endings.

Ganglioside A particular class of glycosphingolipid present in nerve tissue and in the spleen.

Gangrene Necrosis or death of tissue, usually due to deficient blood supply.

g. dry Aseptic gangrene due to cessation of blood supply, the veins remaining patent.

g. diabetic Infected gangrene in diabetics.

g. traumatic Gangrene following extensive injury severing blood supply.

Ganser's syndrome A factitious disorder in which individual mimics symptoms of psychosis.

Gardenella vaginalis A bacteria causing vaginitis.

Gardner's syndrome Familial polyposis of colon, an autosomal dominant condition with propensity for development of carcinoma.

Gargoylism A congenital condition characterized by dwarfism, kyphosis, and skeletal abnormalities with mental retardation.

Garlic An edible strongly flavoured bulb containing chemical allicin, possessing antithrombotic properties.

Garré's disease Chronic sclerosing osteomyelitis.

Gartner's duct A vestigial structure representing the persistent mesonephric duct.

Gas mustard Dichlorethyl sulfide, a poisonous gas used in warfare.

Gasoline A distillation product of petroleum often containing toxic additives like tetraethyl lead or tricresyl phosphate.

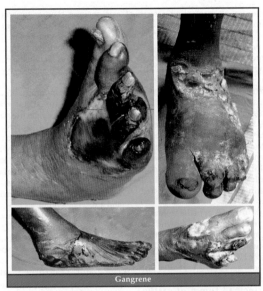
Gangrene

Gastrectomy Surgical removal of a part or total stomach.

Gastro duodenoscopy Visual examination of stomach and duodenum by endoscope.

Gastric analysis Analysis of gastric contents to determine quality of secretion, amount of free and combined hydrochloric acid, absence or presence of blood, bile acid, etc. The test is particularly helpful in cases of Zollinger-Ellison syndrome and gastric malignancy.

Gastric digestion Pepsin secreted in stomach hydrolyzes proteins to proteoses and peptones. HCl is essential for activity of pepsin. It also dissolves collagen, splits nucleoproteins, hydrolyzes disaccharides and kills bacteria. Gastric lipase reduces fat to fatty acids and glycerol.

Gastric glands Tubular glands lying in gastric mucosa that contain peptic cells secreting pepsinogen, oxyntic cells secreting HCl and mucus cell lying at the neck of gland secreting cytoprotective gastric mucin.

Gastric inhibitory polypeptide (GIP) A polypeptide in the cells of duodenum and jejunum which inhibits secretion of gastric juice.

Gastric juice Digestive juice of gastric glands containing HCl, pepsin, mucin, small amount of inorganic salts, intrinsic factor. pH is 0.9 to 1.5, total acidity being equivalent to 30 ml of 1/10 N HCl.

Gastric lavage Emptying out of stomach contents to relieve hiccup; before anesthesia for fear of aspiration and in intestinal obstruction, removal of ingested poisons.

Gastric ulcer Ulcer in the stomach.

Gastrin A group of hormones secreted by antral mucosa that circulating via blood stimulate gastric HCl secretion. Gastrins also affect secretory activity of pancreas, small intestine.

Gastrinoma Tumor of gastrin secreting cells causing Zollinger-Ellison syndrome.

Gastritis Inflammation of stomach characterized by epigastric pain, vomiting and dyspepsia. Gastric mucosa may be atrophic or hypertrophic. Dietary indiscretion, excessive indulgence in alcohol, compylobacter are responsible.

g. acute Manifesting with fever, epigastric pain, vomiting with red angry hyperemic mucosa.

g. hypertrophic SYN Ménétrier's disease; gastric folds are hypertrophic.

Gastrocnemius Larger superficial muscle in the back of lower leg that helps to plantarflex the foot and flex the knee upon the thigh.

Gastrocolic reflex Peristaltic wave in colon induced by entrance of food into stomach.

Gastroenteritis Inflammation of stomach and intestinal tract manifesting with epigastric pain, vomiting, fever and dysentery.

Gastroenterology The branch of medical science dealing with diseases of digestive tract and related structures like esophagus, liver, gallbladder and pancreas.

Gastroepiploic Pertains to stomach and greater omentum.

Gastroesophageal reflux Reflux of acid contents of stomach into lower esophagus due to obesity, hiatus hernia, anticholinergic use, pregnancy, etc.

Gastrografin Diatrizoate meglumine used for radiological examination of GI tract.

Gastro ileal reflex Physiologic relaxation of ileocecal valve resulting from food in stomach.

Gastrointestinal decompression Removal of gas and fluids from GI tract through Kyle's tube.

Gastrojejunostomy Surgical anastomosis between stomach and jejunum.

Gastrolysis Surgical breaking of adhesions between the stomach and adjoining structures.

Gastroptosis Downward displacement of stomach.

Gastrostomy Surgical creation of a stoma in stomach for purpose of introducing food into stomach as in gastroesophageal malignancy.

Gate theory The hypothesis that painful stimuli can be prevented from reaching higher centers for recognition by stimulation of sensory nerves, a key mechanism explaining acupuncture analgesia.

Gaucher cells Large reticulo-endothelial cells with eccentric nucleus seen in Gaucher's disease.

Gaucher's disease A disease due to glycosphingolipid accumulation in RE cells with splenomegaly, bone lesions, skin pigmentation, etc.

Gautt's reflex Blinking of eye following a loud noise-close to ear, a test helpful in people malingering deafness.

Gauss sign Unusual mobility of uterus in early pregnancy.

Gauze Loosely woven cotton.

Gay's glands Large sebaceous circum anal glands.

Geiger counter Instrument for detecting ionizing radiation.

Geiger reflex Contraction of muscles of lower abdomen on stimulation of inner aspect of thigh in females. It corresponds to cremasteric reflex.

Gel Jelly like semisolid state.

Gelasmus Spasmodic laugther of insane.

Gelatin A protein derivative of collagen, used in X-ray films to suspend silver halide crystals, used in capsule making.

Gelatinase An enzyme present in bacteria, molds, and yeasts that liquefies gelatin.

Gelatinous Having consistency of gelatin.

Gelfoam Absorbable gelatin foam, a hemostatic.

Gemfibrozil Lipid lowering agent (mainly triglycerides)

Gemination Development of two teeth or two crowns within a single root.

Gemistocyte Swollen astrocyte with eccentric nucleus seen adjacent to areas of infarct/edema.

Gemmation Cell reproduction by budding.

Gender Sex of an individual.

Gene Basic unit of heredity lying in chromosomes. Their mutation gives rise to new characters.

g. allelic Pairs of genes located at same site on chromosome pair.

g. dominant Gene that expresses without assistance from its allele.

g. histocompatible Gene that controls the specificity of antigenic expression by tissues.

g. recessive Gene that expresses its effect only when present in both chromosomes.

Gene amplification The duplication of regions of DNA to form multiple copies of a specific portion of the original region.

Gene map A map of the human genome, i.e. a map of each cromo-some. Man has 100000 genes that determine the amino acid structure of proteins.

General adaptation syndrome Organism's nonspecific response to stress occurring in 3 stages. 1. alarm reaction with pituitary adrenal hyperactivity to face the stress by fight or flight 2. stage of adaptation when the physical symptoms diminish and 3. stage of exhaustion when body can no longer respond to stress but manifests with stress related emotional disturbances, cardiovascular problems, etc.

Generation 1. The act of forming a new organism 2. Period of time between birth of parents and birth of their children.

Generator pulse Device producing stimuli intermittently, e.g. cardiac pacemaker.

Generic Distinctive, general.

Genesiology The science of reproduction.

Genesis Act of reproducing, generation, origin of any thing.

Gene splicing In genetic molecular bilogy, the substitution of a portion of a DNA is spliced into the DNA of another gene.

Gene therapy Inserting a normal gene into an organism in order to correct a genetic defect.

Genetic code The information system in living cells that determines the amino acid sequence in polypeptides.

Genetic counselling The application of knowledge of genetics in providing advice to parents to have off springs free of hereditary disease.

Genetic engineering The synthesis, modification or repair of genetic DNA by synthetic means.

Genetics The study of heredity and its variation.

Gene transfer Transfer of gene from one person to another for repair of inherited defect in the recipient.

Geneva convention 1864 declaration in Geneva that the sick and wounded victims of war including persons involved in their care like doctors, nurses, ambulance drivers, stretcher bearers are neutral and would not therefore be target of military action.

Genioplasty Plastic surgery of cheek or chin.

Genitalia Reproductive organs.

g. ambiguous External genitalia do not clearly conform to that of male or female.

g. female Labia majora/minora, clitoris, fourchet, vestibular gland, Bartholin's gland, vagina, uterus, two fallopian tubes and two ovaries.

g. male Penis, two seminal vesicles, two ductus deferens, two testes, two bulbourethral glands.

Genitourinary system Organs and parts concerned with urine formation and excretion and reproductive organs.

Genius An individual with exceptional menial or creative capability.

Genome A complete set of chromosomes.

Gentamicin An antibiotic from fungi of genus micro monospora.

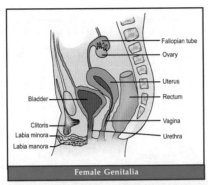

Female Genitalia

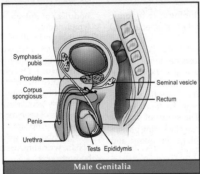

Male Genitalia

Gentian Dried rhizome roots of plant Gentian lutea.

g. violet A dye derived from coaltar. Widely used as a stain in histology, cytology and bacteriology. Also is anti-infective and antifungal.

Genu The knee.

g. valgum Knock knee, a condition in which knees are close to each other and ankles are wide apart (> 5 cm).

g. varum Bowleg, curving out of the legs.

g. recurvatum Hyperextension at the knee joint.

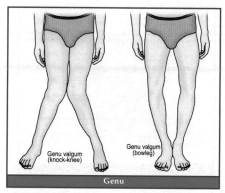

Genu valgum
(knock-knee)

Genu valgum
(bowleg)

Genu

Genus In biology, taxonomic division between species and family.

Geographic tongue Numerous denuded areas on dorsal surface conforming to geographical pattern.

Gerdy's fibers Superficial transverse ligament of palm.

Geriatrics The study of various aspects of aging including physiology, pathology, economic and social problems.

Gerlach's valve Inconstant valve at the opening of appendix into the cecum.

Germ An organism that causes disease.

Germicidal Agent destructive to germs.

Germinal center A light area of lymphocytopoietic cells that occupies the center of lymphatic nodules, of spleen, tonsils and lymph nodes.

Germinal epithelium The epithelium that covers the surface of the genital ridge of an embryo.

Germination Development of impregnated ovum into an embryo or sprouting of spore.

Germinoma Neoplasm arising from germ cells of testes or ovary.

Geroderma Appearance of senility brought about by premature loss of hair, wrinkling of skin, general body atrophy.

Gerotophilia Fondness or love for old.

Gerota's capsule The perirenal fascia.

Gestation Time span from conception to birth, usually 259-287 days.

g. ectopic Fetus develops outside the uterus.

g. interstitial Tubal gestation in which ovum develops in a portion of fallopian tube.

g. secondary Gestation in which the ovum becomes dislodged from the original seat of implantation and continues to develop at new site.

Gestation assessment Assessment of fetal age and maturity by ultrasound.

Gesture A body movement that assists in expression of thoughts (body language).

Ghon's focus Sharply defined peripheral lesion in X-ray chest with hilar lymphadenitis, a feature of primary kochs.

Giant cell A large cell with several nuclei.

Giant cell tumor 1. A connective tissue tumor of bone marrow 2. tumor of tendon sheath 3. epulis 4. chondroblastoma.

Giardia A flagellated protozoa inhabiting intestinal mucosa.

Giardiasis Infestation with *Giardia lamblia*.

Gibbus Humped back, commonly due to compression fracture, collapse.

Gibson's murmur Murmur of patent ductus arteriosus.

Giddiness Light headed sensation.

Giemsa's stain A stain for staining blood smears for differential count and detection of parasitic microorganisms.

Gifford's reflex pupillary contraction upon effort to close eyelids held apart.

Gigantism Excessive physical development due to increased growth hormone secretion, fate fusion of bones (eunuchoid gigantism).

Gigli's saw A wire saw previously used to cut symphisis pubis for delivery of fetus.

g. median rhouboid Diamond shaped inflammation on dorsum of tongue

g. Moeller's Chronic superficial glossitis.

Gilbert's syndrome Hereditary deficiency of glucuronyl transferase with unconjugated hyperbilirubinemia.

Gilles de la Tourette's syndrome A neurological disorder manifesting with muscular coordination, ticks and barks.

Gimbernant's ligament The lateral portion of inguinal ligament forming medial portion of femoral ring.

Gingiva The tissue surrounding the neck of tooth in maxilla and mandible. Gingiva has free edge surrounding anatomic crown of tooth, a labial surface and lingual surface.

Gingivectomy Excision of gingiva in periodontal disease.

Gingivitis Inflammation of gums characterized by redness, swelling and tendency to bleed.

g. necrotizing ulcerative Ulcerative and necrotic gingivostomatitis, usually by fusiform organisms.

Giralde's organ A remnant of wolffian body at posterior side of testicle.

Girdle Structure that resembles a circular belt or band.

g. pelvic Composed of the ileosacral and femoral articulation.

g. shoulder Two clavicles, scapulae and humeral articulation.

Girdle symptoms Feeling of constriction in the chest, as in tabes dorsalis, or cord compression.

Gitter cell A honey combed cell packed with lipid granules.

Gitalin A cardiac glycoside.

Glabella That portion of frontal bone lying between the superciliary arches just above root of nose.

Glacial Resembling ice.

Gland A secretory organ.

g. acinous Glands with secreting units in shape of sacs each possessing a narrow lumen.

g. apocrine Glands in which the secreting cells lose some of their cytoplasmic contents in the form of secretion, e.g. some sweat glands, mammary gland.

g. Bartholin Numerous glands that open into the vestibule of vagina akin to bulbourethral glands of male.

gs. ceruminous Glands in external auditory canal, secreting cerumen.

gs. Ebner's Serous glands of tongue located in the region of valate papillae whose ducts open into the furrows surrounding the papillae.

g. mammary A compound alveolar gland secreting milk. It has 15-20 lactiferrous ducts each one discharging milk through a separate orifice on the surface of the ripple. The dilatation of these ducts form the milk reservoir during lactation.

g. mixed 1. Glands having both exocrine and endocrine function, e.g. pancreas 2. Salivary glands secreting mucus and serous secretions.

g. pineal Tiny conical body lying between two superior quardrigeminal bodies, connected with thalamus.

g. parathyroid 4 in number of size 6 × 4 mm lying at the lower edge of thyroid gland secreting parathormone.

g. prostate Gland surrounding neck of bladder and upper urethra, consists of a median lobe and two lateral lobes, weighing about 20 gm. Secretes thin opalescent slightly alkaline fluid that forms part of semen.

g. sebaceous A simple or branched alveolar gland secreting sebum, the ducts opening into hair follicle.

s.g. of Skene Two glands at the margin of female urethra, opening into lower urethra on either side.

g. thyroid A ductless gland located in the base of neck; below consists of two lateral lobes connected by isthmus. Histologically consists of large number of closed vesicles called follicles lined with tall columnar cells synthesizing T3 and T4.

s. g. Tyson's Tiny sebaceous glands in the inner surface of perpuce and on the glans penis.

g. Zuckerkandl's Accessory thyroid gland between genioglosus muscles.

Glander Contagious disease of horses caused by *Pseudomonas mallei*, transmitted often to man.

Glans The head of the clitoris/penis.

Glanzman's thrombasthenia Congenital abnormality of platelets with easy bruising, prolonged bleeding time and poor clot retraction.

Glasgow Coma Scale A scale for evaluating and quantitating the degree of coma by determining the best motor response, verbal and eye opening to standard stimuli. A score of 9 or greater excludes diagnosis of coma.
It also has prognostic significance in head injury patients.

Glass photochromatic The glass becoming dark on exposure to light and regaining transparency on being away from light

g. bifocal Glasses in which the refractory power of lower portion of glass is for near vision and the upper portion for distant vision.

Glaucoma Raised intraocular pressure which can end in blindness. Narrowing of filtration angle, and sclerosis of canal of Schlemm, ocular diseases are responsible.

Glenoid cavity The socket in scapula that receives head of humerus.

Glenoid fossa The fossa of temporal bone that receives the condyle or capitulum of the mandible.

Gliadin A water insoluble protein present in the gluten of wheat.

Glioblastoma A malignant tumor of neurological cells.

Glioma A sarcoma of neurological origin.

Gliomatosis Formation of glioma.

Glipizide Sulphonyl urea compound for diabetes.

Globulin Simple protein present in blood.

g. antihemophilic A clotting component of plasma, deficient in hemophiliacs.

g. gamma That fraction of globulin responsible for body immunity.

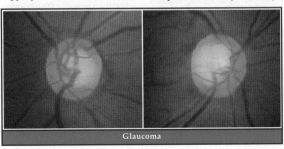

Glaucoma

g. antilymphocyte Globulin from a person who has become immunized to lymphocytes; used as immunosuppressants.

Globus hystericus Sensation of lump in throat in hysterics.

Glomangioma A benign tumor developing from an arteriovenous glomus of skin.

Glomerular disease A group of disorders mostly autoimmune but some secondary (systemic disease, infectious disease, metabolic disease, hypertension, poison, etc.) that involve the glomerulus manifesting with proteinuria, hematuria and hypertension.

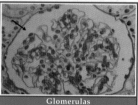
Glomerulas

Glomeruli Cluster of capillary vessels enveloped in Bowman's capsule in cortex of kidney.

Glomerulonephritis A form of nephritis where lesions are confined primarily to glomeruli.

Glomerulopathy Any disease of glomeruli.

Glomerulosclerosis Fibrosis of glomeruli.

Glomoid Similar appearance to glomeruli.

Glomus A small round mass made up of tiny blood vessels and found in stroma containing many nerve fibers.

Glossina Tsetse flies that transmit trypanosomes, agents of trypanosomiasis.

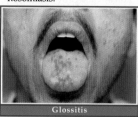
Glossitis

Glossitis Inflammation of tongue; can be acute, painful or chronic, due to infection or avitaminosis (B complex group).

Glossodynamo meter Device for measuring contractile power of tongue muscles.

Glossograph An instrument for measuring tongue's movement during speech.

Glossopharyngeal nerve Ninth cranial nerve carrying taste sensation from posterior third of tongue and distributed to pharynx, meninges, parotids and ears.

Glossotrichia Hairy tongue due to greatly elongated filiform papillae often that give the tongue a hairy appearance, often associated with antibiotic therapy.

Glottis Larynx with the two vocal cords and the intervening space, the rime glottides.

Glucagon Polypeptide hormone secreted by alpha cells of pancreas that raises blood sugar and relaxes smooth muscles of GI tract.

Glucagonoma A malignant tumor of alpha cells of pancreas.

Glucocerebroside A cerebroside with glucose in the molecule, present in tissues in patients of Gaucher's disease.

Glucocorticoid A class of adrenal hormones that are released in response to stress and effect carbohydrate and protein metabolism.

Glucogenesis Formation of glucose from glycogen.

Glucokinase An enzyme in liver that converts glucose to glucose 6 phosphate.

Gluconeogenesis Formation of glycogen from noncarbohydrate sources like amino or fatty acids.

Glucopenia Abnormal low concentration of glucose.

Glucosamine An amino saccharide present in chitin and mucus.

Glucose Called D-glucose, the primary fuel of human body; in tissue either converted to glycogen, or fat or is oxidized to CO_2 and H_2O.

Glucose-6-phosphate dehydrogenase An essential enzyme for pentose-phosphate pathway of glucose metabolism that generates reduced glutathione.

Glucose tolerance test A test performed by giving 1.5 gm/kg wt of glucose to a patient orally in empty stomach and then examining blood samples every ½ hr for 2 hours. The test helps to assess ability of patient to metabolize glucose and is of primary importance in diagnosis of prediabetic states and

hyperinsulinemia.

Glucoside A glycoside that upon hydrolysis yields glucose and additional products, e.g. digitalin, present in digitalis.

Glucosuria Abnormal amount of sugar in urine.

Glucoronic acid An acid that possesses detoxifying action.

Glucuronide Combination of glucuronic acid with phenol, alcohol, etc.

Glutamic acid An amino acid formed during hydrolysis of proteins. It is the only amino acid metabolized by brain.

Glutamine The monoamide of aminoglutaric acid, essential for hydrolysis of proteins.

Glutaminase An enzyme that catalyzes the breakdown of glutamine into glutamic acid and ammonia.

Glutaraldehyde A sterilizing agent effective against all microorganisms.

Glutathione A tripeptide of glutamic acid, cystine and glycine, important for cellular respiration.

Gluten Vegetable albumin, a protein obtained from wheat and other grain.

Gluten free diet Elimination of gluten from the diet by exclusion of all products prepared from wheat, rye, barley and oats.

Gluten induced enteropathy Adult celiac disease manifesting with malabsorption and diarrhea.

Gluburide Sulphonyl urea compound for diabetes mellitus.

Glycerin $C_3H_8O_3$ A trihydric alcohol present in chemical combination in all fats used extensively as a solvent, preservative and emolient.

Glyceride An ester of glycerin compounded with an acid.

Glyceryl The trivalent radical of glycerol.

g. monostearate An emulsifying agent used in preparing creams and ointments.

g. trinitrate Nitroglycerin, agent used in angina pectoris.

Glycorbiarsol An arsenical amebicide

Glycocholic acid Bile acid present in bile, a conjugate of cholic acid and glycine.

Glycogen Polysaccharide; the storage form of carbohydrate in the body (liver and muscle).

Glycogenase An enzyme in the liver that hydrolyzes glycogen to glucose.

Glycogenesis Formation of glycogen from glucose.

Glycogenolysis Conversion of glycogen to glucose.

Glycogen storage disease Inherited disease with abnormal storage of glycogen in the liver.

gsd type I - (von Gierke's disease) Glucose-6-phosphatase deficiency.

gsd type II - Lysosomal alpha glucosidase deficiency

gsd type III - Deficiency of debranching enzymes.

gsd type IV - (Anderson's disease) brancher enzyme deficiency with hepatic failure.

gsd type V- (McArdle's disease) Muscle phosphorylase deficiency.

gsd type VI - Deficiency of liver phosphorylase with growth retardation, hepatomegaly, acidosis and hypoglycemia.

gsd type VII - Deficiency of muscle phospho-fructokinase with weakness and cramping.

Glycolipid Lipid with carbohydrate and nitrogen, but no phosphoric acid; found in myelin sheath of nerves.

Glyconeogenesis *SYN* – gluconeogenesis

Glycophorin Glycoprotein that spans the bilipid layer of erythrocyte membrane, functioning as a channel for passage of anions in and out of red cells.

Glycopyrrolate An anticholinergic drug used in preanesthetic medication to reduce GI and bronchial secretions.

Glycoside A plant product which on hydrolysis yields sugar and additional products.

Glycosphingolipids Carbohydrate containing fatty acid derivatives of ceramide, e.g. cerebrosides, gangliosides and ceramide oligosaccharides. Abnormal accumulation of them in nervous tissue due to deficiency of metabolizing enzymes leads to death.

Glycosuria Presence of glucose in the urine resulting from insulin deficiency, reduced renal threshold, excessive glycogenolysis or adreno pituitary disorders.

Gnat Insects smaller than mosquitoes that include black flies, sandflies and midgets.

Gnathostoma A genus of nematodes that inhabit alimentary tract of domestic animals and occasionally infest man.

Gonosia The perceptive faculty of recognizing persons, things and forms.

Goblet cells A unicellular gland seen in intestinal and respiratory tract, that secretes mucus by rupture of cell wall.

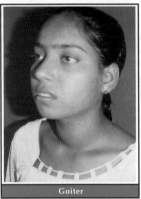
Goiter

Goiter An enlargement of thyroid gland.

g. adenomatous Thyroid enlargement due to adenoma.

g. colloid Thyromegaly with great increase in follicular contents.

g. cystic Cystic thyromegaly; cyst formation being due to degeneration within an adenoma.

g. diffuse Diffuse increase in thyroid tissue in contrast to its nodular form as in adenomatous goiter.

g. endemic Thyromegaly due to iodine deficiency in water in some geographical areas.

g. exophthalmic Grave's disease where antithyroid receptor antibodies play the dominant role with increased TSH and stimulation of thyroid.

g. lingual Hypertrophied aberrant thyroid tissue forming a mass on dorsum of tongue posteriorly.

g. toxic Goiter with excessive production of thyroxine and triodo thyronine.

Gold Yellow metal used as alloy (mixed with copper, silver, platinum for dental use (crown, inlays, orthodontics); sodium thiomalate and thioglucose used in rheumatoid arthritis.

Gold standard A standard with which other tests or procedures are compared.

Golgi apparatus A lamellar membranous structure near the nucleus. In secretory cells it functions to concentrate and package the secretory products.

Golgi cells Multipolar nerve cells in the cerebral cortex and posterior bones of spinal cord.

Golgi corpuscle A sensory nerve ending or receptor found in tendons and aponeureses.

Goll's tract *SYN* — fasciculus gracilis, posterior white column of spinal cord.

Gonad A generic term referring to male and female sex glands (testes and ovary).

Gonadal dysgenesis Congenital disorder with failure of ovaries to respond to pituitary gonadotropin stimulation resulting in amenorrhea, failure of sexual maturation and short stature. Webbing of neck, cubitus valgus may be present. Genetic pattern is 45 XO (*SYN*—Turner's syndrome).

Gonadotrope A gonadotropic hormone.

Gonadotrophic Relates to stimulation of gonads.

Gonadotropin

g. s. anterior pituitary Secreted by anterior pituitary as FSH and LH, called interstitial cell stimulating hormone in male (ICSH)

g. chorionic Produced by chorionic villi of placenta.

Gonadotropin releasing hormone Produced in hypothalamus, it acts on pituitary to cause release of gonadotropic hormones.

Goniometer Apparatus to measure joint movement and angles.

Gonioscope Device for inspecting the angle of anterior chamber of eye and determining ocular mobility and rotations.

Goniotomy Incision at angle of anterior chamber to promote free flow of aqueous into canals of schleim.

Gonococcus Neisseria gonorrhoeae, causative organism of gonorrhea.

Gonorrhea Contagious inflammation of genital mucous membrane manifesting with burning micturition, painful induration of penis in males, vaginitis and cervicitis in females. Can cause salpingo-oophoritis ending in tubal blockage and sterility in female and chronic prostatitis in male. Can spread to blood to involve principally the joints.

Goodell's sign Softening of the cervix during pregnancy.

Goodpasture's syndrome IgA nephropathy with hemoptysis and hemosiderosis.

Goose flesh Transient roughness of skin with contraction of arrector pili muscles, as a reaction to cold or shock.

Good Samaritan Law Legal stipulation for protection of those who give first aid in emergency situation.

Godon's reflex Extension of great toe on pressure to calf muscles, a sign of pyramidal tract disease.

Gorget An instrument grooved to protect soft tissues from injury as pointed instrument is inserted in a body cavity.

Goserelin A synthetic LHRH, used in treatment of prostatic cancer, endometriosis

Gossypol A toxic chemical of cotton seed.

Gouge Instrument for cutting away hard tissue of bone.

Goundou Bilateral hyperostosis of nasal bones.

Gout Hereditary metabolic disease of uric acid metabolism with hyperuricemia and arthropathy.

g. tophaceous Gout marked by development of tophi (deposits of sodium urate) in the joints, external ear and about the finger nails.

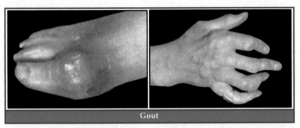

Gout

Gower's sign Clinical sign of muscular dystrophy in childhood. Affected children use their arms to push themselves erect by moving their hands up their thighs.

Gower's tract Spino-cerebellar tract

Graffian follicle A mature follicle of ovary which on rupture discharges the ovum. Within the ruptured graffian follicle, the corpus luteum develops that secrets estrogen and progesterone to help in implantation of fertilized ovum.

Gracile Slender, thin built.

Gracile nucleus Nucleus in medulla oblongata where fasciculus gracilis ends.

Gracilis A long slender muscle on the medial aspect of thigh.

Gradenigo's syndrome Suppurative otitis media with abducens nerve palsy.

Gradient A slope or grade.

Graefe's sign Failure of the upper eyelids to follow a downward movement of the eyeball, a feature of Grave's disease.

Graft Transplanted tissue in a part of body for repair of a defect.

g. allogeneic Graft from genetically non identical donor of the same species as the recipient, (allograft)

g. cadaver Grafting tissue taken from cadaver like cornea, bone, heart, lungs, kidney, etc. soon after molecular death.

g. fascicular Nerve graft with each bundle of nerve stitched separately.

g. full thickness Graft of entire layer of skin without the subcutaneous fat.

g. homologous The donor is of same species as the recipient.

g. isologous Graft in which the donor and recipient are genetically identical, i.e. identical twins.

g. lamellar Very thin corneal graft used to replace superficial opaque corneal layer.

g. pedicle A skin graft that is left attached at one end until the free end has begun to receive blood supply from grafted site.

g. sieve Graft in which a section of skin is removed except for small regularly spaced areas that grow to cover the donor site.

g. thiersch's Graft in which only

epidermis and small amount of dermis is used.

Graham's law The rate of diffusion of a gas is inversely proportional to the square root of its density.

Gram A unit of weight (mass) of metric system equal to 1000 mg.

Gram's method A method for staining bacteria, a heat fixed blood film is stained with gentian violet, rinsed off and, then iodine solution is put and rinsed off and decolorized in 90% ethyl alcohol or acetone. Then the slide is counterstained with carbolfuschsin or safranine. Gram-positive organisms retain violet stain while gram-negative organisms become red.

Grandiose In psychiatry, unrealistic and exaggerated concept of self worth, importance, ability, power and wealth.

Granlocyte macrophage colony stimulates factor: A glycoprotein that stimulation proliferation of neutrophils, monocytes and macrophages; both GCSF and GMCSF helpful in treating chemotherapy induced neutropenia

Granular Of the nature of granules, rough.

Granular cast Coarse or fine granules or casts, sometimes yellowish, soluble in acetic acid; seen in inflammatory and degenerative nephropathies (chronic renal failure).

Granulation Formation of granules, often by outgrowth of capillaries

g. arachnoidal Villus like projections of subarachnoid layer of the meninges that project into the superior sagittal sinus and other venous sinuses of brain. Though these CSF is absorbed into venous systems.

g. exuberant Excessive mass of granulation tissue formed in the process of healing of wound or ulcer.

Granule A minute mass in a cell that has an outline but no apparent structure.

g. acidophilic Granules easily staining with acid dyes, e.g. granules in eosinophils.

g. azurophil Granules that take stain with azure dyes easily, found in lymphocytes and monocytes.

g.s. chromatin Small masses of deeply staining substances suspended within the meshes of lining network of nucleus of a cell.

g. chromophil Granule of chromophil substance present in cytoplasm of neurones (e.g. Nissl)

g.s. metachromatic Granules found in protoplasm of numerous bacteria, irregular in size and stain deeply.

g. Schuffner's Coarse and red granules in parsitized erythrocytes in malaria.

g.s. zymogen Granules present in gland cells esp. secretory cells of pancreas, chief cells of gastric glands and serous cells of salivary gland. They are precursors of enzyme secreted by these glands.

Granulocyte A granular leukocyte, i.e. neutrophil, eosinophil and basophil.

Granulocyte colony stimulating factor A glycoprotein that stimulates or neutrophil proliferation.

Granulocyte macrophage colony stimulating factor A glycoprotein that stimulation proliferation of enutrophils, monocytes and macrophages both GCSF and GMCSF helpful in treating chemotherapy induced Neutropenia

Granuloma A granular tumor or growth of lymphoid and epithelioid cell. It occurs in various infectious diseases like leprosy, yaws, syphilis, etc.

g. dental Granuloma developing at root of a tooth, secondary to pulp infection. It contains chronic inflammatory cells, debris and bacteria.

g. eosinophilic A form of xanthomatosis with eosinophilia and cystic degeneration of bone.

g. inguinale Granulomatous ulcerative disease caused by Donovania granulomatis, a gram -ve coccobacillus.

g. Wegner's A rare disease of unknown etiology characterized by widespread granulomatous lesions of the bronchi, necrotising arteriolitis, and glomerulonephritis.

Granulocytopenia Reduction in blood granulocyte count.

Granulomatosis The development of multiple granulomas.

Granulopoiesis Formation of blood granulocytes.

Granulosa cell tumor Tumor of ovary secreting estrogens, hence feminizing in nature.

Granulosa theca cell tumor Ovarian tumor related to graffian follicle, feminizing in function.

Graphesthesia The ability by which outlines, numbers, words, symbols, traced or written upon skin are recognized.

Grasp To hold.

Grattage Removal of morbid growth by rubbing with a brush.

Gravel Coarse sand; concretions in kidneys, made up of calcium, oxalate, phosphate, uric acid.

Grave's disease Exophthalmic goiter.

Gravid Pregnant

Gravitation Force that draws every particle of matter.

Gravity Property of possessing weight. The force of earth's gravitational attraction.

g. specific Weight of a substance compared with an equal volume of water.

Gray Colour between extremes of black and white.

Gray matter Nervous tissue lying peripherally in brain and somewhat centrally in spinal cord where myelinated fibers do not predominate.

Gray syndrome of the newborn Ashen gray colour, vomiting, cyanosis and flaccidity of newborn when treated with chloramphenicol.

Grinder's disease Chronic lung disease due to dust inhalation (*SYN*-pneumoconiosis).

Gripe Acute infectious disease with fever, malaise, headache, cough and nasal congestion (*SYN*-influenza).

Gripes Spasmodic bowel pain, intestinal colic.

Griseofulvin An antifungal antibiotic given orally.

Grits Coarsely ground corn.

Groin Inguinal region, area between thigh and trunk.

Grommet Ventilation tube placed across the tympanic membrane for equalization of pressure in treatment of retracted tympanic membrane secondary to eustachian block/catarrh.

Groove Long narrow channel.

g. bicipital Groove for long tendon of biceps brachi on anterior surface of humerus.

g. carotid Broad groove on the inner surface of sphenoid bone lateral to the body accommodating carotid artery and cavernous sinus.

g. Harrison's Groove or line extending laterally from xiphoid process, marking attachment of diaphragm, prominent in patients of rickets.

g. malleolar Groove on anterior surface of distal tibia that lodges tendon of tibialis posterior and flexor digitorum longus.

Ground bundle A bundle of short descending nerve fibers surrounding gray matter of spinal cord

Ground itch Skin inflammation in foot due to invasion by larva of hookworm.

Ground substance The material that occupies the intercellular spaces in fibrous connective tissue, cartilage or bone.

Grouping Classification of individual traits according to shared characteristics.

g. blood Classification of blood of different individuals according to agglutinating and hemolyzing properties.

Group therapy A form of simultaneous psychotherapy involving many patients by psychotherapist.

Growing pain Pain in the musculoskeletal system in growing children.

Growth The progressive increase in size or development both physical/mental in a living thing.

Growth hormone Anterior pituitary secretion that regulates human growth; *SYN* – somatotropin.

Grunfelder's reflex Faning of the toes with extension of great toe on pressure over posterior fontanel.

g. suit A type of garment having inflatable compartments over legs and abdomen to prevent pooling of blood.

Guaiacol O-methoxyphenol used as antiseptic, germicidel, intestinal antiseptic and expectorant.

Guanabenz A vasodilator.

Guanadrel Adrenergic blocking agent.

Guanase Enzyme that converts guanine into xanthine

Guanethidine A sympatholytic drug used in hypertension

Guanidine A protein product.

Guanine $C_5H_5N_5O$. An organic compound of animal and vegetable nucleic acids. Uric acid is its metabolic end product.

Guanosine A nucleoside formed from guanine and ribosome, It is a major constituent of RNA and DNA.

Gubernaculum A structure that guides, a cord like structure linking two structures.

g. dentis A connective tissue band connecting unerupted tooth with overlying gum.

g. testis A fibrous band extending from caudal end of fetal testis through the inguinal canal to scrotal sac; playing no role in descent of testis,

Gudden's law In division of a nerve, degeneration in the proximal portion is towards nerve cell.

Guide wire Wire helpful in positioning and manipulating an intravenous or intraarterial catheter.

Guillain-Barré-syndrome Polyneuritis with flaccid muscular palsy following an infectious disease.

Guillotine Instrument for excising tonsils and laryngeal growth.

Guilt Feeling grief for doings what is thought to be wrong.

Guinea pig A small rodent used in laboratory research.

Guinea worm Dracunculus medinensis.

Gum The fleshy tissue covering the alveolar process of jaw.

Gum boil Abscess of jaw.

Gumma Encapsulated granulomatous tumor with central necrosis, characteristic of tertiary syphilis seen in skin, liver, testis, brain and bone.

Gustatory Pertains to sensation of taste.

Gustometry Measurement of sense of acuteness of taste.

Gut The bowel or intestine.

Gut associated lymphoid issue The lymphoid tissue of tonsil, appendix, Peyer's patches, primarily B lymphocytes

Gutta-percha Purified dried latex of certain trees, used in dentistry for root canal treatment.

Guttering Groove in bone.

Guyon's canal A tunnel on ulnars side of wrist formed by pisiform bone and hook of hammate for passage of ulnarx nerve

Guyon's sign Ballotment of kidney.

Gymnophobia Abnormal aversion to seeing a naked body.

Gynandroid Individual having hermaphroditic sexual characteristics to be mistaken for a person of opposite sex.

Gynecoid Resembling female.

Gynecology The study of disease of female reproductive organs including breast.

Gynecomastia Abnormally large mammary tissue in male (> 2.5 cm in dm) often secreting milk.

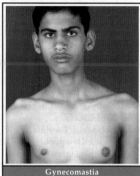
Gynecomastia

Gypsum Hydrated calcium sulfate, used for plaster, dental casting.

Gyrus Convolution of the cerebral hemispheres.

g. angular Gyrus of the parietal lobe that embraces the posterior end of superior temporal sulcus.

g. callosal A large gyrus on the medial surface of cerebral hemisphere lying directly above corpus callosum.

g. dentate Gyrus lying above hippocampal gyrus

g. Hescl's Transverse temporal gyrus.

g. pre central Gyrus immediately anterior to central sulcus containing the pyramidal cells (motor area).

g. post central Gyrus immediately posterior to the central sulcus of cerebrum containing sensory cortex.

g. of Retzius The supra and sub-callosal gyri.

g. supramarginal Gyrus in the inferior parietal lobule twisting about the upper terminus of the sylvian fissure.

g. uncinate Anterior hooked portion of hippocampal gyrus.

H

Habenula A whip like structure; A stalk attached to pineal body of brain; a narrow band like structure.

Habenular commissure A transverse band of fibers connecting the two habenular areas.

Habenular trigone A depressed triangular area located on the lateral aspect of the posterior third ventricle.

Habilitation The process of education and training persons with disability both physical and mental to improve their ability to function in society.

Habit A motor pattern following frequent repetition or an involuntary act that comes as a reflex action.

h. spasm Involuntary spasmodic muscle contraction; *SYN*-tic.

Habituation Act of becoming accustomed to anything from frequent use.

Habitus A physical appearance that indicates a tendency to certain diseases or positioning of internal organs in certain planes.

Hacking cough Recurrent non-productive cough.

Hemogogus A genus of mosquitoes which serves as a vector for yellow fever.

Hailey Hailey disease Benign familial pemphigus.

Hageman factor Blood coagulation factor, helps in kinin synthesis.

Hair A thin keratinized and cornified structure arising from hair follicle. The shaft of hair has 3

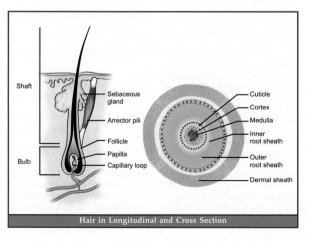

Shaft
Bulb

Sebaceous gland
Arrector pili
Follicle
Papilla
Capillary loop

Cuticle
Cortex
Medulla
Inner root sheath
Outer root sheath
Dermal sheath

Hair in Longitudinal and Cross Section

layers, the outer cortex containing the pigment melanin. Hair of eyebrow has life of 3-5 months and that of head 2-5 years with continuous turnover.

h. auditory An epithelial cell to which are attached delicate hair like processes. These are present in the spiral organ of Corti concerned with hearing and in crista ampularis, macula utriculi and macula sacculi concerned with equilibrium.

h. bamboo Sparse brittle hair with bamboo like nodes. *SYN* — trichorrhexis nodosa.

h. beaded Swellings and constrictions in the hair shaft due to developmental defect; monilethrix.

h. gustatory Fine hair like processes extending from ends of gustatory cells in a taste bud.

h. kinky Short, sparse, kinky hair, poorly pigmented associated with kinky hair disease.

Hair analysis Investigation for chemical composition of hair to exclude toxic chemical intoxication, state of nutrition and monitoring course of certain diseases.

Hair bulb The lower expanded portion of a hair.

Hair follicle An invagination of the epidermis that forms a cylindrical depression extending into subepidermal layer. Sebaceous glands and arrectores pili muscles are attached to these hair follicles.

Hair papilla A projection of dermis extending into hair bulb at the bottom of hair follicle. It contains capillaries through which hair receives its nourishment.

Hair transplantation Technique of transferring skin containing hair follicles from one place to another; done to treat alopecia.

Hairy tongue Tongue covered with hair like papilla with threads of Aspergillus or Candida.

Halazone A chloramine water disinfectant.

Halcinonide A corticosteroid.

Half-life 1. Time required for radioactive substance to reduce to one-half its energy due to metabolism or excretion. 2. Time required for radioactive nuclei undergoing decay to lose half their radioactivity. 3. Time taken by body to inactivate half of the administered drug/chemical (biological half-life).

Half way house A facility to house mental patients who do not need hospitalization but who are not ready for independent living.

Halibut liver oil An oil obtained from liver of halibut fish rich in vit A and vit D.

Halide Compound containing a halogen i.e., bromine, chlorine, fluorine or iodine.

Halitosis Bad breath, offensive breath.

Hallervorden Spatz disease An inherited progressive degenerative disease beginning in childhood manifesting with rigidity, athetotic movements and mental retardation.

Hallucination A sense of false perception.

h. auditory Imaginary perceptions of sounds, usually voices.

h. gustatory Sense of tasting.

h. hypnagogic Pre-sleep phenomena having the same practical significance as a dream but experienced while consciousness persists.

h. olfactory Hallucination involving smell.

h. tactile False sensation of insects creeping under skin.

h. visual Sensation of seeing objects that are not real.

Hallucinogen Drugs that produce hallucination e.g., LSD.

Hallucinosis The state of having hallucinations.

Hallux The great toe.

h. dolorosus Pain in the metatarsophalangeal joint of great toe due to flat foot.

h. rigidus Painful restricted mobility of great toe.

h. valgus Displacement of great toe toward other toes.

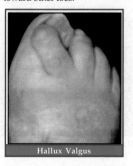

Hallux Valgus

h. varus Displacement of great toe away from other toes.

Halo 1. A circle of light surrounding a shinning body. 2. A ring surrounding the macula.

h. Fick's A colored halo around light, observed in some people wearing contact lens.

h. glaucomatous Visual perception of rainbow like colors due to glaucoma induced edema of cornea.

Halofantrine Antimalarial agent.

Halogen A substance forming salt like chlorine, iodine, bromine and fluorine which combine with metals to form salt and with hydrogen to form acid.

Haloperidol Antipsychotic agent used in schizophrenia.

Haloprogin Halogenated phenolic ether, fungicidal.

Halothane Fluorinated hydrocarbon used as general anesthetic.

Halsted's operation An operation for inguinal hernia, also radical mastectomy

Halsted's suture An interrupted suture for intestinal wounds

Hamartoma Disorganized self-limited, benign growth of normal tissue; when occurring in blood vessels called hemangioma; common to lungs and kidneys.

Hamate bone The medial bone in the distal row of carpal bones of wrist.

Hammer An instrument with rubber cap to tap muscle, tendon or nerve to initiate reflex response.

Hammer finger Flexion deformity of the distal joint of a finger, caused by avulsion of extensor tendon.

Hamstrings The group of three muscles on the posterior aspect of thigh comprised of semi-membranous, semitendinosus and biceps femoris that flex the leg, extend and adduct the thigh.

Ham test Test for diagnosis of paroxysmal nocturnal hemoglobinuria. The red cells lyse in acidic medium.

Hand That part of body attached to forearm at the wrist consisting of 8 carpal bones, 5 metacarpals and 14 phallanges.

Hand-foot-mouth disease Highly infectious coxsackie virus causing painful ulcerative and vesicular lesions of hand and feet.

Handicap Mental or physical impairment preventing or interfering with normal physical and mental activities.

Hand-Schuller-Christian disease A lipid storage disease manifesting with histiocytic granuloma in skull, skin and viscera often with exophthalmos and diabetes insipidus.

Hang nail Partly detached piece of skin at root or lateral edge of finger or toe nail.

Hanger's lines The structural orientation of fibrous issue of skin.

Hanger's muscle Muscular fibers from insertion of pectoralis major over the bicipital groove to the insertion of lattissimus dorsi.

Hangman's fracture Fracture dislocation of upper cervical spine due to judicial hanging.

Hangover Headache, depression, fatigue and irritability present some times after consumption of alcohol or CNS depressant.

Hansen bacillus Lepra bacillus.

Haploid Presence of half the number of chromosomes (i.e., 23) as found in ovum and sperm.

Hapten That portion of an antigen determining its immunological specificity.

Haptoglobin Mucoprotein accepting hemoglobin in plasma on release in hemolytic conditions. Hence haptoglobin is decreased in hemolytic disorders and increased in certain inflammatory conditions.

Hardness Water with less cleansing action due to presence of soluble salts of calcium and magnesium. These compounds precipitate with soap.

Hare lip A cleft in the upper lip due to faulty fusion of median nasal process and the lateral maxillary processes.

Hare lip suture A twisted figure of eight suture used in surgical correction of hare lip.

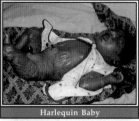
Harlequin Baby

Harlequin fetus Newborn with skin features of ichthyosis with deep red fissures.

Harpoon A device with a hook on the end for obtaining small pieces of tissue.

Harris-Benedict equation Equation for calculating basal body energy expenditure.

Hartman's solution A solution of 0.6 gram NaCl, 0.03 gram KCl, 0.02 gram $CaCl_2$ and 0.31 gram sodium lactate in 100 ml of water used for fluid and electrolyte replacement.

Hartnup disease A disorder of tryptophan metabolism manifesting with pellagra.

Harvey, William British physician who described circulation of blood.

Hashimoto's struma Hashimoto's thyroiditis.

Hashish An extract from flower, stalk and leaves of cannabis saliva, smoked or chewed for its euphoric effect.

Hasner's valve Fold of mucous membrane at the opening of nasolacrimal duct.

h. burn burning sensation behind sternum due to acid reflux

h. failure failure of cardiac contraction to maintain adequate circulation for tissue oxygenation.

h. lung machine a device that maintains function of heart and lung during bypass surgery or valve replacement.

Hassal's corpuscle Spherical bodies with central area of degeneration with surrounding flattened cells, seen in thymus gland.

Haunch The hips and buttocks.

Haustra The sacculated pouches of colon, formed because the longitudinal bands are shorter than the gut.

Haversian canal Minute vascular canals in bone transmitting nutrient vessels.

Haversian gland Minute projections from the surface of synovial tissue into the joint space.

Haversian system Architectural unit of bone consisting of haversian canals, with alternate layers of intercellular matrix surrounding it in concentric cylinders.

Hay fever Allergic rhinitis usually caused by airborne pollens, fungal spores.

Head 1. The part of animal body containing brain and organs for vision, hearing, smell and taste. 2. Proximal end of bone.

Headache Acute or chronic pain over the skull not confined to any nerve distribution.

h. cluster Headache occurring in cluster usually in male soon after falling asleep; akin to migraine.

h. exertional Headache of short duration, appearing after strenuous physical activity, relieved by rest.

h. histamine Headache resulting from ingestion of histamine containing foods.

h. post lumbar puncture Leakage of CSF after lumbar puncture leading to CSF hypotension and headache.

h. tension Contraction of musculotendinous structures of scalp giving rise to a band line compressing around head in situations producing mental strain.

Healing Restoration to normal mental or physical state.

Health A state of complete mental, physical and social wellbeing, not being mere absence of disease or infirmity.

Health certificate An official statement signed by a physician attesting to state of health.

Health education Educational program aimed for improving and maintaining good health.

Health hazard Any substance, condition or circumstances not conducive to good health.

Hearing aid An apparatus amplifying sound, worn by persons with impaired hearing.

Heart A hollow muscular 4-chambered contractile pump in the chest cavity, the principal organ of circulating system.

Heavy chain disease Abnormality of immunoglobulin when excessive quantities of alpha, gamma, mu or epsilon chain are produced causing fever lymphadenopathy, hepatosplenomegaly, malabsorption etc.

Hegar's sign A sign of early pregnancy when in bimanual examination lower part of uterus is easily compressed.

Heimlich maneuver A technique for removing foreign body from trachea and pharynx by giving thrust on victim's upper abdomen.

Heinz bodies Granules in red blood cels due to damage to haemoglobin in splenic disease and haemolytic anaemias.

Heliobacter pylori Motile gram negative bacteria of stomach causing peptic ulcer and MALT lymphoma

Hellin's low A law stating that twins occur once in 80 pregnancines, triplets in 80^2 and guadruplets once in 80^3, pregnancies

HELLP syndrome Occurs in severe preeclampsia with haemolysis, raised liver enzymes, low platelets

Helmet cells A damaged RBC,

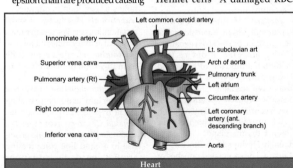

Heart

partially fragmented, seen in some cancers, DIC and G_6 PD deficiency

Helminth A worm, free living or parasitic.

Helweg's bundle A part of extrapyramidal system extending from olivary body to anterior horn cell

Hemagglutinin An antibody that causes clumping of erythrocytes.

Hemangioendothelioma A tumor of endothelial cells lining blood vessels.

Hemangioblast A mesodermal cell that can form either endothelial cell or haemocytoblasts

Hemangioma A benign tumor of blood vessel, with dilated capillaries

Hematemesis Vomiting of blood

Hematin The non protein portion of haemoglobin where iron is in ferric state.

Hematinic A blood forming tonic

Hematochezia Passage of bloody stool.

Hematocrit Percentage of RBCs in volume in a given volume of blood.

Hematoma A swelling due to collected blood.

Hematopoiesis The process of formation of red blood cells

Hematospermia Semen containing blood

Hematosalpinx Retained menstrual blood in the fallopian tube.

Hematuria Passage of blood in urine

Heme An iron containing porotoporphyrin.

Hemiarthrosis A false articulation between two bones.

Hemiballismus Switching or jerking of one side of body

Hemihydrate A compound with one molecule of water for every two molecules of other substance

Hemimelus A fetal malformation with defective development of extremities

Hemipagus Twins joined at thorax

Hemiplegia Paralysis of one half of body.

h. capsular Lesions of internal capsule producing hemiplegia.

Hemisacralization Abnormal development of one half of fifth lumbar vertebra fusing with the sacrum.

Hemispasm Spasm of one side of body or face.

Hemisphere Either half of the cerebrum or cerebellum.

h. dominant Cerebral hemisphere controlling speech usually the left in 90% right handed persons and 15% of left handed persons.

Hemithorax One half of the chest

Hemivertebra Congenital absence or failure of development of half of vertebra.

Hemoagglutination Clumping of RBC.

Hemoagglutinin An agglutinin that clumps RBC.

Hemobilia Blood in bile duct.

Hemochromatosis A congenital disorder of iron metabolism leading to excess iron accumulation in liver, pancreas, and heart. *SYN*-bronze diabetes.

Hemoconcentration A relative or an absolute increase in RBC mass; can be secondary to fluid loss.

Hemocyanin An oxygen carrying blue pigment in the plasma of arthropods and moluscus.

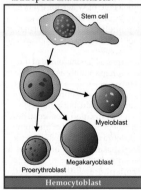

Hemocytoblast

Hemocytoblast The primitive reticuloendothelial stem cell of bone marrow differentiating into various blood components.

Hemocytogenesis Formation of blood cells.

Hemocytology Study of structure and function of blood cells.

Hemodialysis A method of removing poisonous substances, urea, creatinine, etc. from plasma by passing the patient's blood across semipermeable membranes. *SYN* —hemoperfusion.

Hemodialyzer Device used in performing hemodialysis.

Hemodilution Reduction in relative concentration of RBC due to plasma volume expansion.

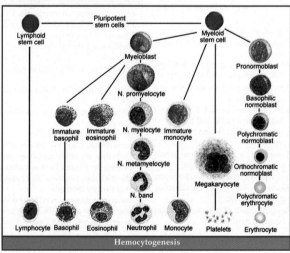

Hemocytogenesis

Hemodynamics Study of blood circulation.

Hemoflagellate Any flagellate protozoan of the blood e.g., trypanosoma, leishmania.

Hemofuscin A brown pigment derived from hemoglobins.

Hemoglobin The iron containing protoporphyrin IX, responsible for carriage of oxygen from lungs to tissues.

h. fetal Fetal hemoglobin contains 2 alfa and 2 gamma chains in globin unit, constitutes the total Hb in fetus and is replaced by adult Hb after birth. Normal concentration in adults is 2%, level is increased in thalassemia minor.

Hb S The hemoglobin of sickle cell anemia which polymerizes on exposure to hypoxic conditions, causes hemolysis and organ dysfunction due to vascular occlusion.

Hb M The iron in HbM is in ferric form and is not able to combine with oxygen (hence called methemoglobin). There is diffuse cyanosis.

Hb AIC Glycosylated Hb where glucose is attached to terminal amino acid of betaglobin chain. Normal level is s 6%. Value above 6% indicates poor blood sugar control.

Hemoglobinemia Presence of free hemoglobin in plasma.

Hemoglobinometer Apparatus for estimating blood Hb.

Hemoglobinuria Presence of hemoglobin in urine.

Hemogram Differential blood count.

Hemolysin Agents destroying blood corpuscles.

Hemolysis Destruction of RBC.

Hemolytic anemia Anemia resulting from haemolysis of red blood cells.

Hemolytic disease of newborn ABO or Rh incompatibility resulting in hemolysis, anemia, jaundice, edema and hepatic enlargement.

Hemolytic-uremic syndrome Characterized by microangiopathic hemolytic anemia, acute nephropathy and thrombocytopenia in children usually preceded by upper respiratory illness or GI upset.

Hemoperfusion Perfusion of blood through substances, such as activated charcoal or ion exchange resins, to remove toxic material. The blood is not separated from the chemical or solution by semipermeable dialysis membrane unlike hemodialysis.

Hemopericardium Accumulation of blood in the pericardial sac.

Hemoperitoneum Accumulation of blood in peritoneal cavity.

Hemopexin A glycoprotein of beta globulin that binds to hemin but not hemoglobin.

Hemophilia A sex linked hereditary disorder of coagulation with prolonged clotting time, repeated hemarthrosis and bleeding from nose or after trivial trauma. There is deficiency of factor VIII.

Hemophilus A genus of bacteria, gram -ve, non motile, requiring

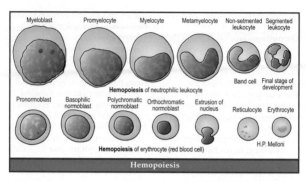

Myeloblast   Promyelocyte   Myelocyte   Metamyelocyte   Non-setmented leukocyte   Segmented leukocyte

Band cell   Final stage of development

Hemopoiesis of neutrophilic leukocyte

Pronormoblast   Basophilic normoblast   Polychromatic normoblast   Orthochromatic normoblast   Extrusion of nucleus   Reticulocyte   Erythrocyte

H.P. Melloni

Hemopoiesis of erythrocyte (red blood cell)

Hemopoiesis

blood factors X or V for their growth.

h. aegyptus Koch Week's bacillus, causative agent of conjunctivitis.

h. ducreyi Causative agent of soft sore.

h. influenzae Causative agent of pneumonitis, meningitis.

h. pertussis Causative agent of whooping cough.

Hemopneumopericardium Blood and air in pericardial cavity due to the injury to trachea or mediastinum.

Hemopneumothorax Blood and air in pleural cavity.

Hemopoiesis Formation of blood cells.

Hemoptysis Expectoration of blood or coughing up of blood.

Hemorrhage Bleeding, either external or internal.

h. antepartum Bleeding after 28 weeks of gestation and before onset of labor.

h. accidental Retroplacental bleeding.

h. postpartum Bleeding in excess of 500 ml after childbirth.

Hemorrhagic disease of newborn Bleeding from nose, umbilical stump in newborn due to inadequate prothrombin synthesis (premature fetal liver/poor bacterial flora).

Hemorrhagic fevers A group of diseases due to arthropod borne viruses like yellow fever, Kyasanur Forest disease.

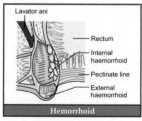

Lavator ani

Rectum

Internal haemorrhoid

Pectinate line

External haemorrhoid

Hemorrhoid

Hemorrhoid Dilated, tortuous veins in the ano-rectal region.

h. external Dilated vein or veins at the junction of anal mucosa with the anal skin.

h. prolapse Prolapse of internal hemorrhoids through the anus.

h. strangulated Painful prolapsed hemorrhoids with cessation in their blood supply by pressure from anal sphincter.

Hemorrhoidectomy Removal of hemorrhoids by surgery, ligation or cryo, etc.

Hemosalpinx Bleeding into fallopian tube.

Hemosiderin Iron containing pigment derived from hemoglobin liberated from disintegrated RBC.

Hemosiderosis Deposition of iron in reticuloendothelial cells of liver principally after multiple blood transfusion as in hemoglobinopathy and hemolytic diseases.

Hemostasis Arrest of bleeding.

Hemothorax Blood in the pleural cavity, either due to trauma, tumor of lungs and pleura, connective tissue disease, etc.

Henderson Hasselbalch equation An equation for expression of pH.

Henöch-Schonlein purpura Allergic purpura with erythema, urticaria accompanied by gastrointestinal and joint symptoms.

Henry's law The weight of a gas dissolved by a given volume of liquid at a constant temperature is directly proportional to the pressure.

Heparin A polysaccharide produced by mast cells of liver and basophils, inhibits conversion of prothrombin to thrombin.

Hepatic coma Impaired CNS function due to liver dysfunction. Coma results from increased serum ammonia, false neurotransmitters and middle molecules, the toxic products of protein metabolism. Common precipitating factors are high protein diet, bleeding into GI tract (varices), infections, electrolyte imbalance, diuretics and drugs. Mousy odor, flapping tremor and EEG changes are characteristic.

Hepatic duct The bile channel from liver that joins with cystic duct to form common bile duct

Hepatic veins The three veins draining right and left lobes of liver into inferior vena cava.

Hepatitis Inflammation of liver; causative agents include viruses (Hepatitis A, B, C, delta agent), bacteria, alcohol, drugs and autoimmune diseases. Common symptoms and signs are nausea, vomiting, jaundice, fever and hepatomegaly.

h. A Average incubation period 4 weeks, acute onset, transmitted by feco-oral route. Rarely leads to chronic liver diseases.

h. B Average incubation period 60 days, slow onset, usually progresses to chronic active hepatitis, spread is by blood and blood product and sexual contact.

h. C Previously designated non A, non B, acute onset, usually spreads

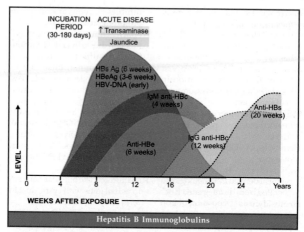

INCUBATION PERIOD (30–180 days)

ACUTE DISEASE
↑ Transaminase
Jaundice

HBs Ag (6 weeks)
HBeAg (3–6 weeks)
HBV-DNA (early)

IgM anti-HBc (4 weeks)

Anti-HBs (20 weeks)

Anti-HBe (6 weeks)

IgG anti-HBc (12 weeks)

LEVEL

0 4 8 12 16 20 24 Years

WEEKS AFTER EXPOSURE

Hepatitis B Immunoglobulins

through blood and blood products, mild course.

h. delta Onset may be acute, usually occurs in those having hepatitis B. Usually self limited.

h. amebic The liver dysfunction is due to a nonspecific reaction to amebic colitis, not true invasion of ameba into liver. Right subcostal pain, tender hepatomegaly, fever and leukocytosis are present.

h. alcoholic History of excessive indulgence in alcohol, with tender hepatomegaly, icterus and marked elevation of SCOT and SGPT.

h. fulminant Rapidly progressive hepatitis with deepening jaundice, liver cell failure and coma.

Hepatitis-associated antigen It was originally applied to hepatitis B surface antigen or Australia antigen. Now other antigens like core antigen (Hbc), 'e' antigen are also identified for diagnosis of hepatitis B infection.

Hepatitis B Immunoglobulin Derived from blood plasma of human donors who have high liters of antibodies against hepatitis B.

Hepatitis B vaccine A recombinant vaccine with hepatitis B surface antigen given as 20 mgm dose-3 doses, to persons at high risk.

Hepatoblastoma Malignant teratoma of liver.

Hepatogenic Having its origin in the liver.

Hepatogenous Originating in the liver.

Hepato-jugular reflux Pressure on the liver or right upper abdomen causes a rise in jugular venous pressure in patients of congestive heart failure.

Hepatolenticular degeneration An autosomal recessive trait with copper deposition in liver, cornea, kidney and brain due to decrease in plasma copper binding protein, the ceruloplasmin.

Hepatolith Biliary concretion in liver.

Hepatology Study of liver.

Hepatoma A primary malignant tumor of liver.

Hepatomegaly An enlargement of liver, may be upward or downward. Commonly due to alcohol, hepatitis, amebiasis, congestive failure, infectious fevers, etc.

Hepato-renal syndrome Kidney dysfunction with uremia secondary to acute or chronic hepatic catastrophe.

Hepatosis Non-inflammatory disease of liver.

Hepatosplenomegaly Enlargement of both liver and spleen; commonly due to enteric fever, malaria, kala-azar, leukemia and lympho proliferative disorders, cirrhosis, portal hypertension, etc.

Herb A plant with soft stem containing little wood, usually seasonal.

Hereditary Genetic characteristic transmitted from parent to offspring.

Heredofamilial Any disease recurring in family members due to inherited defect or other familial factors.

Hering Breuer reflex Reflex inhibition of inspiration resulting from stimulation of lung receptors following lung inflation.

Hering's nerve Afferent nerve fibers from carotid sinus passing to brain via glossopharyngeal nerve. A rise in blood pressure stimulates these nerves to reflexly diminish heart rate.

Heritage The genetic and other characteristics transmitted from parents to offsprings.

Hermaphrodite One possessing genital and sexual characteristic of both male and female. The clitoris is usually enlarged to resemble penis of male.

Hermaphroditism Existence of ovarian and testicular tissue in same individual.

h. false Possession of either testis or ovary but secondary sexual characteristics and external genitalia of opposite sex. *SYN—* pseudohermaphroditism.

Hernia Protrusion of an organ or part of it through a defect in the wall surrounding it.

h complete One in which the organ along with its sac has passed completely through the opening.

h epigastric Hernia of intestine through an opening in the midline above umbilicus.

h. fascial Protrusion of muscular tissue through its covering fascia.

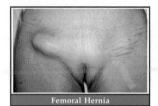

Femoral Hernia

h. femoral Hernia through femoral ring.

h. hiatal Hernia of fundus of stomach through the esophageal hiatus of diaphragm.

h. incarcerated Hernia with complete obstruction of herniating bowel segment.

h. inguinal Herniation of abdominal content (intestine or omentum) through inguinal rings.

h. direct inguinal The hernial sac protrudes through the external inguinal ring in the region of Hesselbach's triangle.

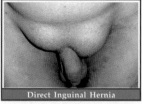

Direct Inguinal Hernia

h. indirect inguinal The hernial sac protrudes through internal inguinal ring and descends along inguinal canal to protrude in external inguinal ring.

h. labial Protrusion of a loop of bowel into the labium majus.

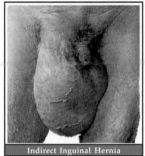

Indirect Inguinal Hernia

h. mesocolic Herniation between the layers of mesocolon.

h. obturator Hernia through obturator foramen.

h. retroperitoneal Hernia into peritoneal sac extending behind the peritoneum into the iliac fossa.

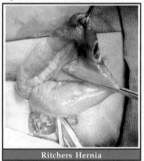

Ritchers Hernia

h. Ritcher's A portion of the wall of the intestinal loop protrudes, the lumen remaining patent.

h. sliding The herniating organ slides in and out of hernial sac.

h. strangulated Irreducible hernia where there is complete cut off blood supply to herniating organ with threatening gangrene.

h. tonsillar Protrusion of cerebellar tonsils through the foramen magnum, causing often compression of medulla oblongata.

h. transtentorial Herniation of uncus and part of temporal lobe through tentorium cerebelli.

Hernial sac The pouch of peritoneum pushed before the hernia and into which it descends.

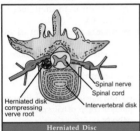

Herniated disk compressing verve root
Spinal nerve
Spinal cord
Intervertebral disk

Herniated Disc

Herniated disc Rupture of nucleus pulposus through annulus fibrosus to protrude into spinal canal.

Herniorrhaphy Surgical repair of hernia.

Herniotomy Surgical correction of irreducible/strangulated hernia by incision over constricting ring.

Heroin An extract of morphine with strong analgesic and addictive potential. Acute intoxication produces euphoria, respiratory depression, hypotension and hypothermia.

Herpangina A coxsackie virus infection with fever, sore throat, and increased salivation. The throat is covered with vesicles.

Herpes Vesiculated eruptions caused by herpes virus.

h. simplex Thin walled vesicles occurring at mucocutaneous junctions. (lips, vagina) or over oral mucous membrane.

h. simplex encephalitis Caused by herpes simplex virus 'B', predominantly involving temporal lobes and is hemorrhagic.

h. zoster Caused by varicella zoster virus with inflammation of posterior root ganglia of cranial or spinal nerves. Painful vesicular eruptions, usually unilateral, distributed over few spinal segments or forehead and eye (trigeminal nerve) are characteristic.

Herring bodies Neurosecretory granules in the terminal nerve endings of hypothalamus and hypophyseal tract.

Hertz An unit of frequency equivalent to one cycle per second.

Hesperidin A chemical present in orange and lemon peel that is hemostatic by strengthening the capillaries.

Hesselbach's hernia Hernia passing through cribiform fascia.

Hesselbach's triangle Triangular space bounded by Poupart's ligament below, outer border of rectus sheath and epigastric artery.

Heterogeneous Composed of different kinds of substances.

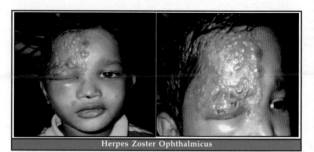
Herpes Zoster Ophthalmicus

Heterogenesis Production of offsprings that have different characteristics in alternate generations.

Heterogeusia Perception of an inappropriate quality of taste when food is chewed.

Heterograft Graft from another individual.

Heterolalia The use of meaningless words.

Heterologous 1. Composed of tissue not normal to the part. 2. A tissue, cell or blood obtained from a different individual/species.

Heterometropia Two eyes with different refraction.

Heterophil An antibody reacting with other than specific antigen.

Heterophonia Change of voice occurring esp. at puberty.

Heterophoria Tendency of the eyes to deviate from their normal position for visual alignment due to imbalance or insufficiency of ocular muscles.

Heterosexual One whose sexual orientation is to members of opposite sex.

Heterosmia Perception of inappropriate smell.

Heterotopia Development of normal tissue at an abnormal location or displacement of an organ from its normal location.

Heterotrichosis Growth of different kinds or colors of hairs on the scalp or body.

Heterotroph An organism like man who requires complex organic food for growth and development.

Heterozygote An individual with different alleles for a given characteristic.

Heubner's disease Syphilitic end arteritis in brain.

Hexachlorphene Polychlorinated phenol, antiseptic disinfectant.

Hexokinase An enzyme catalyzing phosphorylation of glucose; present in muscle tissue and yeast.

Hexose Any monosaccharide of formula $C_6 H_{12} O_6$.

Hexylresorcinol Anthelmintic agent.

Hiatus An opening.

h. semilunaris Groove in the external wall of middle meatus of nose into which frontal sinus, maxillary sinus and anterior ethmoidal cells drain.

Hibernation Condition of remaining asleep and immobile for the winter, especially in animals.

Hibernoma A rare multilobular encapsulated tumor containing fetal fat tissue closely resembling fat stored in the foot pads of hibernating animals.

Hiccough Intermittent spasmodic contraction of diaphragm with closure of glottis, causing a short sharp inspiratory cough.

Hick's sign Intermittent painless uterine contraction occurring after third month of pregnancy.

Hidradenoma Adenoma of sweat glands.

Hierarchy In order of importance.

High blood pressure Blood pressure above the normal range for age. Usually 140/90 mm Hg if below 50 years and above 160/90 if above 60 years.

High residue diet High fiber/cellulose diet (above 30 gm/day) beneficial for colorectal diseases, diabetes and obesity.

Hilton's law A nerve supplying a muscle also supplies the joint that muscle moves and the skin overlying the insertion of that muscle.

Hilton's line A white line at the junction of skin of the perineum and anal mucosa.

Hilton's sac A pit along the external portion of false vocal cord.

Hilum *(SYN— hilus)* 1. The root of lungs at the level of 4th and 5th dorsal vertebra. 2. depression or recess at exit or entrance of a duct into a gland or nerves and vessels into an organ.

Hind gut The caudal portion of entodermal tube giving rise to ileum, colon and rectum.

Hinge joint A joint permitting only flexion and extension in a single axis.

Hip Upper part of thigh formed by femur, ilium, ischeum and pubis.

Hip joint The ball and socket articulation between head of femur and acetabulum.

Hippocampal commissure A thin sheet of fibers passing transversely under posterior portion of corpus callosum.

Hippocampal formation Olfactory structures including hippocampus, dentate gyrus, supra callosal gyrus, diagonal band of Broca and hippo campal commissure.

Hippocampus major Elevation of floor of inferior horn of lateral ventricle.

Hippocampus minor Small elevation on the medial wall of lateral ventricle formed by end of calcarine fissure.

Hippocrates Greek physician who first established the scientific basis of medical practice; hence known as father of medicine.

Hippocratic facies The appearance of face at the time of impending death.

Hippocratic oath The oath Hippocrates exacted from his students which reads like "I will follow that system of regimen which, according to my ability and judgement, I consider for the benefit of my patients, and abstain from whatever is deleterious and mischievous. I will give neither deadly medicine to any one if asked nor suggest any such counsel, and in like manner I will not give to a woman a pessary for abortion. With purity and holiness I will pass my life and practise my art, into whatever houses I enter, I will go into them for the benefit of the sick, and I will abstain from every voluntary act of mischief and corruption, and further from seduction of females or males, of free men and slaves. Whatever in connection with my professional practice, or not in connection with it, I see or hear in the life of men, which ought not to be spoken of abroad, I will not divulge, as reckoning that all such should be kept secret.

"While I continue to keep this oath unviolated, may it be granted to me to enjoy life and the practice of this art, respected by all men in all times. But should I trespass and violate this Oath, may the reverse be my lot."

Hippuric acid Endogenous acid formed in the human body from combination of benzoic acid and glycine and excreted by kidneys.

Hippus Rhythmical and rapid dilatation and contraction of pupil.

Hirschberg's reflex Adduction of foot when sole at base of great toe is stimulated.

Hirschsprung's disease A dynamic megacolon due to failure of development of mysenteric plexus in the rectosigmoid area of colon.

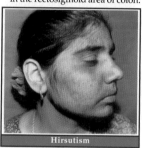
Hirsutism

Hirsutism Excessive hair growth in women.

Hirudicide Any substance that destroys leeches.

His bundle Atrioventricular bundle arising in AV node and ending in the ventricles.

$$HC \equiv\!\!\!= C\text{--}CH_2\text{--}CH\text{--}COOH$$

Histidine

$$HC \equiv\!\!\!= C\text{--}CH_2\text{--}CH_2$$

Histamine

Histamine

Histamine A derivative of histidine that is secreted by mast cells and is responsible for triple response.

Histamine blocking agents H_1 receptor blocking agents are antiallergic and H_2 receptor blockers reduce gastric acid production.

Histamine headache Headache after taking histamine containing foods.

Histidine An amino acid obtained by hydrolysis from tissue proteins.

Histiocyte A phagocytic cell with ameboid activity, present in most connective tissues.

Histiocytosis Abnormal presence of histiocytes in the blood.

Histiocystosis-x A granulomatous destructive disease.

Histochemistry Light and electron microscopy and special chemical tests and stains done to study chemistry of cells and tissues.

Histocompatibility The ability of cells to survive without any immunological influence or interference; important in blood transfusion and tissue transplantation.

Histocompatibility antigens A number of antigens expressed by all nucleated cells which are controlled by genes located in major histocompatibility gene complex (mhc) in chromosome 6.

Histogenesis Origin and development of tissue.

Histoid Resembling one of the tissues.

Histology Study of microscopic structure of cells and tissues.

Histone A class of simple proteins present in cell chromatin.

Histonomy The law governing development and structure of tissues.

Histoplasmosis A systemic fungal infection with histoplasma capsulatum, manifesting as fever, anemia, splenomegaly, leukopenia and pulmonary infiltrations.

Histotomy Cutting of thin sections of tissue for microscopic study.

Histozyme A renal enzyme that converts hippuric acid into benzoic acid and glycine.

Histrionic Theatrical, dramatic.

Hives Eruption of itchy wheals due to allergy; local or systemic.

Hoarseness A rough quality of voice due to simple chronic laryngitis, vocal cord palsy, or infiltration of vocal cords.

Hobnail liver Liver with an irregular surface, usually cirrhosis.

Hochsinger's sign Closure of the fist in tetany when bicep muscle is pressed

Hodgkin's disease A lymphoproliferative disease with painless lymphadenopathy, hepatosplenomegaly, and often relapsing fever. Reed-Sternberg's giant cells in lymph node biopsy are characteristic.

Hoffman's sign Flicking the terminal phalanx of finger causes reflex flexion of other fingers of same hand in pyramidal damage.

Holistic medicine Comprehensive and total care of a patient, taking into account his physical, mental, social, economic and spiritual needs.

Hollenhorst plaques/bodies Atheromanous patches in retinal vessels after dislodgement from carotids

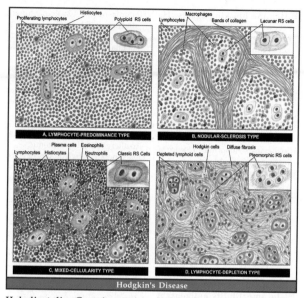

A, LYMPHOCYTE-PREDOMINANCE TYPE

B, NODULAR-SCLEROSIS TYPE

C, MIXED-CELLULARITY TYPE

D, LYMPHOCYTE-DEPLETION TYPE

Hodgkin's Disease

Holodiastolic Covering entire diastole, i.e. closure of aortic valve to closure of mitral valve.

Holoendemic A disease affecting almost all population in a given area. In malaria epidemiology, spleen index rate of $\geq$ 5% in children under 10 implies the disease to be holoendemic.

Holography A method of producing 3 dimensional pictures. The picture obtained is called hologram.

Holoprosencephaly Deficiency in fore brain with CSF accumulation due to trisomy of 13, 14, 15, or 18 chromosomes.

Holorachischisis Complete spina bifida.

Holosystolic Related to entire period of systole.

Holt Oram syndrome Combination upper limb anomaly and congenital heart disease, usually ASD

Holter monitor An ECG recording system capable of recording ECG for 24 hours, particularly useful for recording arrhythmias, and silent ischemia.

Homan's sign Pain in the calf on passive dorsiflexon of great toe, an evidence of deep vein thrombosis.

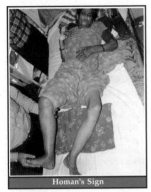

Homan's Sign

Homatropine Antimuscarinic agent used to dilate pupil.

Homeopathy A system of medicine developed by Hahnemann based on the theory "like cures likely", i.e., large doses of a drug that produces symptoms of disease in healthy people will cure the same symptoms in small doses.

Homeostasis. State of equilibrium of internal environment of the body.

Homicide Murder.

Homoblastic Developing from a single type of tissue.

Homocystine A homologue of cystine formed during catabolism of methionine.

Homocystinuria An inherited metabolic disease due to absence of an enzyme essential in the metabolism of homocystine. Clinical features include marfanoid features, mental retardation, subluxation of lens, etc.

Homogeneous Uniform in structure, composition or nature.

Homogenesis Reproduction by same process in succeeding generations uniform.

H1 and H2 receptor blockers Agents that block H_1 and H_2 receptors e.g., terphenadrine and ranitidine respectively.

Hormone The secretion from ductless glands, a substance originating in one organ, gland or body part but acting at a distant site with stimulation or inhibition of activity or secretion of another hormone.

Horn Cutaneous outgrowth composed chiefly of keratin.

horn anterior Gray substance in anterior portion of spinal cord *SYN*—ventral horn.

horn dorsal Posterior projection of gray matter in spinal cord.

horn ofAmmon Hippocampus

Horner's syndrome Myosis, ptosis, enopthalmos and loss of sweating over affected side of face due to paralysis of cervical sympathetic trunk.

Horse power A unit of power equals to 33.000 foot pounds per minute or 745.7 watts.

Horse-shoe shaped kidney A congenital renal abnormality in which both the kidneys are united at their lower poles.

Hospital Institution for treatment of sick and injured.

Hospitalization Admission of a patient into hospital.

Host 1. The organism which nourishes the parasite. 2. The individual receiving the graft in transplantation program.

host definitive The final host in which parasite has sexual maturity and sexual union for reproduction.

host intermediate Host in which parasite undergoes sexual development.

Hostility Manifestations of anger, animosity or antagonism directed towards oneself or others. It may be a symptom of depression.

Hotline A continuously functioning telephone connection.

Hot water bag A rubber or plastic bag for application of dry heat or keeping moist applications warm.

Hour-glass contraction Excessive contraction of an organ at its center resembling hourglass e.g., in malignancy of stomach or gastric ulcer.

House maid's knee Patellar bursitis in house maid due to prolonged kneeling.

House physician An intern or resident responsible for patient care under direction of a senior staff.

Houston's valves Crescent shaped folds of mucous membrane in the rectum.

Howell-Jolly bodies Spherical granules in the erythrocytes seen in asplenia, thalassemia, leukemia etc.

Howship's lacunae Grooves or pits occupied by osteoclasts during bone resorption.

Hubbard tank Tank of suitable size and shape for active and passive underwater exercises.

Huguier's canal Canal in the base of skull through which chorda tympani nerve exits from brain

Huhner's test Aspiration of vagina within an hour of coitus to test for sperm motility in investigation of infertility.

Hum Soft continuous sound.

Human immunodeficiency virus see AIDS.

Human insulin Insulin prepared by recombinant DNA technology using *E. coli*.

Human placental lactogen Placental secretion that helps to prepare the breast for milk secretion.

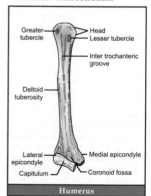

Humerus

Humerus Bone of upper arm that articulates with scapula above and radiusulna below.

Humidity Moisture in the atmosphere.

Humor Any fluid or semifluid substance in the body.

h. aqueous The secretion of cilliary body occupying anterior and posterior chambers of eye. It is absorbed to venous system through canal of Schlemm.

h. vitreous The transparent jelly like substance occupying the space between lens and retina.

Humpback Curvature of spine or kyphosis.

Hunchback Kyphosis with prominent rounded deformity of back.

Hunger A desire to eat with dull pain in epigastrium. Appetite in contrast is pleasant sensation of seeking food to eat to enjoy it.

Hunter's canal Adductor canal.

Hunter's disease Mucopoly-saccharidosis II.

Hunterian chancre Indurated syphilitic chancre.

Huntington chorea Inherited disease of CNS manifesting with chorea, progressive dementia.

Hurler's syndrome A form of mucopolysaccharidosis with skeletal abnormality, cloudy cornea, and often mental deficiency.

Hutchinson Sir British surgeon.

H.'s pupil Widely dilated pupil in CNS disease.

H.'s teeth A feature of congenital syphilis in which the lateral incisors are peg shaped and the central incisors are notched.

H.'s triad In congenital syphilis this diagnostic triad consists of deafness, interstitial keratitis and Hutchinson's teeth.

Hyaline It refers to any alteration within cell or in the extracellular space, which gives a homogeneous, glassy, pink appearance in histologic sections stained with hematoxylin and eosin.

Hyaline Bluish-white glassy translucent cartilage, e.g., semilunar cartilage of knee, thyroid cartilage.

Hyaline cartilage Smooth, pearly true cartilage covering articular surface of bone.

Hyaline casts Pale, transparent casts with homogeneous rounded ends seen in urine in nephropathy.

Hyaline membrane disease A respiratory disease of newborn with poor gas transfer.

Hyalinization The development of an albuminoid mass in a cell or tissue.

Hyalinosis Waxy or hyaline degeneration.

Hyalitis Inflammation of vitreous humor; can be asteroid, punctate and suppurative.

Hyalogen A protein substance in vitreous humor and cartilage.

Hyaloid artery A fetal artery supplying nutrition to the lens. It disappears after birth.

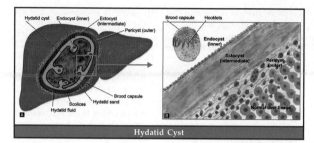

Hydatid Cyst

Hyaloid canal Lymph channel in vitreous extending from optic disk to posterior capsule of lens; contains hyaloid artery in fetus.

Hyaloid membrane Membrane that envelops the vitreous humor.

Hyaluronic acid An acid mucopolysaccharide forming the ground substance of connective tissue; functioning as a binding and protective agent.

Hyaluronidase An enzyme that depolymerizes hyaluronic acid, thereby increases permeability of connective tissues.

Hybrid The offspring of parent that are of different species.

Hybridization Production of hybrids by cross matching.

Hybridoma It is the cell produced by fusion of an antibody producing cell and a multiple myeloma cell. The hybrid cell thus formed can be a source of continuous monoclonal antibodies.

Hydantoin A colorless base, glycolyl urea.

Hydatid A cyst formed in internal organs, commonly lungs or liver by developing larva of E. granulosus.

Hydatid disease The disease produced by the cysts of larval stage of echinococcus.

Hydatidiform mole Degenerative process of chorionic villi with formation of multiple cysts within uterus.

Hydatid of Morgagni Cyst like remnant of mullerian duct that is attached to fallopian tube.

Hydradenitis Inflammation of sweat glands.

Hydradenoma Tumor of sweat gland.

Hydragogue Drug promoting watery evacuation of bowel like sodium sulphate or magnesium sulphate.

Hydralazine Antihypertensive acting through vasomotor center in CNS.

Hydramnios An excess of liquor amnii around the developing fetus.

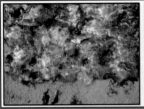
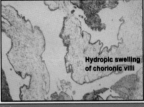

Hydropic swelling
of chorionic villi

H Mole

Hydranencephaly Hydrocephalus due to congenital absence of cerebral hemispheres.

Hydrarthrosis Serous effusion into a joint cavity.

Hydraulics The science of fluids.

Hydriatrics Application of water for treatment *SYN*—hydrotherapy.

Hydrocarbon Compound made of only hydrogen and carbon.

h. acyclic Contains cyclic and straight chain components.

h. aliphatic Contains only cyclic components.

h. aromatic Contains carbon atoms in ring or cyclic fashion.

Hydrocele Fluid accumulation in tunica vaginalis testes or in any sac like cavity.

h. cervical Hydrocele of neck resulting from accumulation of fluid in persistent cervical duct or cleft

h. congenital Hydrocele present since birth resulting in failure of tunica vaginalis to close.

h. encysted Hydrocele in the processus vaginalis with closure of its abdominal and scrotal ends.

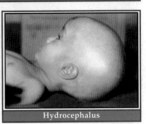

Hydrocephalus

Hydrocephalus Increased content of CSF within the ventricles resulting from decreased absorption of CSF, its increased production or blockage to its circulation resulting from develop–mental anomalies, infection, injury or tumor.

h. communicating Hydrocephalus in which normal communication between 4th ventricle and sub-arachnoid space is maintained.

h. normal pressure Hydrocephalus with normal CSF pressure and without demonstrable block, to CSF circulation.

Hydrochloric acid Produced by oxyntic cells of gastric glands, serves to convert pepsinogen into pepsin,

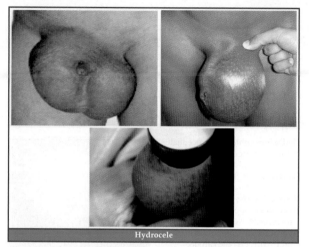

Hydrocele

dissolves and disintegrates nucleo proteins, precipitates caseinogen, hydrolyzes sucrose, inhibits bacterial multiplication, etc.

Hydrochlorothiazide Diuretic.

Hydrochloresis Stimulation of bile secretion with reduced specific gravity, viscosity and total solids.

Hydrocodone Opioid alkaloid, analgesic and hypnotic.

Hydrocolpos Retention cyst of vagina.

Hydrocortisone Corticosteroid hormone produced by adrenal gland.

Hydrocystoma Small sweat gland cysts in the face.

Hydrodiascope Device used in treatment of astigmatism.

Hydroflumethazide A diuretic.

Hydrogen A colorless, odorless and tasteless gas with atomic weight of 1. Three isotopes of hydrogen, e.g. protium, deuterium and tritium have (appx) atomic weights of 1, 2, 3 respectively.

Hydrogenase An enzyme that catalyzes reduction by molecular hydrogen.

Hydrogenation Addition of hydrogen to convert unsaturated fat to solid fat.

Hydrogen donor In oxidation-reduction reactions a substance that gives up hydrogen to another substance.

Hydrogen ion The positively charged hydrogen particle.

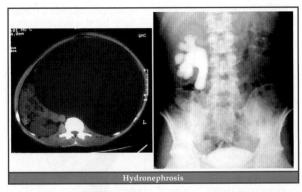
Hydronephrosis

Hydrogen ion concentration The pH value is the negative logarithm of H. ion concentration of a solution, expressed in gram ions (moles) per liter. A solution with pH of 1 is ten times more acid than one with pH of 2 and 100 times more acid than one with pH of 3. A pH above 7 means alkalinity. The blood pH is around 7.35.

Hydrogen peroxide H_2O_2 colorless greasy liquid with irritating odor and acrid taste, decomposes easily liberating oxygen in presence of light 3% solution is a mild antiseptic, germicide and cleansing agent. Used commercially as a bleaching agent.

Hydrogen sulfide H_2S A poisonous, gas with pungent odor of rotten egg.

Hydrolase An enzyme causing hydrolysis.

Hydrolysis Combination of water with salt to produce acid and base or a chemical decomposition in which a substance is split into simpler compounds by addition or the taking up of the elements of water.

Hydrometer An instrument that measures density of liquid.

Hydromorphone An analgesic, opium derivative.

Hydromyelia Distention of central canal of spinal cord with fluid.

Hydromyelocele Protrusion of spinal CSF sac through spinal bifida.

Hydromyoma Cystic uterine fibroid.

Hydronephrosis Collection of fluid in renal pelvicalicyeal system usually due to obstruction to urine flow, ultimately causing atrophy of renal parenchyma.

Hydrophobia Morbid fear for water, synonym for rabies in which attempt to drink water causes spasm of pharynx due to CNS irritation.

Hydrophilic oint Topical ointment that absorbs water and hence is emollient.

Hydrophobophobia Morbid fear of contracting hydrophobia.

Hydropneumatosis Liquid and gas in tissues producing combined edema and emphysema.

Hydropneumopericardium Fluid and gas in pericardial cavity.

Hydropneumothorax Gas and fluid in pleural sac.

Hydrops Edema.

h. endolymphaticus Edema of labyrinth.

Hydropyonephrosis Dilatation of renal pelvis with pus and urine.

Hydroquinone A depigmenting agent.

Hydrostatic densitometry An underwater weighing technique for determination of body components, usually percentage of fat.

Hydrostatic test A test to know if the dead infant has breathed prior to death. If the infants lungs float in water, breathing had been established prior to death.

Hydrosudotherapy Treatment of disease by sweating and hydrotherapy.

Hydrotherapy Scientific application of water in treatment of diseases for following therapeutic objectives. Brief hot tub and shower baths relieve fatigue, cold bath to constrict blood vessels, to reduce

tissue edema after injury. Hot bath dilates blood vessels, encourages perspiration.

Hydrothorax Accumulation of non-inflammatory fluid within thorax.

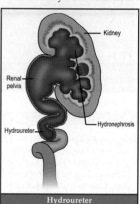

Hydroureter

Hydroureter Distension of ureter due to obstruction.

Hydroxo cobalamin A chemical with activity similar to B_{12}.

Hydroxyapatite Calcium phosphate in combination with calcium carbonate present in the bones; when it combines with fluorine, it becomes decay resistant fluoroapatite.

Hydroxybenzene Phenol.

Hydroxybutyric acid A component of ketone body produced by abnormal metabolism of fat in diabetic ketosis.

Hydroxy chloroquin Antimalarial agent.

Hydroxyproline An amino acid found in collagen.

Hydroxypropyl methyl cellulose A substance used to increase viscosity of solutions.

Hydroxy stibamidine isethionate Antiprotozoal antimonial.

5 *hydroxy tryptamine* Serotonin.

Hydroxyzine An antihistamine.

Hydroxyurea Cytotoxic agent used in leukemia.

Hygiene Study of methods and means of preserving health.

Hygroma A sac containing fluid.

h. cystic A rapidly growing cystic swelling in neck of lymphatic origin.

Hygrometer Instrument for measuring moisture in air.

Hymen A fold of mucous membrane that partially covers the entrance to vagina.

h. annular Hymen with ring shaped opening in the center.

h. biforis Hymen with two parallel openings with a thick septum in between.

h. cribiform Hymen with many small openings.

h. denticulatus Hymen opening has serrated edges.

Hymenitis Inflammation of hymen.

Hymenolepsis A genus of tapeworm.

h. nana Dwarf tapeworm, average length 1" capable of completing life cycle within one host.

Hymenology Science of the membranes and their diseases

Hymenoptera An order of insects that includes ante, bees, hornets and wasps.

Hymenorrhaphy Plastic surgery of hymen to restore it to preruptured state.

Hyoglossus Muscle arising from hyoid bone and inserted into dorsum of tongue. It draws sides down and retracts the tongue.

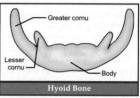

Greater cornu

Lesser cornu

Body

Hyoid Bone

Hyoid bone Horseshoe shaped bone lying at the base of tongue.

Hyopharyngeus Middle pharyngeal constrictor.

Hyoscine hydrobromide Belladona alkaloid having atropine like effect.

Hyper Prefix meaning excessive, beyond.

Hyperacidity Excess of acid in stomach.

Hyperactivity Excessive activity of an organ or entire organism.

Hyperacusis Abnormal sensitivity to sound, e.g. in hysteria.

Hyperalgia Excessive sensitivity to pain.

Hyperalimentation IV infusion of hypertonic solution that contains sufficient amino acids, electrolytes and glucose to sustain life and achieve normal growth and development.

Hyperammonemia Excess of ammonia in blood, e.g., cirrhosis can be congenital either due to deficiency of carbamyl phosphate synthetase or ornithine trans carbamylase that metabolize ammonia.

Hyperamylasemia Increased blood amylase.

Hyperbaric oxygen Oxygen on increased pressure to treat gas gangrene, air embolism, decompression sickness, CO poisoning, nonhealing ulcers, etc.

Hyperbetalipoproteinemia Excessive amount of betalipoprotein in blood.

Hyperbilirubinemia Excessive amount of bilirubin in blood.

Hypercalcemia Excessive amount of calcium in the blood. (12.2 mg%) either idiopathic, or secondary to malignancy, prolonged recumbency, vit D intoxication etc.

Hypercalciuria Excessive excretion of calcium in urine.

Hypercapnia Excess CO_2 in blood.

Hyperchloremia Increased chloride content of blood e.g., hyperchloremic acidosis.

Hyperchlorhydria Excess secretion of HCl in stomach.

Hypercholesterolemia Excessive ($\geq$ 250 mg%) cholesterol in blood; often familial, but usually dietary.

Hyperchromatic Overpigmented.

Hyperchromatopsia Defect of vision in which all objects appear colored.

Hyper corticism Excessive production of adrenocortical hormones.

Hypercyesis Presence of more than one fetus in uterus.

Hyperdontia Presence of more than normal number of teeth.

Hyperemesis Excessive vomiting.

Hyperemesis gravidarum Nausea and vomiting during pregnancy threatening dehydration, and acidosis.

Hyperemia Vascular congestion; can be active as in increased blood flow or passive due to venous stasis.

Hypereosinophilic syndrome Idiopathic persistent hypereosinophilia often with CNS and cardiac involvement.

Hypererethism Excessive irritability.

Hyperergasia Unusual functional activity.

Hyperesthesia Increased sensitivity to sensory stimuli especially pain and touch.

Hyper extension Excessive degree of extension movement in a joint, a feature of collagen disorder.

Hyperferremia Increased iron content of blood.

Hyperfibrinogenemia Increased blood fibrinogen, often threatening spontaneous coagulation.

Hyperglycemia Increased blood sugar as in diabetics.

Hyperglycinemia Accumulation of amino acid glycine in blood manifesting with mental and growth retardation.

Hypergnosia Distorted or exaggerated perception.

Hypergonadism Excessive secretion of sex hormones.

Hyperhidrosis Unusually high sweating, often due to fever, drugs, anxiety.

Hyperhydration Excess amount of water in the body.

Hyperinsulinism Excess of insulin in the body causing hypoglycemia that manifests with hunger, sweating, weakness, convulsion and often coma.

Hyperkalemia Serum potassium exceeding 5 mEq/lit.

Hyperkeratosis Thickening of horny layer of epidermis often due to vitamin A deficiency.

Hyperkinesia Increased muscular movement and physical activity. In children often due to brain dysfunction and phenobarbitone.

Hyperlipemia Excessive quantity of fat in the blood.

Hyperlipoproteinemia Increased lipoprotein content in blood due to increased synthesis or decreased breakdown.

Hypermelanosis Increased melanin content of skin either in epidermis (melanoderma) in which the coloration is brown, or in the dermis in which skin color is blue or slate grey. Conditions responsible for hypermelanosis are ACTH producing tumors, Wilson's disease, biliary cirrhosis, chronic renal failure, etc.

Hypermenorrhea Abnormal increase in duration or amount of menstrual blood loss.

Hypermetabolism Increased metabolic rate seen in hyperthyroidism, fever, following trauma and surgery.

Hypermetria Unusual range of movement as in cerebellar disease.

Hypermetropia Far-sightedness, i.e., the parallel rays fall behind the macula.

Hypermimia Making great number of gestures while speaking.

Hypermnesia Great ability to remember or memorize minute details as in mania or in conditions of temporal lobe stimulation.

Hypermobility Increased range of joint movement due to lax surrounding structures as in Ehlers-Danlos syndrome, Marafan's syndrome.

Hypermorph Large limb length causing high standing height in comparison to sitting height.

Hypernatremia Excess sodium content of blood (150 mEq/lit).

Hypernephroma Renal cell carcinoma.

Hypernormal Abnormal.

Hyperosmia Abnormal sensitivity to odors.

Hyperosmolarity Increased osmolarity of blood (300 mOsms/lit.)

Hyperostosis Abnormal and excessive growth of osseous tissue.

h. frontalis interna Multiple osteomas arising from frontal bone internally into nasal sinuses.

h. infantile cortical Excessive subperiosteal bone growth in the mandible or clavicles.

Hyperoxaluria Increased oxalic acid excretion in urine.

h. enteric Caused by disease or surgical removal of ileum.

h. primary Defective oxalate metabolism causing oxlate calculi in urinary system.

Hyperparathyroidism Increased parathormone secretion, causing osteitis fibrosa cystica, bone pain, renal stone and fracture.

Hyperpathia Hypersensitivity to sensory stimuli.

Hyperphasia Abnormal desire to talk.

Hyperphenylalaninemia Increased phenylalanine in blood.

Hyperphonia Eplosive speech in stammerers.

Hyperphoria Tendency of one eye to turn upward.

Hyperphosphatasemia Raised alkaline phosphatase in blood either due to biliary obstruction or bone destruction.

Hyperphosphatemia Increased blood phosphorus content.

Hyperphosphaturia Increased amount of phosphates in urine.

Hyperphrenia Excessive mental ability as in mania.

Hyperpituitarism Overactivity of pituitary, commonly the anterior lobe producing gigantism/acromegaly.

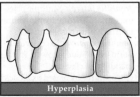
Hyperplasia

Hyperplasia Excessive growth of normal cells with normal tissue architecture.

Hyperploidy Condition having one extra chromosome, e.g. Down Syndrome (trisomy 21).

Hyperpnea Increased rate and depth of breathing,

Hyperpraxia Excessive activity and restlessness.

Hyperprolactinemia Amenorrhea, galactorrhea produced by increased serum prolactin due to hypothalamic pituitary dysfunction.

Hyperprolinemia Excess blood proline level due to inherited metabolic defect.

Hyperproteinemia Excess of protein in plasma, as in multiple myeloma.

Hyperproteinuria Protein excretion in urine exceeding 150 mg/24 hours.

Hyperptyalism Excess salivary secretion.

Hyperpyrexia Body temperature exceeding 106°F. (41.1°C).

h. malignant Hyperpyrexia occurring with inhalant anesthetics and muscle relaxants.

Hyperreflexia Increased tendon reflexes.

Hyper resonance Increased resonance to percussion especially over cavity, bullae, pneumothorax and emphysematous lung tissue.

Hypersensibility Hypersensitivity to a foreign protein or drug.

Hypersomnia Prolonged sleepiness, usually pathological, i.e. narcalepsy.

Hypersplenism Enlarged spleen with enhanced removal of blood components from circulation.

Hypersthenia Abnormal strength or excessive tension of the entire body or part of it.

Hypersthenuria Passage of abnormally concentrated urine.

Hypersusceptibility Unusual susceptibility to a disease, pathological process, parasite or chemicals.

Hypertelorism Abnormal width between two paired organs, usually the eyes.

Hypertension Blood pressure considered abnormally high for an age.

h. essential Hypertension without apparent cause.

h. malignant Severe hypertension with diastolic pressure exceeding 130-140 mmHg. with papilledema.

h. portal Increased portal vein pressure caused by obstruction to portal flow as in cirrhosis, portal vein thrombosis/compression and Budd-Chiari syndrome.

h. renal Hypertension secondary to renal artery occlusion leading to hyperreninemia.

Hyperthecosis Hyperplasia of theca interna of ovary often leading to amenorrhea and hirsutism.

Hyperthelia Presence of more than 2 nipples.

Hyperthermia Unusual high fever; a treatment modality by which foreign protein is introduced into body to raise body temperature.

Hyperthrombinemia Increased thrombin concentration in blood.

Hypertonia Increased vascular/ muscle tone.

Hypertonic Having higher osmotic pressure or having greater than normal tension.

Hypertrichosis Excess growth of hair due to endocrine disease.

Hypertrophy Non tumorous enlargement of an organ or structure due to increase in size or number of cells.

h. concentric The walls of the organ become symmetrically thick without increase in size of cavity.

h. eccentric Regional hypertrophy with dilatation.

h. pseudomuscular An inherited disease affecting boys where the muscles commonly of calf, thigh, buttocks enlarge due to deposition of fat and fibrous tissue. The involved muscles are weak and atrophied with waddling gait and increased spinal curvature.

Hyperuricemia Increased serum uric acid (8 mg%).

Hypervascular Excess vascularity.

Hyperventilation Increased rates and depths of inspiration and expiration.

Hyperviscosity Excess adhesiveness or stickiness property of fluid, commonly blood.

Hypervitaminosis Excessive vitamin content of body tissues, commonly involves fat soluble vitamins like A, D, E and K; usually secondary to excess ingestion.

Hypervolemia Abnormal increase in volume of circulating blood.

Hyphema Bleeding into anterior chamber of eye.

Hypnagogic Induced by sleep; inducing sleep; in psychiatry relates to hallucinations and dreams just before loss of consciousness.

Hypnodontics The application of controlled suggestions and hypnosis to practice of surgery.

Hypnology Scientific study of sleep.

Hypnosis A subconscious condition in which the patient responds to suggestions made by the hypnotist, useful for treatment of phobias, anxiety and chronic pain disorder.

Hypnotics Drugs that cause insensitivity to pain by inducing hypnosis.

Hypnotism An induced sleep like state during which the patient is peculiarly susceptible to the suggestions of the hypnotist.

Hypoacusis Decreased sensitivity to sound stimuli.

Hypoalbuminemia Decreased plasma albumin manifesting with edema, usually due to malnutrition or cirrhosis.

Hypoaldosteronism Decreased plasma aldosterone with hypotension and hyperkalemia.

Hypoalimentation Insufficient nourishment.

Hypobaric Decreased atmospheric pressure.

Hypocalcemia Decreased plasma calcium manifesting with stridor and tetany.

Hypocalciuria Decreased calcium excretion in urine.

Hypocarbia Decreased CO_2 in blood.

Hypocapnea Decreased CO_2 in blood.

Hypocellularity Decreased cell population in any tissue.

Hypochloremia Decreased chloride content in blood.

Hypochlorhydria Decreased HCl secretion in stomach often indicative of malignancy of stomach.

Hypochlorous acid HClO, used as disinfectant/bleaching agent.

Hypochondriac Abnormal and excessive fear of disease.

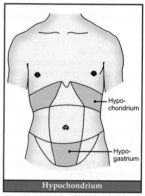

Hypochondrium

Hypochondrium Part of the abdomen below the lower ribs.

Hypochromasia Lack of hemoglobin in RBC *SYN*—hypochromia.

Hypocomplementemia Decreased complement concentration in blood.

Hypocorticism Decreased cortical hormone.

Hypodermic Inserted under the skin.

Hypodontia Absence or poor tooth development.

Hypoersthesia Lessened sensibility to touch.

Hypofunction Decreased function.

Hypogammaglobulinemia Decreased gammaglobulin concentration in blood leading to frequent infections; can be congenital or acquired (AIDS).

Hypogastrium Region below the umbilicus, between the right and left inguinal regions.

Hypogeusia Blunting of taste sensation.

Hypoglossal Situated below the tongue.

Hypoglossal nerve 12th cranial nerve originating in medulla and supplying intrinsic and extrinsic muscles of tongue.

Hypoglottis Under surface of tongue.

Hypoglycemia Decreased blood glucose below 50 mg% manifesting as tremor, sweating, weakness, etc.

Hypoglycemic agents Sulphonyl urea compounds causing a decrease in blood sugar.

Hypoglycemic shock Shock produced by hypoglycemia induced by insulin injection to treat schizophrenia.

Hypokalemia Decreased blood potassium ($\leq 3\,mEq/l$) manifesting with weakness, paralysis and hypotension.

Hypokinesia Decreased motor activity.

Hypolipidemic Reducing lipid concentration.

Hypomagnessemia Decreased plasma magnesium with neuromuscular excitability.

Hypomelanosis Decreased melanin in epidermis, e.g. vitiligo, burn.

Hypomenorrhea Decreased menstrual flow.

Hypomorph Individual with disproportionately short legs.

Hyponatremia Decreased blood sodium concentration (é mEq/L).

Hypoparathyroidism Insufficient parathormone production with hypocalcemia and tetany.

Hypopharynx Lowermost portion of pharynx leading to esophagus and larynx.

Hypophonia Weak voice.

Hypophoria Tendency of one visual axis to fall below the other.

Hypophosphatasia Decreased alkaline phosphatase in serum, usually an inherited metabolic disease manifesting with rickets, osteomalacia, poor dentition etc.

Hypophosphatemia Decreased plasma phosphate concentration.

Hypophyseal Pertains to hypophysis or pituitary.

Hypophysectomy Excision of hypophysis.

Hypophysis The pituitary gland occupying sella turcica.

Hypophysitis Inflammation of pituitary body.

Hypopituitarism Diminished pituitary hormone secretion secondary to pituitary destruction by tumor, infarction, compression resulting in secondary dysfunction of thyroid, adrenal, testis/ovary and growth disturbance in children.

Hypoproteinemia Decreased plasma protein.

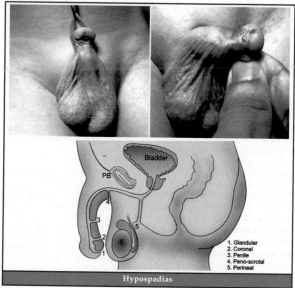

1. Glandular
2. Coronal
3. Penile
4. Peno-scrotal
5. Perineal

Hypospadias

Hypopyon Pus in anterior chamber usually secondary to corneal ulcer.

Hypospadias Abnormal urethral opening, either in the under surface of glans, penile shaft or in perineum.

Hypostasis Diminished blood flow or circulation.

Hyposthenia Weakness, subnormal strength.

Hyposthenuria Secretion of low specific gravity urine.

Hyposthesia Lessened sensibility to touch.

Hypotension Abnormally low blood pressure.

Hypothalamus The portion of diencephalon comprising the ventral wall of third ventricle and adjacent structures responsible for regulation of body temperature, sugar and fat metabolism, and secretion of releasing and inhibiting hormones. It is the principal center for integration of sympathetic and parasympathetic activities.

Hypothenar The fleshy prominence at the base of little finger along innerside of palm.

Hypothermia Subnormal (below 96°F) body temperature, induced for open heart surgery and neurological procedures.

Hypothesis An assumption not proved by experiment or observation.

Hypothrombinemia Deficiency of thrombin in blood.

Hypothyroidism Deficiency of thyroid hormones causing thick coarse hair, dry thick inelastic skin, hoarse voice, obesity, depressed muscular activity, slow pulse and hypercholesterolemia. Mental retardation and growth failure may occur in children (cretinism).

Hypotonia Loss of muscle or arterial tone.

Hypotrichosis Sparse hair.

Hypotrophy Degeneration and atrophy of tissues.

Hypotympanum The part of middle ear below the level of tympanic membrane.

Hypoventilation Reduced rate and depth of breathing.

Hypovitaminosis Condition arising from lack of vitamins.

Hypovolemia Diminished circulating blood volume.

Hypoxanthine A purine derivative formed during protein decomposition to form urea and uric acid.

Hypoxemia Insufficient oxygen content of blood,

Hypoxia Decreased O_2 concentration in inspired air.

Hypsarrhythmia An abnormal EEG pattern in which there is persistent generalized slowing and very high voltage discharge; characteristic of infantile epilepsy.

Hypsiloid U or Y shaped.

Hypsiloid ligament Iliofemoral ligament.

Hypsokinesis Tendency to fall backwards when standing as seen in Parkinson's disease.

Hypsophobia Fear of being at great heights.

Hysterectomy Surgical removal of uterus either by abdominal or vaginal route. It can be subtotal, total or radical. In radical hysterectomy (Wertheim's operation) uterus, tubes, ovaries, adjacent lymph nodes and part of vagina are removed; usually done in stage I and II cancer cervix.

Hysteresis Failure of the manifestation of an effect to keep up with its cause.

Hysteria A conversion disorder in which patient transforms longstanding mental conflict into somatic symptoms. There is no organic disease to account for the symptoms. Patient is amnesic for the period of illness as the primary consciousness reasserts itself.

Hysteric chorea A form of hysteria with choreiform movements.

Hysterography Recording of frequency and intensity of uterine contractions.

Hysterogram X-ray of uterus.

Hysteroid Resembling hysteria.

Hysteromania Nymphomania.

Hysterometry Measurement of size of uterus.

Hysteromyemectomy Excision of uterine fibroid.

Hystero-oophorectomy Excision of uterus and ovaries.

Hysteropia Hysteric visual defect.

Hysterorrhexis Rupture of pregnant uterus.

Hysterosalpingectomy Excision of uterus and tubes.

Hysterosalpingography X-ray visualization of uterus and the tubes by introduction of contrast media.

Hysterosalpingostomy Anastomosis of uterus with the remaining healthy portion of fallopian tube after excision of diseased part.

Hysteroscope Instrument for examination of inside of uterus.

Hysterotomy Incision of uterus as in evacuation of mole, dead fetus or cesarian section.

Hysterotrachelectomy Amputation of uterine cervix.

Hysterotrachelorrhaphy Repair of torn cervix.

I

Iatrogenic Adverse body effect induced by drug, procedure or the doctor.

Ibuprofen A nonsteroidal anti-inflammatory agent.

Ice bag A water tight bag to hold ice for cold sponging over bruised or sprained area.

Ice Solid form of water at temperature of 0°C or below.

Ichnogram A footprint taken while standing.

Ichor Fetid discharge from an ulcer.

Ichthammol A reddish brown viscous fluid acting as an antiseptic, often used in eardressing and skin applications.

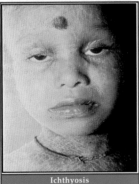
Ichthyosis

Ichthyosis Condition in which skin is dry, scaly resembling fish skin. Ichthyosis vulgaris is hereditary.

Ichthyotoxin Any toxin present in fish.

Ictal Pertains to acute attack of epilepsy or stroke.

Icteric Pertains to jaundice.

Icteroid Resembling jaundice.

Icterus Yellow pigmentation of sclera, mucous membrane and skin due to excess bile sails in blood.

Id. In psychiatry one of the three divisions of psyche, the other two being ego and super ego. The id is the obscure, inaccessible part of our personality that serves as a repository of instinctual drives continually striving for expression.

Idea A mental image, concept.

i. compulsive A persistent obsessional thought.

i. dominant Idea that controls one's thought and action.

i. fixed Idea dominating one's mind and not amenable to change irrespective of evidence to contrary.

i. of reference An impression that the conversations or actions of others have reference to oneself.

Ideal A goal regarded as a standard of perfection.

Ideation The process of thinking or formation of ideas. It is quick in mania but slow in depression, and dementias.

Identical Exactly alike.

Identification 1. The process of determining the sameness of a thing or person with that described or known to exist. 2. A defense mechanism operating unconsciously, by which a person patterns himself after some other person. This plays a major role in personality development

i. dental The use of dental charts, radiographs or records to establish a person's identity.

i. palm and soles Prints of palm and sole used for one's identification.

Identity The physical and mental characteristic by which an individual is known and recognized.

Ideology A philosophy, the science of ideas and thoughts.

Ideomotor Muscular automatic movement regulated by a dominant idea.

Idiocy Severe mental deficiency due to defective mental development, the cause of which may be genetic, vascular or birth asphyxia.

Idioglossia Inability to articulate properly so that the language is not comprehensible.

Idiogram Graphic representation of chromosome karyotype.

Idiolalia Speaking in an unknown self invented language.

Idiomuscular Muscle contraction independent of nerve control.

Idiopathic A disease without recognizable cause.

Idiopathic pulmonary Fibrosis A form of interstitial lung disease with diffuse fibrosis and rapid deterioration.

Idiophrenic Pertaining to or originating in the mind alone.

Idiosyncrasy A peculiar or individual reaction to an idea, action, drug, food or some other substance. Special characteristic by which one person differs from another or reacts differently from another.

Idiot Person with severe mental deficiency.

Idiotropic In psychology turning inward mentally and emotionally, i.e., introvert who is stisfied with his own emotions and is content to live apart from social contacts.

Idiotype In immunology, the specific Fab region of the immunoglobulin to which the specific antigen binds.

Idioventricular A heart rhythm arising from conduction tissue or ventricular muscle without any influence from sinus node.

Idoxuridine Antiviral agent; used for herpes[1] infection of eye in the form of ointment 2%.

IgA Principally present in exocrine secretions like milk, saliva, intestinal secretions and tear. Hence it protects against mucosal invasion by pathogenic organism. IgE is secreted by mast cells and is responsible for allergy, asthma, eczema, etc. IgG is the principal immunoglobulin and is the major antibody against bacteria, viruses and fungi, IgM is formed during early period of antigenic stimulation or infection.

Ileal bypass: A method of treating obesity whereby absorption of nutrients from intestine is decreased from anastomosis of one portion of upper small intestine to another portion down below.

Ileal conduit Method of diverting the urinary flow by transplanting the ureters into an isolated segment of ileum opening into the abdominal wall.

Ileitis Inflammation of ileum.

i. regional A nonspecific chronic granulomatous lesion involving terminal ileum giving rise to pain, weight loss, intestinal obstruction and often fistula formation.

Ileocecal valve A muscular ring at the terminal ileum that regulates passage of food from small intestine to large intestine and prevents reentry of food back into small intestine.

Ileocecostomy Surgical formation of an opening between ileum and cecum.

Ileocolostomy Anastomosis between the ileum and colon.

Ileoileostomy Surgical formation of an opening between two parts of ileum.

Ileorrhaphy Surgical repair of ileum.

Ileostomy Surgical opening of ileum through external abdominal wall.

Ileum Lower 3/5 of small intestine from jejunum to ileocecal valve. Average length 15-31 feet.

Ileus A form of intestinal obstruction due to intestinal muscle paralysis, spasm or obstruction in intestinal lumen, e.g. meconium ileus of newborn.

Iliac crest Upper free margin of hip bone or ilium.

Iliac fascia Transversalis fascia over the anterior surface of iliopsoas muscle.

Iliac region Inguinal region on either side of hypogastrium.

Iliac spine One of the four spines of ilium namely the anterior and posterior inferior spines, and the anterior and posterior superior spines.

Iliotibial band A thick wide fascial layer from the iliac crest to knee joint.

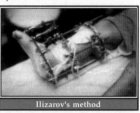
Ilizarov's method

Ilizarov method A method of bone lengthening by distraction up to 1 mm/day by cutting through outer layer but not marrow.

Illness Sickness, ailment.

Illumination Lighting up of a part for examination or of an object under microscope.

i. darkfield A method used to observe spirochetes or colloid particles in which the central or axial light rays are stopped and the object is illuminated by light rays coming from sides.

Illusion Inaccurate perception, misinterpretation of sensory impressions; when an illusion becomes fixed, it is called delusion.

Image A mental picture representing real object or the picture of an object produced by lens or mirror.

i. body The concept an individual has of his or her physical self.

i. double Occurs in squint where the visual axis of eye are not identical.

i. latent In radiology, the image on an exposed film that is invisible because it has not been developed.

i. radiographic An image formed on a fluorescent screen or photographic film by X-ray.

i real Image formed by convergence of rays of light from the object.

Image intensifier Device that increases brightness of an image and permits discrimination of much smaller objects in the image.

Imagery The calling up of events or mental pictures pertaining to sound, smell, taste, etc.

Imagination Formation of mental images of things, persons or situations.

Imaging Production of image of an object by X-ray, ultrasound, magnetic resonance, etc.

Imbalance Loss of balance usually between opposing body forces.

i. autonomic Sympathetic parasympathetic imbalance.

i. vasomotor Excessive vasoconstriction or dilatation.

Imbecile Severe mental deficiency.

Imbed In histology, to surround with a firm substance such as paraffin or colloidium.

Imbibition The absorption of fluid by a solid.

Imbricated Overlapping as tiles.

Imidazole An organic compound with heterocyclic ring as in histamine and histidine.

Imipenem An antibiotic, betalactamase resistant.

Imipramine A tricyclic antidepressant, also used in migraine and enuresis.

Immature Not fully developed or mature.

Immediate Without delay.

Immedicable Incurable.

Immersion foot A form of cold injury due to dampness and cold.

Immersion Placing body or object under water or fluid; in microscopy the act of immersing the objective (lens) in oil.

Immiscible Which cannot be mixed, e.g. oil and water.

Immobilization To make a part or limb immovable by splint, traction, plaster cast.

Immune Protected from or resistant to disease due to development of antibodies.

Immune reaction Reaction of host cells to antigenic stimulation.

Immune response The response of body to substances that are foreign or are interpreted as foreign. Immune response can be cell mediated, humoral or nonspecific.

Immunifacient Making immune.

Immunity State of being protected against disease either by previous infection or by vaccine.

i. acquired Immunity due to active or passive immunization.

i. cell mediated The T cells interact with antigen with a delayed response as seen in graft rejection or infection with tuberculosis, leprosy.

i. natural Immunity conferred by natural inherent factors like race, species.

i. passive Immunity due to transplacental transfer of maternal antibodies, antibodies secreted in milk or injection of hyperimmune specific sera.

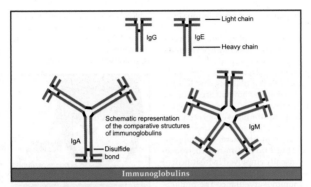

Schematic representation of the comparative structures of immunoglobulins

Light chain

Heavy chain

IgG

IgE

IgA

IgM

Disulfide bond

Immunoglobulins

Immunization The process of rendering a person immune by active (toxoid, inactivated, killed organisms) or passive process.

Immunoassay Assay of concentration of a substance by using the reaction of an antigen with specific antibody.

Immunobiology Study of immune phenomena in biological systems.

Immunochemistry The chemistry of antigen, antibodies and their relation to each other.

Immunocompetence Being capable of developing antibody response stimulated by an antigen.

Immunocompromised Unable to have adequate immunological response because of genetic defect of T and B cells, immunosuppressive drugs or AIDS virus infection.

Immunodiagnosis Use of specific immune response in diagnosing medical conditions.

Immunodiffusion A test method in which antigen and antibody are placed in a gel where they diffuse towards each other and when they meet a precipitate is formed.

Immunoelectrophoresis A method of investigating the amount and character of antibodies and immuno proteins present in body fluids.

Immunofluorescence The use of fluorescein stained or fluorescein labeled antibodies to locate antigen in tissues. The sample is examined in fluorescent microscope.

Immunogen A substance that stimulates formation of antibody.

Immunogenetics The study of genetics by use of immune responses.

Immunogenic Capable of inducing immunity.

Immunogenicity The capability to stimulate antibody formation.

Immunoglobulin Proteins capable of acting with antigens; can be IgG, IgA, IgM, IgD and IgM.

Immunology Study of immunity to disease.

Immunopathology Study of tissue alterations resulting from immune or allergic reactions.

Immunoselection Selective survival of cell populations due to their having least amount of cell surface antigenicity.

Immunostimulant Agent capable of stimulating antibody production.

Immunosuppressant Agent suppressing body immune response, usually employed in treatment of autoimmune diseases.

Immunosurveillance The immune system's recognition and destruction of newly developed abnormal cells arising from mutations. This process eliminates some cancer cells.

Immunotherapy Modalities to enhance immunity.

Impaction Condition of being tightly wedged into a part e.g., tooth impaction, impaction of feces in bowel.

Impairment Any loss or abnormality of psychological, physiological or anatomical structure or function.

Impalpable Not perceptible to touch.

Impedance Resistance met by alternating current while passing through a conductor.

i. acoustic Resistance to the passage of sound waves.

Imperative Obligatory, involuntary.

Imperception Lack of perception, inability to form a mental picture.

Imperforate Without an opening. In imperforate hymen the menstrual

blood accumulates behind to cause hematocolpos. In imperforate anus the infant has absolute constipation.

Impervious Difficult to be penetrated.

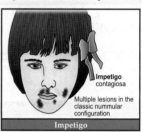

Impetigo contagiosa

Multiple lesions in the classic nummular configuration

Impetigo

Impetigo Inflammatory skin disease marked by formation of pustules which rupture with crust formation, may occur in crops, are contagious.

i. herpetiformis A rare pustular eruption of unknown etiology that occurs especially during pregnancy and in association with hypocalcemia.

Implant To graft, to insert.

i. dental Prosthetic device; endosseous, subperiosteal, mucosal or endodontic.

Implosion A violent collapse inward; opp., (explosion).

Impotency Inability of male to achieve erection, can be anatomic (defect in the genitalia), atonic (paralysis of nervi erigentis), functional or vasculogenic.

Impotent Inability to copulate and procreate.

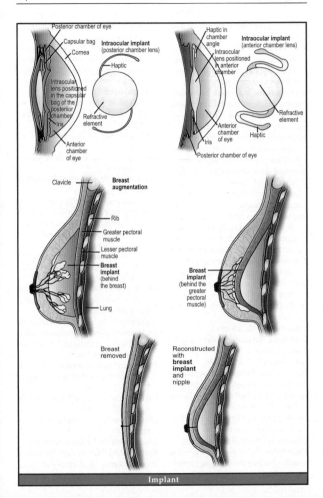

Implant

Impregnate Saturate, to make pregnant

Impression A hollow or depression on surface; effect produced upon mind by external stimuli, the imprint of dental arch.

Impression material Materials appropriate for dental impression work, like plaster of Paris, zinc oxide paste, reversible colloids.

Impression tray A tray to carry impression material to mouth and hold it in opposition to jaw/teeth.

Impulse An incitement of mind; in physiology passage of stimulating/inhibitory wave across muscle or nerve.

Impulsion Idea to do something or commit some act suddenly imposed upon the subject that tortures him until the accomplishment of that act.

Inaction Decrease response or failure of response to a stimulus.

Inactivate To make inactive or to cause loss of activity.

Inadequacy Insufficiency, incompetence.

Inanimate Dull, lifeless.

Inanition Physical debility due to lack of food.

Inapparent Not noticeable.

Inarticulate Without joints, unable to express oneself intelligibly.

Inassimilable Not capable of being utilized by body.

Incarcerated Confined, constricted, constriction as in hernia.

Incarceration Legal confinement.

Incarnatio To grow in (e.g.—toe nails); the process of being converted to flesh.

Inception The beginning, ingestion, intussusception.

Incest Coitus between close relatives.

Incidence The frequency of occurrence of any event or condition over a period of time in a specified population.

Incident A happening, event or occurrence, falling or striking ray of light

Incipient Beginning, coming into existence.

Incise To cut, as with a sharp instrument.

Incisor One of the cutting teeth, that which cuts.

Incisura Indentation at edge of any at structure, e.g. stomach incisura at distal end of lesser curvature.

Incitant The stimulus that sets off a reaction, disease.

Inclination Leaning from normal or from a vertical as in case of tooth, vertebra or pelvis.

Inclinometer Device for measuring ocular diameter from vertical and horizontal lines.

Inclusion Being included or enclosed.

Inclusion bodies Bodies present in the nucleus of cytoplasm of certain cells, e.g. Negri bodies.

Inclusion conjunctivitis *Chlamydia trachomatis* infection of the conjuctiva.

Incoercible Uncontrollable, not able to be held in check.

Incoherent Not coherent or understandable.

Incombustible Unfit for burning.

Incompatible Not being in harmony.

Incompetence Inadequacy in function of a part or organ or commonly a valve (ileocecal, mitral, aortic, pulmonary, venous, etc.).

Incompetent One legally unable to execute; incapable.

Incompetent palatal syndrome Distortion of speech (whinolalia) due to ineffective function of soft palate.

Incontinence Inability to retain urine, feces because of sphincter laxity.

Incontinence stress (urinary) Leaking of urine during coughing, sneezing, laughing, lifting, etc.

Incoordination Inability to produce harmonious, rhythmic muscular movement.

Incorporation Combining two substances to produce a homogeneous mass.

Increment Something added or gained; an addition in number, size or extent.

Incrustation Formation of crusts or scabs.

Incubation Interval between exposure to an infection and appearance of first symptoms; in bacteriology period of culture.

Incubator 1. Enclosed crib in which temperature and humidity are controlled for nursing premature babies 2. Apparatus for maintaining bacterial culture.

Incus The middle of the three oscicles in middle ear.

Indacrinon Uricosuric diuretic.

Indecision Inability to make up one's mind.

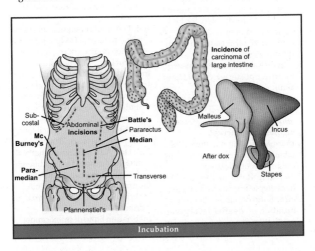

Incubation

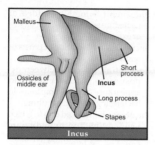

Incus

Indentation A depression or hollow.

Index case In hereditary disease, the initial patient whose condition led to investigation of the disease.

Index The forefinger, the ratio of the measurement of a given substance with that of a fixed standard.

i. cardiac Cardiac output expressed as liters/min divided by body surface area in m².

i. cephalic Skull breadth to length multiplied by 100.

i. cerebral Ratio of greatest transverse to anteroposterior diameter of skull.

i. pelvic Ratio of pelvic conjugate and transverse diameters.

i. phagocytic Average bacteria ingested per phagocyte.

i. therapeutic The maximum tolerable dose of a drug divided by minimum curable dose.

i. thoracic Ratio of thoracic AP diameter to transverse diameter.

i. vital Ratio of number of births to number of deaths in a given population over a stated period of time.

Indican Potassium salt of indoxy-sulfate found in sweat and urine during conversion of tryptophan to indole by action of intestinal flora.

Indicant Some sign or symptom that points to presence of disease.

Indicator In chemical analysis, a substance that can be used to determine pH.

Indifferent Not responsive to normal stimuli, apathetic, neutral.

Indigenous Native to a country or region.

Indigestion Imperfect digestion manifesting as nausea, vomiting heart burn, belching, etc.

Indium A rare metallic element, its isotope ¹¹³I used in scanning.

Indocyanine green A dye used in testing hepatic and renal excretory function.

Indole A solid crystalline substance found in feces, a bacterial decom-position product of tryptophan.

Indolent Inactive, sluggish.

Indolent ulcer Ulcer slow in healing.

Indomethacin Antiprostaglandin agent with anti-inflammatory, analgesic and antipyretic pro-perties.

Induction The process of facilitating labor with oxytoxic drugs.

Inductor Any substance that will cause cells exposed to it to differen-tiate into an organized tissue.

Induration The act of heardening.

Inebriant Any intoxicant; making drunk.

Inebriation State of intoxication.

Inelastic Not elastic.

Inert Not active; in chemistry not able to react with other chemicals.

Inertia 1. Sluggishness, lack of activity. 2. In physics tendency of body to remain in its state uptill acted upon by external force.

i. uterine Absence of uterine contractions.

Infant From time of birth to one year of age.

i. preterm Born prior to 37 weeks of gestation.

i. post term Born after 42 weeks of gestation.

i. term Born between 38-41 weeks of gestation.

Infarct Area of necrosis consequent to cessation of blood supply.

Infarction Formation of an infarct.

Infection Tissue invasion with pathogenic agent that produce injurious effect.

i. acute Infection appearing suddenly.

i. chronic Infection having protracted course.

i. concurrent Existence of two or more infections at the same time.

i. cross Transfer of one disease from one hospitalized patient to another.

i. droplet Infection acquired through microorganisms disbursed to air via breath or nasobronchial secretion.

i. pyogenic Infection by pusforming organisms.

i. lowgrade Mild inflammation without pus formation.

Infectious disease Disease caused by an infecting agent, not necessarily contagious.

Infiltration The process of passing into or through a substance or space.

Infinity Space, time and quantity without limits.

Infirmary A small hospital, a place for care of sick.

Inflammation Tissue reaction to injury with vasodilatation, exudation, leukocyte migration followed by healing.

i. acute Rapid onset and short course.

i. adhesive Inflammation with adhesion of tissue to surrounding structures.

i. catarrhal Inflammation of mucous membrane with excessive mucous secretion.

i. exudative Inflammation with extreme vasodilatation, and large accumulation of blood cells.

i. granulomatous Inflammation with excessive granular tissue production as in tuberculosis, syphilis and systemic fungal infections.

i. hyperplastic Inflammation with excess production of fibrous tissue *SYN*— in proliferative.

i. interstitial Inflammation involving supporting structures in an organ.

i. pseudomembranous Inflammation in which necrotic tissues form a pseudomembrane, e.g. diphtheria.

i. purulent Inflammation with pus formation.

i. ulcerative Inflammation with ulcer formation.

Inflation Distention of a part by air gas or fluid.

Inflator Device used to force air into an organ.

Inflection An inward bending; change of tone or pitch of the voice.

Influenza A viral acute contagious upper respiratory infection.

Influenza virus vaccine Vaccine containing inactivated influenza virus A and B; given every year with different strains of A and B.

Infolding Process of enclosing within a fold.

Informed consent Competent and voluntary permission for a medical test, procedure or medication.

Infra-axillary Below the axilla.

Infra Prefix meaning below, under, beneath.

Infra-red rays Invisible heal rays beyond the red end of spectrum, of 7500-150, 000 AU used for local application of heat and pain relief.

Infracostal Below the ribs.

Infracotyloid Beneath the cotyloid cavity of the acetabulum of hip.

Infraction An incomplete fracture of bone.

Infradentale The bony point between the mandibular central incisors.

Infradiaphragmatic Below the diaphragm.

Infraglenoid Beneath the glenoid fossa.

Infraglottic Below the glottis.

Infrahyoid Below the hyoid bone.

Inframammary Below the breast.

Inframandibular Below the jawbone.

Infraorbital Below the orbit.

Infrapsychic Below the level of consciousness or automatic.

Infrapubic Below the pubis.

Infrascapular Beneath the shoulder blade.

Infraspinous Beneath the scapular spine.

Infratrochlear Beneath the trochlea.

Infundibulum 1. Funnel shaped passage or/structure. 2. Tube connecting the frontal sinus with middle nasal meatus. 3. Stalk of pituitary gland. 4. Peritoneal end of fallopian tube. 5. Upper end of cochlear canal.

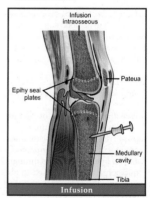

Infusion

Infusion Liquid substance introduced into body vein.

Ingestion Intake of food or the process by which cells take foreign particles.

Ingravescent Becoming more severe.

Ingredient Any unit or part of a complex compound or mixture.

Ingrowing Growing inward.

Ingrown nail Growth of nail edge deep into soft tissues causing pain and inflammation.

Inguinal canal The canal 1½″ long, providing passage for spermatic cord in the male and round ligament of uterus in the female. A potential source of weakness; may serve as site of inguinal hernia and undescended testis.

Inguinal glands Lymph nodes of groin draining from lower limb and perineum.

Inguinal ligament *SYN* — Poupart's ligament. Fibrous band extending from anterior superior iliac spine to pubic tubercle.

Inguinal Pertains to region of groin.

Inguinal region The iliac region on either side of pubes.

Inguinal ring Interior and exterior openings of inguinal canal, termed as internal and external inguinal rings.

Inhalation The act of drawing in the breath, vapor or gas into the lungs.

Inhalation therapy Administration of medicine, water vapor and gases (O_2, CO_2, NO_2).

Inhaler Device for administering medicines by inhalation.

Inherent Natural *SYN*—innate, intrinsic.

Inheritance Something hereditary, acquired through eggs and sperms.

Inhibin A testicular hormone that inhibits LH secretion by pituitary.

Inhibition 1. Restraint of a function. 2. In physiology slowing or stopping the function of an organ.

i. competitive Inhibition by competing with cell receptors.

i. psychic Arrest of an impulse, thought, action or speech.

Inhibitor That which inhibits.

Inhibitrope Person in whom certain stimuli cause partial arrest of function.

Inhomogeneity Lack of uniform quality or consistency.

Iniencephalus Congenitally deformed fetus in which brain substance protrudes through a fissure in the occiput.

Inion External occipital protuberance.

Iniopagus Twins fused at the occiput.

Initials Beginning or commencement.

Initis Inflammation of fibrous tissue.

Inject To introduce.

Injection Forcing a fluid into body via vessel or skin.

i. epidural Injection of anesthetic agent into epidural space.

i. hypodermic Injection of substance beneath the skin.

i. alveolar dental infiltration of anesthetic agent.

i. intra-muscular Injection directly into muscles, e.g. thigh, deltoid, glutei.

i. intra-articular Injection into joint space.

i. z. track An injection technique, the needle taking a Z track to make the injected fluid difficult to track back.

Injectors Instruments used for injection of fluids.

Injury Damage or trauma to some body part.

i. steering wheel Automobile accidents where victims lung and heart are contused by pressure of steering wheel.

Inlay A solid filling made to the precise shape of a cavity of a tooth and cemented into it.

Innate Something natural, belonging from birth.

Innervation Nerve supply, distribution and function of nervous system.

i. collateral Outgrowth of nerves from adjacent nerves, once the original nerve supply is damaged.

i. reciprocal An innervation mechanism by which if flexors are stimulated, the extensors are inhibited.

Innocent Harmless, benign, clinically unimportant.

Innocuous Harmless, benign, without serious effects.

Innominate artery The artery arising on right side from aortic arch and dividing into right subclavian and right common carotid.

Innominate bone The hip bone composed of ilium, ischium and pubis.

Innominate Nameless.

Innominate vein Formed by union of internal jugular and subclavian veins.

Inoculate To inject microorganism, serum or toxic materials into body.

Inoculation The process of being inoculated.

Inoculum Substance introduced by inoculation.

Inocyte Fibroblast.

Inogenesis Formation of fibrous tissue.

Inoperable Unsuitable for surgery.

Inopexia Tendency of blood to coagulate spontaneously.

Inorganic compound A chemical compound without carbon.

Inosemia An excessive amount of fibrin in the blood.

Inositis Inflammation of fibrous tissue.

Inositol A sugar like crystalline substance, a part of vitamin B complex group.

Inotropic Augmenting force of muscular contraction.

Inpatient Hospitalized patient.

Inquest Investigation into circumstances, manner and cause of health.

Insalubrious Not healthy.

Insanitary Not conducive to health.

Insanity Severe mental derangement.

Insatiable Unable to be appeased or satisfied.

Inscription A prescription slip with name of the drug and its doses.

Insect bites and stings The venom of stinging insect, may be more toxic than that of poisonous snake but fortunately the quantity injected is small.

Insecta A class of phylum Arthropoda characterized by three distinct body divisions like head, thorax and abdomen, two pairs of wings and three pairs of jointed legs.

Insecticide An agent destructive to insects.

Insectifuge Insect repellant.

Insecurity Feeling of helplessness, apprehension.

Insemination Fertilization of ovum, semen discharge into vagina during coitus.

Insenescence Process of growing old.

Insensible Without feeling or perception.

Insertion 1. Placement or implanting of some thing into another. 2. distal end of muscle attachment through which it moves a part.

Insidious Used to denote the onset of a disease so silently without patient's awareness.

Insight Self understanding; absence of awareness.

Insipid Lacking in spirit, without taste.

In situ In position, localized, without invasion.

Insolation Heat stroke.

Insoluble Unable to be dissolved.

Insomnia Lack of sleep.

Inspect To examine visually.

Inspection Visual examination.

Inspersion Sprinkling with powder or a fluid.

Inspiration Indrawing of air into lungs.

Inspissate To thicken by evaporation or absorption of fluid.

Insterscapular reflex Scapular muscular contraction following percussion between the scapula.

Instillation Slowly pouring or dropping a liquid into body cavity.

Instinct The inherited tendency for the members of a specific species to react to certain environmental conditions and stimuli in a particular way.

Instruction Directions or command.

Instrumentation The use of instruments.

Insufficiency Inadequacy of function.

i. adrenal Decreased adrenal function.

i. aortic Imperfect closure of aortic leaflets with back flow.

i. cardiac Poor cardiac pump function.

i. coronary Diminished blood flow through coronary vessels.

i. hepatic Hepatic insufficiency with cholemia.

i. mitral Inefficient mitral valve closure with backflow of blood into left atrium during ventricular systole.

i. respiratory Hypoxemia and hypercarbia due to poor pulmonary function.

Insufflate The act of blowing into or pumping air into a cavity/lung as in infants.

Insula Triangular area of the cerebral cortex lying in the floor of the lateral fissure.

Insulator That which insulates.

Insulin Hormone secreted by the beta cells of islets of Langerhans of pancreas.

i. human Synthesized by recombinant DNA technology using *E. coli*.

i. monocomponent Highly purified insulin containing impurity 10 parts per million.

i. isophane (NPH) Intermediate acting insulin with 18-28 hours of action.

Insulin lipodystrophy Atrophy or hypertrophy of skin fat at the insulin injection site.

Insulin pump A battery driven pump delivering insulin subcutaneously into abdominal wall according to preset program.

Insulin shock Hypoglycemic shock due to overdose of insulin.

Insulinase An enzyme that inactivates insulin.

Insulinemia Excess of blood insulin.

Insulinogenesis Production of insulin by the pancreas.

Insulinogenic Pertains to production of insulin.

Insulinoma Insulin producing tumor of pancreas.

Intake Things taken up like food and liquids.

Integration The bringing together of various parts or functions for harmonious working.

Integrator Device for measuring body surfaces.

Integument A covering, the skin.

Integumentary system The skin and its appendages.

Intellect The mind, conscious brain function.

Intelligence quotient A standard score that places an individual in reference to the scores of others within the same age group. This is determined through the subject's answers to arbitrary chosen questions.

Intelligence test A test designed to determine the intelligence of an individual.

Intelligence The ability to think, the capacity to comprehend.

Intemporance Lack of moderation, excess in use of anything.

Intensity The degree or extent of activity, strength, force.

Intensive Related to or marked by intensity.

Intention Goal or purpose, a natural process of healing.

i. first Healing without granulation tissue formation or suppuration.

i. second Healing by adhesion of two granulated surfaces.

i. third Healing by granulation tissue and scar formation.

Insulinoid Resembling or having properties of insulin.

Intention tremor Occurrence of tremor on attempted coordinated movements.

Inter arytenoid Between arytenoid cartilages of larynx.

Inter prefix Means between, midst.

Interradicular bone The alveolar bone between the roots of multi-rooted teeth.

Inter radicular fibers The collagen fibers of periodontal ligament in the interradicular area, anchoring the tooth to alveolar bone.

Interacinar Located between acini of glands.

Interalveolar Between alveoli of lungs.

Interatrial Located between the atria.

Interauricular As above.

Intercadence A supernumerary pulse wave between two regular beats.

Intercalated ducts Short narrow ducts that lie between secretory ducts and the terminal alveoli in the parotid and submandibular glands and in the pancreas.

Intercalated Inserted between.

Intercapillary Between the capillaries.

Intelcarpal Between the carpal bones.

Intercellular Between the cells.

Intercerebral Between the cerebral hemispheres.

Intercilium The space between the eyebrows.

Interclavicular Between the clavicles.

Intercoccygeal Between the segments of coccyx.

Intercostal Between the ribs.

Intercostal muscles, external Outer layer of muscles between the ribs, originating from the lower margin of rib and inserted to the upper margin of next rib below; act to draw adjacent ribs together thereby increasing volume of thorax.

Intercostal muscles, internal Lie beneath external intercostal and function in the same way.

Intercourse Sexual union; social interaction between individuals or groups.

Intercurrent Intervening.

Interdent A specially designed knife used for removing interdental tissue.

Interdentium The space between contiguous teeth.

Interface In computers, a device that enables two normally noncompatible circuits or parts to function together.

Interference Clashing.

Interferon A protein formed by leucocytes and plasma cells in response to viral or other foreign nucleic acids, used in treatment of hepatitis B and C, hairy cell leukemia.

Intergemmal Between taste buds.

Interglobular spaces Gaps in dentin due to failure of calcification.

Intergluteal Between the two buttocks.

Intergyral Between the cerebral gyri.

Interictal Between the two seizure attacks.

Interlamellar Between lamellae.

Interleukin A type of cytokine essential for communication among leukocytes, inflammation and cell mediated immunity. 19 interleukins are identified and their functions defined.

Interleukin I Substance from monocytes and macrophages responsible for acute phase response.

Interleukin II A lymphokine that stimulates growth of T-lymphocytes, often used in treatment of metastatic renal cancer.

Interlobar Between two lobes.

Intermalleolar Between two malleoli.

Intermammary Between two breasts.

Intermarriage Marriage between persons of two distinct populations.

Intermediary metabolism The series of intermediate products formed during process of digestion and excretion.

Intermediary Situated between two bodies; occurring between two periods of time.

Intermediate In between.

Intermedia A substance secreted by pituitary controlling pigmentation of skin in lower animals.

Intermenstrual Between menstrual periods.

Intermission Interval between two paroxysm of disease.

Intermittent Coming and going.

Intermittent fever Fever in which there is complete absence of symptoms between paroxysms.

Intermittent positive pressure breathing Assisted breathing in patients of respiratory failure, myasthenia gravis.

Intermural Between the walls or sides of an organ.

Internal bleeding Hemorrhage especially from G.I. tract.

Internal ear The cochlea, semi-circular canals, vestibule.

Internal injury Any injury not visible from outside.

Internal secretion Secretion of ductless glands.

Internalization The unconscious mental mechanism in which the values and standards of society and one's parents are taken as one's own.

Internatal Between the buttocks.

International classification of diseases A classification code devised by WHO, helpful for international comparison.

International normalized ratio (INR) A system of standoardizing prothrombin time in people on oral anticoagulants. It is derived from calibrations of commercial thromboplastin reagents against a sensitive human brain thromboplastin. A PT ratio of 1.3. to 2 in equivalant to INR of 2-4.

International unit Internationally accepted amount of a substances like vitamins, hormones, vaccines, etc.

Interneuron A neuron situated in between neurons.

Internist Physician specializing in internal medicine.

Internuncial Acting as a connecting medium.

Interocclusal Between the occlusal surfaces or cusps of opposite teeth.

Interoceptive Sensations arising within body itself, not those arising from outside the body.

Interoceptor A receptor activated by stimuli within the body.

Interoinferior Inward and downward position.

Interparietal Between the parietal bones; between the parietal lobes of cerebrum, between walls.

Interpersonal Concerning the relations and interactions between persons.

Interphase The resting stage of a cell between divisions.

Interpolation 1. In surgery transfer of tissue from one site to another. 2. In statistics the calculation of an intermediate value from the observed values.

Interposition The state of being interposed or inserted between.

Interpretation Analysis, significance.

Interradicular Between the roots of teeth.

Intersection Site where one structure crosses another or joins similar structure.

Intersex A person having both male and female sex characteristics but genetically either male or female.

Interspace Space between two similar parts.

Interspinal Between the two spinous processes of the spine.

Interstitial cells of testes Cells of Leydig in seminiferous tubules producing testosterone.

Interstitial cystitis Idiopathic inflammation of bladder.

Interstitial fluid Fluid that surrounds cells.

Interstitial lung disease A large group of diseases, chronic non infectious in nature that hamper oxygen transfer from alveoli to the capillaries.

Interstitial tissue Intercellular connective tissue.

Interstitium Space or gap in a structure or an organ.

Intertransverse Joining the transverse processes of vertebrae.

Intertriginous Having similarity with intertrigo.

Intertrigo Superficial dermatitis of the skin folds.

Intertrochanteric Between greater and lesser trachanter of femur.

Intertrochanteric line Ridge between greater and lesser trochanter of femur.

Intervaginal Between the sheaths.

Interval Space, time or period between two objects or happenings.

i. AV Interval between beginning of atrial systole and ventricular systole.

i. cardio arterial Time between apex beat and radial pulse.

i. isometric Time between onset of ventricular systole and opening of semilunar (aortic-pulmonary) valves.

i. lucid Brief remission of symptoms in head injury and psychosis.

i. PR Period between onset of P wave and beginning of QRS complex. Normal-less than 0.2 sec.

i. QR Period between onset of Q wave and peak of R wave.

i. QRS—QRS duration from beginning of Q wave to end of S wave. Normal 0.12 sec.

i. QT Interval between beginning of Q wave and end of T wave.

Intervention Taking appropriate action.

Intervertebral disc A broad and flat disk of fibrocartilage between the bodies of vertebra.

Intervillous Between the villi.

Intestinal bypass Surgical short circuiting of small intestine to produce controlled malabsorption to treat massive obesity.

Intestinal flora Bacteria present in intestine that synthesize vitamins.

Intestinal gas H_2, methane, CO_2, H_2S and methyl mercaptan produced in GI tract during digestive process.

Intestinal juice Secretion of small intestine containing a number of enzymes like maltase, lipase, peptidase, sucrase, etc.

Intestinal obstruction Blockage of intestinal lumen due to stricture, worms, fibrous band, foreign body, stone, fecolith, etc. producing absolute constipation, abdominal distention, dehydration and pain.

Intestinal perforation Soiling of peritoneal cavity with intestinal content; commonly a complication of enteric fever, tuberculosis or prolonged intestinal obstruction.

Intestinal putrefaction The putrefying effect of intestinal bacteria producing indole, skatole, paracresol, phenol, phenylpropionic acid, phenyl acetic acid, and gases.

Intestinal reflex Intestinal contraction and relaxation above the portion of bowel that is stimulated.

Intestinal tubes Plastic or rubber tubes placed in intestinal tract through nose or mouth to suck gas, fluids or solids.

Intestine The alimentary canal extending from pylorus to anus. The small intestine is 7 meter long and the large intestine 1.5 meter. Cecum is the beginning of large intestine and appendix (3-4" long) is attached to it. The duodenum is 8-10" long; jejunum 9 feet and ileum 14 feet. In the wall of the small intestine are Brunners glands, crypts of Lieberkuhn and Peyers's patches.

Intolerance Unable to bear pain, effects of a drug or other substance.

Intorsion Rotation of eye inward.

Intoxication State of being intoxicated with alcohol, drugs, chemicals.

Intra aortic balloon counterpulsation Placement of an inflatable balloon in aortic root to lower/decrease systolic work of LV and to promote coronary blood flow; useful in treating shock. The balloon is inflated with helium during diastole and deflated during systole.

Intra-atrial Within the atrium.

Intracardiac Within the heart.

Intracath A device for facilitating for introduction of IV catheter. A needle is ensheathed by a catheter and once introduced into vein the needle is withdrawn and catheter remain in place.

Intracisternal Within cistern of brain.

Intracranial Within brain.

Intradural Enclosed by dura mater.

Intragastric balloon Placement of inflatable balloon in stomach to treat obesity.

Intrahepatic Within liver.

Intralocular Within the cavity of any structure.

Intraluminal Within the lumen.

Intramedullary Within the medulla oblongata of brain; within bone marrow; within the spinal cord substance.

Intramural Within the walls of a hollow organ or cavity.

Intraocular Within the eye.

Intraoral Within the mouth.

Intrapartum Occurring during child birth.

Intraperitoneal Inside the peritoneal cavity.

Intrauterine contraceptive device Copper or other metallic device placed within uterus to prevent conception.

Intrauterine Within the uterus.

Intravasation Entry into blood vessels.

Intravenous infusion Injection of colloid or crystalloid solutions into a vein to treat hypovolemia, or maintenance.

Intravenous infusion pump A device to provide constant but adjustable rate of flow of IV solutions.

Intravenous Into a vein.

Intravesical Within urinary bladder.

Intravitreous Within the vitreous of eye.

Intrinsic Belonging to or embedded in, essential nature of a thing.

Intrinsic factor Substance present in the gastric juice that facilitates absorption of vit B_{12}.

Intrinsic muscles Muscles having their origin and insertion entirely within a structure, e.g. intrinsic muscles of eye, tongue and larynx.

Introducer Device for controlling, directing and placing intubation tube within trachea, blood vessels or heart.

Introitus Entrance into a canal or cavity.

Introjection In psychoanalysis, identification of self with another, the victim assuming the supposed feelings of the other personality.

Intromission An insertion or placing of one part into another.

Introns The noncoding region between the coding regions (exons) of the DNA in gene.

Introspection Looking within one's mind.

Introversion Preoccupation with one's self; turning inside out of a part.

Introvert A personality characterized by withdrawal from reality, fantasy formation, as in schizophrenia.

Intubation To insert a tube, e.g. into larynx.

Intuition Knowing something spontaneously in advance.

Intumescence Swelling up or enlarging.

Intussusception Invagination; slipping of one part of intestine into another part below.

Intussusceptum The inner segment of intestine in intussusception.

Intussuscipiens That portion of intestine that receives the intussusceptum.

Induction Ointment rubbed into skin for medicinal effect.

Inulase Enzyme that converts inulin to levulose.

Inulin A polysaccharide found in plants yielding levulose on hydrolysis. Used in study of renal function (GFR).

Invaginate To insert one part of a structure within a part of same structure; to ensheath.

Invalid A sick person confined to bed or wheel chair.

Invasion Entrance of microorganisms into body and their distribution into tissues.

Invasive procedure Procedure in which the body cavity is entered that could interfere with bodily function.

Invasive Tending to spread, e.g. malignant growth.

Invermination Worm infestation.

Inverse square law Law stating that the intensity of radiation or light at any distance is inversely proportional to the square of the distance between the irradiated surface and a point source.

Inversion Reversal of normal relationship; turning inside out.

i. uterine Uterus is turned inside out with internal surface protruding at vagina, a serious complication of placental delivery and causes of postpartum bleeding.

Invert sugar A mixture of levulose and dextrose, formed by inversion of sucrose by the enzyme invertase.

Invertase A sugar-splitting enzyme found in GI tract.

Invertebrate Those species without a backbone.

Investment A covering or sheath.

Inveterate Chronic, firmly seated habit.

In vitro Outside the living body, e.g. tests done in laboratory involving isolated tissue or cell preparation.

In vivo Within the living body or organism.

Involucrum The covering of newly formed bone enveloping the sequestrum in infected bone.

Involuntary Independent, not depending upon volition.

Involution Turning inward, reduction in size of uterus following delivery, the retrogressive change in vital processes after their functions have been fulfilled.

Involutional melancholia Depression visiting men and women between 50-65 years and 40-55 years of age.

Iodameba A genus of ameba seen in GI tract.

Iodide A compound of iodine, e.g., pot iodide.

Iodine A nonmetallic halogen giving violet vapour on melting. Total body content is 50 mg, one third of it being present in thyroid. Daily requirement is 100-150 µg.

i. protein bound That iodine bound to plasma protein.

i. radioactive Isotopes of iodine ^{131}I or ^{125}I, used for thyroid uptake studies, hepatic studies or in treatment of hyperthyroidism and thyroid cancer.

Iodine tincture Preparation of iodine in alcohol and water.

Iodipamide meglumine Agent used for gallbladder X-ray.

Iodism Condition resulting from excess and prolonged use of iodine.

Iodized salt Salt containing 100 mg of sodium or potassium iodide per gram.

Iododerma Dermatitis due to iodine.

Iodoform A compound formed by action of iodine on acetone in the presence of an alkali. Used topically for mild antibacterial action.

Iodohippurate sodium A radio active dye used in renal studies.

Iodophilia Unusual pronounced affinity of polymorphs for iodine in some infections and anemia.

Iodophor Iodine in a solubilizing agent, e.g. povidone iodine.

Iodoquinol Antiamebic agent, can cause subacute myelo-optic neuropathy.

Ion A particle carrying an electric charge. Ions carrying positive charge aggregate near cathode and those with negative charge near anode.

Ion exchange resins Resins that bind to some ions, e.g. cholestyramine.

Ionium A natural radioactive ion of thorium.

Ionization Dissociation of acids, bases and salts into their constituent ions.

Ionometer A device to measure amount of radiation and intensity of rays.

Iontophoresis Introduction of various ions into the skin by means of electricity.

Iopanoic acid Radiopaque dye used for gallbladder studies.

Iophendylate Radiopaque dye used in myelography.

Iothalamate meglumine Radio-opaque material for angiography.

Ipatropium bromide An anti-cholinergic given by inhalation in bronchial asthma.

Ipecac Dried roots of plant ipecacuanha, source of emetine.

Ipodate calcium Radioopaque material for X-ray studies of gallbladder.

Iproniazid Antitubercular drugs.

Ipsilateral On the same side.

Iridalgia Pain in the iris.

Iridauxesis Increase in thickness of iris as in glaucoma.

Iridectome Instrument for cutting iris in iridectomy.

Iridectomy Surgical removal of a portion of iris as in glaucoma, corneal scar.

Iridemia Bleeding from iris.

Irideremia Partial or total congenital absence of iris.

Irides Pleural of iris.

Iridesis Formation of an iris artificially.

Iridium A white hard metallic element.

Iridoavulsion Tearing away of iris.

Iridocapsulitis Inflammation of iris and capsule of lens.

Iridocoloboma Congenital defect or fissure in iris.

Iridocele Protrusion of a portion of iris through a defect in cornea.

Iridocyclectomy Surgical removal of iris and ciliary body.

Iridodesis Ligature of part of the iris to from an artificial one. *SYN* — iridesis.

Iridodialysis Separation of outer margin of iris from its ciliary attachment.

Iridodonesis Tremulousness of iris seen in aphakic eye or subluxated lens.

Iridokinesis Contraction and expansion movement of iris.

Iridoplegia Paralysis of iris.

Iridoptosis Prolapse of iris.

Iridorrhexis Rupture of or tearing of the iris from its attachment.

Iridoschisis Splitting of stroma of iris with disintegration.

Iridotasis Stretching of the iris in the treatment of glaucoma.

Iridotomy Incision of iris for making a new aperture.

Iridotomy Incision of iris.

Iris The organ between lens and cornea.

i. bombe Bulging of iris forwards with annular posterior synechia.

Irish moss A genus of seaweeds.

Irisopsia Visual defect in which coloured circles are seen around lights

Iritis Inflammation, of the iris, with photophobia, lacrimation, irregular pupil, dull-muddy looking iris.

i. plastic Iritis with fibrinous exudate.

Iron A metallic element existing as Ferrous (Fe^{++}) and Ferric (Fe^{+++}) forms, essential part of hemoglobin and myoglobin. Adult requirement of iron is 0.5- 1 mg per day; manganese, copper and cobalt are necessary for proper utilization of iron.

Iron-dextran Injectable form of iron.

Iron storage disease Hemochromatosis.

Irradiation Therapeutic application of X-ray, radium as in malignancy.

Irrational Contrary to what is reasonable or logical.

Irreducible Not capable of being reduced or made smaller.

Irrelevance Unrelated to, in appropriate.

Irreversible Impossible to reverse.

Irrigation Cleansing with fluids.

Irrigator (Device used to flush or irrigate.

Irritability Excitability; impatience.

Irritations Reaction to what is irritating.

Ischemia Lack of blood supply.

Ischiocavernosus An erectile muscle extending from ischium to penis or clitoris.

Ischiococcygeus Coccygeus muscle forming posterior portion of levator ani.

Ischiorectal abscess Collection of pus in ischiorectal fossa.

Ischiorectal fossa Para rectal fat filled fossa bounded laterally by obturator internus and ischial tuberosity, posteriorly by gluteus maximus and medially by levator ani.

Island A structure detached from surrounding structures or a tiny, isolated mass of one kind of cells within another type.

i. of Calleja Groups of densely packed small cells in the cortex of gyrus hippocampus.

i. of Reil The insula, in the floor of sylvian fissure.

i's of Langerhans Clusters of cells in pancreas containing the alpha, beta and delta cells. The alpha cells are dominant and produce insulin.

Ismelin Guanethidine sulphate.

Isoagglutination Agglutination of red blood cells by agglutinin from blood of another person.

Isoagglutinin Antibody in the serum that agglutinates RBC of same species.

Isoantigen A substance present in certain individuals that stimulates production of antibody in other members *SYN*—alloantigen.

Isobucaine hydrochloride A local anesthetic agent.

Isochromatic Having the same color.

Isochromosomes A chromosome with arms that are morphologically; identical and contain the same genetic loci.

Isochronal Taking place at regular intervals or in uniform time.

Isochronia The correspondence of events with respect to time, rate or frequency.

Isocoria Equality in size of both pupils.

Isocytosis Cells of equal size.

Isodontic Having teeth of equal size.

Isoelectric Having equal electric potentials.

Isoelectric period The time or point when no electric energy is produced.

Isoenzyme A form of an enzyme.

Isoetharine hydrochloride A sympathomimetic agent, used as bronchodilator.

Isoflurophate An anticholinesterage drug used to treat glaucoma and atony of intestinal and vesical smooth muscles.

Isogamete A cell which on fusion with a similar cell reproduces.

Isogamy Reproduction resulting from conjugation of isogametes or identical cells.

Isohemaglutin Blood group antibody normally present in blood that causes clumping of incompatible blood.

Isoimmunization Immunization of an individual against the blood of another individual of same species.

Isolation Limitation of movement and social contact of patients suffering from or a known carrier of communicable disease.

Isoleucine An essential amino acid.

Isomer Substances having same molecular formula but different chemical and physical properties, e.g., dextrose is an isomer of levulose.

Isomerase Any enzyme that catalyzes isomerization of its substrate.

Isomerism Compounds with equal number of atoms but with different atomic arrangements.

Isomerization Conversion of a substance to its isomer.

Isometric contraction Contraction without change in muscle length i.e., tension development without any mechanical work.

Isoniazid Antitubercular agent, bacteriocidal, can cause peripheral neuritis.

Isophoria Equal tension of vertical muscles of each eye with visual lines in the same horizontal plane.

Isopropamide Iodide A synthetic antimuscarinic drug with actions similar to belladona.

Isopropyl alcohol C_3H_8O, an alcohol used in medical preparations for external use, antifreeze, cosmetics, and as a solvent.

Isoproterenol A sympathomimetic, used in bronchial asthma.

Iso osmotic Having the same total concentration of osmotically active molecules.

Isosexual Concerning or characteristic of same sex.

Isosorbide dinitrate Antianginal drug.

Isospora A genus of sporozoa e.g., I-hominis, a nonpathogenic protozoa inhabiting small intestine.

Isosthenuria Passage of urine having constant specific gravity; a sign of advanced renal disease.

Isotherapy Treatment of a disease by the same causative agent.

Isotonic Having same osmotic pressure.

Isotonic exercise Contraction of a muscle during which the force of resistance to the movement remains constant throughout the range of motion.

Isotonic solution A solution with osmotic pressure same as that of another solution with which it is compared.

Isotope Elements with nearly identical chemical properties but different atomic weights and electric charges.

Isotretinin A retinoid used in acne.

Isotropic Possessing similar qualities in every direction; having equal refraction.

Isoxsuprine hydrochloride A vasodilator and smooth muscle relaxant.

Issue Offspring.

Isthmoplegia Paralysis of fauces.

Isthmus A narrow passage connecting two cavities, a narrow structure connecting two larger parts, a constriction between two larger parts.

Isuprel hydrochloride Isoproterenol hydrochloride.

Itch Irritation of skin inducing desire to scratch.

i. barbar's Fungus infection of beard area.

i. dhobi Fungus infection of groin and perineum.

i. ground Itching in feet due to penetration by hookworm larva.

i. swimmer's Dermatitis due to swimming in water containing larvae form of schistosomes.

Itraconazole Antifungal agent.

IVY method A method for estimation of bleeding time

Ivy poisoning Poison ivy dermatitis.

Ixodes A genus of ticks.

J

Jacket A bandage usually applied to the trunk to immobilize the spine or correct deformities.

j. procelain Crown restoration with procelain.

j. sayre's Plaster of Paris jacket to support spinal deformity.

Jackscrew A threaded screw used for expanding the dental arch.

Jacksonian epilepsy Focal epilepsy with spasm confined to a group of muscles.

Jacobson Danish anatomist.

j's cartilage Cartilage lying along anterior inferior border of nasal septum.

j's nerve tympanic nerve.

Jacquemier's sign Blue or purple color of vagina in early pregnancy.

Jactitation Restless to and fro movement of body.

Jaegers test types A reading test type for near vision.

Jamais vu Feeling of being placed in a strange environment or unfamiliarity; a feature of temporal lobe epilepsy.

Jame's fiber Preexcitation of ventricles by fibers connecting atria to ventricle or distal. His bundle, bypassing AV node.

Janeway lesion Small painless red blue macular lesions in palms and soles in bacterial endocarditis.

Jargon Speech or writting that includes unfamiliar terms or abbreviations.

Jarvi's snare Snare for removing growth in nasal cavity.

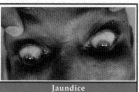
Jaundice

Jaundice Yellow coloration of skin, conjuctiva and mucous membranes due to hyperbilirubinemia.

j. acholuric Jaundice with clear urine i.e., unconjugated hyperbilirubinemia of hemolysis.

j. cholestatic Conjugated hyperbilirubinemia due to stasis of bile excretion, either intrahepatic or extrahepatic.

j. hemolytic Jaundice due to hemolysis.

j. hepatocellular Jaundice due to hepatitis.

j. obstructive Conjugated hyperbilirubinemia with itching due to bile duct stricture, compression or luminal obstruction.

Jaw Maxilla and mandible bearing teeth and forming the framework of mouth.

j. cleft Lack of fusion of the right and left mandible into a single bone.

j. crackling Noise of normal or diseased temperomandibular joint during movement of jaw.

j. dislocation The jaw is pushed downward and forward, occurring due to trauma, following yawning, hearty laugh or chewing large chunks of food.

j. winking Voluntary movement of lower face causing unilateral contraction of orbicularis oculi, seen during the process of recovery from Bell's palsy.

Jejunitis Inflammation of jejunum.

Jejunocolostomy Anastomosis of colon with jejunum.

Jejunoileitis Inflammation of jejunum and ileum as in Crohn's disease.

Jejunorrhaphy Surgical repair of jejunum.

Jejunum The second portion of small intestine next to duodenum, about 8 feet in length, making about 2/5 of small intestine.

Jelly A thick semisolid gelatinous substance.

j. wharton's Soft gelatinous connective tissue that constitutes the matrix of umbilical cord.

Jendrassik's maneuver Facilitation of deep tendon reflexes of lower extremity by hooking the fingers of both hands by the patient and trying to pull them apart.

Jenner Edward British physician who invented cowpox vaccine for immunization against smallpox.

Jenner's stain Eosin methylene blue stain.

Jerk Sudden muscular movement, often as a reflex from tapping of the tendon.

j. ankle Contraction of soleus-gastrocnemius by tapping tendo-Achilles.

j. biceps Contraction of biceps following tapping of biceps tendon at elbow.

j. jerk Taping of mandible when jaw is half open. Vigorous mouth

closure indicates bilateral supra-nuclear cerebral lesions.

j. knee Striking the patellar tendon causes contraction of quadriceps with extension of knee.

Joffroy's sign Absence of facial muscle contraction when eyes turn upward in exophthalmic goiter

Jogger's heel Irritation of fibrofatty tissue of heel in joggers.

Joint An articulation, between two bones. Joints are grouped according to motion: ball and socket (enarthrosis), hinge (ginglymus); condyloid, pivot (trochoid), gliding (arthrodial) and saddle joint. Joints can move in four ways: 1. gliding, in which one bony surface glides on another without angular or rotatory movement. 2. angular 3. circumduction and 4. rotation. Angular movement when occurs forwards or backwards is called flexion and extension and away from the body abduction and towards median plain of body adduction.

j. amphidiarthrodial Joint that is both ginglymoid and arthrodial.

j. ball and socket Rounded end of one bone fits into cavity of another.

j. Charcot's Denervated joint with increased range of movement as in syringomyelia and tabes dorsalis.

j. condyloid Joint permitting all forms of angular movements except axial rotation.

j. hinge Joint having only forward and backward motion.

j. pivot Joint permitting rotation.

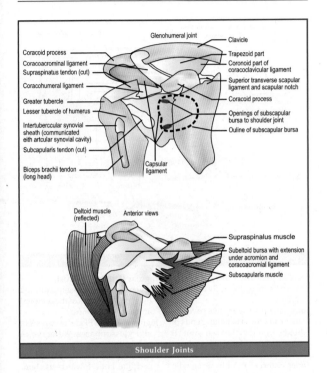

Glenohumeral joint
Clavicle
Coracoid process
Trapezoid part
Coracoacromial ligament
Coronoid part of coracoclavicular ligament
Supraspinatus tendon (cut)
Superior transverse scapular ligament and scapular notch
Coracohumeral ligament
Coracoid process
Greater tubercle
Lesser tubercle of humerus
Openings of subscapular bursa to shoulder joint
Intertuberccular synovial sheath (communicated eith artcular synovial cavity)
Ouline of subscapular bursa
Subcapularis tendon (cut)
Biceps brachii tendon (long head)
Capsular ligament

Deltoid muscle (reflected)
Anterior views
Supraspinalus muscle
Subeltoid bursa with extension under acromion and coracoacromial ligament
Subscapularis muscle

Shoulder Joints

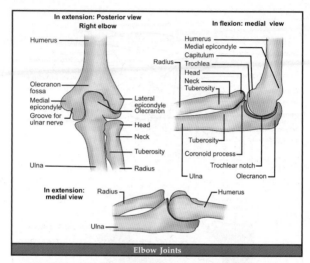

In extension: Posterior view
Right elbow

Humerus

Olecranon
fossa
Medial
epicondyle
Groove for
ulnar nerve

Lateral
epicondyle
Olecranon
Head
Neck
Tuberosity

Ulna

Radius

In flexion: medial view

Humerus
Medial epicondyle
Capitulum
Radius — Trochlea
Head
Neck
Tuberosity

Tuberosity
Coronoid process
Trochlear notch
Ulna
Olecranon

In extension:
medial view

Radius

Humerus

Ulna

Elbow Joints

j. saddle Joint in which the opposing surfaces are reciprocally concavo-convex.

Joint capsule The sac like covering enclosing the articulating ends of bones in a diarthrodial joint. It consists of an outer fibrous layer and inner synovial layer.

Jones criteria USA physician who devised the major and minor criteria for diagnosis of acute; rheumatic fever. The major criteria include: 1. fleeting polyarthritis 2. chorea, 3. erythema marginatum, and 4. subcutaneous nodules.

Joule Work done in one second by current of one ampere against a resistance of one ohm.

Jugular Pertains to throat.

Jugular foramen Opening formed by jugular notches of the occipital and temporal bones.

Jugular ganglion Nodes of vagus root and glossopharyngeal nerve in jugular foramen.

Jugular process Projection of occipital bone towards the temporal bone.

Jugular vein 1. *External* lies superficial to sternocleido mastoid and joins subclavian vein. 2. *Internal* is direct continuation of transverse sinus and joins subclavian vein to form innominate vein. The vein is more prominent during expiration. The height of pulsating

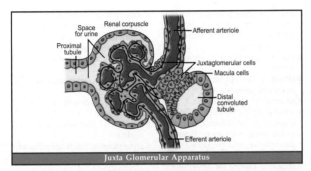

Juxta Glomerular Apparatus

blood column in internal jugular gives an indication of right atrial pressure.

Jugum Ridge or furrow connecting two points.

Junction The place of union of two parts.

j. cementodentinal Interface of dentin and cementum.

j. cementoenamel The boundary line between crown and root of tooth.

j. dento-gingival The interface and zone of attachment between gingiva and enamel of tooth.

j. mucocutaneous Junction between the skin and mucous membrane.

j. mucogingival A scalloped indistinct boundary between coral color gingiva and more vascular oral mucosa.

j. myoneural SYN — motor end plate; where nerve ending meets the muscle.

j. sclerocorneal Outer scleral sulcus where sclera ends and cornea begins.

j. squamocolumnar Line in the cervix where vaginal squamous epithelium meets the columnar epithelium of endocervix, the site for malignancy of cervix.

Jurisprudence The scientific study or application of the principles of law and justice.

j. medical The application of the principles of law as they relate to the practice of medicine.

Jury mast Apparatus for support of head in diseases of spine.

Juster's reflex linger extension instead of flexion when palm of the hand is irritated.

Juvenile Youth or childhood.

Juxta Close proximity.

Juxta-articular Situated close to a joint

Juxtaglomerular apparatus The myoepithelioid cell structure cuffing affarent renal arteriole concerned with production of renin.

Juxtaglomerular cells Myoepithelioid cells resembling those of carotid body in juxtaglomerular apparatus.

Juxtangina Inflamed condition of pharyngeal muscles.

Juxtaposition Positioned side by side.

K

Kader's operation Surgical formation of gastric fistula with the feeding tube inserted through a valve like flap.

Kakidrosis Unpleasant odor of the sweat.

Kakosmia Perception of bad odor that does not exist.

Kakotrophy Malnutrition.

Kala-azar Protozoal tropical disease caused by *Leishmania donovani* manifesting with fever, lymphadenopathy and hepatosplenomegaly with darkening of skin.

Kalimeter Device for determining alkalinity of a substance.

Kalium A mineral (potassium).

Kaliuresis Excretion of potassium in urine.

Kallikrein An enzyme, when activated is a potent vasodilator.

Kanamycin Aminoglycoside antibiotic, used in tuberculosis.

Kanner syndrome Infantile autism.

Kaolin Clay powder containing hydrated aluminium silicate used as adsorbent in diarrhea.

Kaolinosis Pneumoconiosis caused by inhalation of kaolin particles.

Kaposi Hungarian physician.

Kaposi's disease Xeroderma pigmentosum.

Kaposi sarcoma AIDs associated sarcoma of skin.

Kaposi's varicelliform eruption Herpes or vaccinia infection in presence of pre-existing eczema.

Karaya gum Plant product, used as adhesive and bulk laxative.

Karman catheter Catheter used in performing suction curretage of uterus.

Kartagener's syndrome Hereditary syndrome consisting of bronchiectasis, sinusitis and transposition of viscera.

Karyoclasis Fragmentation of cell nucleus.

Karyocyte Nucleated red blood cell, normoblast.

Karyogamy Union of nuclei in cell conjugation.

Karyolysis Destruction of cell nucleus.

Karyopyknosis Shrinkage of nucleus of a cell with condensation of chromatin.

Karyorrhexis Fragmentation of chromatin in nuclear lysis.

Karyosome Irregular clumps of non-dividing chromatin in cell nucleus.

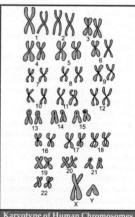

Karyotype of Human Chromosomes

Karyotype A photomicrograph of a single cell in the metaphase to.show chromosomes in descending order of size.

Kasabach Merrit syndrome Capillary hemangioma associated with thrombocytopenic purpura.

Kata (Cata) Prefix meaning down, wrongly, back, against.

Kawasaki disease Mucocutaneous lymph node syndrome; children are the prime victims and run a risk of coronary arteritis with infarction.

Kayser Fleischer ring The green-ring around the cornea due to deposition of copper in descmet's membrane in Wilson's disease.

Kegel exercise An exercise for strengthening the pubococcygeal levator ani muscles in control of urinary and fecal incontinence.

Keinbock's disease Osteochondrosis of lunate bone of wrist

Keith-Wagener-Barker classification A classification of hypertensive changes of retina. Grade I—moderate narrowing of retinal arterioles, Grade II—retinal hemorrhages, Grade III—cotton wool exudates, and Grade IV—papilledema.

Kell blood group One of the human blood groups, composed of three forms of antigens.

Keloid Hypertrophied, raised, firm, thick scar following trauma or surgical incision.

Kelvin scale Temperature scale in which absolute zero is equal to minus 273° on Celsius scale.

Kemadrin Procyclidine hydrochloride, used in Parkinsonism for anticholinergic effect.

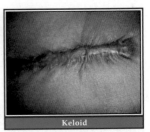
Keloid

Kenalog Triamcinolone hydrochloride.

Kenny treatment Physical therapy for treating poliomyelitis consisting of application of hot moist packs, early muscle education.

Kenophobia Fear of empty spaces.

Kent's bundle Accessory conduction pathway joining atria with ventricles as in WPW syndrome.

Kerasin A cerebroside.

Keratectomy Excision of a portion of cornea.

Keratin A tough protein substance in hair, nail, horny tissue, produced by keratinocytes.

Keratinization The process of keratin formation within keratinocytes and its progress upward through the layers of epidermis to the surface stratum corneum.

Keratinocyte Cell synthesizing keratin.

Keratitic precipitates Inflammatory cells in anterior chamber that stick to inner endothelial surface of cornea.

Keratitis Inflammation of cornea.

k. band White or grey band extending across cornea.

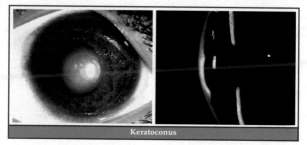

Keratoconus

k. bullosa Formation of large tense blebs on cornea as in trachoma.

k. deep Interstitial keratitis.

k. dendritic Superficial branching corneal ulcer.

k. disciformis Gray disc shaped opacity in the middle of cornea.

k. fascicular Corneal ulcer resulting from phlyctenules that spread from limbus to center of cornea with blood vessels.

k. interstitial Deep non suppurative keratitis with vascularization occurring in syphilis.

k. phlyctenular Circumscribed inflammation of conjuctiva and cornea with accumulation of lymphoid cells, the phlyctenules.

k. sclerosing Triangular opacity in the deeper layers of cornea associated with scleritis.

k. superficial punctate Small gray spots in superficial layers of cornea beneath Bowman's membrane in viral keratitis.

k. xerotic Softening, desiccation and ulceration of cornea with avitaminosis A.

Keratoacanthoma A papular keratin filled lesion resembling squamous cell carcinoma but subsiding spontaneously.

Keratocele Herniation or protrusion of Descemet's membrane through a weakened or absent corneal stroma as a result of corneal ulcer or corneal trauma.

Keratoconjuctivitis Inflammation of cornea and conjuctiva.

k. epidemic viral, self limited but highly infectious keratoconjuctivitis.

k. flash Ultraviolet irradiation induced as in welders and mountaineers.

k. sicca Dryness of conjuctiva with hyperemia and thickened corneal epithelium, occurring in arthropathies.

Keratoconus Conical protrusion of center of cornea without inflammation.

Keratoderma blenorrhagica Prominent hyperkeratotic scaling lesions of palms, soles associated with Reiter's syndrome.

Keratodermia Hypertrophy of stratum corneum of palms and soles of feet.

Keratoma A callosity, a horny growth.

Keratomalacia Softening of cornea as in childhood vit A deficiency.

Keratometer An instrument for measuring curvature of cornea.

Keratometry Measurements of cornea.

Keratomileusis Plastic surgery of cornea in which a portion of cornea is removed, frozen, its curvature is reshaped and then reattached in its place.

Keratomycosis Fungus growth in cornea.

Keratonosis Any non inflammatory disease or deformity of horny layer of skin.

Keratonyxis Surgical puncture of cornea.

Keratopathy band Calcium deposit in superficial layer of cornea and Bowman's capsule, occurring in hypercalcemia or chronic intraocular inflammation.

Keratoplasty Plastic surgery of cornea.

k. optic Replacement of corneal scar with healthy donor corneal tissue.

k. refractive Treatment of myopia or hypermetropia by reshaping corneal curvature either by multiple incision or as in keratomileusis.

k. tectonic Use of corneal tissue to replace that lost due to trauma.

Keratoprotein The protein of hair, nail and epidermis.

Keratorrhexis Rupture of cornea.

Keratoscope Instrument for examination of cornea.

Keratosis Any condition of skin with excessive horny growth.

k. actinic A horny keratotic pre malignant lesion due to prolonged exposure to sunlight.

k. climactericum Circumscribed hyperkeratosis of palms and soles in post menopausal women.

k. follicularis SYN—Darier's disease, characterized by verrucous papular growths that coalesce into plaques affecting face, neck, axillae and scalp.

k. pharyngis Horny projections from tonsils and adjacent lymphoid tissue.

k. pilaris Chronic inflammation of unknown etiology involving hair follicle.

k. punctata Discrete horny projections from sweat pores of palms and soles.

k. senilis Dry harsh skin of aged.

Keratotome A knife for corneal incision.

Keratotomy Incision of cornea.

k. radial Very shallow, bloodless, hairline incisions are made in outer portion of cornea thereby allowing it to flatten; a treatment modality for axial myopia upto 5 diopters.

Keraunophobia Morbid fear of thundering and lightening.

Kerion A lesion secondary to tinea capitis.

Kerley lines Thickening of inter alveolar septa due to pulmonary edema. See — lines kerley.

Kernicterus Bilirubin infiltration of basal ganglia and other areas of

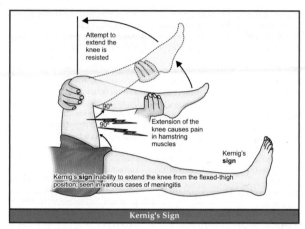

Kernig's **sign** Inability to extend the knee from the flexed-thigh position; seen in various cases of meningitis

Kernig's Sign

brain and spinal cord occurring in erythroblastosis fetalis of newborns when unconjugated hyperbilirubinemia touches 25 mg% or above.

Kernig's sign Reflex spasm and pain in hamstrings when attempting to extend the knee after flexion of hip; a sign of meningitis.

Kerosene A flammable liquid fuel distilled from petroleum. Fumes of it can cause pneumonitis.

Ketamine A nonbarbiturate analgesic-hypnotic substance used IM/ IV.

Ketanserine 5 HT antagonist.

Keto acid Any organic acid containing ketone (CO) radical.

Ketoacidosis Acidosis due to excess of ketone bodies.

Ketoacid uria Presence of ketoacids in urine.

Ketoconazole Systemic antifungal agent.

Ketogenosis Production of ketones.

Ketogenic diet Diet insufficient in calories to produce mild ketosis helpful in some cases of childhood epilepsy.

Ketohexose A nonsaccharide consisting of a six carbon chain and containing a ketone group in addition to alcohol group (e.g. fructose)

Ketolysis The dissolution of ketones.

Ketone A substance containing carbonyl group (C = O) attached to two carbon atoms, e.g. acetone. The ketones are end-products of fat metabolism.

Ketone bodies A group of compounds produced during oxidation of fatty acids and include acetone, beta hydroxy butyric acid and acetoacetic acid.

Ketonemia Presence of ketone bodies in blood in excess quantity.

Ketone threshold Level of ketones in blood above which they appear in urine.

Ketonuria Presence of ketone bodies in urine.

Ketorolac Non opioid analgesic.

Ketose A carbohydrate containing the ketones.

Ketosis The accumulation in the body of the ketones causing acidosis commonly occurring in starvation, high fat diet, pregnancy, uncontrolled diabetes mellitus, following ether anesthesia. They impart a fruity odor to the breath.

17 ketosteroid One of a group of neutral steroids having a ketone group in 17th position, principally produced by adrenal cortex and gonads. They are androsterone, dehydroisoandrosterone, corticosterone, compound E, 11 hydroxy isoandrosterone.

Ketoprofen NSAID group of drug.

Kidney Paired retroperitoneal structures, one on each side of spinal column, wt - 4-6 oz, size 4" long, 2-3" broad. The kidneys in the newborn are about 3 times as large in proportion to body weight as in the adult. The outer cortex contains the glomeruli, 1 million in number. The inner medulla contains the pyramids 8-18 in number made up of collecting tubules being penetrated by cortical substance. Known as columns of Bellini; kidneys are instrumental to the formation of

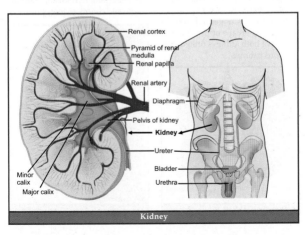

Renal cortex
Pyramid of renal medulla
Renal papilla
Renal artery
Diaphragm
Pelvis of kidney
Kidney
Ureter
Bladder
Urethra
Minor calix
Major calix

Kidney

urine which in 95% water and 5% solids, (urea, uric acid, cretinine, hippuric acid, sodium and potassium); conversion of vit D into active form and secretion of rennin and erythropoitin.

k. artifticial Haemodialysis device that removes wastes like that of kidney.

k. contracted The small kidneys characteristic of chronic glomerulonephritis or interstitial nephritis.

k. fatty Kidney with fatty infiltration causing degeneration of renal substance.

k. flee bitten Arteriosclerotic kidney.

k. floating Displaceable and movable kidney due to weak fascia support.

k. granular Kidney of chronic nephritis where it is small, and of fibrous hard granular texture.

k. horseshoe Congenital malformation where the upper or lower poles of both kidneys united by a fibrous isthmus.

k. polycystic Kidney with multiple cysts, congenital in origin, can be adult onset type or infantile type.

k. sacculated A condition in which renal parenchyma is absorbed leaving behind the distended capsule.

k. sponge Multiple small cysts in the renal parenchyma.

k. wandering Hypermobile kidney.

Kidney failure Diminished function of the kidneys. This may be acute and temporary or may progress to complete loss of renal function.

Kidney stone Calculus present in renal parenchyma, calyx or renal pelvis, composed principally of calcium, urate, oxalate, phosphates and carbonates, ranging from small granular masses to 5 cm or more in diameter. Most common in patients of hyperparathyroidism, oxaluria, gout and chronic pyelonephritis.

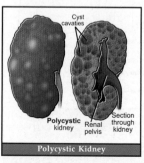

Polycystic Kidney

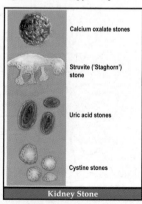

Kidney Stone

Kiesselbachs plexus A rich network of capillaries on the anteroinferior part of nasal septum; the most common site of bleeding in epistaxis.

Kilocycle One thousand cycles as in electricity.

Kilogram One thousand gram.

Kilohertz One thousand cycles as in electricity.

Kilometer 1000 meters, 3281 feet or 0.61 mile.

Kilowatt A unit of electrical energy equivalent to 1000 watts.

Kimmelsteil Wilson syndrome 1 Nodular glomerulosclerosis in longstanding diabetes mellitus with hypertension, edema, retinal lesions, and proteinuria.

Kinanesthesia Inability to perceive extent of movement or direction resulting in ataxia.

Kinase An enzyme that catalyzes the transfer of phosphate from ATP to an acceptor.

Kinematograph Device for viewing photographs of objects in motion.

Kineplasty A form of amputation enabling the muscles of stump to impart motion to artificial limb.

Kinescope Device for conducting refraction of eye.

Kinesiatrics Treatment involving active and passive movements.

Kinesics Systematic study of the body and use of its static and dynamic position as a means of communication.

Kinesiology The study of muscles and body movement.

Kinesthesia Ability to perceive extent, direction and weight of movement.

Kinetic Pertaining to or consisting of motion.

Kinetosis Any disorder caused by motion, such as sea sickness.

Kinin A general term for a group of polypeptides capable of causing smooth muscle contraction, hypotension, hyperpermeability of capillaris and pain.

Kininogen Percursor of kinin.

Kinky hair disease Congenital autosomal recessive syndrome consisting of short, sparse kinky hair, poor physical and mental development, associated with degenerative changes of cerebral gray matter.

Kinomometer device for measuring degree of motion in a joint.

Kinship The descendants from a common ancestor.

Kiotome Device for amputation of uvula.

Kisch's reflex Closure of an eye from stimulation of auditory meatus.

Kite apparatus Apparatus for reeducation of weak muscles and prevention of contractures around forearm, wrist and fingers.

Klebsiella Short mump gram-negative bacilli, encapsulated, nonspore forming frequently causing respiratory infection.

k. pneumonae A species causing pneumonia.

k. rhinoscleromatis Species causing

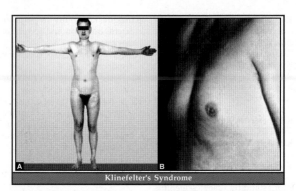
Klinefelter's Syndrome

rhinoscleroma, a destructive granuloma of nose and pharynx.

Klepto To steal.

Kleptolagnia Sexual gratification obtained from stealing.

Kleptomania Impulsive stealing, the motive not being for substantial gain, stolen without prior planning or assistance from others. Stealing provides gratification and mental relaxation.

Kleptomaniac A psychopathic personality suffering from impulsive stealing.

Kleptophobia Morbid fear of stealing.

Klieg eye Conjuctivitis, lacrimation and photophobia from exposure to intense lights as used in making television, film shooting.

Klinefelter's syndrome XXY chromosomal disorder of male manifesting with gynecomastia, tall height, subnormal intelligence, small firm testes.

Klippel's disease Pseudoparalysis due to generalized arthritis.

Klippel-Feil syndrome Congenital anomaly characterized by short wide neck, low hair line, reduction in number of cervical vertebra often with features of upper cervical myelopathy.

Klumpke's paralysis Atrophic paralysis of forearm usually due to birth trauma with stretching, avulsion of brachial plexus.

Kluver-Bucy syndrome Behavioral syndrome usually following bilateral temporal lobectomy, manifesting with hypersexuality, rage, memory deficit, hyperreligiosity, hyperphagia, failure of visual recognition etc.

Knapp's forceps Forceps with roller like blades for expressing trachomatous granulations on .the palpebral conjuctiva.

Kneading A form of massage consisting of grasping, wringing, lifting, rolling, pressing.

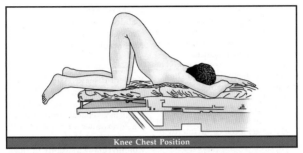
Knee Chest Position

Knee Femero-tibial articulation covered anteriorly with patella.

k. Brodie's A chronic fungoid synovitis of knee joint in which affected parts become soft and pulpy.

k. internal derangement Pertains to a knee with injury to collateral/cruciate ligaments, the menisci, fracture of tibial spine.

k. housemaid Bursitis of bursa anterior to patella due to prolonged kneeling.

k. knock Outward bending of legs allowing the knees to touch each other *SYN* — genu valgum.

k. locked Inability to extend the leg due to torn semilunar cartilage.

Knee cap Patella.

Knee chest position Position in which patient is on knees with thighs straight, head and upper part of chest resting on table and arms crossed in front of head. Employed for sigmoidoscopic examination of colon and rectum, repositioning of retroverted uterus or displaced ovary.

Knee jerk reflex Contraction of quadriceps on tapping ligamentum patellae, while the leg hangs loosely with knee at right angle. The reflex

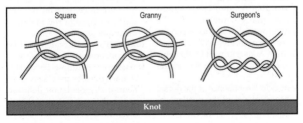

Square	Granny	Surgeon's

Knot

arc is via La-Li Pyramidal tract lesions exaggerate knee jerk and it is absent in lesions of peripheral nerves and anterior horn cells of involved spinal segments.

Knemometry A precise method of determining the length of a limb.

Knob A mass or nodule.

Knot 1. In surgery, the inter-twinning of the ends of a suture, ligature, bandage so that the ends will not slip or get loose. 2. An intertwinning of a cord or cord like structure to form a knob or lump.

k. false An external bulging of the umbilical cord resulting from coiling of umbilical blood vessels.

k. granny A double knot in which the ends of cord do not lie parallel but alternate being over and under each other.

k. Hensen's A knob-like structure at the anterior end of primitive streak.

k. square A double knot in which the ends of second knot are in the same place as the ends of the first knot

k. surgical A double knot in which the cord is passed through the first loop twice.

k. syncytial A protruberance formed by many nuclei of the syntrophoblast and found on the surface of chorionic villus.

k. true A knot formed by the fetus slipping through loop of umbilical cord.

Knuckle Prominence of the dorsal aspect of any of the phallangeal joints.

Kochers reflex Contraction of abdominal muscles following moderate compression of testicle.

Koebner phenomenon Appearance of skin lesion as a result of nonspecific trauma.

Kohler's disease Aseptic necrosis of navicular bone of wrist.

Koilocyte An abnormal cell of squamous epithelium of the cervix, a forerunner of cervical intra epithelial neoplasia.

Koilonychia Dystrophy of finger nails, thinning spooning as in iron deficiency anemia.

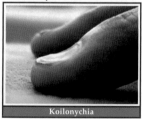
Koilonychia

Koniology Science of dust and its effect.

Koniometer Device for estimating amount of dust in air.

Koplik's spots Small red spots with blue white centers on the oral mucosa opposite the molars, a diagnostic sign of measles.

Korotkoff's sounds Sounds heard in auscultation of blood pressure.

Korsakoff's syndrome Personality characterized by psychosis, polyneuritis, disorientation, delirium, confabulation, a feature of chronic alcoholism.

Krabbe's disease Globoid cell leukodystrophy due to collection of galactocerebrocides in the tissues. Clinically manifesting with seizure, deafness, blindness, and mental retardation.

Kraurosis Atrophy and dryness of skin and mucous membrane — esp. of vulva, malignant degeneration may occur.

Krause's glands Accessory lacrimal glands opening into fornix of eye.

Krause's valves Fold of mucous membrane of the lacrimal sac at the junction of lacrimal duct.

Krause's bulbs Encapsulated nerve endings present in skin.

Krebs' cycle The chain reaction cycle involving oxidation of pyruvic acid and production of ATP.

Krukenberg's tumor A malignant tumor of ovary, usually bilateral and frequently secondary to malignancy of G.I. tract (through peritoneal seedling).

Krypton A gaseous element in the atmosphere.

Kuf's disease Adult form of cerebral sphingo-lipidosis with dementia, retinitis pigmentosa, blindness and myoclonic jerks.

Kugelberg-Welander disease Juvenile spinal muscular atrophy.

Kummel's disease Spondylitis following compression fracture of vertebra.

Kuffer's cells Fixed phagocytic cells lining hepatic sinusoids.

Kuru A progressively fatal encephalopathy probably of slow virus infection spreading by practice of cannibalism.

Kussmaul's breathing Very deep and gasping respiration in acidosis.

Kussmaul's disease Periarteritis nodosa.

Kwashiorkor A severe protein deficiency syndrome in children manifesting with lethargy, dry brittle hair, growth failure, subcutaneous edema, skin changes and hepatomegaly.

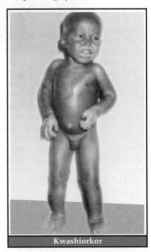

Kwashiorkor

Kyasanur forest disease Tick born encephalitides of South India.

Kyllosis Club foot.

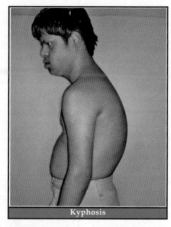
Kyphosis

Kymograph 1. A device for recording movements of a stylus on a moving drum, thus helpful to record respiratory movements, muscle contractions. 2. A radiographic device for recording the range of motion of involuntary movements of the heart or diaphragm.

Kymoscope Device for measuring variations in blood flow and pressure.

Kynurenine An intermediate compound in tryptophan metabolism.

Kyphoscoliosis Forward bending of spine along with increased lateral curvature.

Kyphosis Excessive curvature of spine with convexity backwards. May be congenital or secondary to compression fracture, malignancy *SYN*— humpback.

Kysthitis Inflammation of vagina.

L

LA 50 The total body surface size of a burn that will kill 50% of victims, used for statistical analysis of mortality figures in burn patients.

Labeling The process or procedure followed in using chemical or radioactive labels as an aid in reaching a diagnosis or for experimental study.

Labetalol Both alpha and betablocker used in hypertension.

Labile Unstable, emotions that are easily changeable.

Labioplasty Plastic surgery of labium majus or minus.

Labium A lip shaped structure, a fleshy margin or fold.

Labor The onset of forceful uterine contraction to expel the fetus; divided into three phases, first: from onset of contraction till full dilatation of cervix, second: from full dilatation till delivery of fetus and third: delivery of placenta.

l. arrested Failure of progression of labor.

l. dry Premature rupture of membranes with escape of liquor.

l. false Uterine contractions that do not progress.

l. induced Labor precipitated by drugs, (oxytocics) or artificial rupture of membrane.

l. obstructed Arrest in progress of labor due to cephalo-pelvic disproportion, contraction ring, abnormal fetal position etc.

l. precipitate Rapidly progressing labor threatening fetal and maternal injury.

l. prolonged Extended duration of labor as first phase exceeding 20 hours in nullipara, 14 hours in multipara or cervical dilatation less than 1.2 cm/hr in nullipara and 1.5 cm in multipara.

Labrocyte Mast cells.

Labrum Lip tike structure.

l. acetabulare Triangular rim of fibro cartilage, base of which is fixed to acetabular margin, deepening its cavity.

l. glenoidale A triangular rim of fibrocartilage, the base of which is fixed to circumference of glenoid cavity of scapula.

Labyrinthectomy Partial or complete surgical destruction of labyrinth as in Menier's disease; Techniques employed include injection of absolute alcohol, diathermy, ultrasound, cryosurgery or avulsion of lateral semicircular canal/transtympanic avulsion of utricle.

Labyrinthitis Inflammation of inner ear; can be circumscribed, serous or suppurative.

Labyrinth Any thing twisted or of spiral shape.

l. ethmoidalis Oblong mass of thin walled air cells between two parallel vertical plates of bone.

l. membranous A closed system of communicating sacs in the internal ear, containing endolymph and surrounded by perilymph.

l. osseous The bony cavities in petrous part of temporal bone housing the membranous laby-

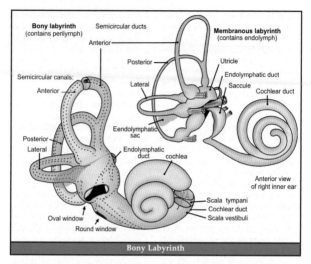

Bony Labyrinth

rinth and connected to middle ear by fenestra vestibuli and fenestra cochleae.

l. vestibularis The portion of membranous labyrinth comprising sacculus, utriculus and their connections and the three semicircular canals.

Laceration Tearing of tissues with ragged irregular margins and surrounding contusion.

l. first degree obstetric Laceration of perineum involving the fourchette, vaginal mucosa, and skin but not underlying fascia and muscle.

l. second degree obstetric Involves underlying fascia and muscle but does not extend to anal sphincter.

l. third degree obstetric Laceration extends to involve anal sphincter.

l. fourth degree obstetric Laceration involves anal sphincter and rectum with rectovaginal fistula.

Lacrimation Production of tears, weeping.

Lactalbumin Proteins in milk that are not precipitated with ammonium sulfate.

B. lactamase Bacterial enzyme that hydrolyzes the B lactam bond antibiotics like penicillin and cephalosporins leading to loss of antibiotic activity.

Lactate dehydrogenase An enzyme catalysing reaction of lactate to pyruvate with liberation of NADH and H^+, helping hereby in anaerobic glycolysis. The enzyme is a tetramer consisting of 2 types of chains, the alfa is predominant in heart muscle and beta in skeletal muscle.

Lactic acid A product of anaerobic glycolysis in muscles and by milk-souring bacteria.

Lactiferrous Capable of producing, transporting or secreting milk.

Lacto bacillus Gram-positive, anaerobic nonspore forming bacilli producing D or L lactic acid in the milk.

Lactoferrin Iron binding protein of milk.

Lactogen Agent stimulating lactation, like prolactin; human placental lactogen is a polypeptide hormone structurally related to human growth hormone and prolactin secreted by placenta. It is essential in maintenance of growth of fetus.

Lactoglobulin A milk protein with a concentration of 3 gm per liter in cow's milk, second only to casein among milk proteins.

Lactose The principal sugar of milk hydrolyzed by B galactosidase to glucose and galactose. Those deficient in this enzyme have discomfort on drinking milk.

Lactose synthetase Enzyme helping in synthesis of lactose, found in mammary glands.

Lactosuria Presence of lactose in the urine.

Lacune A space or cavity between cells or structures.

l. cerebral Hypertensive lipohyalunosis causing minor infarction with lacune formation within cerebral hemisphere (lacunar syndrome).

l. Howship's Bony pits occupied by osteoclasts.

Lag Slowness to act or react, the interval between an expected action or reaction and its occurrence.

l. anaphase A retarded movement of chromosome during mitosis.

l. eyelid Failure of upper eyelid to descend promptly while looking down as in Graves' disease.

l. globe While looking upward, upper eyelid pulls faster than the eyeball is raised, thus exposing the sclera above the iris.

l. jet Altered biological rhythms like sleep, satiety, hunger, after rapid jet transport.

Lagophthalmos Inability to close the eyelids completely as in facial palsy.

Lambda The 11th letter of Greek alphabet; the junction of sagittal and lambdoid sutures.

Lamella Thin plate, layer or sheet as of compact bone.

Lamina A plate or thin sheet of material.

l. dental A flat band of epithelial cells that develops in the embryos along which develop the tooth germs giving rise to primary and secondary dentition.

l. of Rexed Lamination of cells in spinal gray matter marked 1 to 9, arranged in dorsoventral direction and lamina 10 situated centrally.

l. terminally A membrane formed in the developing embryo remaining to adulthood as a thin layer of gray matter extending from superior surface of optic chiasma to rostrum of corpus callosum.

Laminated Arranged in layers.

Laminotomy Division or partial removal of vertebral lamina.

Lamp A device producing light artificially.

l. Eldridge Green Color vision testing device using spectral filters.

l. Finsen Carbon arc lamp utilized for treating lupus vulgaris.

l. Kromayer Mercury quartz ultra-violet lamp for treatment of skin ulcers.

l. Wood's Lamp producing ultraviolet rays at 365 nm giving characteristic fluorescence of some fungi. Infected hairs have bright green fluorescence; *T. versicolor* has gold fluorescence.

Lancet A small surgical blade, used for making small drainage incisions.

Lancinating Sudden sharp transient pain as if tearing into pieces.

Lange's test A gold precipitation test on CSF for diagnosis of CNS syphilis

Langhan's layer The cytotrophoblastic layer of chorionic villi

Languor Lack of vigor, lassitude

Lanolin A waxy fatty secretion of sebaceous glands of the sheep deposited on wool fibers, used as an ointment base.

Lanugo The fine downy hairs devoid of medulla, covering fetus.

Laparoscope An endoscope devised for examination of abdomino-pelvic organs.

Laparotomy Surgical incision abdominal wall for access to abdominal organs.

Larva Motile developing stage of worms, maggots, cater pillars. 1.

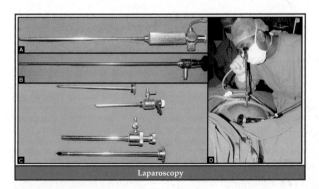

Laparoscopy

fillariform: Infective larva of nematodes.

Larva migrans Migratory phase of the cycle of helminth in an abnormal host/site with random wandering.

l.m cutaneous Linear eruption caused by hookworm larva.

l.m visceral Disorder of visceral larval migration from normal i.e., intestine to liver, heart, lungs, trachea, mouth and back to intestine so that the larva migrate in random with ultimate encapsulation in aberrant site.

Larvicide Medication effective against larval form.

Larvi parous Deposition of hatched larvae than eggs.

Laryngectomy Excision of a part or total larynx.

l. lateral partial Partial laryngectomy for small tumors localized to membranous part of vocal cords.

Laryngismus stridulus Brief nocturnal attack of laryngo spasm.

Laryngitis Inflammation of lining of larynx, may be catarrhal, chronic hyperplastic (often precancerous), chronic non specific, diphtheritic, membranous, (diphtheria, streptococci, pseudomonas).

Laryngocele An air containing pouch, usually bilateral in wind instrument players and glass blowers.

Laryngomalacia A flaccid 3-supraglottic larynx in babies causing inspiratory stridor but with spontaneous cure.

Laryngoplasty Reconstruction of larynx to improve airway as in bilateral abductor palsy.

Laryngoscleroma Rhinoscleroma with laryngeal involvement healing with scarring and distortion.

Laryngoscopy Inspection of interior of larynx.

l. fiberoptic Indirect (mirror) laryngoscopy.

Laryngospasm Spasm of glottic sphincter produced by foreign material, blood, secretion getting access to laryngeal inlet.

Laryngostomy Making an opening into subglottic larynx for relief of upper airway obstruction.

Laryngotracheobronchitis Inflammation of larynx, trachea and bronchi often producing critical respiratory embarrassment in small children chiefly due to subglottic swelling and tenacious secretion usually of viral origin.

Laser Light amplification by stimulated emission of radiation.

l. carbon dioxide Used to remove lesions of skin or other superficial organs.

l. argon Its blue green light causes coagulation of bleeding sites in surgery.

l. neodymium Yag Laser used for capsulotomy, vitrectomy.

Lasigues sign Pain that radiates to leg after hip and knee is extended – an indication of lumbar root compression

Latent Existing but not apparent, dormant.

Latency The period between stimulation application and onset of response.

Lateral On the side of body.

Lateralization The tendency to perform an act predominantly on left or right side of the body.

Lathyrism Spastic paraplegia with sensory impairment due to consumption of khesari dal containing fungus *Lathyrus sativatus.*

Lauric acid A fatty acid found in neutral fat like butter.

Lavage The washing out of hollow organ, e.g. gastric, peritoneal, intestinal.

Law An accepted and tested phenomena.

l. Collin's After removal of a tumor in infancy or childhood if metastasis or recurrence does not develop within period equal to age of patient plus 9 months then risk of such development is small.

l. Courvoisier's Obstruction of common bile duct by a gallstone rarely causes dilatation of gall bladder.

l. Faget's Lack of correlation between body temperature and heart rate in yellow fever.

l. Flatav's The longer ascending and descending tracts of spinal cord tend to be displaced peripherally by shorter axons arriving or terminating at that level.

l. Graham's The rate of diffusion of a gas is inversely proportional to the square root of its density.

l. Laplace The transmural pressure in a free sphere or cylinder is directly proportional to the circumferential tension in the wall; inversely proportional to the radius.

l. Ohm's Voltage across a resistor is equal to current x resistance.

l. Starling's The force of contraction in cardiac muscle is equivalent to fiber length at beginning of contraction.

l. Teevan's Fractures of bones occur in lines of extension and in the line of compression.

Laxative Agent promoting or stimulating bowel movement.

LD 50 The median lethal dose of a substance that will kill 50% of animals receiving that dose.

L-dopa Dihydroxy phenylalanine used in treatment of Parkinson's disease.

L.E. cell (Lupus erythematous cell) a mature polymorph containing phagocytosed nucleus of another cell.

Lead A toxic metallic element, toxicity occurring from intake more than 0.5 mg/day. Any level in blood is abnormal. l encephalitis occurs due to lead ingestion causing rise in ICP, and permanent damage to CNS

Leber's disease Congenital optic atrophy

Lecithin A fatty substance like phospholipids found in blood, bile, brain, egg yolk, nerves, and other animal tissues.

Legg's disease Osteochondritis of upper femoral epiphysis

Legionella *L pneumophila*, a non motile gram -ve rod present in air conditioning system causing pneumonia.

Legionnaires disease A form of pneumonitis caused by gram negative bacillus *Legionella pneunophila*

Leiomyoma A low mitotic benign tumor of smooth muscle cell. Can be seen on skin (dermatomyoma) uterus, seminal vesicles, blood vessels (angiomyoma).

Leiomyosarcoma Malignant tumor of smooth muscle cells.

Leishmaniasis Infectious disease caused by flagellate protozoan parasites and transmitted to man by sandflies.

Leishmanoid Facial cutaneous lesion containing leishmania.

Lemniscus A ribbon, band, bundle of axons.

l. lateral Longitudinal tract of auditory system terminating in inferior colliculus and medial geniculate body.

l. medial Myelinated tract emerging from nucleus gracilis and cuneatus and crossing over to opposite side in medulla and terminating in ventrobasal thalamic nucleus.

l. trigeminal A large band of myelinated axons originating

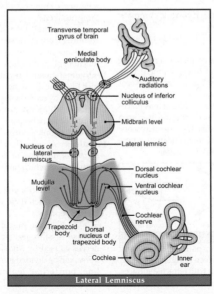

Lateral Lemniscus

from principal trigeminal nucleus and crossing over to opposite side in pons to join medial lemniscus.

Length:

l. cranial Skull length between glabella and inion.

l. crown heel Fetal or infant length from crown to heel.

l. foot Toe to heel length for estimation of age of fetus.

l. sitting Distance between vertex and coccyx.

Lennox-Gestaut syndrome A complex form a early childhood epilepsy poorly controlled with drugs

l. achromatic it corrects chromatic aberration.

l. aplanatic it corrects spherical aberration.

l. bifocal a corrective lens having upper and lower segment with different power for distant and near vision.

l. intraocular Artificial lens places in lens capsule or behind the cornea

l. oilimmersion Used in microscope for higher magnification where sedar wood oil is used.

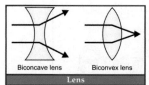

Biconcave lens   Biconvex lens

Lens

Lens 1. Transparent biconvex disk lying between iris and vitreous. 2. A medium with retractile surfaces.

l. aniseikonic Lens that changes the size of an image without altering the focal distance.

l. contact Resin lens fitting directly on cornea.

l. iseikonic A lens that changes size of an object.

l. minus Lens that diverges light rays.

l. photo chromatic Lens that darkens on exposure to ultraviolet light, used in sunglasses.

l. plus Lens that converges light.

Lenticular Pertaining to lens.

Lentiform Shaped like a lentil or lens of eye.

Lentiginosis Presence of lentigens in large numbers.

Lentigo A small brown macule resulting from increased number of meianocyte at dermo-epidermal junction, pleural-lentigines.

Lentigomelanosis Irregular brownish black localized pigmentation produced by senile lentigo.

Lentiasis Bilateral symmetrical hypertrophy of bones of face and cranium of unknown cause.

Lepothrix A superficial *Corynebacterium* infection of axillary or pubic hair in which nodules form on hair.

Leproma A histiocytic cellular reaction characteristic of lepromatous leprosy.

Leprosy Chronic mycobacterial disease of skin and peripheral nerves caused by *Mycobacterium leprae*; can be divided into borderline, borderline lepromatous,

lepromatous, border line tuberculoid and tuberculoid types.

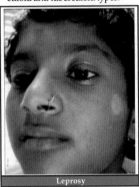

Leprosy

l. borderline Affects persons with moderate degree of cell mediated immunity, can upgrade to tuberculoid or downgrade to lepromatous pole.

l. lepromatous Diffuse bilaterally symmetrical lesions in persons with poor cell mediated immunity.
Bacilli are plenty and well disseminated.

l. lucio A diffuse non-nodular variant of lepromatous leprosy.

l. tuberculoid Few hyposthetic macules, enlarged cutaneous nerves, well developed cellular immunity and few bacteria.

Leptocyte A thinner erythrocyte, appearing hypochromic, seen in iron deficiency anemia, thalassemia, etc.

Leptodactyly Unusual slenderness of fingers.

Leptomeninges Pia-arachnoid membranes together.

Leptophonia A weak thin quality of voice.

Leptoscope An optical instrument used to measure thickness of a thin film.

Leptospira A genus of coiled ectopic spirochete.

Leptospira ictero hemorrhagica A febrile illness caused by leptospira manifesting with hemolysis, jaundice, anemia, bleeding tendency.

Lergotrile Ergot alkaloid.

Leriche's syndrome Atherothrombotic occlusion of aortic bifurcation in pelvic with ischaemic pain in legs, claudication and inpotency.

Lesbian Female homosexual.

Lesch-Nyhan syndrome An inherited form of hyperuricemia in male, mental retardation, self mutilation, aggressive behaviour and renal failure.

Lesion A pathological alteration in structure or function of an organ.

Lethal Deadly, capable of causing death.

Lethargy A state of excessive fatigue, diminished physical and mental activity.

Letterer-Siewe disease Granulomatous destructive disease.

Leucine An essential amino acid.

Leucovorin A calcium salt of folinic acid that counteracts toxic effects of folic acid antagonists.

Leukapheresis Selective removal of leukocytes by hemo-pheresis, useful in treatment of blast crisis or to obtain leukocyte donation.

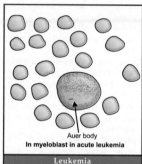

Auer body
In myeloblast in acute leukemia

Leukemia

Leukemia Malignant proliferation of leukocytes and their bone marrow precursors with organ infiltration. Principal types are: acute myeloid, acute lymphoblastic, chronic myeloid, chronic lymphocytic. Acute myeloid has six subtypes- M_1 to M_6 that includes monocytic, myelomonocytic, promyelocytic and erythro-leukemia.

l. aleukemic Peripheral blood picture is normal but there is pancytopenia. Bone marrow puncture yields the excess blast cells.

l. basophilic Marked increase in basophils of blood and marrow, a variant of chronic myeloid leukemia.

l. eosinophilic Peripheral eosinophilia with increased blasts in marrow.

l. lymphosarcoma cell Characterized by numerous large lymphocytes with prominent single nucleoli, a variant of chronic lymphocytic leukemia.

Leukemid A nonspecific cutaneous lesion containing infiltration of leukemic cells.

Leukemoid Resembling leukemia with appearance of immature leukocytes in peripheral blood am leukocytosis. Seen in some infectious diseases.

Leukoblastosis Any malignant disorder of white cells including leukemia and lymphoma.

Leukocyte Nucleated cells of blood and marrow excluding erythrocyte precursors.

Leukocytoblast The earliest recognizable leukocyte precursor.

Leukocytoma Tumorous accumulation of leukocytes including chloroma, granulocytic leukemia and lymphoma.

Leukocytosis Increased number of leukocytes in blood may be lymphocytic, neutrophilic, eosinophilic. It can be seen in newborn, often physiological after exercise, terminal (before death) and toxic (severe infection).

Leukocytotaxis Migration of leukocytes to the site of inflammation and injury.

Leukocytotoxin Any substance that selectively damages leukocytes.

Leukoderma Lack of normal skin pigmentation.

Leukodystrophy Myelin degeneration in white matter of brain and spinal cord consequent to inherited disorders of lipid metabolism.

Leukoencephalitis Encephalitis predominantly involving cerebral white matter.

Leukoencephalopathy Any disease of cerebral white matter; may be hemorrhagic, necrotizing.

Leukoerythroblastosis Presence in the blood of numerous normoblasts together with precursors of granulocyte series.

Leukokoria White reflex of pupil as in retinopathy or any pathological condition posterior to crystalline lens.

Leukoma Dense white scar of cornea.

Leukopathy Punctate leukoderma.

Leukopedesis Migration of lymphocytes through walls of blood vessels.

Leukopenia Abnormal decrease in number of blood leukocytes, (s 4000/cmm).

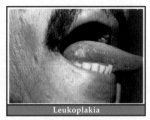
Leukoplakia

Leukoplakia Epithelial hyperplasia with keratosis of mucous membrane appearing as white patch. It chiefly affects gums, lips, cheeks, tongue, larynx, urinary bladder and female genitalia.

Leukopoiesis Formation, growth and maturation of leukocytes.

Leukopsin The colorless product of bleaching of rhodopsin.

Leukorrhea Abnormal white non-bloody discharge from vagina.

Leukotactic Capable of attracting leukocytes.

Leukotaxis Active ameboid, unidirectional movement of leukocytes towards an attractant.

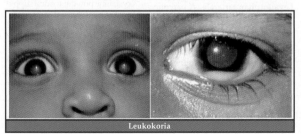
Leukokoria

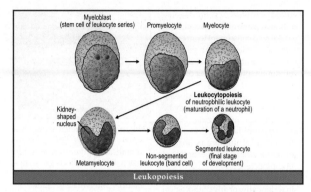

Leukopoiesis

Leukotomy Transorbital frontal lobotomy.

Leukotrienes Mediators of inflammation derived from arachidonic acid. Leukotriene $C_4 D_4 E_4$ play roles in anaphylaxis (slow reacting substance) and B_4 is a chemoattractant and aggregator of neutrophils.

Leuprolide Gonadotropin releasing hormone analog for prostatic carcinoma.

Levallorphan tartarate A narcotic antagonist for treatment of respiratory depression caused by narcotics.

Levamisole The l-form tetramisole, used for treatment of roundworm, hookworm, strongyloides. Also used as an immunopotentiator.

Levarterenol Norepinephrine.

Levator A muscle that raises up the part into which it is inserted.

Levocardia Visceral situs inversus with a normally positioned left sided heart. Such a heart often has aortic arch and valvular malformations.

Levodopa 3-hydroxyl-L-tyrosine, administered orally in parkinsonism and heart failure.

Levorotatory Capable of rotating the plane of polarized light counterclockwise.

Levorphanol Narcotic analgesic similar to morphine.

Levothyroxine L thyroxine; yellow crystalline powder for oral supplement in hypothyroid cases.

Levoxadrol L-isomer of dioxadiol, used as local anesthetic and smooth muscle relaxant.

Levulinic acid 4 oxopentanoic acid, source of aminolevulinic acid which is an intermediate in biosynthesis of porphyrins.

Levulose Levorotatory glucose.

l. forms Slowly growing spherical cells of certain bacterial species that have lost the rigid murien layer.

Lewy bodies Neuronal cells with pigmented inclusion bodies found in substantia nigra in parkinsonism.

L forms Spontaneous variant of bacteria with deficient cell wall.

Lhermitte's sign – sudden electric shock like pain by flexion of neck – a feature of multiple sclerosis, cervical spondylosis and cervical cord tumor

Libido Sexual desire or appetite.

Lichen A tree moss, localized thickening, shinning itchy skin lesion due to continuous friction or rubbing.

Licorice A flavouring agent, demulcent and mild expectorant.

Lidocaine A local anesthetic applied as sprays, creams to skin and mucous membrane.

Lidoflazine A coronary vasodilator.

Lie The relation of long axis of fetus to that of mother; can be longitudinal, transverse or oblique.

Linorenal Pertaining to spleen and kidney.

Life The time span between birth and death.

Ligament 1. Any band of fibrous tissue connecting bones. 2. Any membranous fold sheet or cord like structure that holds an organ in position.

l. acromioclavicular Extends from acromion process of scapula to clavicle.

l. alar Short rounded cords connecting axis to skull base *SYN —* odontoid ligament.

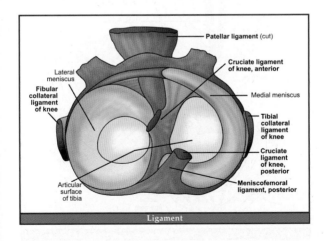

Ligament

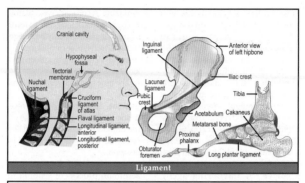

Ligament

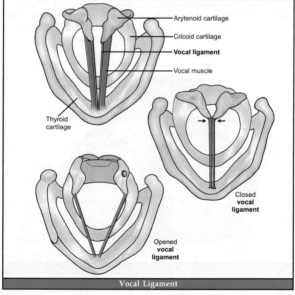

Vocal Ligament

l. alveolodental Periodontal ligament.

l. apical odontoid Ligament extending from apex of odontoid process of axis to anterior margin of foramen magnum.

l. arcuate Median and lateral, that attach diaphragm to first lumbar vertebra and the 12th rib on either side.

l. arcuate median Ligament between crura of diaphragm.

l. broad, of uterus Fibrous sheets of peritoneum extending from uterus to lateral pelvic wall.

l. calcaneofibular Extends from lateral malleolus to lateral surface of fibula.

l. cardinal A sheet of subserous fascia on either side of cervix.

l. Cooper's Suspensory ligament of breast.

l. cricothyroid Extends from superior border of cricoid to inferior border of thyroid cartilage.

l. cruciate of knee One anterior and one posterior crossing each other like *x* that prevent rotation in knee joint.

l. deltoid The medial reinforcing ligament of ankle.

l. falciform A sickle shaped ligament composed of two layers of peritoneum attaching liver to anterior abdominal wall.

l. fibular collateral Attached from lateral condyle of femur to lateral side of heads of fibula.

l. fundiform of penis Fibroelastic tissue adherent to linea alba and pubic symphysis and extending to dorsum of penis.

l. inguinal Rolled inferior margin of external oblique aponeurosis extending from anterior superior iliac spine of ileum to pubic tubercle. *SYN*—Poupart's ligament.

l. lacunar A triangular band extending horizontally from the inguinal ligament to iliopectineal line of pubis.

l. longitudinal anterior and posterior Broad, flat and strong extending from anterior and posterior surface of vertebral bodies, from 2nd vertebra to sacrum.

l. nuchal A broad triangular membranous septum in the back of the neck extending from tips of cervical spinous processes to the external occipital crest. The muscles of neck on either side are attached to it.

l. ovarian A cordlike bundle of fibers between the folds of broad-ligament joining ovary to uterus.

l. palpebral Medial short bands; connecting medial ends of tarsi to the frontal process of maxilla.

l. pectineal A strong aponeurotic band extending from pectineal line of pubis to the lacunar ligament.

l. round of liver Remnant of umbilical vein extending from umbilicus to anterior border of liver *SYN* — ligamentum teres hepatis.

l. round of uterus A fibromuscular cord extending from either side of uterus to labium majus passing through inguinal canal.

l. sacrotuberous A strong triangular ligament extending from tuberosity of ischium to the lateral part of sacrum and coccyx and to the posterior inferior iliac spine.

l. sphenomandibular A band extending from spine of sphenoid bone to the lingula of lower jaw.

l. stylomandibular Condensed band of cervical fascia extending from apex of the styloid process to posterior border of angle of lower jaw.

l. tibial collateral A broad flat membranous band situated medially and posteriorly of knee joint attached to medial condyle of femur and medial surface of tibia.

l. ulnar collateral Thick triangular band of fibers attached above to medial epicondyle of humerus and below to coronoid process of ulna and medial margin of olecranon.

l. uterosacral Fibrous band extending from cervix to sides of sacrum.

l. vestibular of larynx A thin fibrous membrane in the ventricular fold of larynx extending from thyroid cartilage to arytenoid cartilage.

l. vocal The band that extends on either side from thyroid cartilage to vocal process of arytenoid cartilage.

Ligand Any of the molecules or ions, identical or different that bind to same central entity by multiple coordination bonds, e.g., O_2 and N_2 attaching to same iron molecule contained in Hb.

Ligate To tightly tie a thread to compress a vessel, pedicle of a tumor.

Ligation The action to ligate.

l. tubal Both fallopian tubes are tied and cut or crushed for purpose of sterilization.

Ligator Surgical instrument facilitating ligation, superficial or deep.

Ligature A suture tied around a vessel or tube in order to obliterate the lumen. Ligature can be grassline, double, interlocking and continuous type.

Lingula A narrow band of white matter in brainstem connecting nucleus gracilis to inferior cerebellar peduncle, tongue shaped lobule of superior vermix of cerebellum.

Light Electromagnetic radiation of 400-700 nm.

Lightening The descent of fetus deeper into pelvis.

Limb An arm, leg, appendage projecting from trunk.

l. anacrotic Ascending limb of arterial pulse wave.

l. anterior, of internal capsule The most anterior part of internal capsule separating head of caudate nucleus from lenticular nucleus, formed by cortico-spinal fibers.

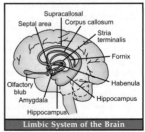

Supracallosal
Septal area   Corpus callosum
Stria terminalis
Fornix
Olfactory blub
Habenula
Amygdala   Hippocampus
Hippocampus
Limbic System of the Brain

Limbic system The parts of brain including hippocampus, amygdala, dentate-gyrus, cingulate gyrus responsible for emotion, arousal, behavior and motor autonomic functions.

Limbus An edge, border or fringe.

Limes zero The largest amount of toxin which when mixed with one standard unit of antitoxin and given to 250 gm guinea pig will produce no reaction.

Lindane Gamma benzen hexachloride, used in pediculosis.

Line A connection between two points or a boundary between two areas.

l. Beau's Superficial transverse depressions in the nail plates appearing after an illness.

l. bismuth Blackline at the gingival margin due to action of bismuth on sulfur of, dental plaques.

l. Camper's Line drawn from base of anterior nasal spine to upper end of tragus of ear.

l. Chamberlain's A line drawn in lateral X-ray of skull from posterior end of hardpalate to the posterior margin of foramen magnum. In normal individual the odontoid process should not lie above this line.

l. cleavage Fine linear clefts in the skin produced by parallel bundles of connective tissue in the reticular layer.

l. Kerley's Thin linear soft tissue densities seen in X-ray chest representing thick interlobular septa. Kerley B lines are located in costophrenic area. A lines are located centrally and C lines are tiny lace like densities in hilum. They are all seen with interstitial pulmonary edema and with pulmonary fibrosis.

l Meyer's An axial line through big toe which when extended posteriorly will pass through center of heel in a normal foot.

l. Nelaton's A line drawn from anterior superior iliac spine to ischial tuberosity, passing above greater trochanter of femur in a normal person.

l. pectinate An uneven horizontal line formed by the continuity between the anal valves and bases of rectal columns 2 cm. above the anal opening. The line represents ectoentodermal junction.

l. Schoemaker's The line joining greater trochanter of femur and anterior superior iliac spine passes normally above umbilicus.

l. simian A transpalmar crease more common to those with Down's syndrome.

l. white of Frankel Line of increased radiodensity in the metaphysis at the provisional zone of calcification; a sign of scurvy.

Linea Along thin mark, ridge, crease or line.

l. alba Midline tendinous band extending from xiphoid process to symphysis pubis, formed by aponeurosis of external oblique, internal oblique and transversalis muscles.

l. nigra Pigmented linea alba of pregnancy.

Lineage The direct descendants of an individual.

Linear Having the properties of a line.

Lingual Tongue shaped process;

l of lung separates cardiac notch from inferior margin of left lung.

l of mandible The mandibular projection giving attachment to sphenomandibular ligment.

l of sphenoid The ridge between body and ala magna of sphenoid.

Linoleic acid An essential fatty acid, precursor of prostaglandin.

Lingulectomy Surgical resection of lingula of left upper lobe.

Linguopapillitis Painful ulcers around the papillae on the tongue margins.

Linguoversion Malposition of tooth towards the tongue.

Liniment An oily medicinal liquid applied to skin by friction as an counter irritant.

Linin Fine thread like achromatic substance of the cell nucleus that interconnects the chromatin grannules.

Lining In dentistry, the coating applied to the walls of a tooth cavity to .protect the pulp from irritation by restorative filling e.g., zinc oxide, eugenol, zinc phosphate and calcium hydroxide.

Linitis Inflammation of cellular tissue of stomach.

l. plastica Extensive thickening of stomach wall due to infiltration by scirrhous carcinoma.

Linkage 1. The force that holds together the atoms in a chemical compound. 2. The relationship existing between two or more genes in the same chromosome.

Linseed The oil acts as a demulcent and laxative.

Lip Any projecting labrum, fleshy parts surrounding mouth opening.

l. cleft Notch, furrow or open space in upper lip developmental in origin.

Lipase Enzyme that catalyzes hydrolysis of fat.

Lipectomy Excision of subcutaneous adipose tissue.

Lipemia Increased turbidity of plasma due to increased lipids.

Lipid Any natural compound soluble in apolar but insoluble in polar solvents. Lipids contain fatty acids, one chain alcohols, steroids or sphyngolipids.

Lipid A The endotoxic component of lipopoly saccharide consisting of glucosamine disaccharide.

Lipidosis Disease state with abnormal lipid storage by RE cells, e.g. metachromatic leukodystrophy (sulfatide); Niemann-Pick disease (sphingomyelin), gangliosidosis, cerebral lipidosis.

Lipoadenoma A tumor with mixture of glandular and fat tissue, e.g. parathyroid adenoma.

Lipoatrophy Atrophy of subcutaneous tissue at sites of insulin injection.

Lipoblast A polyhedral cell with small lipid droplets which becomes a fat cell.

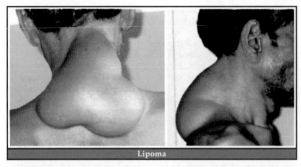
Lipoma

Lipoblastomatosis A benign lobulated tumor of fetal fat cell, may be localized or diffuse.

Lipodermatosclerosis A brawny pigmented fibrosis of the skin and subcutaneous tissue of lower leg resulting from venous stasis.

Lipodystrophy A condition due to abnormal fat metabolism.

l. acquired generalized Loss of body fat, accelerated linear growth hepatomegaly, nephrotic syndrome insulin resistant hyperglycemia hypertriglyceridemia (*SYN*—Laurence syndrome).

Lipofuscin A brown pigment, partially soluble in fat, occurring in nerve and muscle cells.

Lipogranuloma A granulomatous inflammation of the subcutaneous fat.

Lipogranulomatosis A rare metabolic disorder in which ceramides and gangliosides accumulate as a result of ceramidase deficiency.

Lipohyalin Lipoid material sometimes seen in hyalinized beta cells of pancreatic islets of Langerhans in diabetes.

Lipofuscin A golden brown lipid containing pigment representing indigestible residue of cellular lysosomal activity.

Lipoma A benign growth of mature adipose tissue cells.

l. arborescens A lipomatous transformation of synovium producing a villous form.

l. of corpus callosum Calcified lipoma with typical radiological appearance.

l. diffuse symmetrical of neck (Madelung disease) diffuse benign adipose tumor of neck.

l. lumbosacral Overlies a spina bifida.

l. spermatic cord As it extends into scrotum, often resembles hernia.

Lipomatoid Resembling lipoma

Lipomatosis Presence of multiple or diffuse lipomas.

l. dolorosa Presence of multiple painful lipomas.

Lipophilic Fat soluble.

Lipophore A pigmented cell whose color is caused by lipochrome pigment.

Lipopolysaccharide Any substance made up partly from lipid and partly from polysaccharide e.g., bacterial cell wall which is highly antigenic.

Lipoprotein Compounds of lipid and protein.

l. high density Contains 50% protein, 25% phospholipid, 20% cholesterol, and 5% fat, originate both in liver and intestine, function in cholesterol transport, have longer half life and are cardio-protective.

l. low density Contains more of cholesterol and lipids and little triglyceride high blood level is atherogenic.

l. very low density Density 1.006 mg/ml. Contains 50% fat, 25% cholesterol and 20% phospholipid.

Lipoprotein lipase The enzyme that catalyzes hydrolysis of fat into fatty acids and glycerol. VLDL is hydrolyzed in this way. The enzyme lies bound to capillary wall by glycosaminoglycan.

Liposarcoma Malignant tumor of adipose tissue common to soft tissue and retroperitoneum. It can be well differentiated, myxoid (embryonal), round cell, pleomorphic or mixed.

Liposis Diffuse fatty infiltration of body tissues. *SYN*— adiposis.

Liposome A small vesicular structure which forms spontaneously when phospholipids are placed in water.

Liposuction Or suction lipotomy – where subcutaneous fat is suctioned out through cannula.

Lipoteichoic acid The teichoic acid found in bacterial membranes.

Lipotropin Any hormone that causes release of fatty acids from fat.

β *lipotropin* A single chain poly-peptide hormone with 91 amino acids, functions as a prohormone for endorphins, encephalins and MSH.

γ *lipotropin* Single chain polypeptide hormone with 58 amino acids, physiologic property unknown.

Lipovaccine Vaccine prepared by suspending the microorganisms in vegetable oil so that absorption is delayed.

Lipoxygenase An oxidising enzyme for linoleate group.

Lipping A bony spur.

Liquefaction Becoming liquid, often due to hydrolysis.

Liquid A fluid state.

Liquor The fluid secreted by choroid plexus of ventricles, ovarian follicles.

Lisch nodule Melanocytic hamartoma from iris.

Lisencephaly Failure of cerebral gyri to develop with smooth brain surface

Listeria Small gram-positive aerobic rods, e.g. *L. monocytogenes* causing meningitis, septicemia, abscess.

Listerosis Infection with *Listeria* organisms.

Lithagogue Agent that enhances removal of stone/calculus.

Lithectasy Extraction of bladder stone through previously dilated urethra.

Lithiasis Formation of stones; renal, biliary, conjunctival.

Lithium A silvery, soft element, the carbonate form used for manic depressive disorder.

Lithocholic acid Bile acid, found conjugated with taurine and glycine.

Lithogenesis Formation of calculi.

Litholysis Fragmentation or dissolution of stones.

Litholyte An instrument designed to administer stone dissolving agents directly inside bladder.

Lithopedion A retained calcified fetus.

Lithotomy An incision into a duct or organ for removing stone.

Lithotony Formation of bladder fistula for stone removal.

Lithotresis Drilling holes into calculus for its removal.

Lithotripsy Breaking up of gall/urinary stones by shock waves, delivered directly or extra corporeally.

Lithotrite Surgical instrument designed to crush or fragment stones and help their removal.

Lithuria Passage of excess urate or uric acid in urine.

Litmus A natural pigment from lichens whose principle is azolitmin.
It is used as pH indicator being red at pH and blue at pH 8.3.

Litter 1. A stretcher for transporting the invalid. 2. A group of animals produced at one birth by a multiparous mammal. Also called brood.

Livedo A discoloration, skin erythema that follows a reticular pattern of the cutaneous vascular network.

l. reticularis Circulatory disorder of unknown origin causing constant bluish discoloration on large areas of extremity.

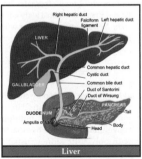

Liver

Liver Largest glandular organ in the body. Weighing 1200-1600 gm. (1/40 of body wt), located in right upper quadrant below right dome of diaphragm; major functions are secretion of bile, synthesis of plasma protenis, fibrinogen, prothrombin; detoxification, metabolism of carbohydrate, fat and protein and storage of glycogen.

l. amyloid Large pale gray waxy looking liver due to deposition of amyloid. Amyloid deposits appear as an amorphous eosinophilic substance, in the space of Disse, between hepatocyte and sinusoidal endothelial cells.

l. cirrhotic biliary Deeply bile stained nodular liver caused by autoimmune damage to small bile ducts (primary biliary cirrhosis) or obstruction to bile outflow.

l. cirrhotic Scarred nodular liver, post hepatitis, alcoholic.

l. brimstone Enlarged bright yellow liver of congenital syphilis.

l. Indian childhood cirrhosis Enlarged firm liver with a leafy edge

l. fatty Yellow soft greasy liver with increased cytoplasmic fat within hepatocytes.

l. frosted Liver with hyaline thickening of its capsule due to chronic perihepatitis.

l. nutmeg Liver affected by chronic vascular congestion as in CHF.

l. polycystic Liver with multiple congenital cysts, often associated with polycystic kidney, usually asymptomatic.

Lividity A black and blue discoloration of skin such as caused by contusion.

Lividomycin Aminoglycoside antibiotic.

Loa A genus of filarial nematode transmitted by blood sucking flies.

Loa-loa The thread like eye worm of Africa causing blindness and calabar swelling. The microfilarae with nuclei extending right upto tail are found only during day.

Lobe 1. A fairly well defined portion of an organ or gland bounded by structural borders such as fissures, sulci or septa-2. Projecting fibro fatty lobule of human ear. 3. One of the main divisions of crown, formed from distinct point of calcification.

l. azygos An occasional small triangular lobe on the mediastinal surface at the apex of the right lung.

l. caudate A small lobe of liver situated posteriorly between the inferior venacava and fissure for ligamentum venosum.

l. frontal The portion of each cerebral hemisphere bounded behind by central and below by lateral sulci.

l. limbic Cingulate and para-hippocampal gyri, as well as underlying hippocampal formation, and dentate gyrus, the oldest portions of cerebral cortex.

l. occipital Most posterior portion of each cerebral hemispheres, bounded anteriorly by parieto occipital sulcus and the line joining it to the preoccipital notch.

l. olfactory A general term usually denoting olfactory bulb, tract, trigone plus anterior perforated substance.

l. parietal Upper central portion of each cerebral hemispheres between the frontal and occipital lobes and above the temporal lobes, separated from frontal lobe by central sulcus.

l. median of prostate The portion of prostate between ejaculatory ducts and urethra, forming the superior

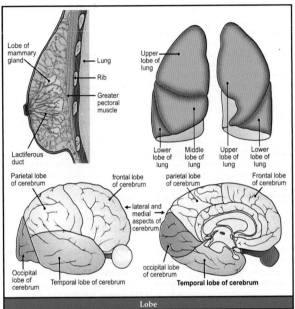

Lobe

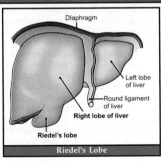

Riedel's Lobe

part of posterior surface of prostate, only becomes obvious when enlarged and enlargement causes bladder neck obstruction.

l. flocculonodular Oldest division of cerebellum made up of the midline nodules and two stalk like flocculi located in the poste–rior and ventral surface of cerebellum. It is functionally related to vestibular nerve and nuclei.

l. piriform A portion of the anterior and ventromedial face of temporal lobe composed of the terminal extensions of the lateral olfactory striae, the uncus and the anterior part of parahippocampal gyrus.

l. pyramidal of thyroid gland An inconstant, narrow cone-shaped lobe of thyroid, arising from upper border of isthmus, often attached to hyoid bone by a fibrous band.

l. Riedel's A tongue shaped mass of tissue often extending downward from right lobe of liver.

l. quadrate A small lobe on inferior surface of liver-between gall-bladder and ligamentum teres.

l. temporal A long lobe on outer side and inferolateral surface of cerebral hemispheres bounded above by lateral sulcus.

Lobeline Ganglionic stimulant.

Lobotomy Incision of a lobe.

l. prefrontal A psychosurgical procedure with division of fibers connecting prefrontal and frontal lobes with thalamus. Also called prefrontal leukotomy.

Lobulated Consisting of or divided into lobules.

Lobule A small lobe.

Lobulet A very small lobule or a section or subdivision of lobule.

Lobulization The process by which homogeneous tissue is changed into a tabulated state.

Localization 1. Determination of site of a morbid process. 2. Restriction of a process to an area.

Localizer A visual training instrument used in the treatment of amblyopia.

Lochia Discharge from uterus following childbirth.

l. alba Light colored uterine discharge consisting of leukocytes.

l. rubra Bloody uterine discharge immediately after delivery.

Lochiometra Retention of lochia (blood and mucus) within uterus.

Lochiorrhea Excessive vaginal discharge after child birth.

Lockjaw Trismus, a symptom of tetanus.

Locomotion Movement from place to place.

Locomotor Relating to motion.

Loculated Divided into many loculi.

Loculation 1. A tissue or structure having numerous small cavities. 2. formation of small cavities.

Loculus A small cavity.

Locum tenens One who temporarily assumes place of another.

Locus A place or spot, as the specific site occupied by a gene in the chromosome.

l. ceruleus A bluish gray area in the floor of fourth ventricle.

l. histocompatibility One of the genes located within major histocompatibility complex that specifies transplantation antigens or immune response functions.

l. operator A regulator locus that governs the transcription of adjacent structural genes of the operon and is the binding site of a repressor protein molecule.

Loeffler's syndrome Disorder lasting less than a month, characterized by transient infiltrates in lungs, low fever and eosinophilia.

Loeffler's disease Also called eosinophilic endomyocardial disease with eosinophilic coronary arteritis, congestive cardiac failure, eosinophilia and multiple systemic emboli.

Logopathy Speech disorder.

Logoplegia Paralysis of speech.

Logorrhea Excessive uncontrolled speech, i.e., logomania.

Loin The part of back and sides of body between the ribs and the pelvis.

Loop A bend in a cord or cord like structure, the arched dermal ridges in dermatoglyphics.

l. capillary Capillaries in the dermal papillae.

l. gamma The reflex arc involving gamma efferent fibers arising in muscle spindles.

l. of intestine One of several U-shaped flexures formed by jejunum and ileum.

l. Lippe's S-shaped intrauterine contraceptive device.

l. Meyer's The portion of geniculo-calcarine radiation that loops

around inferior horn of lateral ventricle.

l. of recurrent laryngeal nerve The arching of recurrent laryngeal nerves after their origin from vagus in the chest. The left one hooks below the arch of aorta behind attachment of ligamentum arterisoum and then up the left side of trachea while the right one hooks around first part of subclavian artery.

Loperamide A meperidine congener, intestinal smooth muscle relaxant.

Lophophorine An extreme toxic alkaloid found in cactus.

Lophotrichous Bacteria possessing multiple flagella at one pole only.

Lorazepam A benzodiazepine anxiolytic.

Lorbamate A cyclopropane carbamate ester used as muscle relaxant.

Lorcainide Antiarrhythmic agent, for ventricular tachycardia.

Lordosis Abnormally increased forward curvature of lumbar spine. Also called sway back or saddle back.

l. compensatory Lordosis secondary to pelvic obliquity/deformity.

Loss

l. dissociated sensory Pain and temperature severely lost with preservation of touch as in syringomyelia or central cord tumors.

l. hearing 1. Sensory neural due to ageing or autoimmune 2. Conductive due to disease of middle ear or external ear.

Lotion Medicated liquids for external application or cosmetic liquid preparations, e.g. benzyl benzoate, I. calamine, (calamine, zinc oxide, glycerin, bentonite, calcium hydroxide).

Loudness The intensity of noise or sound.

Loupe Small magnifying lens.

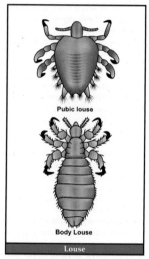

Pubic louse

Body Louse

Louse

Louse Small flat bodied parasitic insect, e.g., body louse, crab louse, head louse, pubic louse).

Low birth weight Birth weight less than 2500 gm.

Lowe's syndrome Oculo-cerebrorenal syndrome.

Lovastatin Ester of methyl butanoic acid, given orally for increased LDL and cholesterol.

Loxapine A tricyclic anti-psychotic agent with tranquillizing properties.

Loxotomy Surgical amputation by means of an oblique incision.

Lozenge A tablet, often diamond shaped, containing medication in a flavoured and sweetened base.

L.S. ratio Ratio of lecithin to sphingomyelin in amniotic fluid of fetus; an indicator of fetal lung maturity.

Lubb-dupp First and second heart sound auscultatory appearance.

Lubricant Agent used to reduce friction.

Lucanthone hydrochloride Antischistosomial drug.

Lucid Easily understood, clear, able to think properly.

Luciferase An enzyme which catalyzes the transfer of an electron from luciferin to oxygen with emission of light, (bioluminescence of fire flies, glow worms and bacterial fungi).

Lucifugal Avoiding light.

Ludwig's angine Suppuration in subcutaneous tissue of upper neck below submandibular gland.

Luetic Syphilitic.

Lugol's solution Strong iodine solution

Lumbago Pain in lumbar region.

Lumbar Pertaining to loins.

Lumbarization Fusion between the transverse processes of the lowest lumbar and adjacent sacral vertebra.

Lumbosacral Pertaining to lumbar portion of spine and the sacrum.

Lumbrical Resembling an earth worm, lumbrical muscles of hand.

Lumbricoid Earthworm like appearance.

Lumen The cavity within tubular structure; the SI unit of luminous flux.

Luminescence Emission of infrared, visible light or ultraviolet by matter from any cause except incandesence.

Luminiferous Capable of transmitting light.

Lumpectomy Localized excision of breast lump.

Lunate Moon or crescent shaped, semilunar.

Lunacy Major mental illness.

Lung Paired organ of respiration in the chest enveloped by pleura. Subserving the function of oxygen uptake and CO_2 elimination.

l. farmer's Extrinsic allergic alveolitis occurring in farmers due to inhalation of moldy hay manifesting with cough, dyspnea and fever. Repeated exposures lead to pulmonary fibrosis.

l. honey comb Small multiple areas of radiolucency with intervening borders of soft tissue density as seen in interstitial pulmonary fibrosis.

l. post perfusion A condition of atelectasis, pulmonary arteriovenous shunting and consolidation following cardiopulmonary bypass.

l. uremic Pulmonary edema with butterfly appearance of lung in X-ray due to circulatory overload and uremic dysfunction of LV.

Lupoma A small granulomatous nodule characteristic of lupus vulgaris.

Lupus Resembling wolf.

l. discoid A disease confined to skin, marked by scaly rash usually in butterfly pattern over nose and cheeks, sometimes extending to scalp but no visceral involvement.

l. pernio Sarcoid lesions of the hands and face, especially the ears and nose resembling frost bite.

l. vulgaris Redbrown nodular skin lesions of face in tuberculosis.

l. systemic Chronic autoimmune disease marked by an erythematous rash on face and other areas exposed to sunlight with vasculitis involving kidneys, brain and arthritis. Antinuclear antibodies to double stranded DNA and native DNA nucleohistone are diagnostic.

l. drug induced Similar to systemic lupus induced by drugs like procainamide and hydralazine but without renal and brain involvement.

Luteal Relating to corpus luteum of ovary.

Lutein A yellow pigment, closely related to xanthophyll occurring in luteal cells of corpus luteum.

Luteinization Transformation of granulosa cells into lutein cells in the ovary. Other cells may undergo luteinization including theca cells, celomic cells and cervical cells.

Luteoid Acting like progesterone.

Luteolysis Involution or destruction of corpus luteum.

Luteoma Growth of lutein cells of ovary during third trimester with regression after parturition, often may secrete androgens.

Luteotropic Promoting development, maturation or hormonal secretion of corpus luteum.

Lutetium Element No 71, isotopes used in nuclear medicine.

Lutembacher's syndrome Congenital cardiac abnormality with ASD and mitral stenosis.

Lutheran blood group Antigens of red blood cells, specified by lugene that react with antibodies designated as anti Lu^a and anti Lu^b, first detected in serum of an individual who had received many transfusions and who developed antibodies against erythrocyte of a donor named Lutheran.

Lux A unit of illumination, equal to one lumen per square meter.

Luxation Dislocation.

Lye Sodium potassium hydroxide.

Lying-in Confinement of a woman during childbirth.

Lyme disease A spirochetal disease transmitted by ticks characterized by erythema chronicum migrans, fever, myalgia, lymphadenopathy, arthritis, pericarditis, myocarditis, and CNS involvement.

Lymph A transparent or slightly opalescent fluid containing lymphocytes, which flows through lymph channels and enters finally into venous system via thoracic ducts.

Lymphaden Lymph node.

Lymphadenectasia Enlargement of lymph nodes with excessive lymph.

Lymphadenectomy Surgical excision of lymph nodes.

Lymphadenia Chronic overgrowth of lymphoid tissues.

Lymphadenitis Inflammation of lymph nodes.

Lymphadenography X-ray examination of lymph nodes.

Lymphadenoma A tumor made of lymphoid tissue.

Lymphadenomatosis Presence of numerous enlarged lymph nodes.

Lymphadenopathy A diseased state of lymph nodes.

Lymphadenosis Generalized enlargement of lymph glands and lymphatic tissue, may be benign (e.g., infectious mononucleosis) or malignant.

Lymphagogue An agent that increases formation and flow of lymph.

Lymphangiectasia Abnormal dilatation of lymphatic vessels.

l. intestinal Dilatation of intestinal lymphatic with subsequent protein losing enteropathy, steatorrhea and diarrhea. It may be congenital due to hypoplasia of thoracic duct or acquired due to inflammation or malignancy of lymphatics. Small intestinal biopsy is diagnostic with dilated lacteals in intestinal villi.

Lymphangiectasis Dilatation of lymph vessels.

l. pericaliceal Multiple lymphatic cyst formation around calyces.

l. pulmonary A congenital condition of lung in which there is multiple small cystic dilatations in the lymphatic network, associated with neonatal respiratory distress and death.

Lymphangiectomy Surgical excision of lymphatic vessel.

Lymphangioendothelioma A tumor composed of small masses of endothelial cells and aggregation of tubular structures thought to be lymphatic vessels.

Lymphangiography X-ray visualization of lymphatic vessels after injection of contrast medium.

Lymphangioleiomyomatosis A proliferation of lymphatic and smooth muscle cells typically affecting lung and lymph node, a lesion of women in reproductive age, with honey combing and respiratory insufficiency.

Lymphangioma A benign growth composed exclusively of lymph vessels lined by a single layer of endothelial cells. The lesion is often congenital, can be subtyped into capillary, cavernous and cystic. The latter two are most frequent in cervical, mediastinal and retroperitoneal regions of infants (hygroma); capillary lymphangioma is difficult to identify from hemangioma.

Lymphangiomyoma A growth composed of bundles of smooth muscle tissue about endothelium lined lymph spaces, commonly seen in mediastinum and retroperitoneum with chylothorax.

Lymphangioplasty Surgical replacement or repair of damaged or destroyed lymphatic vessels.

Lymphangiosarcoma Malignant tumor of lymphatic tissue, mainly associated with chronic lymph stasis usually secondary to radical mastectomy.

Lymphangitis Inflammation of lymphatic vessels.

l. carcinomatosa Growth of carcinoma in lymphatics or lymphatic obstruction by carcinoma.

Lymphatic Relating to lymph, lymph node or lymph vessel.

Lymphectesia Dilatation of lymph vessels.

Lymphedema Chronic unilateral or bilateral swelling of extremities caused by obstruction of lymph vessels or disease of lymph nodes, usually congenital, **type I**: autosomal dominant, associated intestinal protein loss and pleural effusion (Millroy's disease), **type II**: slowly progressive form with onset around puberty.

l. praecox Lymphedema occurring in girls approaching puberty.

Lymph node A rounded body consisting of accumulations of lymphatic tissue found in the course of lymphatic vessels.

Lymphoblast An immature cell, the precursor of lymphocyte, also known as lymphocytoblast/ immunoblast.

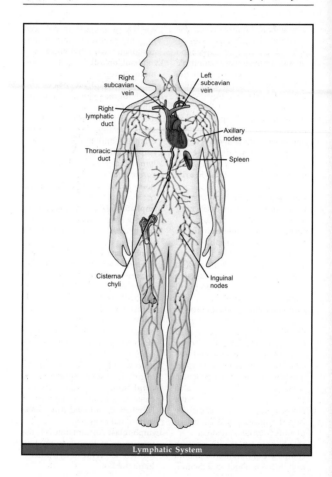

Lymphatic System

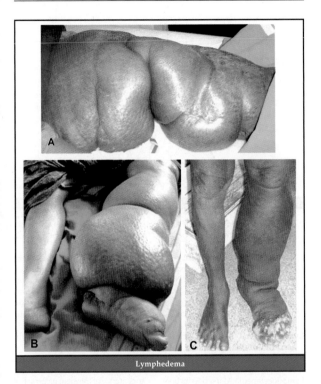

Lymphedema

Lymphoblastoma A form of malignant lymphoma, composed mainly of lymphoblasts.

Lymphocytosis Development of multiple cystic lymphangiomas.

Lymphocyte A white blood cell derived from lymphoid tissue constituting 25-33% of white blood cells in peripheral blood. It has a round nucleus with well condensed chromatin, no nucleolus, and agranular cytoplasm staining pale blue.

l. B Derived from bone marrow, involved in humoral immunity. They recognize antigens irres-

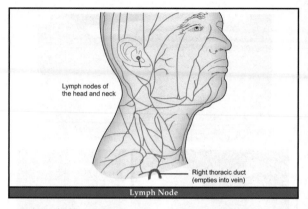

Lymph nodes of the head and neck

Right thoracic duct (empties into vein)

Lymph Node

pective of MCH molecule and transform to plasma cells to secrete antibodies on antigenic stimulation. They are thymus independent.

l. T. Thymus derived lymphocyte, that has been exposed to antigen on an antigen presenting cell. They play large role in cellular immunity. Can be helper cells, killer cells, suppressor cells or null cells.

Lymphocytoma A tumor of low grade malignancy arising in a lymph node, composed mainly of mature lymphocyte.

Lymphocytopenia Marked reduction in number of circulating lymphocytes.

Lymphocytosis Greater than normal number of lymphocytes in peripheral blood.

l. acute infectious An acute benign infectious disease of obscure etiology in children with headache, upper respiratory symptoms, and lymphocytosis.

Lymphocytotoxin A complement fixing antilymphocyte antibody.

Lymphoepithelioma A malignant tumor derived from epithelium around tonsils and nasopharynx containing abundant lymphoid tissue.

Lymphogenous Producing lymph, originating from lymph.

Lymphogranuloma venereum A chlamydial infection marked by appearance of transient ulcer on the genitalia, and enlargement of lymph node in the groin. Can lead to urethral and rectal strictures, rectovaginal fistula.

Lympokine A hormone like factor produced by sensitized lymphocytes when they come in contact with antigen to which they were sensitized, acts as an intercellular messenger to regulate immunologic and inflammatory responses.

Lymphokinesis 1. Circulation of lymph through lymphatic vessels and nodes. 2. Movements of endolymph in the membranous labyrinth of the internal ear.

Lymphoma Malignant disease of lympho reticular system.

l. Burkitt's Malignant lymphoma involving extra-nodal sites like jaw, orbit, abdominal viscera, and ovaries, the most common childhood tumor of tropical Africa. Possibly caused by EB virus and linked to falciparum malaria.

l. histiocytic Lymphoma composed of histiocytes. (poorly differentiated lymphocytic lymphomas).

l. lymphocytic A malignant lymphoma composed of lymphocytes. The pattern may be nodulas or diffuse, and the cells may be poorly differentiated, well differentiated.

l. prolymphocytic The cells are larger and have less condensed nuclear chromatin.

l. sclerosing A lymphoma with prominent stromal component.

l. signet ring cell Cells with a large cytoplasmic vacuole of immunoglobulin which displaces the nucleus to periphery.

l. stem cell Composed of large basket like cells.

Lymphopoietin A soluble factor required for maturation of lymphocytes.

Lymphorrhea Flow of lymph from ruptured lymph channel.

Lymphotaxis The induction of lymphocyte movement.

Lymphotoxin Substance destructive to lymphocytes.

Lymphotrophic Attracted to lymphatic system.

Lynestrenol A semisynthetic progestin.

Lyon hypothesis: One X chromosome in female is inactivated during embryogenesis and forms Barr body.

Lyophilic Dispersing or dissolving easily because of affinity for solvent.

Lyophobic Difficult to disperse because of poor affinity for solvent.

Lypressin Vasopressin with lysine in place of arginine in position 8. An antidiuretic and vasopressor.

Lyophilize To separate a solid from solution by rapid freezing and dehydration under vacuum.

Lysergic acid diethylamide A hallucinogen, can induce chromosomal changes.

Lysine One of the twenty amino acids. It is an essential amino acid deficient in plant proteins.

Lysin Any substance capable of causing lysis.

Lysis 1. Destruction of cell by specific lysin. 2. gradual recovery from an acute disease.

Lysochrome A lipid soluble pigment that is suitable for staining fat.

Lysogen An antigen that stimulates the formation of specific lysin.

Lysogeny A form of viral parasitism in which viral DNA becomes incorporated in a (bacterial) cell genome, without destroying the cell, thereby permitting transmission of virus to subsequent bacterial generations.

Lysokinase An activator agent of fibrinolytic system.

Lysolecithin A lecithin without unsaturated fatty acid residue. It is strongly hemolytic, a good detergent.

Lysosome A membrane limited cytoplasmic organelle containing hydrolytic enzymes capable of breaking down most of the constituents of living matter.

Lysozome An antibacterial enzyme present in tear, sweat, saliva and nasal secretion.

Lyssa virus A genus of rhabdo virus e.g. rabies virus

M

Macaca mulata The rhesus monkey of South East Asia frequently used as laboratory animal.

Mace Chloracetophenone, the component of tear gas.

Macerate To soften a solid or tissue by soaking the tissue in enzyme/acid. 2. The autolysis of fetal tissue after fetal death.

Machine A device for accomplishing a specific objective.

m. heart-lung A combination of pump and oxygenator to affect extracorporeal circulation and oxygenation of blood during open heart surgery.

m. Holtz A machine for developing high voltage static electricity by multiplication of an induced charge.

m. panoramic rotating An X-ray machine capable of radiographing all the teeth and surrounding structures by using a reciprocating motion of the tube and extra oral film.

m. van-de Graaf An electrostatic machine that produces high potential, used for generating high voltage X-rays.

m. Wims Hurst's A machine that converts mechanical energy into electrical energy by electrostatic action.

Macroamylase A form of amylase that occurs as a complex joined to a serum globulin.

Macrobrachia Unusually long arm.

Macrocephalus Unusually large head.

Macrochilia Unusually large lips, usually due to distended lymph spaces.

Macrochiria Unduly enlarged hands.

Macrocrania Abnormal general enlargement of head.

Macrocryoglobulinemia Presence of cold precipitin in blood.

Macrocyte Red blood cell 2 micron larger than normal RBC, also called megalocyte.

Macrocytosis A condition in which red blood cells are larger than normal, e.g. Vit. B_{12} and folic acid deficiency.

Macrodactylia Abnormally large digits.

Macrodont Abnormally large tooth; a skull with dental index ≥ 44.

Macrodontia The condition of having large teeth.

Macroencephaly Malformation and increase in size and weight of brain due to proliferation of glia with small ventricles and mental retardation.

Macrogamete The female gamete, larger egg fusing with microgamete, leading to zygote formation.

Macrogametocyte The mother cell producing macrogamete.

Macroglia The astrocyte and oligodendrocyte, the two neuro glial elements of ectodermal origin.

Macroglobulin Plasma globulin with molecular weight of 1000000, increased in multiple myeloma, cirrhosis, collagen disorders.

Macroglobulinemia Plasma cell myeloma, a disorder with excessive production of IgM with anemia and bleeding; also called Walden-Strom's macroglobulinemia.

Macroglossia Enlarged tongue.

Macrogyria Congenital malformation in which the cerebral gyri are large due to few sulci.

Macrolides A group of antibiotics having moleces made up of large ring lactones, e.g. erythromycin.

Macromelia Enlarged limbs.

Macromolecule Any molecule composed of several monomers.

Macrophage A large mononuclear cell that ingests degenerated cells, widely distributed in body but greatest accumulation in spleen where they remove senescent RBC. In brain and spinal cord known as microglia and in the blood as monocyte.

m. alveolar A cell that moves on the alveolar surface of lung engulfing airborne particles reaching the alveoli.

Macropsia Condition of seeing objects larger than their actual size.

Macroscopic Visible with naked eye.

Macrostomia Abnormally large mouth.

Macrotia Abnormally large ears.

Macula A small area differing in appearance from surrounding structure.

m. corneae A moderately dense white opacity of cornea.

m. communis The thickened portion of the medial wall of the auditory

vesicle in the embryo, eventually dividing to form macula sacculi and macula utriculi.

m. densa That portion of distal convoluted tubule of the kidney in contact with the wall of afferent arteriole just before the latter enters the glomerulus, it contains cells that are tall and narrow, secreting renin.

m. retinae A small yellow oval depression on the retina 2 disc diameter lateral and slightly below the optic disc containing fovea centralis.

m. sacculi The oval neuroepithelial sensory area in the medial wall of the saccule that houses the terminal filaments of vestibular nerve.

Maculation The formation of macules or spots on the skin.

Macule A non elevated discolored lesion on the skin.

Maculocerebral Relating to brain and macula lutea of retina.

Maculoerythematous Both red and spotted.

Maculopapular Spotted and elevated.

Maculopathy Any disease of macula of retina.

Mad Suffering from mental disorder, rabid, angry.

Maddox rod Multiple parallel cylindrical rods of glass fused side to side and shaped into a trial lens used for testing of squint and fusion.

Madelong deformity Subluxation of distal radioulnar joint secondary to abnormal growth and curvature of distal radius.

Madarosis Loss of eye lashes.

Madurella A genus of fungi causing maduramycosis.

Maduramycosis A chronic disease affecting feet with draining sinuses discharging yellow to black granules.

Maffucci's syndrome A combination of multiple cutaneous hemangiomas and dyschondroplasia.

Magaldrate Hydroxy magnesium aluminate, an antacid.

Maggot A legless soft bodied larva of various insects, common housefly, developing in dead organic matter.

Magma 1. A paste like preparation of any organic matter. 2. Finely divided material supended in a small quantity of water.

Magnesia Magnesium oxide, it neutralizes acids to give soluble magnesium salts.

Magnesium Element number 12, the silvery white metal, one of the principal cations governing electrochemical properties of living system.

m. carbonate $MgCO_3$, insoluble in water, used as laxative and antacid.

m. citrate Used as laxative.

m. hydroxide Insoluble in water, used as laxative and antacid.

m. oxide also called magnesia (see above).

m. sulphate $MgSO_4$ Effective cathartic, antiarrhythmic and anti-

epileptic, useful in certain poisonings.

Magnetic resonance imaging (MRI) A form of imaging using electromagnetic energy, visualizes brain contents better and can image large sized vessels without use of contrast material

Magnetism 1. The properties of mutual attraction, or repulsion produced by magnet or electric current. 2. Study of magnet and their properties. 3. The force exhibited by a magnetic field.

Magneton A unit of measure of the magnetic movement of an atomic or subatomic particle.

Magnification An enlargement of an object by an optical element or instrument.

Mahaim fibers Conduction tissue connecting proximal av bundle to septal myocardium causing ventricular pre-excitation.

Maim To disable, mutilate, cripple by injury.

Main French for hand.

m. d' accoucheur The characteristic position of hand produced by tetany.

m. en crochet Permanent flexion of the fourth and fifth fingers, resembling the position of a person's hand while crocheting.

m. en griffe Permanent extension of metacarpophallangeal joints.

m. en lorgnette Opera glass hand; shortening of fingers and transverse folding of skin caused by absorption of phallanges.

Mainlining Term used by drug addicts denoting IV injection of heroin or other drugs.

Majocchis' disease Annular telangiectatic purpura.

Major histocompatibility complex A group of genes on chromosome 6 that code for antigens that determine tissue and blood compatibility. Class I MHC antigens are HLA-A, HLA-B, HLA-C, present on all nucleated cells; class II antigens axe HLA-DR, HLA-DQ and HLA-DP present on lymphocytes and antigen processing cells.

Majority The age at which a person becomes legally entitled to full civil rights of an adult. It is 18 in UK, 21 in India, USA, Canada and 20 in Japan.

Mal French for disease.

Mala Latin for cheek bone, cheek.

Makeshift Denoting a shunt from a large variceal collateral vessel to a systemic vein when a standard shunt cannot be employed. Employed for portal hypertension.

Malabsorption Impaired or incomplete absorption of nutrients by the intestine.

m. lactose Lactase deficiency, mostly inherited, commonly manifesting in adults, with pain and diarrhoea after lactose ingestion. Unabsorbed lactose is converted to butyric and lactic acid by colonic bacteria, that causes pain. Lactose being hyperosmolar draws fluid to add to stool volume.

m. syndrome Manifests with pallor, potbelly, bleeding tendency, weakness due to malabsorption of nutrients, caused by any disease.

Malachite green Green crystalline substance used as a pH indicator.

Malacia Softening of tissues.

m. cordis morbid softening of heart.

Malady Illness.

Malaise A vague general discomfort or feeling ill.

Malakoplakia The formation of soft, fungus like growths on the mucous membrane of a hollow organ, esp. urinary bladder.

Malalignment 1. Incorrectly aligned fractured parts. 2. Displacement or abnormal position of tooth.

Malar Relating to cheek or cheek bone.

Malaria An infectious disease caused by any of the four plasmodia, transmitted by mosquitoes of the genus anopheles, manifesting with chill and fever, anemia, splenomegaly.

m. falciparum Caused by *plasmodium falciparum*, the parasite develops within small vessels of internal organs frequently blocking them. Fever paroxysm often occurs daily and is often continuous. Patient can have cerebral, gastrointestinal, renal and pulmonary complications. Also known as malignant tertian.

m. malarae Caused by *plasmodium malarae*, Fever paroxysm occurs on every third day.

m. quotidian A form in which paroxysms occur daily, can be caused by combination of *plasmodium vivax* and falciparum or two generations of falciparum.

m. relapsing A type in which exoerythrocytic cycle persists in liver with relapse e.g., in vivax and ovale infection.

m. vivax Caused by plasmodium vivax or ovale, the fever paroxysm occurring every other day.

Malassizia furfur Fungus that causes tinea versicolor.

Malate Salt of malic acid.

Malathion Insecticide.

Male Sex of an individual containing organs that produce spermatozoa, with one X and one Y chromosome.

Malformation A defect or deformity.

m. Klippel - Feil Short webbed neck due to malformation of cervical vertebrae.

m. Mondini Congenital deafness due to hypoplasia of latter part of cochlea.

Malfunction Abnormal or inadequate function.

Malic acid An intermediate in carbohydrate metabolism, present in unripe apples, cherries, tomatoes etc.

Malignant Denoting any disease resistant to treatment, and of fatal nature. In case of tumor it denotes uncontrollable undifferentiated growth and dissemination.

Malinger To pretend to be ill, for personal gains.

Malingerer Who pretends to be sick.

Malleable Pliable, capable of being made into small sheets.

Malleation A spasmodic movement.

Malleolar Relating to one or both prominences on either side of ankle.

Malleolus One of the two projections on either side of ankle.

Malleus The club shaped and most lateral of the three auditory ossicles involved in sound transmission across middle ear. It is attached to tympanic membrane and articulates with incus.

Mallory Weiss syndrome Laceration of lower esophagus with hematemesis following severe retching and vomiting.

Malnutrition Faulty nutrition due to inadequate diet, metabolic abnormality, wrong proportions of items etc.

Maloclusion Abnormal contact opposing teeth.

m. close bite When jaws are closed edges of anterior mandibular teeth extend lingually towards the gum.

m. open bite When the jaws are closed, the opposing teeth fail to establish contact.

m. Taussig-Bling A congenital malformation characterized by the aorta arising from morphological right ventricle and pulmonary trunk over riding an anterior inter ventricular communication.

Malonic acid It competitively inhibits the oxidation of succinate to fumarate.

Malonyl-coenzyme A Formed from acetyl COA, helpful in fatty acid biosynthesis.

Malpractice Improper, unskillful, or negligent treatment of an individual by a medical man.

Malpighian body Renal corpuscle.

Malrotation Developmental failure of rotation in the normal direction and to normal degree, most common to digestive tract.

Malt Grain, especially barley, containing dextrin, maltose, glucose and some enzymes.

Maltase Digestive enzyme promoting conversion of maltose to glucose.

Maltose $C_{12}H_{22}O_{11}$; a sugar formed by action of a digestive enzyme on starch.

Malunion Faulty union of fractured bones.

Mamma Breast, rudimentary in male and but containing milk producing glands in female.

Mammal Vertebrates that nourish their offspring with milk.

Mammoplasty Plastic surgery of breast; can be augmentative (increase in size by implants) or reductive.

Mammary Relating to breast.

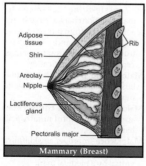

Mammary (Breast)

Mammila Nipple, nipple like protruberance.

Mammiloplasty Reparative surgery of nipple.

Mammilate Having nipple like structures.

Mammogram X-ray of mammary gland.

Mammography A soft tissue X-ray technique for visualization of female breast; used to detect non-palpable lesions and identify palpable lesions.

Mammotrophic Promoting development, and growth of mammary glands.

Mandelate Salt of mandelic acid.

Mandelic acid Urinary antibacterial agent.

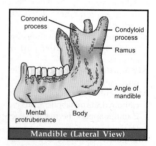

Mandible (Lateral View)

Mandible The horseshoe shaped bone of lower jaw in mammals. Articulating with skull at temporomandibular joint and housing the lower teeth.

Mandibullectomy Removal of lower jaw.

Maneuver A skillful movement.

m. Bracht's In obstetrics, maneuver used in breech extraction whereby breech is allowed to deliver spontaneously upto umbilicus and then the fetal body is held anteriorly toward mother's abdomen to facilitate delivery of vertex.

m. credes A method of expressing the placenta in which body of uterus is vigorously squeezed inorder to produce placental separation.

m. Heimlich A maneuver done to dislodge food stuck in throat obstructing airway. Standing at the back of the victim the rescuer places both the arms around him, making a fist with one hand and grasping it with the other hand presses the fist sharply upwards below the ribcage to cause a forced expiration to dislodge the foreign body.

m. Hippocratic A maneuver to restore proper position of dislocated shoulder. The operator places his foot in patient's axilla and pulls the arm downwards.

m. Phalens A method of bringing out or accentuating symptoms of carpal tunnel syndrome by forced flexion of affected wrist for 30-60 seconds or applying BP cuff to the arm and inflating it above systolic pressure for one minute.

m. Pinard Method of fetal extraction in frank breech presentation; two fingers are passed along fetal thigh to push it away from midline and flex the leg, the foot then easily grasped and brought down and out.

m. Prague A procedure used in breech delivery in which the finger is hooked over shoulder of fetus to exert traction and allow engagement of the head.

m. Scanzoni's Rotation of fetal head with mid forceps from posterior to anterior position.

m. Sellick's Application of pressure on cricoid cartilage to occlude the esophagus posteriorly thereby preventing acid regurgitation especially in patients requiring intubation with full stomach.

m. Valsalva 1. Forced expiration against closed glottis to increase pressure within lungs. 2. Forced expiration with mouth closed and nose pinched to open up auditory tubes.

Manganese Element no. 25, an essential micronutrient.

Manganous Bivalent salts of manganese.

Mange Scabies.

Mania Emotional disorder characterized by excitement, hyperactivity and garrulousness.

Maniac Emotionally disturbed individual with violent behavior.

Manifestation Display of characteristic signs and symptoms of a disease.

m. neurotic The use of various defense mechanisms like conversion, dissociation, depression in an attempt to resolve emotional conflicts.

m. psychotic Loss of contact with reality, personality disintegration.

Manikin An anatomic model of human body for practice of certain manipulations as those of obstetrics and dentistry.

Manipulation Treatment by skillful use of hand in reducing dislocation or changing the fetal position.

Manna The dried sugary exudate of ash tree, rarely used as a laxative.

Mannerism Distinctive characteristic or behavioral trait.

Mannitol An alcohol, $C_6H_{14}O_6$, derived from fructose, used in preparation of dietetic sweets and as an osmotic diuretic.

Manometer An instrument for measuring pressure of liquid and gases.

Mansonia A genus of mosquitoes transmitting filaria.

Mantoux test A intracutaneous test to know exposure of an individual to tuberculosis. 0.1 ml of PPD is injected and result in read after 72 hours. Induration and erythema more than 10 mm in diameter indicates positive test.

Manubrium A structure that resembles a handle but when used alone refers to manubrium sterni.

Manus Latin for hand.

Mantle A covering.

Maple syrup urine disease An autosomal recessive disorder marked by deficient oxidative decarboxylation of alpha keto acids; the urine has characteristic maple syrup odor and the symptoms soon after birth are hypoglycemia, hypotonia, convulsion, etc. Also known as branched chain ketonuria.

Mapping In genetics, locating the position and order of gene loci on a chromosome by analyzing the frequency of recombination between the loci.

Maprotiline Tricyclic antidepressant.

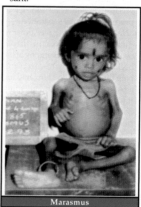
Marasmus

Marasmus Protein calorie malnutrition in young children with progressive wasting, wizened face, shrunken eyeballs but alerted mind.

Marble bone disease Abnormally calcified bone with spotted appearance in X-ray.

Marcus-Gunn's phenomenon Closing of the eyes when mouth is closed and exaggerated opening of the eyes when mouth is opened. *SYN*— Jaw winking syndrome.

Marfan's syndrome Autosomal dominant trait with defective formation of elastic fibers marked by abnormally long slender extremities, spidery fingers, high arched palate, lax joints, aortic regurgitation, MVP and dislocation of lens.

Margin The edge or border of a structure or organ.

m. of safety A measure of drug safety based on the dose required to produce an effective, therapeutic response in most individuals versus the dose required to produce toxic effects in few individuals. It is similar to but not same as therapeutic index.

m. ciliary of iris The border of iris attached to ciliary body.

m. costal The curved lower portion of thoracic wall formed by the cartilages of the seventh through tenth ribs.

m. falciform The lower lateral border of saphenous opening in fascia lata of thigh.

m. free gingival The part of gum, not attached to tooth.

m. orbital Margin of orbit bounded by frontal bone superiorly, zygomatic bone laterally, maxilla inferiorly and the process of maxilla and frontal bone medially.

m. pupillary of iris The border of iris forming edge of pupil.

Margination Adhesion of leukocytes to the interior of capillary wall during early stages of inflammation.

Marginoplasty Plastic surgery of eyelid border.

Marijuana The dried, chopped leaves, flowers and stems of the common hemp plant *canabis sativa,* smoked or eaten to induce euphoria.

Marie Strumpel disease Ankylosing spondylitis.

Mark A blemish, a spot

m. port wine Congenital discoloration of skin, usually on the face varying from pink to purple.

Marker 1. A characteristic factor by which a cell or molecule can be identified or a disease can be recognized. 2. A general term for any trait that helps to throw light on the genetic nature of a disorder.

Marmot Ticks that transmit rocky mountain spotted fever.

Maroteax Lamy syndrome A form of mucopolysaccharidoses characterized by dwarfism, chest deformity, knock knee, stiff joints, cloudy cornea, short hands and fingers, inherited as autosomal recessive and there is excessive dermatan sulphate excretion in urine.

Marrow The meshy material filling the medullary cavities of bones.

m. red Marrow in the cancellous or spongy bones of sternum, ribs, iliac crest, vertebrae and ends of long bones. Concerned with formation of blood.

m. yellow The fatty marrow in center of long bones.

Marsupialization Surgical procedure for eradication of cyst in which the sac is incised, and its edges are stitched to the edges of external incision e.g., pilonidal cyst.

Masculine Relating to characteristics of male sex.

Maser A device that converts incident electromagnetic radiation of various frequencies into a beam of highly amplified monochromatic radiation.

Mask 1. A covering for the face and nose to prevent spread of infection. 2. An expressionless appearance of face, e.g. Parkinson fades. 3. A metal frame covered with gauze placed over face for giving inhalation anesthesia. 4. To cover metal parts of a denture with an opaque material.

m. BLB An oxygen mask used at high altitudes, having a combination of inspiratory and expiratory valves in a rebreathing bag.

m. Venturi Mask that develops a constant concentration of oxygen, using the Venturi principle of entrainment of air to dilute the flow of pure oxygen.

Masking 1. The introduction of noise in one ear for the purpose of excluding that ear from a hearing test given to the other ear. 2. The opaque material placed over the metal or any other part of a dental prosthesis.

Masochism 1. A form of sexual perversion where satisfaction is dependent upon physical torture. 2. The infliction of physical or psychological pain upon oneself to relieve guilt.

Masochist 1. The passive partner in practice of masochism. 2. One who for psychological purposes exposes himself unnecessarily to sufferings.

Mass A collection of tissue; in pharmacology, a soft pasty mixture of drugs suitable for rolling into pills.

m. inner cell An aggregation of cells that stick together and collect at embryonic pole of the blastocyst.

m. lateral of atlas The solid parts of first cervical vertebra (atlas) on either side, articulating above with occipital condyles of skull and below with the axis.

Mass psychogenic illness Psychogenic illness in a group of people at one time e.g. vanishing phallus, decreasing and disappearing breast in females (tarantism).

Massage Rubbing body parts for therapeutic goals.

m. Cardiac Rhythmic manual compression of heart either by thoracotomy (open cardiac massage) or by pressure applied to sternum (closed cardiac massage).

m. carotid sinus Massage of carotid sinus at the angle of jaw for treatment of SVT or identification of tachycardia.

m. prostatic Massage of prostate through rectum to express its secretions into prostatic urethra (examination for gonococci).

Masseter Muscle of lower jaw used for chewing.

Masseur A person trained in or who practises the art of massage.

Mast cell A large tissue cell resembling basophil but does not circulate in the blood. Mast cell degranulation by antigens produces immediate hypersensitivity.

Mastectomy Surgical excision of breast.

m. extended radical Mastectomy that includes removal of chest muscles, axillary lymphnodes and the internal mammary chain of lymph nodes.

m. Halstead radical Removal of breast, chest muscles and lymph nodes of axilla.

m. modified radical Removal of breast and axillary lymphnodes without removal of pectoralis muscle.

m. total Removal of breast only.

Master two sep test A test to evaluate angina when patient goes up and down two steps 9″ high

Masticate To chew.

Mastication The process of chewing.

Mastigophora The subphylum bf protozoa that includes leishmania and trypanosomas; organisms with one or more flagella and a single nucleus.

Mastitis Inflammation of the breast.

m. chronic cystic Fibrocystic disease of breast.

m. interstitial Inflammation of connective tissue of breast.

m. phlegmonous Diffuse breast inflammation tending to abscess formation.

m. plasma cell Benign condition characterized chiefly by dilatation and occlusion of mammary ducts with indurated mass of secretion and plasma cells.

Mastochondroma A benign breast tumor composed chiefly of cartilaginous tissue.

Mastocytogenesis The formation of mast cells.

Mastocytoma A nodule resembling a tumor, composed chiefly of mast cells.

Mastocytosis Disorder characterized by yellow, brown macules and papules on skin due to skin infiltration by mast cells.

Mastodynia Pain in the breast.

Mastoid 1. Resembling a breast or nipple in shape. 2 The downward projection of the temporal bone located behind the ear.

Mastoidectomy Removal of mastoid air cells indicated for persistent or recurrent mastoiditis not controlled by antibiotics.

m. conservative The operation does not interfere with sound conducting system of middle ear.

m. modified radical The pars tensa of tympanic membrane and attached handle of malleolus are spared.

m. radical Done by trans meatal or transmastoid routes with tympanectomy and excision of all diseased tissue of middle ear and mastoid leaving intact the postero-superior bony canal wall to facilitate subsequent tympanoplasty.

Mastoiditis Inflammation of mastoid process of temporal bone.

m. Bezold's Mastoiditis leading to destruction of mastoid tip and abscess formation deep to the fiber of sternomastoid muscle.

m. masked Mastoiditis in the absence of overt physical signs like swelling and tenderness over mastoid process.

Mastomenia Vicarious menstruation from breast.

Mastoptosis Dropping or pendulous breasts.

Mastoplastia Hypertrophy or enlargement of the breast.

Masturbation Self-manipulation of genitals to achieve sexual gratification.

Materia Latin for substance or matter.

m. alba White deposit on teeth or dental appliance.

m. medica The science concerned with drugs.

Material The substance of which something is made or composed.

m. impression Substances used for taking impressions like plaster of paris, hydrocolloid compounds.

Maternal Relating to mother.

Maternity Pertaining to pregnancy, the state of being pregnant.

Mating The union of male and female for reproduction.

m. assortative Mating that is not random but involves individuals of specific characteristics which may be similar or dissimilar.

m. random Mating without regard to genetic constitution of mate.

Matrilineal Relating to inheritance of traits through the maternal line rather than the paternal.

Matter Any thing that occupies space

m. gray nerve tissue containing cell body of neurons on external surface of brain or inner surface of spinal cord.

m. white Consists of nerve fibers occupying periphery of spinal cord.

Maturation 1. The process of becoming mature. 2. A stage of cell division in which chromosome is halved.

Mature Complete in natural development, the reproductive cell which has undergone meiosis.

Matrix 1. The inter cellular substance in a tissue. 2. The mold for dental restoration in the form of thin steel or plastic strip surrounding tooth.

m. bone The ground substance of bony tissue which is composed of protein and mucopolysaccharide. As the bone matures, the content of collagen fibers and bone salt increases.

m. cartilaginous A basic, homogeneous basophil substance of embryonic skeletal tissue in the center of which articular cartilage develops.

m. mesangial A mesh in the space between the renal glomerular loops, formed from material similar to that of capillary basement membrane. The phagocytic mesangial cells are dispersed in this matrix. The matrix is permeable to substances of higher molecular weight which aggregate to form deposits.

Matron The chief nursing officer in a hospital.

Mattress ripple Mattress containing transverse inflatable tubes linked in a series to pump so that alternate tube is inflated. Thus the area of compression between skin and mattress changes that prevents formation of decubitus ulcer/bedsore.

Maurer's dots Coarse stippling of red cells in falciparum infection

Maxilla The upper jaw bone supporting upper teeth and taking part in the formation of orbit, nasal cavity, and hard palate.

Maximum 1. The greatest quantity, value or degree. 2. The height of a fever or any acute state.

m. glucose transport The maximum rate at which kidneys can reabsorb glucose (300 mg/min).

m. tubular (Tm) The maximum ability of renal tubules either to excrete or secrete a substance.

May Hegglin anamaly An autosomal dominant blood disorder with presence of Dohle bodies in granulocytes and platelet

Maze An intricate labyrinth of walled pathways frequently used to study the learning process in laboratory animals.

Mazindol A CNS stimulating agent with properties similar to amphe-tamine, hence used as anorexogenic agent.

Mc Ardle's disease Glycogen storage V due to deficiency of myophosphorylase C

Mc Burney's point A point 1-2 inches above anterior superior iliac spine on a line between ilium and umbilicus

Mc Donald's rule A formula for determining expected height of fundus

Meal Food.

m. Boyden Meal used to test the evacuation time of gall bladder; it consists of flour, egg yolks, and milk mixed with sugar.

m. test Bland food given before analysis of gastric secretion.

Mean An average of a set of values.

m. arythematic The ratio of the sum of the terms in a statistical series to their number.

m. geometric A value indicating the central tendency of a statistical series of 'n' terms, equal to the positive 'n'th root of their products.

m. harmonic For a given set of values, the reciprocal of the mean of the reciprocals of the individual values.

Measles Highly contagious disease caused, by paramyxo virus occurring in young children with fever, coryza, koplik spots, erythematous maculopapular rash spreading from head to trunk to limbs, often complicated by meningitis, carditis.

Measure 1. The dimensions, quantity, capacity like length, area, volume, etc. 2. The act of determining such dimensions, quantity or capacity. 3. A device used for measuring like graduated glass, tape.

Measurement The act of measuring.

m. skin fold Skin fold measurement by caliper for assessing body fat percentage.

Meatometer Apparatus for measuring urinary meatus.

Meatoplasty Reconstructive surgery usually of external auditory meatus.

m. Stacke's A type of meatoplasty used in final stage of radical mastoidectomy where a large rectangular flap of meatal skin is turned back to line the floor of mastoid cavity.

Meatorrhaphy Enlarging the urethral meatus by suturing the urethral membrane to glans penis.

Meatotomy An incision of a meatus to increase its diameter.

Meatus An opening to a canal, or passage in the body.

m. external acoustic S shaped canal of external ear, upto tympanic membrane lined by skin which continues on to the tympanic membrane.

m. internal acoustic A short canal above the anterior part of jugular foramen in the petrous part of temporal bone transmitting facial, intermediate, and vestibulo-cochlear nerves and the labyrinthine vessels.

m. medial nasal The passage under cover of middle nasal. Into its anterior end or infundibulum the frontonasal duct opens while near the roof is the opening of maxillary sinus.

m. superior nasal A short narrow passage located partly under superior nasal choncha into which the posterior ethmoidal sinuses open by single aperture.

Mebendazole A benzimidazole given for hookworm, roundworm, trichuriasis and enterobiasis.

Mebeverine A smooth muscle relaxant used for gastrointestinal motility disorder like IBS.

Mebutamate Orally acting hypo–tensive agent.

Mecamylamine An orally acting ganglion blocking agent rarely used to treat severe hypertension.

Mechanics 1. The branch of physics concerned with the interaction of force and matter.

m. body mass The study of action of muscles on body in motion and in rest.

Mechapion Device used to measure output of an x-ray tube in roentgens.

Mechanism 1. An aggregation of parts that interact in order to perform a specific or common function. 2. The means by which an effect is obtained

m. association Mental process through which the memory of past experiences may be related to or compared with present ones.

m. cough A mechanism for expulsion of foreign material from respiratory tract, consisting of short inspiration, closure of glottis, forced expiration with opening of glottis with a air flow rate of 3000 to 4000 ml/sec.

m. counter current Mechanism essential to the production of an osmotically concentrated urine; it involves two basic processes, counter current multiplication in loop of Henle and countercurrent exchange in vasa recta.

m. defense A psychic structure, usually unconscious, which serves as a protection against awareness of conflicts and anxiety.

m. investing The structures that surround a tooth and provide retention including periodontal membrane, cementum, alveolar bone and gingiva.

m. pressoreceptive Mechanism whereby pressor receptors in carotid sinus and aortic arch respond to change in blood pressure.

m. proprioceptive Process by which body regulates its muscular movement and maintains its equilibrium.

m. reentrant A fundamental mechanism of arrhythmogenesis in which cardiac tissue is reexcited by the same impulse for one or more cycles.

Mechlorethamine Alkylating agent used in treatment of lymphomas.

Meckel's diverticulum The persistent proximal end of yolk sac present in 2% people 2″ long and 2′ above ileocaecal junction

Meclizine Drug used in treatment and prevention of motion sickness.

Meclocycline A topically applied antibiotic closely related to chlortetracycline.

Mecloqualone A compound with hypnotic and sedative properties.

Meconism Opium addiction or opium poisoning.

Mecometer Instrument used to measure newborn infant.

Meconium The odorless, sticky greenish black semisolid intestinal content of fetus. It is replaced by feces within 2 days of birth.

Medallion A circumscribed red, scally patch, characteristic of pityriasis rosea.

Medazepam A week tranquilizer, anxiolytic agent.

Medial 1. Towards the midline 2. relating to tunica media or middle layer.

Median In statistics denoting the middle value in a distribution i.e., the point in a series at which half of the plotted values are on one side and half on the other.

Mediastinitis Inflammation of mediastinum.

Mediastinography X-ray visualization of mediastinum by injection of NO_2.

Mediastinoscope An endoscope to visualize superior mediastinum, introduced through a small suprasternal incision.

Mediastinum 1. The central space in chest bounded anteriorly by sternum, posteriorly by vertebral column and laterally by pleural sacs. 2. Any septum or partition between two parts of an organ.

m. anterior That portion of lower mediastinum located in front of heart behind the sternum. It contains thymus gland, few lymphnodes and loose areolar tissue.

m. lower The part of mediastinum below the plane of manubriosternal joint in front and lower border of 4th thoracic vertebra behind. It is divided into anterior, middle and posterior.

m. middle It contains the heart, pericardium and the emerging great vessels.

m. posterior It contains esophagus, thoracic duct, thoracic aorta, vagus and lymphnodes

m. superior It lies above the pane of manubrio sternal articulation and contains aortic arch and its branches, superior venacava, brachiocephalic veins, left recurrent laryngeal nerve, thoracic duct, thymus, vagus nerve and some lymph nodes.

Medicament A remedy, healing agent.

Medicate To treat disease with medicine, to impregnate with a medicinal substance.

Medicated Treated medically, permeated with a medicinal substance.

Medicine A drug: The art and science dealing with the maintenance and restoration of health.

m. adolescent The branch of medicine dealing with care and treatment of individuals from onset of puberty to the age of 19.

m. aviation A specialized branch of medicine dealing with physiologic, pathologic psychologic conditions which occur in fliers, and people transported in air. It helps in selection of aircraft personnel, air transport of sick and wounded.

m. behavioral The applications of the principles of learning and learning theory to treat those disorders caused at least in part by psychologic factors as if they were behavioral. Specific techniques are applied to reverse the expressions of maladaptive functioning whether purely psychologic as in phobias or partly physiologic as in faulty patterns of learned autonomic nervous system response leading to cardiovascular disease.

m. clinical The study and practice of medicine at bed side, as opposed to theoretical and laboratory investigations.

m. community Medicine dealing with community health care and their solution as a whole rather than individual health problem e.g., preventive medicine, public health services.

m. family Medical speciality dealing with first patient contact, long term care, and a broad responsibility to all members of the family irrespective of age.

m. folk Treatment of disease at home with remedies and techniques passed from generation to generation.

m. emergency A branch of medicine that specializes in providing immediate diagnosis and treatment of those who are acutely or often suddenly ill or severely injured.

m. environmental The study of environmental aspects related to health and their modification for better health.

m. experimental Study of disease process and various therapies in animal models.

m. forensic The application of medical knowledge and skill to the solution of problems encountered in administration of justice.

m. geriatric Medicine dealing with diagnosis, treatment and prevention of disease in elderly.

m. holistic An approach to health care based on theory that health is the result of harmony between body, mind and spirits and that stress of any kind including physical, psychological and social pressure is inimical to health.

m. internal The branch of medicine which deals with the diagnosis and nonsurgical treatment of diseases.

m. nuclear Application of nuclear energy in the diagnosis and treatment of disease e.g., use of radioisotopes.

m. occupational A branch of medicine dealing with prevention of disease and injury among people at work. It has two functions: to ensure suitability of an individual for particular work and to identify and control health and safety hazards in the work.

m. oral The study and treatment of diseases of soft tissues of mouth.

m. perinatal A specialized branch of medicine dealing with the management of mother and fetus during pregnancy and the infant immediately after delivery.

m. physical and rehabilitation The branch of medicine concerned with use of physical agents and modalities including electricity light, heat, sound, mechanical devices and physical activity, in the diagnosis, treatment and prevention of disease.

m. space A special branch of aviation medicine which deals with the stresses imposed on man by projection through and beyond the earth's atmosphere, flight in interplanetary space and return to earth. Such stresses include the agravic state, exposure to radiation and isolation.

m. tropical The medical speciality concerned with diseases and disorders contracted in tropic or which exhibit unique characteristics in tropical countries.

Medico A medical student, a combining form meaning medical.

Medicolegal Pertaining to a matter that involves both medicine and law.

Medionecrosis Necrosis of middle layer (tunica media) of an artery.

Meditation (transcedental) (TM) An exercise of contemplation that induces a temporary hypometabolic state, a sense of well being, and a feeling of complete relaxation; this hypometabolic state is associated with change in physiologic function including a reduction in oxygen consumption, a decrease in cardiac output and altered EEG activity.

Medium 1. A material in which a substance, an impulse, or information is transported. 2. A material, in which interaction takes place. 3. Culture medium.

m. apathy's An aqueous medium for mounting slide preparations directly from water. It is used when dehydration with alcohol and xylene would be detrimental.

m. Bavister's A simple culture medium in which hamster and human eggs can be fertilized in vitro.

m. brain-heart-infusion A liquid culture medium containing peptone and infusion solids of calf brain and beef heart for growing fastidious bacteria.

m. clearing A medium used to make histologic specimens transparent or translucent.

m. contrast In radiology, a substance of different radio-opacity from that of the organ or tissue studied, to allow X-ray demonstration of contour or lumen. When the substance is more radiopaque than tissue it is positive contrast; e.g. barium sulphate, iodine, when the substance is less radiopaque than tissue — negative contrast e.g., air.

m. Neal and Nicolle A saline rabbit's blood medium suitable for culture of leishmania donovani.

Medls part forms the floor of fourth ventricle. It contains central nuclei of glossopharyngeal, vagus, accessory and hypoglossal nerves and regulates life sustaining cardiovascular and respiratory reflexes.

m. ovary The central vascular portion of ovary with loose elastic tissue, smooth muscle fibers and a mass of contorted blood vessels.

m. renal The inner part of kidney containing renal pyramids, the bases of which face outwards abutting on cortex whereas the apex is directed inwards appearing as renal papillae projecting into minor calyx. Each pyramid is composed of renal tubules.

m. of bone The soft material filling the cavities of bones composed of hemopoitic tissue.

Medullary Relating to or resembling the medulla or marrow.

Medullated Having a myelin sheath, having a medulla.

Medullization The replacement of bone by marrow tissue.

Medulloblast An undifferentiated cell of embryonic neural tube. It is rounded, poor in cytoplasm without processes found in middle layer of neural tube and is derived from germinal cells of inner ependymal layer.

Medulloblastoma A rapidly growing malignant brain tumor composed of poorly differentiated small preneuroglial cells that tend to form pseudo rosettes. Common to children, arising from cerebellar vermis and floor of fourth ventricle.

m. desmoplastic A variant of medulloblastoma appearing in elderly and with abdundant reticulin fibers and fibrous stroma.

Medulloepithelioma A tumor of eye, primarily of children, characterized by formation of multilayered sheets of undifferentiated cells resembling primitive medullary epithelium of optic vesicle. The malignant form resembles retinoblastoma.

Mees lines Transverse white lines in finger nails in arsenic exposure

Mefenamic acid An agent with analgesic, anti-inflammatory and antipyretic properties.

Mefexamide A CNS stimulant, used to treat fatigue and depression.

Mefloquine Antimalarial agent, schizonticide.

Mefruside A diuretic with use similar to chlorthiazide.

Megabecquerel A unit of activity in radionuclide equal to 10^6 becquerel. Symbol —MBq.

Megacolon Abnormally large colon, either segmental or total, manifesting with constipation.

m. acquired Enlargement is secondary to an associated disease. There is neither aganglionosis nor any other congenital motor abnormality.

m. congenital An autosomal recessive condition characterized by marked dilatation of colon proximal to a narrowed segment which is devoid of ganglionic cells in submucosal (Meissner's) and myenteric (Aurbach's) plexuses. This aganglionic area is unable to relax properly during normal peristaltic activity *SYN*—Hirschprung's disease.

m. toxic Gross colonic dilatation in complicated ulcerative colitis, Crohn's disease, infectious colitis.

m. idiopathic Megacolon without a known causes but related probably to laxative abuse.

Megadyne Unit of force equal to 1 million dynes.

Mega electron volt (mev) One million electron volts.

Megaesophagus Abnormal enlargement of lower esophagus.

Megakaryoblast A primitive cell of megakaryocyte series with a large oval or kidney shaped nucleus and scanty cytoplasm. It develops into a promegakaryocyte and finally then to megakaryocyte.

Megakaryocyte A giant cell with usually multilobed nucleus, (upto 100μ.) the precursor of platelets.

Megaloblast Large nucleated erythrocyte precursor seen m bone marrow in vit B_{12} and folic acid deficiency.

Megaloblastoid Having some features resembling megaloblastic maturation. An erythrocyte precursor is said to be megaloblastoid when nuclear chromatin condensation is in clumps but with a prominent parachromatin, i.e. open, transparent, unstained cleft are prominent in the nucleus and the contours of nucleus are irregular.

Megalocornea A sex-linked recessive disorder in which the central corneal diameter is enlarged without increased intraocular pressure.

Megalocystis An abnormally enlarged or distended bladder.

Megaloglossia Macroglossia.

Megalomania A psychopathologic condition in which the individual has unfounded conviction of his great importance and power.

Megaloureter Abnormally dilated ureter in absence of obstruction.

Megavitamin A vitamin dose far in excess of daily recommended dose.

Megavolt A unit of electromotive force equal to one million volts.

Megavoltage Electromotive force in the range of 2-10 mev. used in radiotherapy.

Megestrol acetate A synthetic progestin used as antineoplastic agent in palliation of metastatic endometrial cancer.

Meglumine A substance used in the preparation of radio opaque compounds.

Meiosis The reduction cell division during maturation of sex cells in which two nuclear cell divisions occur in quick succession thus forming four gametes each containing half the number of chromosomes.

Meig's syndrome Poly serositis associated with ovarian fibroma.

Meissner's corpuscle An encapsulated end organ of touch found on hairless portion of skin

Melalgia Pain in the lower extremity.

Melancholia A condition characterized by severe depression as manifested by loss of pleasure in all activities, early morning awakening, anorexia and feeling of guilt.

m. involutional A major depression occurring in the involutional period, i.e. 40-55 years in female and 50-65 years in males. Its characteristic triad of symptoms are delusions of guilt or poverty, obsession with death, and delusional fixation on gastrointestinal functioning all within a setting of depression and agitation.

Melanic Having a dark color.

Melanin The natural pigment of hair and skin formed by oxidation of tyrosine via dopa and dopaquinone to a complex polymeric material.

Melanomeloblastoma Benign tumor of anterior maxilla, usually occurring in infants.

Melanoblast A derivative of neural crest which differentiates in an embryo into a melanocyte.

Melanocyte A cell capable of forming melanin, mature pigment cell.

Melanocytoma A benign pigment deposit on optic disk occurring especially in black persons.

Melanoderma Any abnormal dark pigmentation of the skin predominantly resulting from accumulation of the pigment melanin.

Melanogenemia The presence in blood of substances that produce melanin.

Melanoginesis The formation or production of melanin by living cells.

Melanoma Any benign or malignant melanocytic tumor.

m. acral lentiginous A malignant melanoma occurring on palms, soles, nail beds and characterized by a lentiginous growth of atypical melanocytes in the epidermis, elongated rete ridges and acanthosis.

m. lentigo maligna An irregularly shaped, flat patch with various shades of brown, blue, red, white and tan, typically occurring in sun exposed skin and old people.

m. malignant Malignant tumor of melanin producing cells commonly in the skin, uveal tract of eye, oral mucosa, vagina, lung, meninges. Metastasis are typically widespread at unusual sites like heart and small bowel. Tumor can be nodular, i.e., spreading vertically and rapidly exhibiting deep dark brown discoloration or may be superficial spreading type with irregular borders.

Melanomatosis Presence of numerous melanomas.

Melanonychia Black discoloration of nail.

Melanopathy Any disease characterized by black discoloration of skin.

Melanophage A phagocytic cell that engulfs the melanin particles.

Melanophore A pigment cell carrying melanin.

Melanoplakia Pigment patches on tongue and oral mucosa.

Melanoprotein A protein complex with melanin.

Melanosis Abnormal deposits of dark pigment in various organs.

Melanosome A single melanin containing organelle that has finished synthesizing melanin.

Melarsoprol A trivalent arsenic containing antiprotozoal drug for trypanosomiasis.

Melasma Cloasma affecting cheeks, forehead and lips.

Melatonin A hormone believed to be secreted by pineal gland. It has action opposite to that of MSB. It stimulates aggregation of melanosomes in melanophores, thus lightening the skin.

Melena Black tarry stool due to GI bleed.

m. spuria Melena in breast fed babies where blood originates from fissures in mother's nipple.

Melioidosis An infectious disease primarily affecting rodents. Caused by *Pseudomonas pseudomalleli,* often transmitted to man via open wounds, manifesting with fever, pneumonia and metastatic abscess formation.

Melitis Inflammation of cheek.

Mellitum Any pharmaceutical preparation having honey as excipient.

Mellitus Latin for honeyed.

Melphalen A phenylalanine analogue of nitrogen mustard, an antineoplastic agent for multiple myeloma.

Melomelia A condition of unequal conjoined twins in which both normal limbs and rudimentary accessory limbs are present.

Melorheostosis A rare disease of long bones where new born formation resembles a candle with wax dripping down the sides

Membrane A thin sheet of tissue that covers a surface, envelops a part, lines a cavity, divides a space or connects two structures.

m. abdominal Peritoneum.

m. alveolocapillary The blood air barrier in the lungs consisting of alveolar epithelium, basal lamina and capillary endothelium.

m. anterior limiting Bowman's membrane.

m. atlanto occipital Anterior and posterior membranes extending from border of foramen magnum to the atlas.

m. basement A thin transparent non cellular layer under the epithelium of mucous membranes and secreting glands.

m. basilar of cochlear duct Membrane extending from the osseous spiral lamina to the basilar crest of cochlea, forming the floor of the cochlear duct and supporting the spiral organ of corti.

m. Bowman's One of the five layers forming the cornea, consisting of fine inter woven fibrils.

m. Brusch's Basal lamina of choroid in contact with the pigmented layer of retina.

m. cell A delicate structure about 90 Å thick that encloses a cell. Composed of mucopolysaccharides and lipids, regulates the movement of substances in and out of cell.

m. cricothyroid A broad thin membrane originating from upper border of cricoid cartilage and extending to the vocal process of arytenoid cartilage and to the thyroid cartilage.

m. Descemet's One of the five layers of cornea covering the posterior surface of substantia propria, also called posterior limiting membrane and is extremely thin, elastic, transparent and homogeneous.

m. diphtheritic Yellowish gray leathery exudate on the mucous membrane of upper respiratory tract seen in diphtheria.

m. dialysis A semipermeable cellulose membrane separating blood from dialysate in hemodialysis.

m. external limiting The third of ten layers of retina, it has the form of chicken wire.

m. s fetal Extraembryonic membranes concerned with respiration, excretion, nutrition, and protection of embryo. They include amnion, chorion, allantois, yolksac, decidua and placenta.

m. glassy A prominent basal lamina in the ovary separating the epithelial layer of follicle from the surrounding connective tissue stroma.

m. glomerular filtration The capillary wall of the renal corpuscle permitting ultrafiltration of blood.

m. hyaline Like the eosinophilic homogeneous, transparent membrane lining the alveoli in premature infants afflicted with hyaline membrane disease.

m. internal limiting The last of ten layers of retina forming the inner limit of retina and outer limit of vitreous.

m. mucous Membrane lining tubular structures and consisting of epithelium, basement membrane, lamina propria and lamina muscularis.

m. obturator Membrane that almost completely closes the obturator foramen except superiorly where the membrane is deficient, forming lower boundary of obturator canal. The obturator externus and internus muscles partly arise from this membrane.

m. perineal The inferior layer of the fascia of urogenital diaphragm.

m. periodontal Dense white cartilaginous connective tissue that attaches root of tooth to alveolar bone.

m. post synaptic The portion of cell membrane at the site of synapse, sensitive to neurotransmitter substances.

m. presynaptic The cell membrane of an axon at the site of the synapse through which neurotransmitter substances pass into the synaptic cleft.

m. secondary tympanic The membrane closing the round window between blind end of scala tympani and the middle ear chamber.

m. Reissner's Vestibular membrane of cochlear duct.

m. semipermeable A membrane which permits the passage of water and small molecules but not large molecules and colloidal matter.

m. serous The outer most coat lining the external walls of body cavities and reflected over exposed surfaces of protruding organs.

m. suprapleural A dense tent shaped fascial layer attached from the inner part of first rib and costal cartilage to the transverse process of seventh vertebra, thus closing the thoracic inlet.

m. synovial The connective tissue membrane that lines the cavity of a synovial joint and produces the synovial fluid.

m. tectorial of cochlear duct A delicate gelatinous membrane in spiral organ of corti.

m. Toldt's The anterior layer of fascia of kidney.

m. thyrohyoid A broad fibro elastic sheet that fills the interval between the hyoid bone and thyroid cartilage.

m. tympanic (TM) The membrane separating the external ear from the middle ear cavity, kept tense by tensor tympani. The displacement of tympanic membrane (vibration) during ordinary conversation is only that of the diameter of molecule of hydrogen.

m. undulating An organelle of locomotion of certain flagellate parasites consisting of a fin like extension of the limiting membrane with a wave like flagellar sheath.

m. urogenital The anterior part of cloacal membrane in the embryo.

m. vaginal The hymen.

m. Zinn's The anterior layer of iris comprising a layer of flattened endothelial cells.

Membranelle A minute membrane composed of fused cilia, seen in some ciliate organisms.

Membranocartilaginous Partly membranous and partly cartilaginous.

Membraniform Having the appearance of a membrane.

Membrano cranium The primitive precursor of skull in embryo.

Membranoid Like a membrane, as in appearance or quality.

Membranous Being or having properties of a membrane.

Membroid A capsule of membranous composition which is resistant to the action of gastric secretions but dissolves in small intestine, hence used for enteric coating of drugs to be delivered in small intestine.

Memory 1. To remember; the persistence of the effects of experience on the behavior of living organism which includes learning, retaining, recalling and recognizing. 2. That portion of computer in which instructions and data are stored.

m. iconic The hypothesized first stage of visual memory formation in which a faint copy of visual input persists very briefly allowing a longer interval for extraction of information.

m. immunologic The capacity of immune system to mount a vigorous and sustained response to a subsequent exposure to a particular antigen than was mounted to initial exposure. This memory is retained by a subpopulation of T lymphocytes (memory cells).

m. kinesthetic Memory of movement rather than event.

m. long-term The hypothesized substage of memory process in which information is stored in a relatively permanent way for the rest of life.

m. retrograde The memory for events prior to a trauma or other incident that has affected one's memory.

m. short term A hypothesized substage of memory process not exceeding 25 minutes per event.

Menacme The height of menstrual activity in a woman life.

Menadione (Vit. K_3) Methyl naphthoquinone, parent substance of various forms of vitamin K.

Menadiol sodium diphosphate A synthetic derivative of menadione.

Menadione sodium bisulfite The water-soluble form of menadione, used in the treatment of hemorrhage consequent to hypoprothrombinemic states.

Menaquinone Any of the several substituted menadiones with Vitamin K activity.

Menarche Appearance of first menstrual period.

Mendelevium Radioactive element (Md), atomic number = 101.

Menetrier's disease/syndrome A disease of unknown etiology characterized by large gastric rugae, and pseudo-polyps which may be associated with ulcer like symptoms, bleeding or idiopathic hypoproteinemia, *SYN* — Hypertrophic gastritis.

Meniere's disease/syndrome Paroxysmal labyrinthine vertigo with deafness and tinnitus, due to unexplained increase in endolymphatic pressure.

Meninges The three membranes that cover the brain and spinal cord; consisting of dense fibrous outer dura mater, thin innermost pia mater and trabeculated middle arachnoid mater. The last two are grouped as leptomeninges.

Meningitis Inflammation of meninges; can be cerebral, spinal or cerebrospinal. Pachymeningitis involves dura mater while leptomeningitis involves pia arachnoid but the latter is more common.

m. acute aseptic Viral infection with CSF lymphocytic pleocytosis; any toxic state, parameningeal infective process.

m. acute septic Bacterial meningitis with pus formation, e.g. meningococcal, pneumococcal, *E. coli* meningitis.

m. basal Meningitis largely restricted to base of brain occurring in subacute, chronic or inadequately treated bacterial meningitis or in granulomatous processes like tuberculosis, sarcoidosis, syphilis.

m. carcinomatosa Widespread or diffuse metastatic carcinoma in the meninges.

m. eosinophilic Occurring in parasitic infection or malignancy,

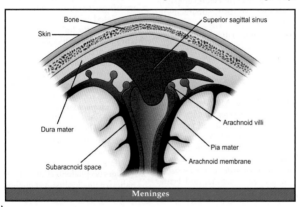

Meninges

(labels: Bone, Skin, Superior sagittal sinus, Dura mater, Arachnoid villi, Subarachnoid space, Pia mater, Arachnoid membrane)

e.g. rat lung worm, parago-nimiasis, schistosomiasis, gnatho-stomiasis, etc. with CSF eosinophilia but benign and self-limited.

m. gummatous Meningitis occurring in tertiary stage of syphilis with gumma formation in pia or dura mater, manifesting as increased intracranial pressure or basal meningitis.

m. mollarets Acute meningitis with CSF pleocytosis and presence of abundant large endothelial cells in CSF; rapid spontaneous remission.

m. neonatal Acute septic meningitis of neonates caused by gram -ve organisms mainly *E. coli.*

m. tuberculous Occurs due to hematogenous spread or rupture of cortical tuberculoma into CSF. Sub-acute onset with chronic course, often with encephalomyelopathy, cerebral arteritis, subarachnoid adhesions.

Meningioma Tumor of meninges, especially from dura where ara-chnoid villi are numerous. Usually benign, producing symptoms due to compression or bone erosion, can undergo sarcomatous changes.

m. anaplastic Meningioma with anaplastic features but not sarcoma.

m. angiomatous Small and large vascular channels predominate.

m. hemangioblastic Resembles hemangioblastoma of cerebellum.

m. olfactory groove Gives rise to unilateral anosmia, and Foster Kenedy syndrome.

m. parasagittal Causes spastic paraparesis of legs.

Meningiomatosis Presence of multi-ple meningiomas.

Meningism A group of symptoms and signs suggesting meningitis but without identifiable pathologic lesion of meninges. Occurs in children suffering from febrile infections like pneumonia, tonsil-litis, systemic viral infection.

Meningocele A congenital sac like skin covered protrusion of meninges through a defect in skull or vertebral column. Common to mid occipital area or lumbosacral area.

Meningococcemia Presence of meningococci in blood, often asso-ciated with petechial rash, cardio-vascular collapse and meningitis/ (waterhouse-Fredrichson syndrome), chronic persistent meningococcemia may be associated with lowgrade fever, rash and arthritis.

Meningoencephalitis Inflammation of brain and meninges.

m. primary amebic Caused by Naegleria or Acanthameba, infec-tion travelling via cribiform plate with fatal course in a week.

m. trypanosomal Subacute or chronic meningoencephalitis predomi-nantly involving the base of brain caused by *Trypanosoma gambiensae or rhodesiense.* Producing sleeping sickness and dementia.

Meningoencephalomyelitis Combi-nation of meningitis, encephalitis and myelitis.

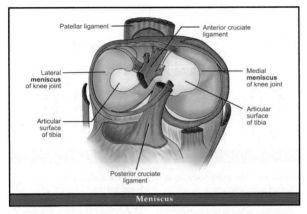

Labels: Patellar ligament — Anterior cruciate ligament — Lateral **meniscus** of knee joint — Medial **meniscus** of knee joint — Articular surface of tibia — Articular surface of tibia — Posterior cruciate ligament

Meniscus

Meningoencephalomyelopathy Any disease involving brain, meninges and spinal cord.

Meningoencephalomyeloradiculo-neuritis Inflammation of brain, spinal cord, meninges, nerve roots and peripheral nerves.

Meningocyte A mesenchymal epithelial cell of subarachnoid space.

Meningoencephalopathy A diffuse disorder of function of brain and meninges; commonly relates to toxic and metabolic encephalopathies.

Meningomyelitis Inflammation of spinal cord and its covering membranes.

Meningomyelocele A protrusion of spinal cord and associated meninges through a developmental defect in spinal canal.

Meningo-osteophlebitis Periosteitis that is associated with inflammation of venous sinuses and meninges.

Meningovascular Concerning meninges and adjacent blood vessels.

Meniscectomy Surgical removal of semilunar cartilage especially of knee.

m. arthroscopic Removal of a part of damaged meniscus through arthroscope.

Meniscus A crescent shaped structure; one of the fibrocartilaginous discs of knee joint.

m. lateral A nearly circular crescent shaped fibrocartilage attached to lateral articular surface of upper end of tibia.

m. medial A crescent shaped fibrocartilage attached to medial surface of upper end of tibia.

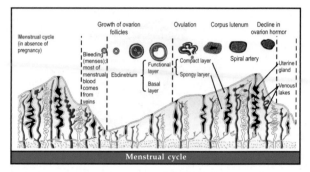

Menstrual cycle

Menolipsis The temporary cessation of menstruation.

Menometrorrhagia Abnormal bleeding during or between menstrual periods.

Menopause The normal physiologic cessation of menstruation commonly between 45 and 50 years of age. Frequent symptoms include hot flushes, headache, vulvar discomfort, painful sexual intercourse and mental depression.

m. artificial Cessation of menopause by irradiation or surgical removal of ovaries.

m. premature Early menopause, idiopathic or secondary to pituitary disease, systemic illness.

Menorrhagia Excessive or prolonged menstruation, *SYN*—hypermenorrhea.

Menoschesis Suppression of menses.

Menostasis Amenorrhea.

Menses Periodic bloody discharge from uterus, called menstruation.

Menstrual Relating to menses.

Menstruation The periodic discharge from uterus of a non clotting bloody fluid at 4-5 weeks interval.

m. anovulatory Menstruation not preceded by ovulation.

m. vicarious Bleeding from sites other than uterus occurring at the time of normal menstruation.

Mensual Monthly.

Mensuration Measurement by immediate comparison.

Mental 1. Relating to mind. 2. relating to chin.

Mentation Mental activity.

Menthol Peppermint camphor, an organic compound derived from pippermint oil or prepared synthetically. It provides a sensation of coolness in mucosal membranes by stimulation of cold receptors.

Mentoanterior In a face presentation, having the fetal chin pointing anteriorly in relation to maternal pelvis.

Mentoplasty Plastic operation on chin.

Mentoposterior In face presentation, having fetal chin pointing posteriorly in relation to maternal pelvis.

Mentotransverse In face presentation, having the fetal chin pointing laterally in relation to maternal pelvis.

Mentum The anterior prominence of mandible produced by mental protruberance; the chin.

Mepacrine An anthelmintic for tapeworm and giardiasis, also an antimalarial agent.

Meparfynol A colorless liquid with unpleasant burning taste, often used as a short acting hypnotic.

Mepazine A phenothiazine compound, used for pre or post-operative sedation and anxiety.

Mepenzolate bromide An anticholinergic agent used for hypermotility of colon.

Meperidine A synthetic narcotic analgesic, with spasmolytic properties and high addiction potential.

Mephenesin An agent used for skeletal muscle relaxation.

Mephenoxalone A skeletal muscle relaxant, also has mild anxiolytic properties.

Mephentermine An adrenergic agent used as a nasal decongestant or in certain hypotensive states to augment vascular tone.

Mephenytoin Anticonvulsant agent for focal, jacksonian, grandmal and psychomotor seizure.

Mephobarbitol Long acting barbiturate with anxiolytic and anticonvulsant properties.

Mepivacaine An analogue of lidocaine for local anesthesia, peripheral nerve block or epidural block.

Meprednisone A synthetic glucocorticoid used to treat corticosteroid responsive diseases, allergic conditions.

Meprylcaine A local anesthetic for infiltration and nerve block anesthesia.

Mepyramine malleate An antiallergic.

Mequidox An antibacterial agent.

Meralgia Pain in the thigh.

m. Paresthetica is troublesome tingling, pricking or numbness in lateral aspect of thigh due to compression of lateral femoral cutaneous nerve while it passes beneath or through the inguinal ligament just medial to anterior superior iliac spine.

Meralein sodium A water soluble topically applied antibacterial agent.

Meralluride A mercurial salt of succinamic acid used as a parenterally administered diuretic.

Merbromin Topically used antibacterial and antiseptic Syn-Mercurochrome.

Mercaptan Any substance containing the radical-SH bound to carbon, analogous to alcohol and phenols but containing sulfur instead of oxygen. Used in dentistry as an elastic impression compoud.

Mercaptoethanol Most commonly used reagents containing thiol group.

Mercaptoethylamine A component of coenzyme A, used in treatment of radiation sickness and chronic leukemia.

2-Mercaptoimidazole A thiourea group of antithyroid drug, five times more potent than methylthiouracil.

Mercaptomerin sodium A mercurial diuretic given SC/IM.

Mercaptopurine 6-Purinethol, A hypoxanthine and adenine analogue used as antineoplastic agent for its potent inhibitory effect on DNA synthesis.

Mercapturic acid An S-aryl-N acetyl cysteine found in the urine after ingestion of aromatic halogen compounds.

Mercurialism Poisoning by mercury or its compounds.

Mercuric Bivalent mercury.

Mercurous Monovalent mercury.

Mercury A heavy, silvery poisonous metallic element liquid at room temperature, atomic No. - 80, used in thermometer.

Mercury197 (^{197}Hg) A radioactive mercury isotope used in brain tumor localization and in the study of renal function.

Meridian A line surrounding a spherical body passing through both poles or half of such circle containing both poles.

Merocrine Denoting secretory cells that remain intact during discharge of secretory products as those in the salivary glands.

Merotomy Cutting into parts.

Merozoite The product of asexual schizogony of a protozoan in the body of host; in malaria merozoites are liberated from rupture of RBC to invade fresh RBC or form gametocyte, the sexual form in man, infective to mosquito.

Merocyte An incompletely isolated cell found in the vicinity of the yolk of a fertilized ovum during segmentation. Its nucleus is generally derived from accessory spermatozoa.

Meroencephalus Developmental absence of any parts of brain.

Merogony The development of only a portion of an egg. If the egg contains only male pronucleus, the development is called andromerogony and if only female pronucleus gynomerogony.

Merology Study of rudimentary tissue.

Meromycin One of the two proteins — heavy meromycin and light meromycin formed by enzymatic digestion of muscle protein mycin.

Merphalon A racemic mixture of melphalan and medphalan; antineoplastic drug.

Mersalyl sodium A mercurial diuretic given parenterally.

Mesangiolysis Degeneration of mesangial cells and matrix secondary to radiation and some snake toxins.

Mesangium The framework of glomerulus which arises from

vascular pole and extends into intercapillary spaces. It contains matrix and mesangial cells which are phagocytic in nature.

Mesarteritis Inflammation localized to tunica media of vessel.

Mescaline A hallucinogenic alkaloid.

Mesaortitis Inflammation of muscular coat of aorta.

Mesaxon A supporting cell membrane that completely encloses the axon like a jelly roll, forming a myelin lamellae.

Mesencephalon The embryonic midbrain; the second cephalic dilatation of neural tube that develops into corpora quadrigemina, the cerebral peduncles and aqueduct of Sylvius.

Mesenchyme Embryonic connective tissue consisting of an aggregation of cells in close contact by means of long processes thus forming a loose network (stellate cells).

Mesenchymoma A rare benign or malignant tumor consisting of two or more clearly identifiable mesenchymal elements in addition to fibrous tissue.

Mesenteritis Mesenteric inflammation.

m. retractile Chronic mesenteritis resulting in progressive fibrosis and nodular thickening with retraction and distortion of intestinal loops, related to retroperitoneal fibrosis.

Mesentery A double layer of peritoneum attaching various organs to body wall and conveying to them their blood vessels and nerves; commonly referred to peritoneal fold attaching small intestine to the posterior body wall.

m. primitive Double layered embryonic membrane formed by union of the two opposing splanchopleuric layers when the abdominal wall closes off and the peritoneal cavity develops. The dorsal part of primitive mesentery becomes common dorsal mesentery.

m. common dorsal A double layer partition of visceral splachnic mesoderm which divides the embryonic coelem into halves, suspends primitive digestive tube from body wall and carries the blood supply to tube.

m. persistent common A condition in which the embryonic dorsal mesentery retains the primitive attachments between the mid dorsal body wall and the G.I. tract.

m. ventral A fold of peritoneum which extends from the ventral wall of fore gut towards diaphragm and anterior abdominal wall.

Meshwork Network.

Mesial Situated in, near, or towards the midline or apex of dental arch.

Mesoappendix A triangular fold of peritoneum around the vermiform appendix, attaching the latter to posterior surface of the mesentery of the ileum. The artery to appendix runs along the free margin of this fold.

Mesocardium The double layer mesoderm attaching the embryonic heart to the wall of pericardial cavity.

Mesiobuccal Pertaining to the mesial and buccal surface of tooth.

Mesiobucco-occlusal Relating to the mesial, buccal and occlusal surfaces of posterior tooth.

Mesioclusion Malocclusion in which the lower dental arch is anterior to the upper.

Mesiodens An accessory tooth located between two upper incisors.

Mesiodistal Denoting the plane of a tooth from its mesial surface across to its distal surface distal surface.

Mesiolabioincisal Relating to the mesial, labial and incisal surfaces of an anterior tooth, usually denoting the point angle formed by junction of three surfaces.

Mesiolinguo-occlusal Relating to mesial, lingual and occlusal surfaces of posterior tooth.

Mesio-occlusal Relating to mesial and occlusal surface of posterior tooth, usiully denoting the line angle formed by junction of two surfaces.

Mesioversion 1. Position of tooth closer to midline than normal, 2. Position of jaw anterior to its normal position.

Mesmerism A form of hypnosis.

Mesoblast The mesoderm in early stage of development, the middle of three germinal layers of embryo.

Mesocecum The mesentery of cecum.

Mesocephalic Denoting a skull having cephalic index between 75-80; intermediate between dolichocephalic and brachy cephalic.

Mesocolon The double layer of peritoneum attaching colon to posterior abdominal wall. Only the transverse colon and sigmoid colon have actual mesentery.

Mesocolopexy Surgical procedure in which the mesocolon is fixed or resuspended to prevent ptosis or torsion of transverse colon.

Mesocoloplication A surgical procedure of folding back the mesocolon on itself and stitching in place in order to restrict mobility of transverse colon.

Mesocord An umbilical cord, a segment of which is bound to placenta by an accessory fold.

Mesocortex The cerebral cortex of the cingulate and retrosplenial gyri that does not pass through a six layered developmental stage.

Mesocyst A rare peritoneal fold that suspends gallbladder from its fossa on the liver.

Mesoderm The middle of primary germ layers, in between outer ectoderm and inner entoderm. From this layer are derived the majority of skeletal system, the circulatory system, the musculature, the excretory system and most of the reproductive system in vertebrates.

Mesoduodenum A part of the primitive midline dorsal mesentery in relation to embryonic duodenum.

Mesoepididymis A fold of tunica vaginalis that connects the testis to the epididymis.

Mesogastrium That part of primitive dorsal mesentery which is related to developing stomach and becomes greater omentum.

Mesognathic Having an average jaw to head relationship or gnathic index between 98-103.

Mesomelia The relative shortening of middle segments of limbs.

Mesometrium The portion of broad ligament below mesovarium.

Mesomorph A person having a body build with prominent musculature and heavy bony structure.

Mesognathion The part of maxilla bearing the lateral incisor.

Meson Subatomic paricle with mass a in between that of electron and proton.

Mesonephroma Rare ovarian tumor believed to be formed from displaced mesonephric tissue.

Mesonephros An intermediate excretory organ of the embryo, it is replaced by permanent metanephros (kidney). While its ductal system is retained in male as epididymis and deferent duct and in female as tubules of epoophoron. Also known as wolfian body.

Mesorchium A thick fold of peritoneum which connects the developing testis to the mesonephric fold in embryo. It contains testicular vessels and nerves.

Mesorectum A short peritoneal fold investing the upper part of rectum and connecting it to sacrum.

Mesoridazine Antipsychotic agent.

Mesosalpinx The upper free portion of broad ligament investing the fallopian tube.

Mesosigmoidopexy Attaching the sigmoid mesocolon to anterior abdominal wall to prevent sigmoid volvulus or rectal prolapse.

Mesosome A convoluted membranous body derived from invagination of plasma membrane in some bacteria functioning the cellular respiration.

Mesotendon The connective tissue fold of synovial membrane extending from a tendon to the wall of its synovial tendon sheath.

Mesothelioma A benign or malignant tumor arising from the mesothelial lining of one of the coelomic cavities, commonly pleura or peritoneum, consisting of epithelial and spindle cell elements.

Mesothelium Epithelial cells of mesodermal origin which line the serous cavities, also found as secretory epithelium of kidney and mesothelium of anterior chamber of eye.

Mesovarium A short thick peritoneal fold that attaches ovary to posterior layer of broad ligament and permits passage of blood vessels and nerves to ovary.

Messenger 1. The RNA that carries the information coded in DNA sequence to the site of protein biosynthesis where it specifies the order of aminoacid residues. 2. The mediator of an effect.

Mestranol An estrogen used in preparation of oral contraceptive.

Mesurpine HCl A vasodilator and smooth muscle relaxant.

Meta Prefix means 1. changed in form, or position transformed, 2. after, behind, following 3. next to.

Meta analysis A statistical procedure for combining data from a number of studies and their analysis

Metabiosis The dependence of an organism upon the preexistence of another for its development.

Metabolic rate The rate of utilization of energy calculated from oxygen consumption

m rate basal The metabolic rate when body in at complete rest. It is 1 cal / kg / hour or 40 cal/m² / hour

Metabolism A general term applied to chemical processes taking place in the living tissues for maintenance of life.

m. acid-base The processes influencing hydrogen ion concentration in the body.

m. aerobic Metabolic activity dependent upon oxygen.

m. intermediary The chemical changes associated with the synthesis of cellular components from food materials and their degradation.

Metabolite A substance taking part in or produced by metabolic activity.

m. secondary Any of the compounds produced by many microorganisms not subserving growth.

Metabutethamine Used in dentistry as a local anesthetic for nerve block/infiltration anesthesia.

Metacarpus The five bones of hand between the carpus and the phallanges.

Metacentric Pertaining to chromosome with centromere in the middle.

Metachromasia 1. The property by which some cells stain in a colour different from the dye with which they are stained 2. The property through which a single dye stains different tissues in different colours.

Metachromatic Term applied to cells and dyes exhibiting metachromasia.

Metacercaria The encysted stage of a digenetic trematode which occurs in the tissues or on the surface of intermediate host such as snail. This stage is usually infective or is the transfer stage to definitive host.

Metachrosis The ability to change color.

Metacresol A local antiseptic.

Metacryptozoite A member of second or subsequent generation of the extra erythrocytic, tissue dwelling malarial parasite; it develops from sporozoites.

Metacyesis Extrauterine pregnancy.

Meta female A female with 3 X chromosomes (trisomy X) usually short statured, mentally retarded and obese.

Metagonimus A genus of small flukes which may infect man upon eating fish containing the larvae.

Metakinesis The separation of two chromatids of a chromosome during the anaphase of mitosis.

Metal Any of the several chemical elements that share a group of characteristic properties, are good conductors of electricity, malleable and liberate cations.

m. heavy Any metal 5 times or more heavier than water.

m. noble Metal that can neither be oxidized by heat nor can be easily dissolved, e.g. gold, silver, platinum.

m. rare earth Any metal with atomic no. 57 through 71.

Metaldehyde A polymer of acetaldehyde formerly used as an antiseptic.

Metalloenzyme An enzyme having a metal ion as an integral part of its active form, e.g., cytochrome (Fe^{2+} Fe^{3+}). Cytochrome oxidase (Cu^{2+}, Cu^2) or alcohol dehydrogenase (Zn^{2+}).

Metallophil A cell or tissue which stains with metallic salts, e.g., reticular cells.

Metalloprotein A protein with metal ion bound to it. Many enzymes are metalloproteins.

Metamale A male with one x chromosome but 2y chromosomes; usually

tall, lean, often having tendency towards aggressive behavior.

Metamere One of a series of homologous body segments, e.g. earthworm.

Metamerism The state of having a series of structures arranged in a repetitive pattern.

Metamorphopsia Distortion of visual image as in parietal lobe disease, retinal lesion or intoxication.

Metamorphosis A change in form or structure as in the development of certain insects from larva to adult.

m. retrograde The gradual degeneration of certain structures through lack of use, as eyes of certain deep sea dwelling fish.

Metamyelocyte An immature granulocyte, an early stage of granulocyte derived from myelocyte with kidney shaped nucleus and finely granulated cytoplasm containing azurophilic granules.

Metanephrine One of the catabolic products of epinephrine excreted in urine.

Metanephros The permanent kidney in the human fetus, formed caudal to mesonephros close to termination of cloaca. It is composed of metanephric duct (primitive ureter) and the metanephrogenic tissue.

Metaneutrophil Not staining normally with neutral dyes.

Metaphase The second stage of cell division by mitosis during which the chromatids are aligned along the equatorial plate of cell and attached by spindle fibers to centromere.

Metaphysis The line of junction of epiphysis with diaphysis (shaft).

Metaplasia The abnormal transformation from one differentiated adult tissue to another type adult tissue within a given organ.

m. agnogenic myeloid Extramedullary hematopoisis especially in the spleen in myelofibrosis.

m. apocrine A metaplasia of breast epithelium to apocrine sweatgland epithelium as in fibrocystic disease.

m. intestinal The transformation of gastric mucosa into a glandular epithelium typical of intestine with goblet cells and Paneth cells as seen in chronic atrophic gastritis.

m. squamous The transformation of an epithelium, usually mucosal or glandular to a stratified squamous epithelium. It is a common adaptation to injury as in ciliated columnar epithelium of bronchus in consequence to chronic cigarette smoking.

Metaplexus The choroid plexus of fourth ventricle.

Metaproterenol A potent beta-adrenergic stimulant used as bronchodilator.

Metarminol A compound with vasopressor activity used to treat acute hypotension.

Metarhodopsin An intermediate formed in retina from degradation of lumirhodopsin. It is unstable and degrades to scotopsin and trans retinene.

Metarminol Sympathomimetic agent.

Metarteriole That part of terminal arteriole that is surrounded by an additional layer of smooth muscle cells and acts as the final control of blood flow to capillary bed.

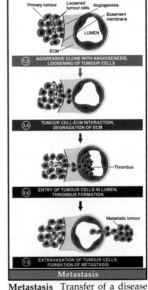

Metastasis Transfer of a disease from its primary site to a distant location either by blood, lymphatic channel, CSF flow, etc.

m. osteoblastic Metastasis which is bone forming, e.g. carcinoma prostate.

m. osteoclastic Destruction of bone at metastatic site.

m. paradoxical Metastasis in a direction other than that of expected flow of blood or lymph.

Metatarsus The anterior portion of foot between the toes and the instep. Composed of 5 cylindrical bones.

m. adductus A deformity where front part of foot is drawn towards the midline.

m. varus A fixed deformity in which the distal part of the foot is rotated on longitudinal axis of the foot so that plantar surface of ball and toes tend to face the sagittal plane of the body.

Metathalamus That portion of thalamus composed of medial and lateral geniculate bodies.

Metathesis The deliberate moving of a pathologic process to a site where it will be less troublesome.

Metathrombin A thrombin-anti-thrombin complex formed during clotting and is inactive.

Metaxalone Orally administered smooth muscle relaxant.

Metazoa A subkingdom of animals comprising all multicellular organisms having specialized cells producing a different type of tissue.

Metazoonosis A type of zoonosis requiring both a vertebrate and an invertebrate host stage in the life-cycle of causative organism.

Metencephalon The more rostral part of brain in embryo that develops into cerebellum and pons.

Meteorism Distention of intestine with gas.

Meter (m) Measure of length equal to 39.37 inches or 100 cm.

Metergoline An ergot alkaloid derivative.

Metestrus The period of regression immediately following the period of sexual desire (estrus) in, the mating season.

Metformin A structural analogue of in phenformin, hypoglycemic agent.

Methacholine A derivative of acetyl choline with only muscarinic effect.

Methacycline A semisynthetic antibiotic of tetracyclic group given orally.

Methadone A synthetic narcotic analgesic with morphine like effect. It is used in opium withdrawal and as a maintenance treatment in heroin addicts.

Methallenestril A synthetic non-steroidal estrogenic agent.

Methamphetamine A sympathomimetic amine similar to amphetamine; used as a CNS stimulant.

Methandriol Anabolic steroid.

Methandrostenolone A compound of methyl testosterone with anabolic and androgenic properties.

Methane CH_4 Marsh gas, the simplest hydrocarbon.

Methanol Methyl alcohol, prepared synthetically or from distillation of wood. Toxic and causes blindness when drunk.

Methantheline bromide An anticholinergic agent used to suppress gastric motility and secretion.

Methapyrilene Antihistaminic of medium potency and short duration; used as fumarate or hydrochloride.

Methaqualone A sedative and hypnotic, chronic use can lead to psychologic and physical dependence.

Metharbital A barbiturate used as anticonvulsant for grandmal, petitmal and myoclonic seizures.

Methazolamide An agent inhibiting carbonic anhydrase, hence used in glaucoma; given orally.

Methemalbumin A complex of plasma albumin with heme released from hemoglobin when there is intravascular hemolysis.

Methemoglobin A derivative of hemoglobin with oxidized iron, hence incapable of carrying oxygen.

Methemoglobinemia Methemoglobin greater than 1%. of total hemoglobin in blood; therefore causing cyanosis.

m. enterogenous Conversion of ingested nitrate to nitrite by intestinal bacteria and its absorption causing hemoglobin oxidation to methemoglobin.

m. hereditary Hereditary disease due to deficiency of RBC methemoglobin reductase.

m. toxic Methemoglobinemia resulting from exposure of Hb to toxic drugs, or their metabolites and nitrites. The drugs most commonly responsible are phenacetin, sulfone (dapsone), phenazopyridine etc.

Methemoglobin reductase Enzyme that converts methemoglobin to Hb.

Methenamine $C_6H_{12}N_4$ Used in treatment of infections of urinary tract because of its slow hydrolysis to formaldehyde. Hippurate and mandelate salts are in use.

Methetoin An analog of phenytoin used as oral anticonvulsant.

Methicillin sodium A semisynthetic derivative of penicillin given IM. in infections resistant to penicillin G.

Methimazole Potent, widely used antithyroid drug. It acts by interfering with incorporation of iodine.

Methiodal sodium Iodine containing contrast for urinary tract.

Methionine One of the essential amino acids, the main biologic donor of methyl groups for protein synthesis.

Methisazone A synthetic antiviral agent, not in use.

Methixene hydrochloride Anticholinergic agent used orally in gastrointestinal hypermotility and spasm.

Methocarbamol A muscle relaxant, given orally, IM and SC.

Method A set form or mode of procedure, a systemic way of performing an examination, test or operation.

m. Abbott's A technique for correction of scoliosis.

m. agar diffusion A method for estimating drug sensitivity or concentration by measuring the diameter of area of growth inhibition around a deposit of drug on a heavily seeded plate.

m. Bell's A vertical tooth brushing technique in which the bristles of a soft multituft brush are swept from teeth to gums.

m. Cajal A histologic technique for demonstrating the presence of astrocytes in nervous tissue by using gold chloride.

m. Castel A histochemical method to demonstrate arsenic or bismuth in the tissue.

m. Charter's A vibratory tooth brushing technique in which the bristles of a hard two rowed brush are applied at 45° to the long axis of teeth directed towards biting surfaces.

m. Copenhegen A technique of artificial respiration developed by Danish Army in which the patient lying prone inspiration is induced by extension of arms and expiration by pressure on the scapula.

m. Crede 's A method of expressing the placenta in which the body of the uterus is vigorously squeezed in order to produce placental separation.

m. Dickinson's A technique to control post partum hemorrhage. The uterus is lifted superiorly out of pelvis and is compressed against vertebral column.

m. Esbach's A method for semi-quantitative estimation of protein in the urine by using picric acid precipitation.

m. Fick Measurement of cardiac output using Fick principle.

m. Fone's A tooth brushing technique with the teeth in occlusion and the head of the brush describing large circles over the teeth and gum.

m. immunofluorescence Any method in which a fluorescent labelled antibody is used to detect the presence or determine the location of corresponding antigen.

m. Lee - White A method of determining the coagulation time of venous blood by placing it in tubes of standard bore at body temperature.

m. India Ink A method for visualizing spirochetes and yeast or other fungi.

m. Manchester A method for repair of bilateral congenital cleft lip.

m. Nissl's A histologic technique that demonstrates the presence of aggregated RNA or Nissl's granules in neurones.

m. Radioactive balloon A method of radioactive exposure to bladder wall by placing the radioactive material in the balloon of Foley's catheter.

m. rhythm Birth control by avoiding sexual intercourse for 4 days before and 4 days after the approximate date of ovulation.

m. Shick's A method of producing immunity to diphtheria by injecting a mixture of toxin and antitoxin of that disease.

m. Westergreen A method for estimating the sedimentation rate of redblood cells in the blood; 4.5 ml of venous blood is mixed with 0.5 ml of 3.8% sodium citrate and is pippetted into a standard 2 mm bore 300 mm long pippette, filled upto zero mark and kept in upright position for 1 hour to record the fall of RBC column. Normal value for male in 0-10 mm and for female is 0-20 mm.

m. **Wintrobe** The determination of ESR by measurement of sedimentation at one hour and correction for hematocrit value by a standard table.

Methohexital sodium Short acting barbiturate used IV like pentothal sodium.

Methotrexate A potent folic acid antagonist used as cytotoxic agent and immunosuppresant.

Methotrimeprazine A phenothiazine with potent analgesic properties used in obstetric analgesia, and as a preanesthetic medication.

Methoxamine An adrenergic vasopressor, often used in supraventricular tachycardia.

Methoxsalen A psoralen compound used in association with ultraviolet exposure to enhance repigmentation in vitiligo. It is also used to precipitate a phototoxic response in the treatment of psoriasis.

Methoxychlor An insecticide used to control mosquito larva and flies.

Methoxyphenamine An adrenergic agent used as bronchodilator.

Methoxyflurane A colorless non explosive liquid used as a slow anesthetic.

Methoxypromazine A phenothiazine tranquilizer.

Methscopolamine A quaternary derivative of scopolamine with anticholinergic actions; used as gastrointestinal sedative.

Methsuximide An anticonvulsant for petit mal and psychomotor epilepsy.

Methyclothiazide A thiazide antihypertensive diuretic.

Methylal Dimethoxy methane, anesthetic and hypnotic agent.

Methylchloride A refrigerant, used in spray form for local anesthesia, also same property by m. iodide.

m. methacrylate An acrylic resin for dental use.

m. salicylate An antipyretic, analgesic, used in pain killing ointments.

Methyl orange Used as an indicator with a pH range of 3.2-4.4 (yellow at 3.2 and pink at 4.4).

Methyl red Used as an indicator, red at 4.4 and yellow at 6.

Methylate To combine with methyl alcohol or the methyl radical.

Methyl cellulose A bulk forming cellulose derivative with laxative properties. Used for constipation, as appetite suppressant in management of obesity, and in ophthalmic solutions/ointment.

Methyl benzenethonium chloride A topical antiinfective agent.

Methylcholanthrene One of the carcinogenic polycyclic hydrocarbons of coaltar.

Methyl dopa Sympathetic activity inhibitor used in treatment of hypertension.

Methylene blue Methyl thionine chloride, an aniline dye formerly used as urinary antiseptic; now used in treatment of methemoglobinemia, as an antidote for cyanide poisoning, as a staining agent for basophilic and metachromatic substances.

Methylene green A synthetic metachromatic dye used to distinguish mast cell granules.

Methyl ergonovine maleate An oxytocic agent used to induce uterine contraction to reduce post partum hemorrhage.

Methylene dioxyamphetamine (MDA) A hallucinogen commonly referred as the love drug.

Methyl glucamine ditrizoate An organic compound used as a contrast medium in the making of X-ray transparencies.

Methyl malonic aciduria Elevation of methyl malonic acid in blood with excessive excretion in urine. Caused due to congenital enzymatic deficiency or B_{12} deficiency.

Methyl malony CoA Formed from propionyl CoA, helpful for utilization of fatty acids.

Methyl methacrylate Acrylic resin used to make denture bases, artificial teeth, crowns and restorations.

Methyl phenidate Mild psychomotor stimulant, used to treat hyperkinetic children, and narcolepsy.

Methyl prednisolone Methylated analog of prednisolone given orally as immunosuppressant.

Methyl salicylate A colorless oily liquid with strong odor used in perfumes and as counter irritants.

Methyl testosterone Orally given androgenic steroidal agent as a replacement therapy for androgen deficiency states.

Methyl tetrahydrofolic acid An intermediate subserving as a donor of methyl group to homocystine to form methionine.

Methyl violet Dye for staining amyloid.

Methyprylon A compound with sedative and hypnotic properties.

Methysergide A serotonin receptor antagonist used as vasoconstrictor in migraine.

Metitepine 5 HT antagonist.

Metmyoglobin Oxidized (Fe^{3+}) myoglobin.

Metocurine A derivative of tubocurarine which is more potent and longer acting.

Metolazone A diuretic acting on proximal and distal tubules.

Metopagus Equal conjoined twins with the union at forehead.

Metopion The craniometric point at which a line joining the frontal eminences intersects the median sagittal plane.

Metopism The persistence in the adult of the frontal or metopic suture.

Metoprolol A betaadrenergic antagonist used in treatment of hypertension and angina pectoris.

Metorchis A genus of flukes in animals, occasionally transmitted to man.

Metratonia Lack of uterine tone after childbirth.

Metrectomy Hysterectomy.

Metrifonate A drug effective against bladder flukes *(Schistostoma hematobium).*

Metritis Inflammation of uterus.

Metrizamide A nonionic radiographic contrast agent.

Metrizoate sodium A contrast medium for coronary angiography.

Metrizoic acid A compound used as contrast medium in diagnostic procedures.

Metromalacia Necrosis and softening of uterus.

Metronania Unusually small size of uterus.

Metronidazole A nitroimidazole compound used for treatment of amebiasis, trichomoniasis, anaerobic infections.

Metrodynamo meter Instrument used to measure the strength of uterine contractions.

Metropathia hemorrhagica Excessive prolonged bleeding from uterus associated with cyst formation in the endometrium.

Metroptosis Prolapse of uterus.

Metrorrhexis Rupture of uterus.

Metrostaxis Continuous oozing from uterus.

Metyrapone An inhibitor of adrenocortical steroid C-ll betahydroxylation, administered orally or IV as a diagnostic test to determine the capability of pituitary to increase production of corticotropin.

Mexilentine Antiarrhythmic drug.

Mevalonic acid A product of methyl valeric acid produced in the pathway of biosynthesis of sterols.

Mevinolin HMG CoA reductase inhibitor used as lipid lowering agent.

Micelle 1. A submicroscopic unit of a protoplasm. 2. A molecular aggregate as that of a colloid often formed by action of detergents on a hydrocarbon in water.

Miconazole Antifungal, topically used 2%.

Micro One million the (10^6); very small, minute.

Microabscess A small abscess usually less than a mm, often multiple.

m. of Munro One of the characteristic lesions of psoriasis consisting of focal accumulation of polymorphonuclear leukocytes in the upper layer of epidermis.

m. Pautrier's Focal collection of atypical T lymphocytes in the epidermis in mycosis fungoides.

Microadenoma A small (≤ 10 mm diameter) non malignant glandular tumor, as associated with Cushing's disease.

Microaerophil An anaerobe that can tolerate low O_2 tension.

Microaerosol A suspension in the air of minute particles of 1-10 μ.

Micro albuminuria Excretion in urine of less than 100 μgm per minute of albumin.

Microanalysis Analysis using small amounts of material than classical methods of chemical analysis that involves weighing precipitate material.

Microaneurysm An aneurysmal dilatation affecting small arteries arterioles and capillaries; a feature of diabetes mellitus, thrombotic thrombocytopenic purpura. Diabetic microaneurysms of retina with exudates and hemorrhages constitute characteristic features of diabetic retinopathy.

Microangiography Magnification roentogenography of small blood vessels that have been opacified by injection of contrast medium.

Microangiopathy A disease process affecting small blood vessels.

m. diabetic Thickening of capillary basement membrane, in the retina, kidney, heart with micro aneurysm formation.

Microbiology Branch of science concerned with microorganisms subdivided into virology, bacteriology, mycology, protozoology and phycology.

Microbe A microorganism, a one celled plant.

Microbalance A scale designed to weigh minor amounts of material.

Microcephaly Abnormal smallness of head.

Microblast A small nucleated red blood cell.

Microcirculation Blood circulation in arterioles, capillaries and venules.

Micrococcoceae A family of gram positive spherical bacteria that characteristically divide in more than one plane to yield irregular clusters.

Micrococcin A naturally occurring antibiotic obtained from particular strain of Micrococcus. It has antitubercular activity.

Microcoria An abnormal smallness of pupil.

Microcurie A unit of activity of radionuclides equal to 10^{-6} curie, 3.7×10^4 becquerels.

Microcyte A small red blood cell at least 2 μ smaller than normal, as seen in iron deficiency.

Microcytosis Condition in which RBCs are abnormally small.

Microdactyly Abnormally small fingers.

Microdontia Abnormally small teeth.

Microfilaria A prelarval or embryonic form of filarial worms.

Microgamete The smaller male element in the conjugation of cells of unequal size.

Microgametocyte The mother cell that produces microgametes.

Microgamy Conjugation between two young cells in certain protozoans.

Microgenia Abnormal smallness of chin.

Microglia The smallest neuroglial cell, the macrophage of brain and spinal cord that remove cellular debris in CNS.

Microglossia Small tongue.

Micrognathia Abnormal smallness of jaw, especially the lower jaw producing bird like profile.

Microgram Unit of weight equivalent to 10^{-6} gram.

Microgyria Abnormally small cerebral convolutions.

Microinvasion The earliest stage in the spread of carcinoma to adjacent tissue.

Microlith A small calculus.

Micrometer One millionth of a meter.

Micrometer An instrument containing a microscope for accurate linear measurement of very small units of length.

Micronize To pulverize or reduce material to particles of very small size.

Micronutrient Any essential dietary constituent like vitamins and minerals required by body in small quantities.

Microorganism Any single celled organism.

Microphage A small phagocyte, especially polymorphonuclear leukocyte capable of digesting bacteria.

Microphonics Electrical potentials generated in the cochlea by passage of sound waves.

Micropipette A pipette calibrated for accurate delivery of very small quantities less than 0.5 ml.

Micropore A submicroscopic break in the membrane of a protozoan cell or microbe through which exchange of materials, pinocytosis occur.

Microprobe An ultrafine probe used for exploration and fixation of tissues in microsurgical procedures.

Micropsia Perception of objects as smaller in comparison to their actual size. It occurs in retinal detachment, temporal lobe epilepsy, delirium and drug intoxication.

Microradiograph A recorded image obtained by microradiography, used in high resolution imaging of thin objects like tissue sections.

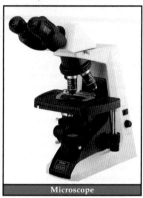

Microscope

Microscope An optical instrument used for viewing magnified images of small objects.

m. acoustic A device in which ultrasound distorts a reflective surface, which is then optically scanned to produce an image.

m. dissecting A compound microscope with two sets of eye pieces and objectives constructed to present a nonreversed, stereoscopic image of three dimensional objects.

m. electron A microscope that uses electrons rather than visible light to irradiate clear magnified images; capable of magnifying objects having dimensions smaller than wavelength of light.

m. interference A microscope in which emerging light is split into two beams which pass through the object and are recombined in the image plane where transparent and refractile specimen details become visible as intensity differences occur; useful in the examination of living or unstained cells.

m. laser A microscope in which LASER beam is focussed on microscopic field, causing it to vaporize; the emitted radiation is analyzed by a microspectrophotometer.

m. operating A microscope used in operating room for magnifying the surgical field.

m. phase contrast A microscope that makes use of the relationship between two paths of light 1. light that enters microscope objective through the specimen and 2. light that enters objective after being diffracted by the specimens; all points of divergence between these two paths of light reveal a specimen or object whose lack of contrast would make it invisible under other types of illumination.

m. polarizing A microscope especially equipped to polarized light and to examine the alterations of polarized light by the specimen, useful in identification of crystals.

m. electron scanning A microscope where specimen is examined point by point by an electron beam and an image is formed on television screen from the secondary electrons given off the surface.

m. ultraviolet A microscope whose energy source is electromagnetic

radiation with a wavelength of 180-400 nm.

m. X-ray A microscope which uses a beam of X-ray instead of light with the image.usually being recorded on photographic film.

Microscopic Extremely small.

Microscopy The study of objects using a microscope.

Microsecond One millionth of a second.

Microsection A thin slice of tissue prepared for examination under a microscope.

Microsome A fragment of endoplasmic reticulum with associated ribosomes.

Microspectrography Study of composition of an object, especially of cellular constituents using a spectroscope. That makes a photographic record of the spectrum.

Microspectrophotometer An instrument used to measure the absorption, reflection or emission of light by objects under a microscope, especially used for spectral analysis of individual cells.

Microsporidiosis Intracellular spore forming protozoa causing human disease in HIV patients

Microstomia Disproportionately small oral orifice.

Microtia Abnormally small auricle or pina.

Microtome A mechanical device used for preparing histologic sections for microscopic examinations; can be m. freezing or m. rotary.

Microtomography A technique for rotating a small sample in an electron microscope through 90 degrees, processing the data by computer and displaying three dimensional images.

Microtonometer An instrument for measuring the partial pressure of gases in minute quantities of material.

Microtubule A small, hollow, cylindrical structure found in the cell cytoplasm. During cell division they increase greatly in number to form the mitotic spindle, play an important role in intracellular movements and in maintaining shape of the cell.

Microvilli Submicroscopic finger like projections on the surface of cell membrane which greatly increase the surface area.

Microvolt One millionth of a volt, 10^{-6} volt.

Microwave Any electromagnetic radiation having a very short wavelength between 1 mm and 30 cm wavelength 1 mm are in infrared region and that beyond 30 cm are radio waves. Sources of emission include radar, cathode ray tubes, induction furnaces, and electrotherapy devices. Microwave exposure can cause cataract.

Micturition The act of urination.

Midazolam A benzodiazepine.

Midbrain The part of brain developing from embryonic mesencephalon, divided into three parts;

tectum, (quadrigeminal plate), tegmentum (cephalic continuation of pontine tegmentum) and the crus cerebri.

Middle lobe syndrome A form of chronic atelectasis marked by collapse of middle lobe of the lung resulting from compression of bronchus by enlarged lymphnodes/tumor. Symptoms include chronic cough and recurrent respiratory infections. *SYN* — Brock's syndrome.

Midfoot The middle portion of foot consisting of navicular, cuboid and cuneiform bones.

Midgut 1. The small intestine comprising jejunum and ileum. 2. The middle segment of embryonic intestine, precursor of stomach to transverse colon.

Midpelvis The area of pelvis extending from the posterior inferior aspect of symphysis in a line through ischial spines to sacrum intersecting it at S_2 or S_3 vertebra.

Midwife A woman who attends women during delivery.

Midwifery Practical obstetrics.

Migraine A recurrent hemicranial intense headache associated with nausea, vomiting and visual disturbances.

m. abdominal Episodic abdominal pain, nausea, vomiting in migraine sufferers.

m. complicated An attack of migraine accompanied by prolonged aphasia, hemiplegia, hemianopia, epilepsy etc.

Composition of Milk (per 100g)		
	Human	Cow's
Protein	2 g	3.5 g
Carbohydrate	7 g	5 g
Fat	4 g	3.5 g
Calcium	25 mg	120 mg
Phosphorus	16 mg	95 mg
Iron	0.1 mg	0.1 mg
Thiamine	17μg	40 μg
Riboflavin	30 μg	150 μg
Nicotinic acid	170 μg	80 μg
Ascorbic acid	3.5 μg	2.0 μg
Vitamin A	170 IU	150 IU
Vitamin D	1.0 IU	1.5 IU
Calories	70	66

m. facioplegic Transient unilateral facial palsy occurring during attack of migraine.

m. hemiplegic Migraine in which recurrent attacks of hemiplegia occur.

m. ophthalmoplegic Oculomotor palsy occurring during an attack of migraine.

migraine equivalant Symptoms produced by migraine like mechanism but without an associated headache e.g., transient partial loss of vision.

Migration Passing from one part of body to another.

Mickulicz's disease Benign bilateral swelling of the lacrimal and salivary glands associated with dryness of mouth and reduced, lacrimation, identical to Sjogren's syndrome.

Mickulicz's syndrome Painless bilateral enlargement of salivary and lacrimal glands with dryness of mouth and decreased lacrimation as in sarcoidosis.

Miliaria Skin eruption due to retention of sweat in sweat follicles. *SYN* — sweat fever, summer eruption; can be m. papulasa, profunda, rubra and even pustular types.

Miliary Of the size of a millet (2 mm diameter).

Milieu Environment, surroundings.

Milium A minute whitish or yellowish papule on the skin caused by retention of fatty material (sebum) or densely packed keratin.

m. colloid A degenerative disorder of dermal connective tissue with yellowish translucent plaques.

Milk The secretion of mammary glands.

m. adapted Cow's milk made similar to human milk by reducing casein and increasing the ratio of unsaturated to saturated fatty acids.

m. homogenized Milk treated mechanically after pasteurization to breakdown the fat globules into small parts.

m. witch's A few drops of milk expressed from newborn's nipple during first few days of life.

Milk alkali syndrome Hypercalcemia without hypercalciuria or hypophosphaturia induced by prolonged ingestion of large quantity of milk and soluble alkali as in therapy of peptic ulcer.

Milking A manual or mechanical technique for removing fluid from body part.

Milk-leg Colloqial term for a painful swollen leg due to leg vein thrombosis occurring in post-partum period.

Milkman's syndrome Osteoporosis with multiple fractures as seen in post menopausal women.

Milk teeth Deciduous teeth.

Millard-Gubler syndrome Paralysis of facial muscles on one side and extremities on opposite side by brain stem lesions.

Millicurie A measure of radioactivity; one thousandth of a curie.

Milliequivalent A quantity equal to 10^{-3} of the equivalent weight of an element or compound.

Milligray A unit of absorbed dose in the field of ionizing radiation equal to 10^{-3} gray.

Millimeter One thousandth of a meter.

Milligram One thousandth of a gram.

Millimicrogram One billionth of a gram, biller called a nano gram.

Milling in The placing of abrasives between the occlusal surface of dentures, used to perfect the occlusion.

Milliosmole One thousandth of an osmole; the osmotic pressure exerted by the concentration of a substance in solution; expressed as milligrams per kilogram divided by atomic weight for an ionized substance or divided by molecular weight for nonionized solute. Normal plasma osmolality is 280-300 mOsm/kg.

Millirad A unit of absorbed dose of ionizing radiation equivalent to 10^{-3} rad, 10^{-5} Gray.

Millirem A unit of radiation dose equivalent to 10^{-3} ren 10^{-5} joule/kg, 10^{-5} silvert.

Milliroentgen A unit of ionization exposure equal to 10^{-3} roentgen; 2.58×10^{-7} coulomb/kg.

Milrinone Sympathomimetic, cardiac stimulant.

Milroy's disease Familial and congenital swelling of subcutaneous tissues usually confined to extremities with large accumulation of lymph.

Milwaukae brace Brace extending from chin upto pelvi's, meant to correct scoliosis

Mimesis State in which one disease presents the symptoms of another.

Mimetic Of or relating to mimesis.

Mimicry The imitation of one species by another in an adaptation tending to improve its chances of survival.

Minaserine 5 HT antagonist.

Mind The organized total of psychological processes and contents that allow the individual to respond to external and internal stimuli in an integrated and dynamic way, relating response of present to both past and future of the individual. The principal processes of mind are perceiving, learning, thinking, remembering, feeling and behaving with intelligence.

Mineral Any naturally occurring homogeneous inorganic substance, having a characteristic crystalline structure and chemical composition.

Mineralization The conversion of organic material to inorganic material.

Mineral corticoid One of the steroids in the adrenal cortex that act principally on renal retention of sodium and excretion of potassium, e.g. aldosterone.

Minim A unit of fluid measure; about a drop or l/60th of a dram.

Minimum Smallest amount or size.

Minimal brain dysfunction syndrome A complex of symptoms that involve impairment of some or all of the following functions: language, perception, memory, concentration, and motor functions.

Minimal change disease A form of nephrotic syndrome in which minimal or no glomerular abnormalities are, noted by light microscopy but fusion of foot processes of podocytes in electron microscopy.

Minocycline A semisynthetic antibiotic of tetracycline group used for acne.

Minoxidil Vasodilator; used for alopecia locally as 2% solution.

Miopus Unequal conjoined twins united at head in such fashion that face of one member is rudimentary.

Miosis Marked constriction of pupils, can be spastic or paralytic.

Miotic Any agent causing miosis.

Miracidium A free swimming ciliated larva of a trematode that penetrates a small intermediate host where it develops into a sporocyst.

Mirror A polished surface that forms optical images by reflection.

m. head A concave mirror worn on a headband or spectacle frame used for focussing a beam of light.

m. laryngeal A circular plane mirror used to examine the interior of larynx and hypopharynx.

Miscarriage Spontaneous abortion.

Miscarry To give birth to a nonviable fetus.

Misce Mix, a direction given in pharmacy.

Miscible Capable of being mixed.

Misdiagnosis Wrong diagnosis.

Misogyny Hatred of women.

Misophobia Abnormal fear of contamination.

Mistura Mixture; used in pharmacy.

Mite Any of various minute arachnids that are often parasitic on man and animals; they may infest food and propagate disease.

Miticide An agent for killing mite.

Mithramycin An antineoplastic antibiotic given IV in testicular malignancy and hypercalcemia.

Mitigate To make or become milder.

Mitochondria A double membrane cytoplasmic organelle, self reproducing, present in cell cytoplasm of all living cells; responsible for energy production (ATP), Each cell has several hundreds of mitochondria, each of 15.00 Å length.

m. giant Unusually large mitochondria produced due to nutritional deficiency, toxic influences or effects of electromagnetic fields.

Mitogen Agent promoting cell mitosis and lymphocyte transformation.

Mitogenesis The induction of mitosis in a cell.

Mitosis Multiplication or division of a cell that results in formation of two daughter cells normally receiving the same chromosome and DNA as that of original cell.

Mitomycin A group of antibiotic substances produced by species of streptomyces and differentiated as mitomycin A, B, and C. Mitomycin C inhibits cell division by blocking the cross linking of DNA strands; hence used as antineoplastic agent in lymphomas and solid tumors.

Mitotane Antineoplastic agent.

Mitral Left atrioventricular valve.

Mitral valve The bicuspid valve between left atrium and left ventricle with a orifice of 2.5 cm

Mitral valve prolapse The mitral valve prolapses into left atrium during systole causing regurgitation

Mitralization Straightening of left cardiac border due to enlarged left atrial appendage and pulmonary artery in mitral stenosis.

Mittelschmerz Inter menstrual pain specially at the time of ovulation.

Mixture 1. An aggregation of two or more substances that are not chemically combined 2. A pharmaceutical preparation consisting of an insoluble substance suspended in a liquid by viscid material such as sugar, glycerol etc.

m. Brompton A mixture of cocaine hydrochloride and morphine hydrochloride given orally to patients for relief of cancer pain.

m. Vincent's A combination of sodium hypochlorite and boric acid used for covering surgical or traumatic wounds.

M. mode A motion B mode tracing of ultrasound to visualize moving structures.

Mnemonic The use or devising of techniques to facilitate memory.

MNS blood groups A system of erythrocyte antigen determined by the allelic genes, M.N. and S; the grouping is primarily used to solve identification problems such as disputed paternity and genetic linkage, population studies.

Mobility The capacity for movement.

m. electrophoretic The velocity at which ions of a substance migrate in an electric field.

Mobilization A process or an operation whereby an object or a substance is freed or made mobile.

m. chromosome The conjugative transfer of part or all of a bacterial chromosome, resulting from integration of plasmid that codes for transfer of itself.

m. stapes The transmeatal operative mobilization of the stapes as ankylosed in otosclerosis, thereby restoring hearing loss.

Mobius sign Convergence weakness of eyes occurring in exophthalmic goiter.

Mobius syndrome A congenital disorder characterized by bilateral paralysis of both external recti and hypotrophy of facial musculature due to agenesis of ganglion cells in the brainstem of occulomotor and facial nerve nuclei.

Modality 1. Any of the several forms of therapy 2. Any of the main forms of sensation.

Mode In statistics, the value occurring most often.

Model 1. A three dimensional shape representing a likeness of some existing structure 2. In dentistry, positive reproduction of the dentition and adjoining structures.

m. disease The artificial creation of an abnormality in an experimental animal in order to allow further study of the entity.

m. study A replica of teeth and adjoining oral structures used as diagnostic aid.

m. Danielli-Davson A representation of the molecular arrangement of the components of cellular membranes in which the lipid layer separates two protein layers. The lipids are phospholipids and are arranged in two monomolecular layers with their hydrophobic tails towards the inside of membrane and their hydrophilic phosphates towards surface protein.

m. Waston-Crick A molecular model which represents the structure of deoxyribonucleic acid as a soluble helix with right handed coiling. The two strands of helix are composed of antiparallel strands of polynucleotides.

Modifier Agent that alters form, or character without transforming; e.g., in genetics, a gene which alters the phenotic effect of another gene.

Modiolus The central pillar or column of bone around which the spiral canals of cochlea turn.

Modulation The changes that take place in response to changes in the environment.

Moiety One of two, more or less equal parts. One of two or more main components, such as the groups of atoms in a complex molecule.

Molality The amount of substance of a solute divided by mass of the solvent; expressed in mole per kg.

Molar Any of the most posterior teeth in jaw.

Molarity The concentration of a substance expressed in moles per liter.

Mold 1. Any fungus having a cottony appearance, usually growing on decaying material. 2. A receptacle for shaping any cast material. 3. to shape.

Molding 1. The process of shaping 2. The changes in shape of the fetal head as it passes through the birth canal.

Mole 1. Intrauterine mass. 2. Pigmented cellular nevus; circumscribed pigmented growth on skin. 3. gram molecule.

m. carneous A spontaneous abortion in which the ovum is surrounded by a capsule of clotted blood.

m. hydatidiform A developmental anomaly of placenta consisting of a nonmalignant mass of clear vesicles resembling bunch of grapes formed from cystic swellings of chorionic villi. The moles may cause uterine enlargement disproportionate to period of gestation.

Molecular Relating to or consisting of molecules.

Molecular weight The sum of the atomic weights of all the atoms making up a molecule.

Molecule The smallest unit of a substance which can exist in a free state and still retain the chemical properties of the substance.

m. cyclic A molecule that appears in organic compounds and whose atoms are arranged in a ring or polygon.

Molimen The effect exerted in the performance of bodily function, often applied to pre- and perimenstrual dyscomfort.

Molindone Antipsychotic agent.

Molluscum A skin disease marked by the presence of soft rounded tumors.

m. contagiosum An infectious disease of skin marked by small wart like lesions containing a substance resembling curd, usually of viral etiology.

Molt To cast off.

Molybdenum Element No. 42, a silvery white hard metal required for many animal enzyme function.

Moment of death That point in time when an individual is declared dead. This determination is based on criteria which are defined by law and which differ according to situation. For autopsy and burial purposes, criteria include the clinical judgement that respiration and circulation have ceased and rigor mortis has started. For organ transplantation brain death is employed even though functional circulatory and respiratory activities may persist.

Momentum The product, of mass and velocity of a body, an index of quantity of motion.

Momism The state of being excessively dependent on or subordinate to one's mother.

Monad A free swimming solitary unicellular flagellate organism.

Monarthritis Arthritis of single joint.

Monarticular Denoting a single joint.

Monaural Relating to one ear.

Monday disease The return of symptoms after a weekend away from work, as in the case of an allergic reaction to a substance encountered while at work.

Mondor's disease Inflammation of the subcutaneous veins of the chest and breast, usually extending from epigastric region to the axilla and occurring in both sexes.

Mongolism Down syndrome due to trisomy 21.

Mongoloid Having characteristics or resembling mongolism.

Monilethrix Beaded hair, an anomalous condition in which the hair shaft exhibits nodosities or points of thickening alternating with normal or constricted areas.

Monilia A genus of molds or fungi, commonly known as fruit molds, now called *Candida*.

Moniliasis Infection with any fungus of genus monilia.

Moniliform Having the shape of a necklace.

Monitor 1. To keep close watch over 2. An apparatus used to record or display data.

m. apnea An alarm system for alarming attendants to the occurrence of apnea commonly in a premature infant.

m. cardiac Continuous display of cardiac rhythm in a screen to detect irregularities in the heart rhythm.

m. electronic fetal An electronic instrument monitoring fetal heart rate and patterns of uterine contraction.

Monkey rhesus Macaca mulatta widely distributed in India and China; easily raised in captivity, hence amply used in medical and biological research.

Monoamine Compound containing only one amine group.

m. oxidase An enzyme that catalyzes the oxidation of a wide variety of physiologic amines into aldehydes and ammonia. It is important for catabolism of epinephrine and tyramine.

Monobenzene The monobenzyl ether of hydroquinone used as ointment to cause hypopigmentation in the treatment of hyperpigmentation.

Monoblast An immature cell of monocytic series, 18-22 μ in diameter, having many nucleoli, formed primarily in spleen and lymphoid tissue.

Monochromatic Having one colour.

Monocrotic Forming a smooth single crest on the downward line of a curve. e.g. pulse.

Monocular Relating to, having, or used by one eye.

Monocyte A large mononucleated white blood cell 15-25 μ with a round kidney shaped or lobulated nucleus and gray-blue cytoplasm. It is the largest cell in blood film and on leaving blood it becomes macrophage.

Monocytosis Abnormal increase in number of monocytes in blood.

Monograph A detailed written account of one particular subject or a small area of a special field of learning.

Monohybrid A cross between parents that differ in one character.

Monoiodotyrosine (MIT) An amino acid formed by iodination of tyrosine at C_3, the first step in production of thyroxin.

Monokine A hormone like factor produced by activation of monocytes; acts as an intercellular messenger to regulate immunologic and inflammatory responses.

Monolepsis The appearance in offspring of the characteristic of one but not the other parent.

Monomer A single unit or molecule which can polymerize with similar units to form a chain or polymer.

Monomania Pathologic preoccupation with only one idea.

Monomorphic Having but one shape, unchangeable in size and form.

Mononeuritis Inflammation or degeneration of a single nerve trunk or some of its branches.

m. multiplex Neuritis involving single nerves at several distant sites, usually vascular origin (PAN).

Mononuclear Unicellular.

Mononucleosis EB virus infection marked by fever, sore throat, splenomegaly, lymphadenopathy and peripheral atypical lymphocytosis. *SYN*— kissing disease; similar symptoms also occur in post transfusion patients.

Monophasia Disorder in which the individual's vocabulary is limited to a single word or sentence.

Monoplegia Paralysis of one limb.

Monorchid An individual with only one testis.

Monosaccharide A carbohydrate which cannot be further broken down, simple sugar.

Mono sodium glutamate (MSG) The sodium salt of glutamic acid with one sodium ion per molecule used as a food flavoring agent, causative agent for chinese restaurant syndrome.

Monosome A chromosome without its homologous chromosome.

Monosomy Condition in which one chromosome of a pair of homologous chromosomes is missing.

Monostotic Pertaining to or involving a single bone.

Monosynaptic Pertaining to a neural pathway like reflex are containing only a single synapse.

Monotrichous Possessing a single flagellum.

Monoxide An oxide containing only one oxygen atom.

Monozygotic Denoting idential twins, or twins formed by division into two of the embryo derived from a single fertilized egg.

Mons In anatomy, a slight prominence, or elevation.

m. pubis The fleshy prominence formed by a pad of fatty tissue over the symphysis pubis in female.

m. ureteris A slight prominence at the wall of the bladder at the entrance of ureter.

Monster A congenitally severely deformed individual.

Montage In EEG, an arrangement of electrodes applied to the scalp in such a way that the electrical activity of entire brain or of a particular area can be recorded simultaneously.

Monticulus Protuberance e.g. m.cerebelli

Mood A prevailing emotional state of mind.

Moraxella Short, aerobic, gram-negative bacteria.

Morbid Diseased, pathologic, pertaining to or affected by disease.

Morbidity The condition of being diseased; within a given population, the number of sick persons or cases of disease recorded as of a stated point in time or over a stated period. Thus morbidity can be expressed as the number of new cases arising (incidence) or the number of cases existing whether old or new (prevalence).

Morbilliform Resembling the skin eruption of measles.

Morbus Latin for disease.

Mordant A substance used in bacteriology to fix a dye or stain.

Morgan (m) The unit of map distance on a chromosome.

Morgue A place where dead bodies are kept pending identification, autopsy or burial/cremation.

Moribund Dying; Close to death.

Morioplasty Surgical restoration of parts lost through injury or disease.

Morning sickness Nausea and vomiting occurring particularly in the morning during first trimester of pregnancy

Morning stiffness Joint and muscle stiffness on awakening, a features of inflammatory arthropathy e.g. rheumatoid disease

Moro reflex A reflex of healthy newborn. When the surface on which infant lies is struck, there is rapid abduction and extension of arms followed by adduction (embrace reflex, startle reflex)

Morphea A circumscribed form of scleroderma presenting as a central atrophic lesion with a pigmented border occurring chiefly on the chest, face or neck.

Morphine The principal alkaloid of opium; white, crystaline, insoluble in water, alcohol and ether; potent narcotic analgesic, can cause respiratory depression. Repeated use causes physical dependence and addiction. Used as morphine sulfate or tartarate.

Morphogenesis The embryonic differentiation of cells leading to formation of characteristic structure or form of the organism or its parts.

Morphologic Relating to structure or form of organism.

Morphology 1. The study of configuration or structure of living organism. 2. The form or structure of an organism.

m. colonial The form of bacterial colony including such important features as size, shape, colour, surface, texture, opacity and friability.

Morquio's syndrome A form of mucopolysaccharidosis characterized by dwarfism, knock knee, pectus carinatum, flat vertebra, corneal clouding, deformed wrist and hands. There is excess excretion of keratin sulfate in urine and the disease is autosomal recessive, also called mucopolysaccharidosis IV.

Mors Latin for death.

Mortal Subject to death, deadly.

Mortality The quality of being mortal. The death rate.

m. neonatal Death during first month or four weeks of life.

m. perinatal The combined mortality from still births and deaths in first week of life.

m. reproductive The total mortality related to reproductive function, and associated diseases.

Morrhuate sodium The oily salt used as sclerosing agent and is injected into veins.

Mortification Gangrene or necrosis, death of a part.

Mortar A small receptacle in which substances are crushed or pulverized with a pestle.

Mortification Gangrene.

Morton's disease/syndrome Congenital short hypertrophied second metatarsal

Morton's neuralgia Pressure in lateral plantar nerve due to collapse of transverse plantar arch

Morton's neuroma A neuroma of inter metatarsal nerve

Mortuary A funeral home where bodies of deceased are prepared for cremation SYN— morgue.

Morula A cluster of cleaving blastomeres resulting from early division of zygote; a stage in the development of the embryo prior to the blastula.

Morulus The lesion characteristic of yaws, resembling a mulberry or raspberry.

Mosaic 1. In genetics an individual whose cells consist of at least two geno typically distinct populations that arose after fertilization through somatic mutation or somatic non-disjunction.

Mosaicism The state or situation of being mosaic.

m. chromosomal The state of being mosaic for a morphologic variation in karyotype.

m. erythrocyte The presence of two distinct populations of erythrocytes in the blood of one individual being not the result of blood transfusion or chimerism.

m. gonadal In genetics, the presence in a gonad of a germ cell line that is genotypically distinct from that comprising rest of individual.

Mosquito Blood sucking winged insects of family culicidae, responsible for transmission of malaria, dengue, etc.

Mother surrogate One who replaces an individual's mother in emotional feelings. A mother who bears offspring of another.

Motile Having capacity to move spontaneously.

Motion Movement.

Motion sickness A condition marked by nausea, dizziness, and often vomiting and headache, induced by some movement as in travel by aeroplane, train, bus or ship.

Motilin A gastrointestinal peptide of 22 amino acids located in enterochromaffin cells, chiefly of duodenum and upper jejunum that stimulates gastric and colonic motility.

Motility The capacity for spontaneous movement.

m. segmental Regularly spaced ring like contractions of small intestine.

Motivation An incentive to act or the reason for an attitude; an inner state of a person that serves to arouse, maintain and guide behavior towards a goal.

Motor Carrying or transmitting an impulse to a peripheral effector organ of the nervous system, either to elicit a response or to inhibit it 2. Producing movement.

Mottling 1. A condition marked by spotty coloration 2. Macular lesions of varying shades and hues.

Moulage The making of a mold of a bodily structure, especially for identification, prosthetics and teaching models.

Mount To prepare slides of tissues for microscopic examination.

Mound anal A small midline swelling in front of the anal opening of an embryo formed by union of anal tubercles.

Mountain sickness (Monge's disease) Rapid climbing to high attitude (>9000 ft.) causes headache and sleeplessness due to anoxia

Mounting A dental laboratory procedure in which a maxillary or mandibular cast is attached to an articulator.

Mouse A small rodent.

Mouse pox A viral disease of mice, also called ectromelia.

Mouse peritoneal A discrete, small calcific density seen in abdominal X-ray representing an appendix epiploica or a small piece of omentum which is twisted, necrosed and calcified.

Mouse pleural A round soft tissue density seen in chest X-ray representing a fibrin body in the pleural space.

Mouth The body opening through which one takes food.

m. tapir The characteristic pouting appearance of lips seen in facio scapulohumoral muscular dystrophy.

Mouth trench Necrotizing ulcerative gingivitis.

Mouthwash A solution for rinsing the mouth, having antibacterial, astringent or deodorant properties.

Movement 1. Change of place or position. 2. the act of defecation.

m. ameboid Locomotion of cells like leukocytes or amebas resulting from protoplasmic streaming into pseudopodia.

m. brownian Erratic motion of microscopic particles suspended in a liquid or gas resulting from collision with molecles in the suspending medium.

m. cardinal The six cardinal positions of eye.

m. ciliary Rhythmic movement of cilia of epithelial cell or protozoa.

m. circus The movement of an excitation wave, continuing uninterrupted around a ring of muscle or through the wall of the heart responsible for tachyarrhythmias.

m. dystonic Slow and often bizarre involuntary movement with alteration of posture.

m. Frenkel's A system of exercises used in the treatment of Parkinsonism and ataxia to increase precision and spontaneity of movement.

m. conjugate (of eyes) Movement of both eyes in one direction.

m. involuntary Involuntary contraction of one or more muscle groups producing movement of a limb or body part, e.g. tremor, chorea, athetosis, tics, myoclonus, dystonia and hemiballismus.

m. morphogenic The changes in position and displacement of cells and groups of cells, the folding and rearrangement of layers of cells and any alteration in position of structures or organs during development of an embryo.

m. passive Movement of body or any of its parts effected by an external force.

m. rapid eye (REM) The short quick movements of eyes during sleep which last from 5-60 minutes and associated with dreaming.

m. saccadic Rapid abrupt movement of eyes as occurs in changing fixation from one point to another.

m. streaming The characteristic movement of the protoplasm of certain white cells and unicellular organisms.

Moxa A small mass of combustible material placed near the skin and ignited to produce counter irritation.

Moxalactam A cephalosporin group antibiotic.

Moxibustion Counter irritation by means of a moxa.

Muciferous Secreting or producing mucus.

Mucilage In pharmacology, a thick viscous liquid, a water solution of the mucilaginous principles of certain vegetable substances.

Mucin A substance secreted by mucous membranes containing mucopolysaccharide which raises the viscosity of medium around it.

Mucinase Any of several enzymes that break down the mucin or glycosaminoglycan.

Mucinemia The presence of mucin in blood, often occurring in metastatic malignancies of GI tract or the ovaries.

Mucinosis An abnormal accumulation of mucopolysaccharides in the skin.

m. follicular An inflammatory disorder characterized by infiltrated cutaneous plaques with scaling and loss of hair. Histologically there is accumulation of mucopolysaccharides in the sebaceous glands and the outer root sheath of hair follicle.

Mucocele 1. An intrasinus cystarising from mucosal lining. 2. An enlarged cavity containing mucus. 3. Mucus polyp.

Mucocartilage Cartilaginous tissue with a soft mucoid matrix as found in central nucleus pulposus of the intervertebral disk.

Mucoclasis The surgical removal or destruction of the inner lining of any hollow organ.

Mucocyte An amorphous extracellular basophillic metachromatic mass averaging 100 µ found in white matter of normal and abnormal brains; probably artifactual, derived from precipitation of myelin during tissue fixation.

Mucocutaneous Relating to both mucous membrane and skin; especially the line of meeting of these two tissues in lips, nose, vaginal and anal orifices.

Mucocutaneous lymph node syndrome (Kawasaki disease) Condition affecting mainly infants and young children; marked by fever, conjuctivitis, reddening of oral cavity and lips, cervical lymphadenopathy, peeling of hands and feet. Coronary arteritis with infarction is a complication and aneurysms in coronary circulation may occur.

Mucoenteritis Inflammation of intestinal mucous membrane.

Mucoid Resembling mucus.

Mucolipidosis Any inborn error of metabolism that has characteristics of both mucopolysaccharidosis and sphyngolipidosis. 4 distinct types of disease known and are autosomal recessive.

Mucoperiosteum Periosteum having a mucous surface.

Mucopolysaccharidase Enzyme that catalyzes hydrolysis of polysaccharides.

Mucopolysaccharide Polysaccharide that forms chemical bonds with water. It is thick, gelatinous and forms intercellular ground subtance. It is found in mucous secretions and synovial fluid. *SYN* — Glycosaminoglycan.

Mucopolysaccharidosis (MPS) A group of inherited disorders with accumulation of mucopolysaccharides in reticuloendothelial system, intimal smooth muscle cells and fibroblasts within body; manifesting with coarse facies, mental retardation, corneal clouding, skeletal dysplasia, joint stiffness, etc.

MPS IH is known as Hurler syndrome. It is due to deficiency of the enzyme alpha-L-iduronidase with accumulation of heparan sulphate and dermatan sulphate.

MPS IS Scheie's syndrome. It is a variant of *MPS IH* but without mental retardation.

MPS IHS It is intermediate between MPS IH and MPS IS.

MPS II Hunter syndrome. It is due to deficiency of L-iduronosulphate sulphatase. Unlike *MPS IH* there is no corneal clouding.

MPS III Sanfilippo syndrome. Corneal clouding is absent and skeletal growth is normal.

MPS IV Morquio's syndrome The deficient enzyme is N-acetyl galactosamine-6-sulphatase. Distinguishing features, are dwarfism, kyphoscoliosis, cardiac lesions and joint hypermobility.

MPS VI Maroteaux Lamy syndrome. Deficient enzyme is N-acetyl galactosamine-4-sulphatase. Clinically it is similar to *MPS IH* but there is no mental retardation.

MPS VII The deficient enzyme is beta-glucoronidase.

Mucoprotein A complex of protein and mucopolysaccharide.

m. Tamm-Horsfall It is secreted in renal tubules (not from plasma) and is contained in most urinary casts.

Mucopurulent A mixture of mucus and pus.

Mucor A genus of fungi seen on dead or decaying matter; often causes infection of external ear, skin and respiratory passage.

Mucosa A mucous membrane with epithelial lining, basement membrane, and often lamina propria. It may contain goblet cells, may be keratinized and the covering epithelium may be stratified squamous, columnar or pseudo stratified columnar depending upon location.

Mucosin Mucin found in thick sticky mucus.

Mucositis Inflammation of mucous membrane.

Mucous colitis *SYN* — irritable bowel syndrome.

Mucoviscidosis *SYN* — cystic fibrosis.

Mucus A viscid secretion containing mucin, leukocytes, epithelial cells, etc. secreted by mucous membrane.

Muller Heinrich German anatomist.

M.'s muscle 1. Circular fibers of ciliary muscles. 2. Superior tarsal muscle of eyelid.

M's trigone Portion of tuber cinereum folding over optic chiasm.

Multi Prefixe indicating many or much.

Multifactorial The result of many factors.

Multifocal Concerning many foci or locations.

Multiform Having many forms. *SYN— Polymorphic.*

Multigravida A woman who has been pregnant two or more times. *SYN —multipara.*

Multinodular Containing many nodules.

Multiparity Condition of having borne more than one child.

Multiple endocrine neoplasia (MEN) An inherited disease involving hyperplasia/malignancy of multiple endocrine glands.

MEN I *SYN —Wermer's Syndrome* Tumors of parathyroids, pancreatic islets and adrenal cortex.

MEN II Pheochromocytoma, parathyroid hyperplasia, medullary carcinoma thyroid.

Multiple personality Condition in which the subject may develop more than one personality.

Multiple sclerosis (MS) An autoimmune demyelinating disorder due to decrease in suppressor T lymphocyte function, manifesting with visual loss, gait disorder, motor dysfunction and bladder bowel disturbance. Multiple sites of involvement in brain and spinal cord common.

Mummification Drying and shrivelling of body; mortification producing a dry hard mass.

Mumps A febrile viral disease characterized by inflammation of salivary and parotid glands.

Munchausen syndrome A psychiatric disorder in which patient feigns illness by self-mutilation.

Muramidase *SYN*—lysozyme. An enzyme richly present in leukocytes. Level increased in leukemias.

Murmur A soft blowing or rasping sound heard during cardiac auscultation; produced due to excess blood flow through normal valves or normal flow through diseased valves.

m. Austin Flint A mid or late mitral diastolic murmur heard in aortic regurgitation due to partial closure of mitral valve due to aortic regurgitant jet.

m. Carey Coomb Diastolic murmur of mitral valvulitis in rheumatic fever.

m. Cruveilhier Murmur heard in abdominal wall due to portosystemic shunting.

m. Durozeiz Systolic and diastolic murmurs heard over femoral artery in aortic insufficiency.

m. Gibson Continuous machinary murmur of patent ductus arteriosus.

m. Graham Steell's Early diastolic murmur of pulmonary insufficiency in pulmonary hypertension.

m. Still's Benign functional midsystolic murmur of children.

Murphy's sign Pain and catch in right hypochondrium to pressure during deep inspiration in acute cholecystitis.

Musca domestica The common house fly transmitting cholera, typhoid, amebic/bacillary dysentery, and other diseases.

Muscae volitantes Black floaters in visual field due to vitreous opacities.

Muscarine A toxic poison found in fungi.

Muscle Contractile tissue of mesodermal origin with properties like irritability, conductivity, and elasticity. Can be smooth, striated and cardiac. Smooth muscles (involuntary muscle) are found to line GI tract, bronchi, urinary and genital ducts, gall bladder, urinary bladder. The cells are fusiform or spindle-shaped with one central nucleus. Striated (skeletal) muscles are under conscious control. The muscle fibers are grouped into bundles called fasciculi and each cell or fiber has multiple nuclei. Denervation causes complete

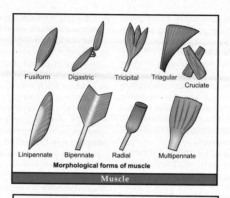

Morphological forms of muscle

Muscle

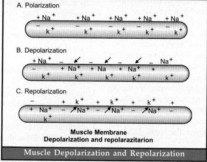

A. Polarization

B. Depolarization

C. Repolarization

Muscle Membrane
Depolarization and repolarazitarion

Muscle Depolarization and Repolarization

paralysis of striated muscle but not of cardiac or smooth muscle.

m.'s antigravity Muscles that pull the skeleton against force of gravity to maintain erect posture.

m.s articular Muscles attached to capsule of a joint.

m. axial Muscle of head and trunk.

m. extrinsic Muscle whose origin is outside the part it moves.

m. intrinsic Muscle having its origin and insertion within the same structure, e.g. tongue, eye, limb.

m. papillary Muscle within ventricle of heart from which arise the chordae tendinae.

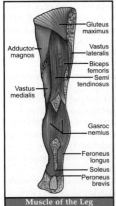

Muscle of the Leg

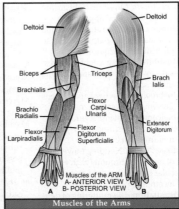

Muscles of the Arms

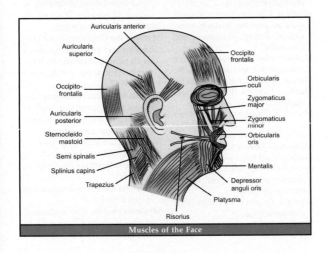

Muscles of the Face

m. pectinate Muscle in right atrium giving it a ridged appearance.

Muscle cramp Painful contraction of muscle, idiopathic or due to electrolyte imbalance.

Mushbite Making a dental impression by asking the patient to bite into a soft wax.

Mushroom Umbrella-shaped fungus growing on decaying material.

Musicomania Intense love for music.

Musk Oily perfumed secretion of male musk deer.

Musset's sign Nodding movement of head synchronous with ventricular contraction as in gross aortic incompetence.

Mussitation The muttering of delirium or moving of the lips without production of sound.

Mustard Powder of mustard seeds used as counter-irritant, rubefacient, emetic, stimulant, and condiment.

Mutagen Any agent that causes gene mutation, e.g. ionizing radiation.

Mutant A variant of genetic structure.

Mutase Enzyme that accelerates oxidation-reduction reactions.

Mutation Change in genetic structure; can be natural or induced by drugs, chemicals and radiation.

Mutilation Destruction, maiming.

Mutism Unable to speak.

m. akinetic Condition in which patient can neither speak nor can move body parts.

Myalgia Pain in the muscles often with tenderness.

Myasis Infestation with larva of flies or maggots.

Myasthenia Weakness of muscles.

m. gravis An autoimmune disease with extreme muscle weakness due to presence of acetyl choline receptor antibodies.

Mycetes The fungi.

Mycetism Poisoning from eating fungi.

Mycetoma A suppurative condition due to actinomycetes and fungi.

Mycobacterium A genus of acid-fast organism causing leprosy and tuberculosis. They are grampositive, nonsporeforming and non motile rods.

m. atypical Forms of mycobacteria causing mild but resistant form of tuberculosis in man. They are *M. avium-intracellular, M. kansasii, M. chelonei, M. marinum, M. xenopi,* etc.

Mycology Science of fungi.

Mycoplasma Organisms in between bacteria and viruses, responsible for atypical pneumonia, urethritis; common forms are — *M. hominis, M. orale, M. salivarium.*

Mycosis fungoides A malignant disease of RE system of skin, with intense itching and lymph node and internal organ involvement.

Mydriasis Dilatation of pupils.

Mydriatic Drug/agent causing pupillary dilatation, e.g. atropine, belladona.

Myelatelia Defective development of spinal cord.

Myelencephalon The embryonic hindbrain giving rise to medulla oblongata.

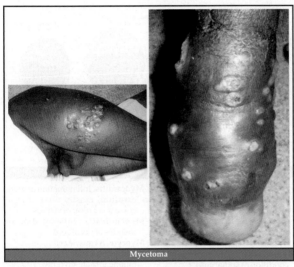

Mycetoma

Myelin The complex lipid-protein sheath around axons in nervous system.

Myelinosis Fatty degeneration during which myelin is produced.

Myelitis Inflammation of spinal cord.

Myeloblast Immature white cell precursor of marrow from which develop myelocytes and eventually granulocytes.

Myelocele Protrusion of spinal cord through a defect in spinal arch — usually spina bifida.

Myelocyte A leuckocyte precursor in bone marrow.

Myelo diastasis Destruction and disintegration of spinal cord.

Myelofibrosis A condition where bone marrow is replaced by fibrous tissue.

Myelogram 1. X-ray of spinal canal after injection of radiopaque material into spinal sub-arachnoid space. 2. Differential count of bone marrow cells.

Myelolysis Dissolution of myelin.

Myeloma A tumor originating from marrow element.

m. multiple A plasma cell tumor with multiple lytic bone lesions and increased paraprotein in blood and urine.

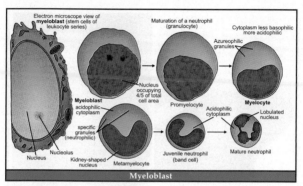

Electron microscope view of **myeloblast** (stem cells of leukocyte series)

Maturation of a neutrophil (granulocyte)

Cytoplasm less basophilic more acidophilic

Azureophilic granules

Nucleus occupying 4/5 of total cell area

Myeloblast acidophilic cytoplasm

Promyelocyte

Acidophilic cytoplasm

Myelocyte

Lobulated nucleus

specific granules (neutrophilic)

Nucleolus

Nucleus

Kidney-shaped nucleus

Metamyelocyte

Juvenile neutrophil (band cell)

Mature neutrophil

Myeloblast

Myelomalacia Abnormal softening of spinal cord.

Myelomeningocele A condition where spinal cord along with meningeal covering protrudes through the spinal defect.

Myelopathy Any pathological condition of spinal cord.

Myelopoiesis Development of bone marrow.

Myeloproliferative Concerning proliferation of bone marrow elements.

Myeloradiculitis Inflammation of spinal cord and nerve roots.

Myenteric reflex Intestinal contraction above and relaxation below the point of stimulatioin.

Myerson's sign Inability to stop blinking on tapping the forehead as in Parkinson's disease.

Myoblast Embryonic cell developing into muscle fiber.

Myocardial infarction Death of myocardium usually due to coronary thrombosis or spasm.

Myocarditis Inflammation of myocardium, mostly viral, due to coxsackie group of viruses.

Myochorditis Inflammation of muscles of vocal cord.

Myocyte A muscle cell.

Myodynamometer Device for determining muscle strength.

Myoepithelial cells Spindle-shaped contractile cells found between glandular elements and basement membrane of sweat, mammary and salivary glands.

Myoepithelium Tissue containing contractile epithelial cells.

Myofilament Electron microscopic picture of muscle showing thick *myosin* and thin *actin* filaments, essential for muscle contraction.

Myoglobin The respiratory pigment in muscle tissue that serves as oxygen carrier.

Myograph Instrument for graphic recording of muscle contraction.

Myoma A tumor containing muscle tissue.

Myonectomy Removal of myomatous tumor, generally of uterus.

Myometrium The muscular layer of uterus.

Myonecrosis Death of muscle tissue.

Myopathy Any disease or abnormal condition of striated muscle; may be an acquired or hereditary.

Myope One suffering from myopia or short sightedness.

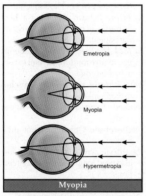

Emetropia

Myopia

Hypermetropia

Myopia

Myopia Short sightedness, the parallel rays passing through optical axis are focussed in front of retina. Can be axial (elongation of eye ball), curvature or lenticular types. Corrected by use of minus lens.

Myoplasm The contractile part of the muscle cell.

Myorrhaphy Suture of a muscle wound.

Myosin The contractile protein of myofibrils constituting about 65%

of muscle prbteins. Myosinogen is the precursor of myosin.

Myositis Inflammation of striated muscle.

m. ossificans Calcification and osteoblastic invasion of muscle hematoma, commonly after supracondylar fracture of elbow.

Myotonia Tonic spasm of a muscle.

m. congenita SYN — Thomsen's disease. A hereditary disease with tonic spasm of muscle induced by voluntary movements.

m. dystrophica Hereditary disease characterized by myotonia, muscle atrophy and cataract.

Myringa The tympanic membrane.

Myringitis Inflammation of tympanic membrane.

Myringoplasty Plastic surgery of tympanic membrane usually for closure of perforation.

Myringotomy Incision of tympanic membrane as to relieve pain in acute otitis media.

Mythophobia Abnormal fear of making an incorrect statement.

Myxedema A condition resulting from hypofunction of thyroid; commonly autoimmune or due to iodine lack, dyshormonogenesis.

Myxoma Tumor composed of mucous connective tissue similar to that present in embryo or umbilical cord. It is soft, gray, lobulated, translucent and incompletely encapsulated.

Myxovirus Family of viruses, the common member being influenza virus.

N

Nabothian cyst Retention cysts of the nabothian glands in the cervical canal, usually associated with ectropion.

Nadolol A beta-blocker, used in hypertension.

Naegele German obstetrician (1777-1851).

n. obliquity Anterior parietal presentation of fetal head in labor.

n. pelvis An obliquely contracted pelvis.

n. rule The method of counting expected date of delivery by counting 90 days backwards from LMP and adding 7 days to that date.

Nafcillin A semisynthetic penicillinase resistant penicillin.

Nafoxidin Antiestrogen.

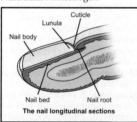

The nail longitudinal sections

Nail

Nail A modified epidermal structure forming flat plate on dorsal aspect of terminal phallanx.

n. eggshell A condition in which the nail plate is soft and semi-transparent, bends easily and splits at the end, a feature of leprosy, hemiplegia.

n. hang Broken epidermis at the edge of nail.

n. ingrown Growth of nail edge into the soft tissue.

n. intermedullary Surgical rod inserted into the intermedullary canal to fix the fracture.

n. Smith-Peterson A three flanged nail used to fix fracture neck of femur.

n. spoon Nail with depressed centre and raised borders, feature of iron deficiency *SYN* — koilonychia.

n. biting A form of neurosis where free edge of nail is bitten down by the patient.

n. fold The groove in the cutaneous tissue surrounding the nail except at its free edge.

nail-patella syndrome Onychoosteodysplasia.

Naked Exposed to view; without cloth.

Nalbuphine Opioid receptor antagonist.

Nalidixic acid Urinary antibiotic; also used for gastrointestinal infections.

Nalorphine Narcotic antagonist.

Naloxone Narcotic antagonist.

Naltrexone Narcotic antagonist.

Nandrolone decanoate Anabolic steroid.

Nanism Dwarf like body build.

Nano - 10^{-9} or one billionth part.

Nap Short sleep.

Nape Back of neck.

Naphazoline hydrochloride Topical vasoconstrictor, ingredient of nasal and eye drops.

Naphthalene A coaltar derivative, used as antimoth agent.

Narcissism Sexual pleasure sought by observing one's own naked body; self-admiration.

Narcoanalysis A form of psychotherapy where the subconscious is exposed after light anesthesia.

Narcolepsy Recurrent attacks of uncontrollable desire to sleep but easily awakenable.

Narcotic An agent that in moderate doses relieves pain but in higher doses causes coma and respiratory paralysis.

Narcotism State of stupor induced by a narcotic.

Nasal feeding Feeding through a tube passing through nose.

Nasal index The greater width of nasal aperture in relation to a line from the lower edge of nasal aperture to the nasion.

Nasal reflex Inducible sneezing from irritation of nasal mucosa.

Nascent Just born, beginning; substance being set free from a compound.

Nasion The point where sagittal plane intersects frontonasal suture (root of nose).

Nasmyth's membrane Epithelial membrane that envelops the enamel of a tooth after birth.

Nasogastric tube Tube inserted through nose into the stomach for feeding or stomach wash.

Nasomental reflex Percussion on side of nose causing contraction of mentalis muscle with elevation of lower lip and wrinkling of skin of the chin.

Nasopharynx Part of pharynx situated above the level of soft palate.

Natal Relating to birth.

Natamycin Topical antibiotic.

Nates Gluteal region *SYN* — buttocks.

Native Born with, inherent.

Natriuresis Excess excretion of sodium in urine.

Natural killer cells Large T-lymphocytes that bind to cells infected with viruses and kill them and often kill tumor cells; the most natural defence against tumor/viral infection.

Naturopathy A therapeutic system that employs natural forces as light, heat, air and water to cure ailments rather than drugs.

Nausea Unpleasant epigastric sensation preceding vomiting.

n. gravidarum Morning sickness of pregnancy.

Nauseant Provoking nausea.

Navel The depressed scar in the center of abdomen *SYN* — umbilicus.

Navicular Shaped like a boat.

Near death experience The feeling of an after life while coming close to death.

Near drowning The survival in an immersion incident that could have been fatal

Near point Closest point of near vision with maximum accommodation. It is 3" at 2 yrs and recedes to 40" at 60 years.

Nearsighted Only able to see clearly the near objects; *SYN*—myopia, corrected by concave lens.

Nebula Very thin scar on cornea.

Nebulizer An apparatus for producing fine spray or mist.

Necator A genus of nematode hookworms, includes *N. americanus.*

Neck That part of body lying between shoulders and the head.

n. femoral The thick compact portion of femur joining head with the shaft.

n. of mandible The narrow area below the articular condyle where are attached the lateral pterygoid muscle and the articular capsule.

n. surgical of humerus The narrowed portion of humerus below the tuberosity; more prone for fracture.

n. wry SYN — torticollis; muscle contraction involving sternocleidomastoid, the neck rotated to opposite side.

Necklace of Casal Ring of pigmented reddened skin around the neck in pellagra.

Necrobiosis Degeneration and swelling of collagen in the dermis, common to diabetics.

Necromimesis A delusion in which one believes to be dead.

Necrophilia Sexual intercourse with dead; abnormal interest in corpses.

Necrosis Death of tissue following cut-off in blood supply, physical or chemical injury, infection, etc.

n. coagulation Necrosis where the necrosed area is converted to a homogeneous mass.

Necrotizing Causing necrosis.

Needle A pointed instrument for stitching, puncture or ligature; can be straight, curved, double curved or sigmoid

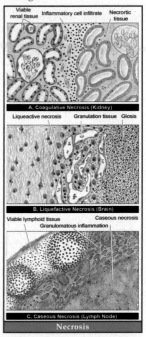

A, Coagulative Necrosis (Kidney)

Viable renal tissue — Inflammatory cell infiltrate — Necrortic tissue

B, Liquefactive Necrosis (Brain)

Liqueactive necrosis — Granulation tissue — Gliosis

C, Caseous Necrosis (Lymph Node)

Viable lymphoid tissue — Caseous necrosis — Granulomatous inflammation

Necrosis

n. atraumatic a needle of smaller diameter than the suture material

Negativism Behavioral disorder in which patient does opposite to suggested action or does not do it at all, a sign of dementia.

Negri bodies Aggregations in nerve cells as in rabies.

Neisseria Gram -negative bacteria, lie in pairs, e.g. *N. gonorrhoeae, N. meningitidis, N sicca* and N. *catarrhalis* (last two cause respiratory infection and often endocarditis).

Nelton's line Line from anterior superior iliac spine to tuberosity of ischium.

Nematoda Spindle shaped or rounded worms.

Neocerebellum The posterior lobe of cerebellum that develops last and is concerned with integrations of voluntary movements.

Neodymium A silvery rare earth metal used in LASER.

Neogenesis Regeneration of tissue.

Neologism A new work or phrase or a new meaning put to an old work/phrase; a feature of mental diseases.

Neomycin An aminoglycoside antibiotic isolated from streptomyces, toxic to kidney and eighth cranial nerve but effective against many gram +ve and -ve bacteria, particularly resistant tubercle bacilli.

Neon A rare inert gas.

Neonate First six weeks after birth.

Neoplasia The development of neoplasms.

Neoplasm A tumor or new growth.

n. benign Growth having a definite capsule and non-infiltrating.

n. malignant Growth that lacks a capsule, infiltrates surrounding structures or has distant metastasis, or recurs after surgery.

n. organoid Neoplasm resembling some organ in its structure.

Neostigmine Cholinergic drug used for myasthenia; bromide and methyl sulfate salts are used.

Neostriatum Caudate nucleus and putamen together.

Neothalamus The lateral and dorsomedial parts of thalamus.

Nephrectomy Removal of kidneys.

Nephritis Inflammation of kidneys involving glomeruli, tubules and interstitial tissue singly or combinedly, can be acute/chronic; interstitial, salt losing (Chrohn's syndrome).

Nephritogenic Causing nephritis.

Nephrocalcinosis Deposit of calcium in renal tubules.

Nephroid Resembling kidney.

Nephromere The intermediate mesoderm of embryo from which kidney develops.

Nephropathy Any diseased condition of kidney including inflammatory, degenerative, arteriosclerotic lesions, e.g. analgesic nephropathy, hypokalemic nephropathy, membranous nephropathy, etc.

Nephropexy Surgical fixation of mobile kidney.

Nephroptosis Downward displacement of kidney.

Nephrosclerosis Arteriosclerosis of kidney vessels resulting in ischaemic atrophy and fibrosis of kidney.

Nephrosis Non-inflammatory degenerative disease of kidney, e.g. lipoid nephrosis manifesting as nephrotic syndrome.

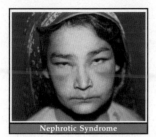

Nephrotic Syndrome

Nephrotic syndrome A symptom complex with leakage of protein in urine due to damage to capillary wall of glomeruli.

Nephrotomography Tomography of kidney after injection of radiopaque dye to opacity the kidneys.

Nerve Bundles of nerve fibers connecting CNS or spinal cord with various parts of body.

n. adrenergic Sympathetic nerves that liberate noradrenaline at the neuro effector synapse.

n. afferent Any nerve that transmits impulses from periphery towards centre.

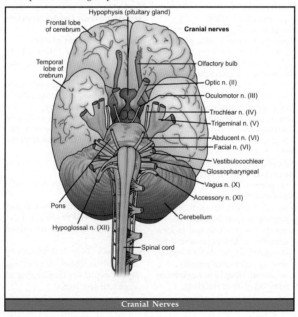

Cranial Nerves

n. cholinergic Parasympathetic nerve liberating acetylcholine for impulse transmission.

n. cranial Nerves emerging directly from brain stem.

n. efferent Nerves that transmit impulses from center towards periphery.

n. mixed Nerve contains both motor (efferent) and sensory (afferent) fibers.

n. secretory Nerve that stimulates secretion from glands.

n. spinal 31 pairs of peripheral nerves, 8 cervical, 12 thoracic, 5 lumbar, 5 sacral, 1 coccygeal.

Nerve gas Gaseous material (usually organophosphorus compound aerosolized) used in war that also penetrates through the skin, protection is by gas mask and charcoal lined suits.

Nerve growth factor A protein necessary for growth and maintenance of certain nerves.

Netilmicin Amino glycoside antibiotic.

Neural crest A band of cells along the neural tube of embryo from which cells forming cranial, spinal and autonomic ganglia arise.

Neural fold One of two longitudinal elevations of the neural plate of embryo that unite to form the neural tube.

Neuralgia Sharp pain along the course of nerve.

n. geniculate Neuralgia characterized by pain in distribution of facial nerves.

n. glossopharyngeal Severe pain in the back of throat, tonsils and middle ear along the distribution of glossopharyngeal nerve.

n. Morton's Neuralgic pain of third and fourth metatarsal.

n. occipital Neuralgia involving upper cervical nerves.

n. trigeminal Neuralgia involving the gasserian ganglion or one or more branches of trigeminal nerve.

Neural plate A thickened band of ectoderm along the dorsal surface of an embryo.

Neural tube Tube formed from fusion of neural folds.

Neural tube defect Defective closure of neural tube during embryogenesis leading to defects like spina bifida, anencephaly, meningocele, meningomyelocele.

Neurasthenia Psychiatric illness with unexplained chronic fatigue and lassitude.

Neurilemma The schwann cell sheath around myelin in peripheral nervous system that contributes to regeneration of nerve fibers by producing growth factors and serving as a tunnel for growth of nerves fiber.

Neurilemmoma A firm encapsulated fibrillar tumor of peripheral nerve

Neurinoma A peripheral glioma arising from endoneurium.

Neuritis Inflammation of nerve; inflammatory or degenerative.

Neuroblastoma A malignant tumor of neuroblasts in children giving rise to cells of sympathetic nervous system; especially adrenal medulla.

Neurocirculatory asthenia Functional circulatory and nervous disturbance with precordial pain and fatigue.

Neurodermatitis Cutaneous inflammation with itching mostly due to emotional disturbances.

Neuroepithelium Specialized epithelial structure forming the gustatory cells, olfactory cells, hair cells of inner ear, rods and cones of retina.

Neurofibril Tiny fibrils in the cytoplasm of nerve cell body.

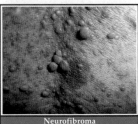
Neurofibroma

Neurofibroma Tumor of connective tissue around nerve.

Neurogenesis Growth and development of nerve tissues.

Neurogenic Originating from nervous tissue or happening due to nervous dysfunction.

Neuroglia Supporting tissue of nervous system, includes astrocytes, microglia, Schwann cells, satelite cells, ependyma, etc. All except microglia are of ectodermal origin.

Neurohypophysis Posterior lobe of pituitary secreting oxytocin and vasopressin.

Neurokeratin The type of keratin found in myelinated nerve fibers.

Neuroleptic Synonymous with antipsychotic.

Neuroleptic malignant syndrome Catatonic rigidity, stupor, sweating and hypertheremia occurring with use of astipsychotic agents

Neurolysis Stretching of a nerve to relieve tension; release of a nerve from fibrous tissue.

Neuroma cells Any tumor composed of nerve.

Neuromatosis Multiple tumors of nerve tissue.

Neuromyesthenia Muscular weakness consequent to emotional disorder.

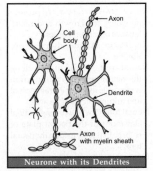
Neurone with its Dendrites

Neurone A nerve cell; consisting of cell body and its processes, i.e. axons and dendrites.

n. afferent Neurone conducting impulses to the brain and spinal cord.

n. associative Neurone coordinating impulses between sensory and motor neurons.

n. efferent Neurones conducting impulses away from brain and spinal cord.

n. lower motor Neurone with cell body in anterior gray column.

n. upper motor Neurone with cell body in motor cortex.

n. preganglionic Neurone of autonomic nervous system whose cell body lies in central nervous system and axon terminates in peripheral ganglia.

n. postganglionic Neurone whose cell body lies in an autonomic ganglion and its axon terminates in effector organ.

Neuronitis Inflammation of nerve cell.

Neuropathy Any disease of nerves.

n. entrapment Nerve inflammation secondary to entrapment in a closed constricting space, e.g. median nerve in carpal tunnel of wrist.

n. hypertrophic Inflammation with thicking of nerves as in Refsum disease.

Neurophysin Proteins that bind oxytocin and ADH, secreted by posterior pituitary.

Neuropraxia Trauma to a nerve followed by loss of conduction even though anatomical integrity is maintained.

Neuroradiology Branch of medical science utilizing radiography for diagnosis of neurological diseases.

Neurosis A minor mental disease where person's insight is maintained.

n. anxiety Neurosis where vague anxiety or apprehension interferes with effective functioning.

n. obsessional Neurosis where obsession dominates.

Neurosyphilis Syphilis affecting the nervous system.

n. meningovascular The meninges and the cerebral blood vessels are affected the most with ischemia, infarction, hydrocephalus.

Neurotensin Tridecapeptide from hypophysis stimulating pituitary.

Neurotic Person suffering from neurosis.

Neurotmesis Nerve injury with complete loss of function in absence of anatomical disruption.

Neurotransmitter Chemical substance released by stimulation of presynaptic neurone that excites or inhibits target cell, e.g. acetyl choline, dopamine, norepinephrine.

Neutral Neither alkaline nor acidic, indifferent.

Neutralization The process of counteracting the effects of any harmful agent/substance.

Neutral point A pH of 7.0 which is neither acid nor alkaline.

Neutral red An indicator dye.

Neutron Electrically neutral particle equal in mass to proton.

Neutrophil A leukocyte staining easily with neutral dyes.

Nevus Congenitally discolored localized area of skin; vascular skin tumor due to hyperplastic blood vessels.

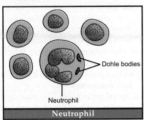

Neutrophil

n. junctional Nevus in the basal layer of epidermis appearing as nonhairy pigmented area, with high malignancy potential.

Niacin Nicotinic acid used for pellagra.

Niche A depression or recess on a smooth surface, e.g. ulcer niche.

Nicking Compression of retinal vein at the site crossed by artery.

Niclosamide Anthelmintic.

Nicotinamide adenine diphosphate (NADP) An enzyme that accepts electrons.

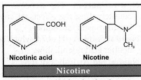

Nicotinic acid   Nicotine

Nicotine

Nicotine Alkaloid of tobacco, a vasoconstrictor, stimulant and addictive agent.

Nidus Focus of infection, nest like structure.

Niemann-Pick disease A disturbance of sphingolipid metabolism characterized by hepatosplenomegaly, lymphadenopathy and mental deterioration.

Nifedipine Calcium channel blocker.

Nightblindness (nyctalopia) Inability to see in dark due to deficient rhodopsin or its slow regeneration after exposure to light, a feature of retinal pigmentary degeneration or vitamin A deficiency.

Nightmare A bad dream accompanied by fear.

Night sweat Profuse sweating during night sleep, e.g. diabetes, with hypoglycemia due to excess insulin, chronic debilitating diseases (tuberculosis), rickets.

Nigrostrial Bundle of nerve fiber connecting corpus striatum with substantia nigra.

Nihilism A delusion in which everything in unreal or does not exist

Nikethamide Respiratory and CNS stimulant.

Nikolsky's sign Spreading of a pemphigus bleb by application of mild pressure due to easy epidermal separation.

Nimodipine Calcium channel blocker.

Nipple The conical protruberance at center of breast containing erectile tissue and pierced by milk ducts.

Niridazole Anthelmintic used for guinea worm and schistosomiasis.

Nissl bodies Chromophil granules in cell bodies and dendrites of neurones composed of RNA.

Nit Egg of louse or any parasitic insect.

Nitazoxanide A drug used in treatment of amoebiasis

Nitrate Salt of nitric acid.

Nitrazepam Benzodiazepine, anxiolytic.

Nitrendipine Calcium channel blocker.

Nitric oxide A vasodilator gas produced by vascular endothelium. It also inhibits aggregation, activation and adhsion of platelets

Nitrite Salt of nitrous acid, an antispasmodic and smooth muscle dilator.

Nitroblue tetrazolium test A test of ability of leukocytes to transform nitroblue tetrazolium from a colorless state to deep blue, a test of leukocyte bacterial killing ability.

Nitrofurantoin Urinary antibacterial agent.

Nitrofurazone Topically used antibacterial agent.

Nitrogen mustards Antilymphoid agents used in treating lympho-sarcoma, rheumatoid arthritis, leukemia, nephritis. Agents in this group are cyclophosphamide, mechlor ethamine, melphalan and chlorambucil.

Nitrogen balance The difference between the amount of nitrogen ingested and excreted per day.

Nitrogen narcosis Increased nitrogen concentration in body tissues with euphoria, impaired motor ability and co-ordination as in divers and submarine troops.

Nitroglycerin Any nitrate of glycerol used for vasodilatation in angina pectoris as 2% ointment or tablets; be kept in tinted glass (not plastic) container without cotton plug.

Nitromersol Topically used mercurial antiseptic.

Nitrous oxide Inhalation anesthetic used in conjuction with oxygen *SYN* — laughing gas.

Nocardiasis Infection with gram-positive aerobic bacteria (often acid fast to be confused with tubercle bacillus), causing pulmonary infection or foot infection (madura-mycosis).

Nociceptive reflex Reflex initiated by painful stimuli.

Nocturia Urination at night.

Nocturnal emission Involuntary semen discharge during sleep.

Nocturnal penile tumescence Penile erection during sleep, a normal phenomenon, when present excludes organic causes of impotency.

Nodal points A pair of points situated on the axis of optical system.

Nodal rhythm Cardiac rhythm originating at AV node.

Nodding Falling forward of the head.

Node A small swelling or constriction.

n. AV The mass of Purkinje fibers at lower end of interatrial septum giving origin to bundle of His.

n. Bouchard's Bony enlargement of proximal interphallangeal joint in osteoarthritis.

n. Heberden's Nodes in terminal interphallangeal joints of hand in osteoarthritis.

n's of Ranvier Constriction of myelin sheath along the course of medulated nerve fiber.

n's Osler Tender nodes in pulp of finger and toes in subacute bacterial endocarditis.

n's of Parrot Osteophytes around anterior fontanel in congenital syphilis.

n. Schmorl's Prolapse of nucleus pulposus into vertebral body.

n. Singer's Small white nodes on vocal cords due to vocal abuse.

n. Sinoatrial Node in the wall of right atrium near entry of SVC acting as the pacemaker of heart.

Nodule A small node; collection of cells.

n. Aschoffs Myocardial nodule with central fibrinoid necrosis with surrounding epithelioid cells, a feature of rheumatic carditis.

Noma (cancrum oris) A gangrenous infection spreading from mucus membrane of mouth to skin in under nourished children

Nomogram Representation by graphs, diagrams or charts of the relationship between numerical variables

Non compos mentis Mentally incompetent

Nonoxynol A spermicide.

Noonan's syndrome Congenital pulmonary stenosis with skeletal abnormalities.

Norepinephrinc Vasopressor hormone secreted by adrenal medulla.

Norethandrolone An anabolic steroid.

Norethindrone Progestational agent.

Norfloxacin A quinolone with broad spectrum antibacterial activity.

Norgestrel A progestational agent.

Normetanephrine A metabolite of epinephrine.

Normoblast Type of nucleated red blood cell during erythropoisis.

Normochromasia Normal staining capacity of tissue.

Normocyte Averaged size RBC.

Normosthenuria Urine of normal amount and specific gravity.

Normotensive Normal blood pressure.

Norplant Levonogestrel implant for contraception

n. see saw nystagmus in which the interning eye moves up and the opposite eye moves down

Norrie's disease Sex linked blindness with retinal malformation, vitreous opacity, often with hearing loss and mental retardation.

Nortryptyline Tricyclic antidepressant.

Norwalk agent A virus implicated in gastroenteritis.

Noscapine Antitussive opium alkaloid.

Nose The organ of olfaction, also warms, moistens and filters the air. Orifices of frontal, anterior ethmoid and maxillary sinuses open into middle meatus while posterior, ethmoid and sphenoid sinuses open into superior meatus.

Nosocomial Hospital acquired infection.

Nosology The science of classification of diseases.

Nosophilia An abnormal desire to be ill.

Nostalgia Homesickness.

Notch Depression, narrow gap.

n. acetabular Notch on the inferior border of acetabulum.

n. aortic Notch of aortic valve closure in pulse tracing.

n. sciatic Two in number, greater and lesser sciatic notches on hip bone.

Notifiable disease All communicable and contagious diseases to be notified to local health authorities under the starutes of law.

Notochord The axial skeleton of embryo, its remnant in adult is nucleus pulposus of intervertebral disk.

Novocain Procaine hydrochloride.

Noxious Harmful.

NREM sleep Nonrapid eye movement sleep.

Nuck's canal A peritoneal pouch extending into labium in female, homologous to processus vaginalis of male.

Nuclear antigen Antigenicity of nuclear materials in some connective tissue disorders.

Nuclear magnetic resonance When certain atomic nuclei with odd number of protons or neutrons or both are subjected to strong magnetic field they absorb and reemit electromagnetic energy. Application of a radio frequency pulse causes deflection in the net magnetization vector and image production. The technique is useful for imaging of brain, soft tissue and heart.

Nuclear medicine Medicine dealing with diagnostic, therapeutic and investigative aspects of radionuclides.

Nucleic acid A complex product consisting of pentose, phosphoric acid, purines and pyrimidines.

Nucleolus A spherical body within the nucleus.

Nucleoprotein Combination of nucleic acid with protein found in cell nuclei.

Nucleoside Glycoside formed by union of pentose sugar with purine or pyrimidine.

Nucleotide Compound containing phosphoric acid, pentose sugar and purine/pyrimidine.

Nucleosidase Enzyme causing hydrolysis of nucleoside.

Nucleus The central vital portion in a cell which controls metabolism, reproduction and transmission of cell characteristic.

n. ambiguous Nucleus of 9th and 10th cranial nerves in the medulla.

n. caudate The comma shaped constituent of basal ganglia.

n. cuneate Nucleus in lower medulla in which end the fibers of fasciculus cuneatus.

n. Deiters Lateral vestibular nucleus.

n. Dentate The large nucleus in lateral part of cerebellar lobe giving rise to fibers of superior cerebellar peduncle.

n. Edinger Westphal Nucleus in midbrain giving rise to parasympathetic fibers to innervate cilliary muscles and sphincter iris.

n. emboliform Nucleus in cerebellum lying in between dentate and globose nuclei.

n. fastigial Nucleus in medullary portion of cerebellum.

n. gracilis Nucleus in lower portion of medulla where fibers of fasciculus gracilis terminate.

n. habenular Nucleus in diencephalon functioning as olfactory correlation center.

n. pulposus The central gelatinous remnant of notocord in intervertebral disks.

Null hypothesis The hypothesis that the observed difference between two groups of patients studied is accidental.

Nullipara A woman who has not produced a viable child.

Numb Dead, insensible.

Numular Shaped like a coin.

Nurse Person providing health care.

Nursery Newborn care center.

Nutrient Food constituents supplying body with essential elements of metabolism.

Nutriment Nutritious substance.

Nutrition The process involved in assimilation and utilization of food.

Nutritious Providing nutrition.

Nux vomica Poisonous seed containing strychnine.

Nyctalopia Night blindness as seen in avitaminosis A and retinitis pigmentosa.

Nyctamblyopia Poor night vision without any other eye changes.

Nyctaphonia Hysterical loss of voice only at night.

Nyctophilia Abnormal preference for darkness.

Nyctophobia Abnormal fear of darkness.

Nylidrin Peripheral vasodilator.

Nymph Wingless immature stage in developmental cycle of insects.

Nympha Labia minora.

Nymphomania Abnormal and excessive sexual desire in a female.

Nystagmograph Apparatus for recording nystagmus.

Nystagmus Involuntary to and fro movement of eye ball.

n. fixation Nystagmus only occurring on fixation of eyes.

n. latent Nystagmus that occurs only when eye is closed.

n. miners Nystagmus in those working in darkness.

n. optokinetic Nystagmus occurring while looking at moving objects.

n. rhythmic Nystagmus where eyes move slowly in one direction and then are jerked back to original position.

Nystalin Antifungal agent.

Nyslen's law The law that states that rigor mortis begins with muscles of mastication and then progresses down.

O

Oat A cereal used as food.

Oat meal Porridge of oat.

Obduction Autopsy.

Ober test A clinical test for tightness of iliotibial band

Obese Fatty.

Obesity Weight in excess of 20% than the ideal weight for height, age and sex.

o. endogenous Obesity caused by metabolic abnormality within the body.

o. exogenous Obesity due to excess food calori intake.

o. hypothalamic Obesity resulting from hypothalamic dysfunction, i.e. regulation of eating behavior.

Obfuscation Mental confusion.

Object Anything visible or appealing to senses.

Objective sign In reaching a diagnosis, a sign that can be seen, heard or felt by the examining doctor.

Objective symptoms Symptom apparent to physical means of diagnosis.

Obligate Necessary

Oblique Slanting or diagonal.

Obliquity The state of slanting.

o. Litzman's Inclining of fetal head with posterior parietal bone presenting.

o. Naegele's Inclining fetal head with oblique biparietal diameter in relation to pelvic brim.

Oblongata Oblong, e.g. medulla oblongata.

Obscure Hidden, indistinct.

Obsession A mental state where one is occupied with uncontrollable desire, idea or emotion even though he knows fully about it.

Obstetrics Branch of medicine dealing with child birth, puerperium and management of pregnancy.

Obstipation Complete constipation without passage of flatus and feces.

Obstructive lung disease A group of diseases which cause increased resistance to passage of air in and out of the lungs, e.g. asthma, chronic bronchitis, etc.

Obstruent Blocking up.

Obtundent A soothing remedy.

Obturator Anything that closes a cavity or opening.

Obturator foramen An opening in the membrane.

Obturator muscle Muscle in the pelvis that rotates the thigh outwards.

Obturator sign Inward rotation of hip so as to stretch obturator internus, causes pain in acute appendicitis.

Occipital bone Bone in hind part of skulll between parietal and temporal bones.

Occipital lobe Posterior lobe of cerebral hemisphere shaped like a three sided pyramid.

Occiput The back part of skull.

Occlusion State of being closed.

Occult Hidden, concealed.

Occult blood test Examination of stool for microscopic hemorrhage.

Occupational therapy Therapy aimed at making a patient independent and able for self care, and prevent disability.

Occupational neurosis Neurosis that develops in certain persons in particular occupations.

Ochlesis Any disease caused by over crowding.

Ochlophobia Abnormal fear of populated places or crowds.

Ochronosis An inborn error of metabolism marked by dark pigmentation of cartilage, ligaments and skin with black coloration of urine due to excretion of homogentisic acid.

Octamethyl-pyrophosphoramide Anticholinesterage insecticide.

Octapeptide Peptide with eight amino acids.

Octogenarian A person in his/her eighties.

Octopanine An adrenergic transmitter.

Oculocardiac reflex Slowing of pulse following pressure on eye ball.

Oculo-cerebro renal syndrome A sexlinked syndrome characterized by cataract, mental retardation, amino aciduria, vitamin D resistant rickets, etc.

Oculogyric crisis Involuntary upward gaze fixation lasting for minutes to hours in post-encephalitic parkinsonism.

Oculomotor nerve The third cranial nerve arising from midbrain and supplying extrinsic muscles of eye excluding lateral rectus and superior oblique.

Odaxesmus Biting of tongue, lip or cheek during attack of epilepsy.

Odogenesis The generation of axons from proximal severed end.

Odontalgia Toothache.

Odonterism Chattering of teeth.

Odontitis Inflammation of tooth.

Odontoblast The dentin forming cells in dental papilla or pulp chamber.

Odontocele An alveodental cyst.

Odontoclasis Fracture of tooth.

Odontoclast A class of cells that bring about resorption of roots of deciduous teeth.

Odontodynia Toothache.

Odontogenesis The formation/development of teeth.

Odontograph Equipment to determine the degree of uneveness of enamel.

Odontoid Tooth like.

Odontoid process Tooth like projection from 2nd cervical vertebra.

Odontology The art and science of V dentistry.

Odontoma Tumor originating from dental tissue.

o. ameloblastic Tumor of dental tissue containing enamel, dentine and odontogenic tissue but does not form enamel.

o. composite Odontoma in which epithelial and mesenchymal cells are completely differentiated producing enamel and dentin.

o. follicular Odontoma crepitating to pressure with excessive number of dental follicles.

Odontosis Development of teeth.

Odor Any smell.

Odorant Anything that stimulates the sense of smell.

Odoriferous Perfumed.

Odorous Having fragrance.

Odynophagia Dysphagia.

Oedius complex Abnormally intense love of child for opposite sex parent.

Ogilvie's syndrome Acute intestinal pseudoobstruction.

Ohm Unit of electrical resistance equal to current of 1 ampere produced by potential difference of one volt across the terminals.

Ohm's law The strength of an electric current expressed in amperes is equal to the electromotive force expressed in volts divided by resistance.

Oikofugic Having a compulsion to leave home.

Oikophobia Morbid dislike for home.

Ointment A medicated fatty soft substance for external application.

Oleic acid Fatty acid.

Oleogranuloma Granuloma formation at the site of injection of oily substances.

Olfaction The act of smelling.

Olfactometer The apparatus for testing power of sense of smell.

Olfactory area Area in hippocampal convolution and uncus of brain.

Olfactory bulb Enlarged upper end of olfactory tract.

Olfactory membrane Membrane in the upper part of nasal cavity containing olfactory receptors.

Olfactory nerves Fine unmyelinated fibres arising from olfactory mucosa and ending in olfactory bulb after piercing cribiform plate.

Olfactory tract The tract that extends from olfactory bulb to the anterior

perforated substance where it divides into olfactory striae.

Olfactory trigone Small triangular area between lateral and medial olfactory striae.

Oligemia Low blood volume.

Oligo Small or few.

Oligodendroglia The neuroglial cell with long slender processes which maintains the myelin sheath.

Oligodendroglioma A malignant tumor of CNS, frequently calcified arising from oligodendrocytes.

Oligohydramnios Less than normal amniotic fluid, a feature of post maturity.

Oligomenorrhea Scanty or infrequent menstruation.

Oligosaccharide Compound made up of small number of monosaccharides.

Oligospermia Diminished sperm count.

Oligotrophy Inadequate nutrition.

Oliguria Decreased formation of urine.

Olivary body A rounded mass of nerve tissue in anterolateral portion of medulla oblongata.

Ollier's disease Chondrodys–plasia.

Ollier's layer The deepest layer of periosteum containing bone forming osteoblasts.

Olophonia Malformed vocal apparatus with production of unnatural speech.

Olsalazine A drug to treat ulcerative colitis

Omalgia Neuralgic pain around shoulder.

Omental bursa The cavity in greater omentum.

Omentopexy Fixation of omentum to anterior abdominal wall.

Omentum A double fold of peritoneum attached to stomach, the portion attached to greater curvature of stomach extending to envelop the intestines is called greater omentum and the portion extending from lesser curvature of stomach to transverse fissure of liver is called lesser omentum.

Omeprazole Proton pump inhibitor, used in peptic ulcer; Zollinger-Ellison syndrome.

Ommaya reservoir A mushroom shaped reservoir with a self sealing plastic dome and attached to a catheter. The reservoir is implanted under the skin flap in skull and catheter is put into lateral ventricle useful for measuring CSF pressure and administration of drugs.

Omnivorous Eating both meat and vegetables.

Omohyoid Concerning scapula and the hyoid bone, the muscle attached to these two structures.

Omphalitis Inflammation of umbilicus.

Omphalocele Congenital umbilical hernia.

Omphalophlebitis Inflamed umbilical veins.

Omphalorrhexis Rupture of umbilicus.

Omphalotomy Cutting of umbilical cord after birth.

Onanist Person practising coitus interruptus.

Onanoff's reflex Contraction of bulbocavernosus muscle on pressing the glans penis.

Onchocerca volvulus Oncocerca invading the eye and causing blindness in Africa.

Oncogene Genes that can cause tumor formation.

Oncogenesis Tumor initiation and growth.

Oncology The branch of medicine dealing with tumors.

Oncotic pressure The osmotic pressure exerted by proteins in plasma.

Oncovin Vincristine sulphate.

Ondine's curse Primary alveolar hypoventilation due to reduced responsiveness of respiratory center to CO_2.

Oneirology The scientific study of dreams.

Oneiroscopy Dream analysis for study of one's emotional state.

Oniomania An irrepressible urge to spend money.

Onlay A graft applied to the surface of tissue, e.g. bone graft applied to bone.

Ontogeny The history of development of an individual.

Onychia Inflammation of nailbed with loss of nail.

Onychodystrophy Maldevelopment of a nail.

Onychograph Device that records capillary blood pressure under the finger nail.

Onycholysis Losing and detachment of nail.

Onychomycosis Fungal infection of nails.

Oocyst Encysted form of zygote in certain sporozoa.

Oocyte Primitive ovum.

Oogenesis Growth and maturation of ovum.

Oogonium The primordial cell from which an oocyte originates.

Ookinesis Mitotic phenomena taking place within an ovum during maturation and fertilization.

Ookinete Motile zygote of plasmodia.

Oophorrhaphy Suture of displaced ovary to pelvic wall.

Oospore A spore formed by the union of opposite sexual elements

Opaque Not transparent; not allowing light rays to pass through.

Open heart surgery Surgery on heart or its blood vessels requiring cardiopulmonary bypass.

Open reduction Exposure of fractured ends of a bone for bringing reunion by suitable reduction.

Operant conditioning Conditioning or influencing behavior by rewarding for certain desired acts.

Operation The act of operating, i.e. incision, excision, suture.

o. ablative Operation where a body part is removed.

o. radical Operation involving removal of large part of an organ.

Opercular Concerning a covering structure.

Operculitis Inflammation of gingiva over a partly erupted tooth.

Operculum Any covering.

Operon A term used in genetics to mean a group of linked genes and regulatory elements functioning as an unit for transcription.

Ophiases A form of baldness of scalp.

Ophidism Poisoning from snake bite.

Ophritis Inflammation of eyebrow.

Ophthalmia Inflammation of the eye.

o. gonococcal Severe purulent conjunctivitis.

o. neonatorum Severe purulent conjunctivitis of newborn, usually gonococcal.

o. sympathetic Uveitis of healthy eye following trauma to other eye.

Ophthalmic nerve A branch of trigeminal, having only sensory function.

Ophthalmitis Inflammation of eye.

Ophthalmodynamometer Instrument for measuring pressure in ophthalmic arteries.

Ophthalmodynia Pain in the eye.

Ophthalmologist A doctor who practises in the treatment of diseases of eye.

Ophthalmometer Instrument for measuring errors of refraction, size of eye and anterior curvature.

Ophthalmoplegia Paralysis of ocular muscles.

o. externa Paralysis of extraocular muscles.

o. interna Paralysis of iris and ciliary body.

o. nuclear Paralysis of 3rd, 4th and 6th cranial nerves due to a lesion involving their nuclei.

o. Parinaud's Paralysis of conjugate deviation of eyes in upward direction.

Ophthalmoscope Instrument for examination of fundus and retina.

Opiate receptor Specific receptors on cell surfaces to which combine the opiates, endorphins and encephalitis for mediating their effects.

Opioid Synthetic narcotics or endogenous substances with opium like activity, e.g. encephalins and endorphins.

Opisthion The craniometric point at the middle of the lower border of foramen magnum

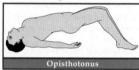
Opisthotonus

Opisthotonus A form of tetanic spasm where the body bends backwards.

Opium Substance derived from juice of unripe capsules of poppy.

Oppenheim's disease SYN— myotonia congenita characterized by poor muscular development in the limbs.

Opponens digiti minimi Intrinsic muscle of hand that helps apposing little finger to thumb.

Opponens pollicis Muscle that places thumb opposite the little finger.

Opsin One of the colorless proteins in rods and cones.

Opsonin A substance present in blood that prepares bacteria for phagocytosis.

Opsonize To render microorganisms susceptible to phagocytosis.

Optical center The point where the secondary axes of a refractory system meet and cross the principal axis.

Optical index A constant applied to objectives for purpose of comparison taking into account the focal length.

Optical isomerism Substances having similar structural formula but differing rotation of polarized light.

Optic atrophy Atrophy of optic nerve head with sharply demarcated chalky white optic disc.

Optic axis The imaginary line passing through center of cornea and posterior pole of retina.

Optic canal The groove at the apex of orbit through which pass optic nerve and ophthalmic artery.

Optic chiasma The commissure anterior to hypophysis where there is partial decussation of fibers of optic nerve.

Optic disk The posterior pole in retina where the fibers from ganglion cell converge to form optic nerve.

Optic neuritis Involvement of optic nerve due to inflammation, degeneration, demyelination resulting in visual loss.

Optic radiation The geniculocalcarine tract connecting lateral geniculate body with area 17 and 19 of calcarine cortex.

Optics Branch of science relating to properties of light, its refraction, reflexion and relation to vision.

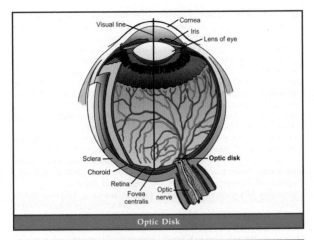

Optic Disk

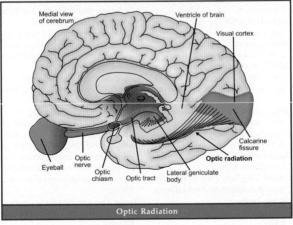

Optic Radiation

Optic tract The visual path from optic chiasm to lateral geniculate body.

Optic vesicle The embryonic evagination of diencephalon giving rise to pigmentary and sensory layers of retina.

Optimal Most desirable.

Optokinetic Relating to eye movements in relation to movement of objects in visual field.

Optokinetic nystagmus Nystagmus occurring when moving objects traverse the field of vision or vice versa.

Optometer Instrument for measuring refractive error of eye.

Optometry Measurement of visual power.

Oral contraceptive Contraceptives taken by mouth.

Ora serrata Portion of retina behind ciliary body.

Orbicularis oculi The ring muscle of eye, causing its closure.

Orbicularis oris The ring muscle of mouth, causing pursing of lips.

Orbit The bony socket containing the eye formed by frontal, sphenoid, ethmoid, maxillary and palatal bone.

Orbital cellulitis Inflammation of soft tissue of orbit usually following sinusitis causing proptosis and diplopia.

Orbital index Orbital height to orbital breadth X100.

Orbital lobe Part of frontal lobe that rests on orbital plate of frontal bone.

Orchic Testis.

Orchiopexy Surgical fixation of testis.

Orchitis Inflammation of testis.

Ordinate The vertical line of the two coordinates.

Organelle Special structures of a cell, e.g. mitochondria.

Organic 1. Pertains to living organisms, 2. In chemistry pertaining to compounds of carbon, 3. Physical not mental or psychogenic.

Organic acid Any acid containing carboxyl group.

Organic brain syndrome Diffuse impairment of brain function.

Organic disease Disease with recognizable structural changes in organs and tissues.

Organic murmur Murmur due to structural changes in heart valves.

Organism Any living entity capable of carrying on life process.

Organize To undergo organization, i.e. repair process with growth of fibroblasts and capillaries.

Organizing pneumonia Pneumonia where the exudate undergoes organization and cicatrization rather than resorption.

Organogenesis The formation and development of body organs from embryonic tissue

Organoid Resembling an organ.

Orgasm The intense pleasure of sexual intercourse at climax with pelvic throbbing, contraction of levator ani and anal sphincters to culminate in seminal ejaculation.

Orifice An opening or entrance to a cavity.

Origin The starting point.

Ormond's disease Retroperitoneal fibrosis

Ornithine An amino acid in the urea cycle.

Ornithosis Psittacosis contracted from birds other than parrots.

Oropharynx Portion of pharynx below the level of soft palate.

Orosomucoid An acidic muco protein from nephrotic urine.

Orotic acid A pyrimidine precursor.

Oroya fever Bartonellosis.

Orphenadrine Antispasmodic antitremor drug.

Ortalani's sign Slipping of femoral head back to acetabulum with a snapping sound when congenitally displaced hip in full abduction is tapped.

Orthochromatic Having normal staining characteristics.

Orthodontics The branch of dentistry dealing with malocclusion and its treatment.

Orthograde Walking or standing in upright position.

Orthopedics That branch of surgery dealing with corrective treatment of deformities, diseases of locomotor apparatus.

Orthophoria Normal balance of eye muscles, i.e. parallel.

Orthopnea Difficulty in breathing in lying down but not in sitting or upright position.

Orthopraxis Mechanical correction of deformities

Orthoptics The training meant for making visual responses normal like esophoria.

Orthosis Any device added to the body to stabilize or immobilize the body part, prevent deformity or assist with function

Orthostatic Standing upright.

o. albuminuria Albuminuria when assuming erect position.

o. hypotension Fall in blood pressure while assuming erect position.

Orthostat Device for straightening curvatures of long bones.

Orthotics Science of orthopedic appliance and their use.

Orthotopic In the natural or normal position.

o. transplantation Transplantation of an organ from a donor into its normal anatomical position in recipient.

Os Bone, mouth.

Oscillation A swinging or vibration.

Oscilopsia A form of visual aberration where stationary objects appear to move to and fro leading to blurred vision.

Oscilloscope A cathode ray vacuum tube to reflect oscillations of electromotive forces.

Osgood-Schlatter disease Osteochondritis of tibial tubercle.

Osler-Rendu-Weber disease Hereditary hemorrhagic telangiectasia.

Osler's disease Polycythemia vera.

Osler's node Painful indurated red areas on finger pulp in acute bacterial endocarditis.

Osmol The quantity of a solute existing in solution as molecules, commonly stated in grams, that is osmotically equivalent to one mole of an ideally behaving electrolyte.

Osmometer Instrument for measuring osmotic pressure.

Osmophobia Abnormal fear of odors.

Osmoreceptors Hypothalamic receptors that respond to changes in osmotic pressure of blood and hence influence ADH secretion.

Osmosis The passage of solvent through a membrane from a dilute solution into a more concentrated one.

Osmotic fragility The susceptibility of RBCs to lyse in hypotonic solutions.

Osmotic pressure The pressure developed when two solutions of different concentrations of some solute are separated by a semi-permeable membrane.

Osseous Bony.

Ossicle A small bone, particularly that in middle ear.

Ossification The formation of bone.

Ossifucent Breaking down and softening of bone.

Ossifying fibroma A benign tumor from connective tissue of bone.

Osteitis Inflammation of bone.

o. carnosa Inflammation of bone with excess of granulation tissue formation.

o. condensans: ilii Formation of opaque sclerotic bone in the ileum adjacent to sacroiliac joint causing low back ache; of unknown etiology.

o. deformans Paget's disease.

o. flbrosa cystica Generalized bone demineralization with large osteoporotic areas resembling cyst as in hyperparathyroidism.

o. fragilitans Osteogenesis imperfecta.

o. fungosa Inflammatory hyperplasia of medulla of bone with new ossification of fungoid granulation tissue.

Osteoarthrosis Degenerative joint disease.

Osteoblast Cells of mesenchymal origin concerned in the formation of bony tissue.

Osteoblastoma Malignant tumor of osteoblasts *SYN*—Osteosarcoma.

Osteochondral Composed of both bone and cartilage.

Osteochondritis dissecans A joint disease characterized by partial or complete detachment of a fragment of articular cartilage and underlying bone.

Osteochondrodysplasia Abnormal development of bony and cartilaginous structures.

Osteochondrodystrophy Morquio's syndrome.

Osteochondroma Benign hamartomatous tumor of bone or cartilage.

Osteochondromyxoma An osteochondroma with myxoid component.

Osteochondrosarcoma An osteosarcoma with significant myxosarcomatous element.

Osteochondrosis A process involving ossification centers with avascular necrosis followed by slow regeneration.

Osteoclasis The fracture of a long bone without resorting to open surgery for correcting deformity.

Osteoclast Multinucleated cells responsible for bone remodelling.

Osteoclast activating factor A lymphokine that causes bone resorption IL-1 is an OAF.

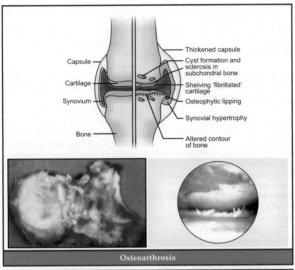

Osteoarthrosis

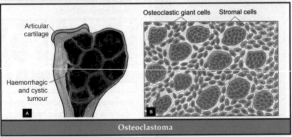

Osteoclastoma

Osteoclastoma Giant cell tumor.
Osteocyte A mesodermal bone forming cell of marrow
Osteodiastasis Separation of bone without true fracture.

Osteodystrophy Defective bone formation.
Osteofibroma A benign bone tumor with fibrous tissue component.
Osteogenesis imperfecta Autosomal dominant disease characte-

rized by hypoplasia of bone and cartilage leading to fracture with minimal trauma, hypermobility, blue sclera.

Osteogenic sarcoma A malignant tumor composed of mesenchymal anaplastic cells with varying elements of osteogenesis, osteolysis, telangiectasis and bone cyst formation.

Osteoid The young hyaline matrix of true bone in which calcium is deposited.

Osteoid osteoma A benign hamartomatous tumor of bone composed of a nidus of well vascularized tissue with pain.

Osteolysis Bone resorption/degeneration.

Osteoma Benign bony tumor arising from membranous bones.

Osteomalacia Failure of ossification due to fall in serum calcium.

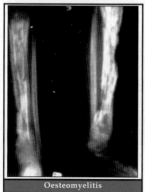
Oesteomyelitis

Osteomatosis Presence of multiple osteomas.

Osteometry The study of proportions and measurement of skeleton.

Osteomyelitis Inflammation of marrow and hard tissue of bone.

Osteonectin A glycoprotein present in the noncollagenous portion of bone matrix

Osteopathy A school of healing art which teaches that the body is a vital mechanical organism whose structural and functional integrity are coordinated and interdependent.

Osteopenia Less bone tissue than normal.

Osteopetrosis A familial disease characterized by excessive radiographic density with a tendency towards fracture and obliteration of marrow cavity.

Osteophyte A bony outgrowth.

Osteopoikilosis Disease of unknown etiology with ellipsoidal dense foci in all bones of body.

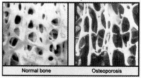
Normal bone   Osteoporosis

Osteoporosis Absolute decrease in quantity of bone tissue with enlarging marrow cavity and haversian spaces.

Osteosclerosis Abnormal increase in density of bone.

Osteosis Metaplastic bone formation.

Osteotome An instrument for cutting bone.

Osteotomy Cutting of a bone.

Osteotropy Nutrition of bony tissue.

Ostium A mouth or aperture.

Otic Pertaining to ear.

Otic capsule The cartilage capsule that surrounds developing auditory vesicle and later fuses with the sphenoid and occipital cartilage.

Otitis Inflammation of the ear.

Otitis externa Inflammation of external ear.

Otitis interna Inflammation of internal ear.

Otic ganglion The nerve ganglion immediately below foramen ovale of sphenoid bone giving rise to post ganglionic parasympathetic fibers to parotid gland.

Otitic hydrocephalus Hydrocephalus associated with chronic ear infection, esp. mastoiditis.

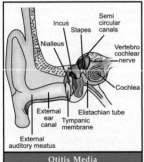

Otitis Media

Otitis media Inflammation of middle ear.

Otocleisis Occlusion of ear.

Otogenic Originating or arising within the ear.

Otolaryngology Speciality dealing with diseases of ear, nose and larynx.

Otolith Calcareous concretions within membranous labyrinth.

Otology The science of ear and its diseases.

Otomycosis Fungal infection of ear canal.

Otorhagia Discharge of blood from the ear.

Otorrhea Discharge from external auditory meatus.

Otosclerosis A disease characterized by new bone formation around oval window with immobilization of foot plate of stapes and hence conductive hearing loss.

Otoscope Instrument for visualization of external ear and the tympanic membrane.

Ototoxic Agents toxic to the neural process of hearing.

Ouabain A digitalis glycoside, rapid acting.

Ounce An unit of measure equivalent to 28 grams.

Outer nuclear layer The layer of retina which contains rods and cones.

Outflow In neurology trans–mission of efferent impulses.

Outgrowth Growth or development from a pre-existing structure or state.

Outline The shape.

Outpouching Evagination.

Ovale malaria Malaria caused by *Plasmodium ovale* with the red blood cells and trophozoites both being often oval in shape.

Ovalocyte Elliptocyte.

Ovarian agenesis Failure of development of ovaries. *SYN*—Turner's syndrome.

Ovarian follicle An ovum and the granulosa cell surrounding it occupying the cortex of ovary.

Ovarian graft A portion of ovary implanted commonly to abdominal wall to preserve hormone secretion.

Ovarian hormones 1. Follicular hormones-estradiol, estrone, and estriol 2. luteal hormone-progesterone.

Ovarian ligament The terminal portion of genital ridge uniting the caudal end of embryonic ovary with the uterus.

Ovarian plexus A network of veins in the broad ligament or nerve plexus around the ovary.

Ovariocele Hernia of the ovary.

Ovariocyesis Ovarian pregnancy.

Ovary The glandular female reproductive organ giving rise to ova.

Overbite The extent to which the upper anterior teeth overlap the lower during occlusion.

Overriding The extent of overlapping of broken ends in a fracture.

Overweight Excessive weight of an individual by more than 10% than permissible for sex and age.

Oviparous Producing eggs.

Ovoid Egg shaped.

Ovotestis Ovarian and testicular tissue combined in the same gonad.

Ovulation The maturation and discharge of ovum.

Ovum The female germ cell.

Oxalate Any ester or salt of oxalic acid.

Oxalic acid An acid found in plants and vegetables, used as reagent.

Oxaloacetic acid A participant in citric acid metabolic cycle.

Oxalosis An inborn error of metabolism due to impaired glyoxylic acid metabolism with overproduction of oxalic acid and deposition of calcium oxalate in body tissues.

Oxaluria Presence of oxalic acid or oxalates in urine.

Oxandrolone An anabolic steroid

Oxazepam A benzodiazepine, tranquilizer.

Oxethazaine Gastric mucosal anesthetic.

Oxidase Enzyme that promotes an oxidation reaction.

Oxidation An increase in positive valence of an element or decrease in negative valence occurring due to loss of electrons; the process of combining with oxygen.

Oxime Any compound resulting from action of hydroxylamine upon an aldehyde or ketone.

Oximeter Photoelectric instrument for measuring degree of oxygen saturation of blood.

Oxprenolol A beta-blocker used in coronary artery disease.

Oxtriphylline A drug that resembles theophylline in action

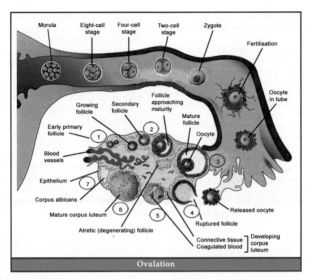

Ovulation

Oxycephaly A condition where head is conical in shape.

Oxycodone A narcotic analgesic, dihydro hydroxy codeinone.

Oxygen The colorless and odorless gas that supports combustion and essential to animal life. It constitutes one-fifth of atmosphere, eight-ninth of water and one-half of earth's crust.

Oxygen saturation Oxygen content divided by oxygen capacity expressed in volume per cent.

Oxygen tent A transparent air tight chamber, enclosing patient's head and shoulder, in which oxygen content can be maintained at a higher level.

Oxygen toxicity Progressive respiratory failure with inhalation of more than 100% oxygen for prolonged period

Oxyhemoglobin Hemoglobin combined with oxygen.

Oxyhemoglobin dissociation curve A curve that shows the relationship between partial pressure of oxygen and percentage saturation of haemoglobin

Oxylalia Rapid speech.

Oxymetazoline A vasoconstrictor used topically to reduce nasal congestion.

Oxymetholone An anabolic steroid.

Oxymorphone A semisynthetic narcotic analgesic.

Oxyntic Secreting acid, e.g. parietal cells of stomach.

Oxyopia Unusual acuity of vision.

Oxyphenbutazone A metabolite of phenyl butazone used for its analgesic-anti-inflammatory property.

Oxyphenisatin A cathartic.

Oxyphenonium bromide An anticholinergic agent used in peptic ulcer and gastrointestinal hypermotility or spasm.

Oxypurinol A xanthine oxidase inhibitor, used in gout.

Oxytetracycline An antibiotic of tetracycline group from *Strep-* *tomyces rimosus* where the hydrogen atom of tetracycline is replaced by a hydroxyl group.

Oxytocin An octapeptide secreted by posterior pituitary, causes uterine contraction and promotes lactation.

Ozena A form of atrophic rhinitis with crusting, bleeding and offensive odor

Ozone O_3. An allotropic form of oxygen, a powerful oxidizing agent, used as disinfectant.

Ozonide A compound of ozone with certain unsaturated organic substances that exert bactericidal effect from liberation of nascent oxygen.

P

Pachhionian bodies Pedunculated fibrous tissue growths along longitudinal fissure of cerebrum.

Pacemaker 1. Electronic device that controls rate and rhythm of heart 2. The specialized cells in right atrium that generate impulse.

p. wandering A form of arrhythmia where the origin of cardiac impulse shifts from place to place.

Pachyderma Unusual thickening of skin.

Pachydermatocele A pendulous state of skin with thickening; usually due to large neurofibroma.

Pachymeniagitis Inflammation of dura mater.

Pachyonychia Abnormal thickening of nails.

Pachysomia Pathological thickening of soft parts of body.

Pacing code A three letter code for describing pacemaker type and function. The first letter indicates the heart chamber paced (V = ventricle, A = atrium, D = dual), the second letter indicates the chamber from which electrical activity is sensed and the third letter indicates the response to sensed electrical activity.

Pacinian corpuscle Encapsulated sensory nerve endings of skin and internal organs sensitive to deep pressure.

Pack A dry or moist; hot or cold blanket or sheet used for therapeutic purpose.

Packed cell Blood containing cellular elements only, devoid of plasma.

Pa CO$_2$ Partial pressure of CO$_2$ in arterial blood.

Pad Cushion of soft material used to apply pressure, or support on an organ.

Paget's disease Skeletal disease of elderly with thickening, softening and bending of bones.

P's disease of breast Carcinoma of mammary ducts.

Pagophagia A form of pica where patient loves eating ice.

Pain Sensory and emotional experience associated with irritation/inflammation of tissue.

p. girdle A constricting cord like pain around the waist in spinal cord disease

p. growing Joint and limb pain in growing children but certainly not related to somatic growth

p. hunger Epigastric pain due to hunger

p. referred Pain arises from an area other than where it is felt; e.g. anginal pain referred to arm and shoulder due to same somatic inervation

Paint Castellani's A germicide containing phenol, resorcinol, boric acid etc.

Palatal reflex Soft palate contraction during attempt of swallowing.

Palate Roof of the mouth separating it from nasal cavity.

Palatine arches Two arch like folds of mucous membrane (glossopalatine and pharyngopalatine) that form the lateral margin of faucial and pharyngeal isthmuses.

Palatine artery Branch of maxillary artery, supplying palate and pharynx.

Palatoglossus Muscle that arises from sides and undersurface of tongue and inserted to palatine aponeurosis. It acts as a constrictor of faucial isthmus by raising the root of tongue.

Palatography Recording of movement of palate during speech.

Palatopharyngeus Muscle that arises from thyroid cartilage and pharyngeal wall and inserted into aponeurosis of soft palate. It constricts pharyngeal isthmus and raises larynx.

Palatorrhaphy Operation for cleft palate.

Paleocerebellum The oldest portion of cerebellum that includes flocculi, and part of vermis concerned with equilibrium, and locomotion.

Paleothalamus Medial older parts of thalamus.

Palilalia Rapid repetition of same words and phrases.

Palinal Moving backward.

Pallidectomy Surgical or cryogenic/laser destruction of globus pallidus.

Pallor Paleness.

Palm Anterior surface of hand from wrist to fingers.

Palmar reflex Grasping reflex in infants that disappears after 4-5 months of age.

Palm-Chin reflex Contraction of superficial muscles of eye and chin on scratching of thenar eminence of the same side. *SYN*— Palmo mental reflex.

Palmitic acid A long chain fatty acid found in palm oil.

Palpable Perceptible to touch.

Palpation Examination by application of hand or fingers.

Palpebra An eyelid.

Palpebral Commissure. The union of the eyelids at each end of palpebral fissure.

Palpebral fissure Opening between the eyelids.

Palpebral ligament The medial and lateral ligaments that fix the two ends of tarsi to the orbital wall.

Palpitation Rapid throbbing pulsation of heart.

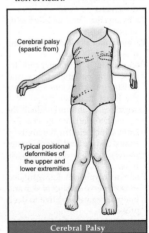

Cerebral palsy (spastic from)

Typical positional deformities of the upper and lower extremities

Cerebral Palsy

Palsy Paralysis/loss of ability to act.

p. Bell's Lower motor facial palsy.

p. bulbar Paralysis of lower cranial nerves.

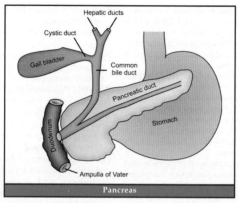

Pancreas

p. cerebral Nonprogressive palsy of childhood from developmental defect of brain, or birth asphyxia or trauma.

p. Erb's Palsy of C_5C_6 due to lesion of brachial plexus.

p. shaking Paralysis agitans.

Palynology Study of spores and pollens.

Pampiniform Convoluted like a tendril.

Pampinocele *SYN* — varicocele; swollen dilated veins of pampiniform plexus of spermatic cord.

Panangitis Inflammation of all the three layers of a blood vessel.

Panarteritis Inflammation of all the three coats of an artery.

Pancarditis Inflammation of all the three layers of heart, i.e. pericardium, myocardium and endocardium.

Pancoast's syndrome Tumor of lung apex that erodes into brachial plexus to produce Horner's syndrome.

Pancolectomy Surgical excision of entire colon.

Pancreas A compound acinotubular gland in front of L_1L_2 vertebra behind the stomach, secretes hormones like insulin, glucagon and digestive enzymes.

p. annular A portion of pancreas encircles duodenum.

p. divisium The two portions of embryonic pancreas have failed to fuse

Pancreatic juice 500-800 ml of alkaline pancreatic secretion per day containing enzymes like trypsinogen, amylopsin, lipase etc. Secretin and cholecystokinin secreted by duodenum stimulate pancreatic secretion.

Pancreaticoduodenostomy Surgical creation of an artificial tract between pancreas and duodenum.

Pancreatin A mixture of pancreatic enzymes like amylase, lipase and proteases.

Pancreatitis Inflammation of pancreas.

p. calcareous Pancreatitis accompanied by pancreatic calcification.

p. chronic Scarred pancreas due to chronic inflammation.

Pancreatolith Calculus within pancreas.

Pancreozymin Polypeptide that stimulates pancreas to secrete insulin; also found in brain.

Pancuronium bromide Neuromuscular blocking agent.

Pancytopenia Reduction in all cellular elements, i.e. RBC, WBC, platelets in blood.

Pandemic Disease widely prevalent in population.

Pandiculation Yawning and stretching of limbs as on awakening from sleep.

Panic Sudden anxiety, terror or fright.

Panic attack Acute intense anxiety with sweating, palpitation, nausea, chest pain and feeling of approaching death.

Panniculitis Inflammation of fatty connective tissue.

Pannus Vascularization around cornea.

Pansinusitis Inflammation of all paranasal sinuses, i.e. maxillary frontal, ethmoidal.

Pantalgia Pain over entire body.

Pantamorphia Malformation involving entire body.

Panting Shallow rapid breathing.

Pantograph A device that reproduces figures or drawings.

Pantopaque Iophendylate, a radiographic contrast for myelography.

Pantothenic acid A member of vitamin B complex group found in yeast, liver, eggs etc.

PaO2 Partial pressure of oxygen in arterial blood.

Papain Proteolytic enzyme from papaya.

Papanicolaou test A study for detection of cancer from examination of cells shed from abnormal mucosal growths.

Papaverine Smooth muscle relaxant.

Papilla Small elevation, nipple like.

p. circum vatiate Large papilla near base of tongue.

Papaverine

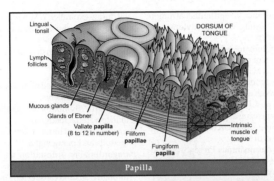

Papilla

p. filiform Small papilla at tip of tongue.

p. interdental Triangular shaped gingiva between the teeth.

p. lacrimal Small elevation at inner end of eyelid through which lacrimal duct opens.

p. of hair A conical portion of dermis through which capillaries enter into hair root.

p. of Vater Elevation in medial wall of second part of duodenum through which pancreatic and common bile duct open.

p. renal Apex of renal pyramids.

Papillary muscle The two muscle groups in each ventricle of heart connecting to free margin of A-V valves.

Papilledema Edema of optic nerve head.

Papilliform Resembling papilla.

Papillitis Inflammation of optic nerve head.

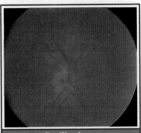

Papilloedema

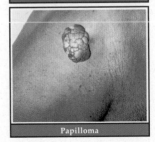

Papilloma

Papilloma Benign epithelial tumors including wart, condyloma and polyp.

Papillomatosis Widespread formation of papillomas.

Papovavirus The group includes polyoma virus, papilloma virus which are incriminated in cancer.

Pappus The fine downy beard hair appearing at puberty.

Papule Solid circumscribed elevation of skin.

Papulosquamous Presence of papules and scales.

Papyracens Parchment like, dead mumified fetus

Para-aminobenzoic Used as sunscreen.

Para amino hippuric acid Derivative of amino benzoic acid used for testing renal excretory function.

Para amino salicylic acid Bacteriostatic antituberculous agent.

Paracentesis Cavity puncture for draining fluid.

Paracentral Near to center.

p. lobule Cerebral convolution on medial surface serving as motor area of leg.

Parachromatism Defective color perception.

Paracoccidioido mycosis Chronic granulomatous fungal disease of skin.

Paradigm An example that serves as a model

Paradox Absurd, inconsistent with logic, conflicting

Paradoxical respiration 1. Seen in open pneumothorax where lungs fill during expiration 2. Moving up of diaphragm during inspiration in diaphragmatic palsy.

Paraffin Hydrocarbon derivative of petroleum.

p. liquid Mineral oil.

p. soft petrolatum Used for making creams and ointments.

Paraganglia Sympathetic ganglia akin to adrenal medulla.

Paraganglioma Tumor of adrenal medulla and paraganglia.

Paragonimiasis Infestation with fluke *P. westermanni,* transmitted through crabs and causing lung infection.

Paragranuloma Benign form of Hodgkin's disease only limited to lymphatic system.

Para influenza virus A group of viruses causing acute upper respiratory infection.

Parakeratosis A partial keratinization process where keratinocytes still contain nuclei.

Paraldehyde Colorless liquid polymer of acetaldehyde used as a hypnotic, analgesic and anticonvulsant.

Paralexia Difficulty in comprehension of vocal/printed matter with substitution of meaningless words.

Paralax Displacement of objects by change in observer's position.

Paralysis Loss of muscular function usually due to nerve dysfunction; may be spastic or flaccid.

p. agitans Parkinson's disease characterized by rigidity, akinesia, tremor and gait disorder.

p. Bell's Lower motor facial palsy.

p. crossed Paralysis of one side of body and opposite side of face, a feature of lesion in brainstem.

p. familial periodic Flaccid palsy usually on awakening due to disturbances in serum potassium.

p. hysteric Apparent paralysis due to psychiatric conflict.

p. Erb's Paralysis of muscles of upper arm due to C_5C_6 root lesion.

p. Klumpke's Birth injury causing paralysis of arm and hand muscles (Policeman's hand in bribe).

p. Pott's Tuberculosis of spine causing paraplegia.

p. pseudobulbar Upper motor palsy of cranial nerves due to central lesion.

p. Saturday night Compression of radial nerve in spiral groove (usually due to alcoholic binge on saturday night).

p. Todd's Transient muscular palsy (upto 24 hours) following epilepsy, due to neuronal exertion.

Paralytic ileus Intestinal palsy with distention of abdomen, vomiting and obstipation.

Paramagnetic Anything attracted by a magnet.

Paramedian Close to midline.

Paramedic A trained person to assist doctor.

Paramedical Supplementary to medical profession like occupational, speech and physiotherapy.

Paramethidione Anticonvulsant.

Parametritis Inflammation of parametrium.

Parametrium Loose connective tissue around uterus.

Paramnesia Use of words without meaning or recall of events that never occurred.

Paramyotonia Increased muscle tone and poor relaxation after contraction.

Paramyxoviruses Includes measles, mumps, parainfluenza and respiratory syncytial virus.

Paranasal Sinuses Frontal, maxillary, ethmoidal and sphenoidal sinuses.

Paraneoplastic syndrome Symptoms of multiple organ dysfunction in a patient of cancer (lung, kidney) without actual metastasis.

Paranoia Paranoid schizophrenia.

Paranoid Ideas of persecution, suspicious thinking.

Paraphasia Misuse of spoken words or word combinations.

Paraphilia A psychosexual disorder that includes festishism, transvestism, pedophilia, voyeurism which mean bizarre acts for sexual excitation.

Paraphimosis Inflamed or narrowed prepuce unable to be retracted over glans and strangulating it.

Paraphrasia Unintelligible speech due to incorrect and jumbling up of words used.

Paraplegia Paralysis of both legs.

p. dolorosa Extremely painful paraplegia due to pressure of a neoplasm on nerve roots and spinal cord.

p. Pott's Tuberculosis of spine with paraplegia.

Paraprotein Abnormal plasma protein like macroglobulin, myeloma protein.

Parapsoriasis Itchy, scaly red skin disease

Parapsychology Psychology that deals with extrasensory perception, telepathy, psychokinesis

Paraquat A weed killer that when ingested causes liver, renal and pulmonary damage.

Parasite Organism living at expense of another organism.

p. external Parasite living on outer surface of host, e.g. lice, fleas, ticks etc.

p. facultative Parasite capable of living independent of the host at times.

Parasitemia Presence of parasite in the blood.

Parasitize To infest with a parasite.

Parasitology The study of parasites and parasitism.

Parasternal Adjacent to sternum.

Parasympathetic nervous system The preganglionic fibers arise from midbrain, medulla and sacral portion of spinal cord through 3rd, 7th, 9th and 10th cranial nerves and S2-S4 somatic nerves to synapse with postganglionic neurones located in autonomic ganglia. Parasympathetic stimulation causes smooth muscle contraction, increased glandular secretion (except that of sweat) and slowing of heart.

Parasympathomimetic Agent that produces actions similar to parasympathetic stimulation.

Parasympatholytic Agents that have actions opposite to parasympathetic stimulation.

Parasystole Ectopic rhythm from ventricle.

Parathion Insecticide, toxic to humans.

Parathormone Parathyroid hormone controlling calcium and phosphorus metabolism.

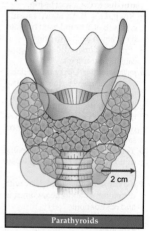

2 cm

Parathyroids

Parathyroids 4 small glands lying in neck adjacent to thyroid whose extirpation leads to hypocalcemia, carpopedal spasm, and tetany.

Paratrichosis Abnormality of hair or its growth pattern.

Paratyphoid fever A less severe form of typhoid caused by salmonella paratyphi.

Paraurethral Close to urethra.

Paravertebral Close to or alongside vertebra.

Paravesical Close to urinary bladder.

Paraxial On either side of body axis.

Parazoon An animal that lives as parasite on another animal.

Paregoric 1. Soothing 2. Tincture opium used for diarrhea.

Parenchyma The functional portion of an organ.

Parent A father or mother.

Parenteral Any route other than alimentary canal.

Paresis Partial or incomplete paralysis.

Paresthesia Sensation of numbness, pricking, needling, tingling due to irritation of a nerve or its central connections.

Parietal Forming wall of a cavity or outer shell.

p. cells Large cells or oxyntic cells secreting HCl in stomach.

Perinaud's syndrome Paralysis of vertical gaze due to subthalamic bleed.

Pari passu Side by side, occurring at the same time/rate.

Parity Carrying pregnancy upto viability (28 weeks gestation).

Parkinson's disease See paralysis agitans.

P's facies Expressionless mask like face.

Parodontitis Inflammation of tissues around a tooth.

Paromomycin Aminoglycoside antibiotic used to treat amebiasis.

Paroniria Terrifying dreams.

Paronychia Infection of nail margin soft tissue.

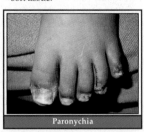
Paronychia

Paronychosis Growth of nail in an abnormal position.

Paroophoron Vestigial structure consisting of minute tubules, the remains of caudal group of mesonephric tubules, homologous to paradidymis of male.

Parosmia Perversion of sense of smell where agreeable odors are considered offensive and vice versa.

Parosteal Connected to or arising from outer layer of periosteum.

Parotid duct The duct of parotid gland 2" long opening into mouth opposite 2nd upper molar.

Parotid gland One of the salivary glands near angle of mouth secreting saliva.

Parotitis Inflammation of parotid gland.

Parovarium Vestigial remains of mesonephric tubules located in mesosalpinx between the ovary and fallopian tubes.

Paroxysm Periodic recurrence of symptoms.

Paroxysmal cold hemoglobinuria Autoimmune hemolysis due to hemolysins occurring in syphilis and some viral infections, manifesting with chill, abdominal pain and fever with hemoglobinuria.

Parrot's node Bony outgrowths on the skull of infants with congenital syphilis.

Pars flaccida A portion of ear drum that is not taut *SYN* — Sharpnell's membrane.

Pars tensa Tightly stretched larger portion of tympanic membrane.

Parthenogenesis (Parthenos = virgin). Reproduction arising from unfertilized female egg.

Particle A tiny fragment or very minute piece.

p. alpha A charged radioactive particle of low penetrability.

p. beta A high speed electron emitted during decay of an atom.

p. Dane HBsAg, serum hepatitis capsular antigen.

Parturient Concerning childbirth.

Parturition Delivery or childbirth.

Parvo virus A group of viruses similar to adenovirus; pv B_{19} causes erythema infectiosum or fifth disease

Passion Great emotion or zeal usually concerning sexual excitement.

Passive exercise Exercise to muscle given by an assistant or machine.

Passive smoking Inhaling smoke by persons around the smoke.

Passivity Dependence upon others, not willing to take responsibility.

Pasteurella The organism of plague

P. multocida is a gram negative coccobacillus that causes cellulitis, pneumonia, meningitis

Pasteurization The process of sterilizing a fluid without changing its chemical composition.

Past pointing Inability to place fingers at a selected point in space, a feature of cerebellar disorder.

Patella The sesamoid bone infront of knee in the tendons of quadriceps femoris

p. alta high positioned patella

p. baja low positioned patella

p. bipartite patella developing from two centers of ossification, mistaken for fracture

Patellar ligament The extension of quadriceps femoris tendon beyond inferior pole of patella to be attached to tuberosity of tibia.

Patellar reflex Contraction of quadriceps on tap on patellar ligament.

Patent Open.

Patency The state of being open.

Patent ductus arteriosus Persistent communication between aorta and pulmonary artery after birth.

Paternity test Group of tests (blood group, HLA) done to determine if a particular individual has fathered the specific child in question.

Pathetism Winning over and exploring some one's mind by suggestion.

Pathogen Any microorganism capable of causing disease.

Pathognomonic Discrete or characteristic symptom of a disease.

Pathology Branch of medical science dealing with nature and cause of disease and the functional/structural changes caused by the disease.

p. experimental Study of disease process induced artificially usually in animals.

p. surgical Study of surgically removed tissues for studying disease.

Pathophysiology Study of changes in physiology by the diseased process.

Patient One who is ill or sick, physically or mentally.

Patient-controlled analgesia A system of controlling pain by drugs whose delivery is controlled by the patient himself; usually helpful in obstetric pain of labor by epidural catheter drug delivery.

Patulous Open, spread apart.

Paul-Bunnel Test Test for heterophil antibody in patients of infectious mononucleosis.

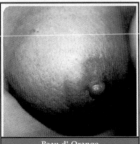
Peau d' Orange

Peau d' orange Dimpled skin resembling orange as in carcinoma breast.

Pectin A carbohydrate obtained from peel of citrous fruits and apple pulp used as astringent.

Pectineal line The ridge of pubis bone.

Pectineus The quadrangular muscle at upper and inner thigh acting as a flexor and adductor of thigh.

Pectoralis Pertains to breast; the muscles on anterior chest wall.

p. major Triangular muscle attached to upper humerus that draws the arm forward and downward.

Pectoriloquy The distinct transmission of vocal sounds to ear through the chest wall as in consolidation.

Pectus The chest or thorax.

p. carinatum Abnormal prominence of sternum as in rickets *SYN*—Pigeon chest.

p. excavatum Abnormal depression of sternum.

Pedesis Brownian movement of particles in a system, may be liquid or gas.

Pediatrics Medical science dealing with children below 14 years of age.

Pedicle The stem that attaches the tumor to the organ.

Pedicle flap The skin flap used in plastic surgery which carries its blood supply.

Pediculosis Infestation with lice.

Pedigree The tree or chart involving one's ancestors as used for genetic analysis.

Pedodontist Dentist practising pediatric dentistry.

Pedograph Imprint of foot on paper.

Peduncle A connecting band of nervous tissue.

p. cerebellar inferior Connects spinal cord and medulla with cerebellum.

p. cerebellar middle Channel for pontocerebellar fibers.

p. cerebellar superior Connects cerebellum with midbrain.

p. cerebral A pair of white bundle connecting cerebrum to midbrain; the pathway for descending corticospinal and corticonuclear projection.

Pegrete The downward extension of thickened epidermis between the dermal papillae.

Pel-Ebstein fever Cyclic fever occurring in Hodgkin's disease.

Pelger-Huet anomaly A congenital inherited anomaly of neutrophils which have coarse chromatin in the nuclei but function in normal manner.

Peliosis Purple patches on skin and mucous membrane. *SYN* — purpura.

Pellagra Avitaminosis due to want of nicotinic acid manifesting with diarrhea, dermatitis and dementia.

Pellet A tiny pill.

p. cotton a small rolled cotton ball particularly useful in dentistry

Pellicle Scum, film on surface of liquid

Pelotherapy Therapeutic use of mud or hay to treat disease by application on body.

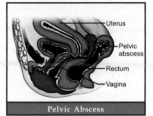

Pelvic Abscess

Pelvic inflammatory disease Infection of fallopian tubes, broad ligament and supporting tissues of uterus.

Pelvic inlet Upper pelvic entry, i.e. space between sacral promontory and upper aspect of symphysis pubis.

Pelvic outlet Lower pelvic outlet outlined by tip of coccyx, ischial tuberosities and lower margin of symphysis pubis.

Pelvic rock An exercise to strengthen the abdominal muscles and reduce the risk of backache during pregnancy

Pelvimetry Measurement of pelvic dimension manually or by X-ray.

Pelvis The structure formed by iliac bones, sacrum and coccyx.
Inlet A-P diameter =11 cm.
Diagonal conjugate = 13 cm.
True conjugate =11 cm.
Transverse diameter =11 cm.
Outlet AP diameter = 11 cm.

p. android Male type pelvis with shallow sacral hollow.

p. anthropoid Long narrow pelvis.

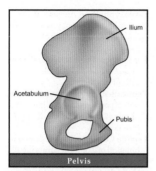

Pelvis

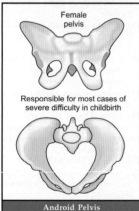

Female pelvis

Responsible for most cases of severe difficulty in childbirth

Android Pelvis

p. contracted Pelvis in which one or more diameters are less so as to impede birth of fetus.

p. funnel shaped Pelvis with normal inlet but markedly contracted outlet.

p. Naegeles Obliquely contracted pelvis.

p. Otto Pelvis in which head of femur extends into pelvic cavity due to depressed acetabulum.

Pemphigus A bullous disease that appears suddenly on normal skin and disappears leaving pigmented spots.

p. erythematous Erythematous macules and blebs resembling lupus erythematosus and perphigus vulgaris.

p. foliaceus Pemphigus with a chronic course and purulent bulous fluid from beginning.

p. vegetans Pemphigus with pustules instead of bullae followed by warty vegetations.

p. vulgaris Common form of bullous pemphigus with bilateral distribution.

Pemphigoid Skin lesion similar to pemphigus.

Penetrance The frequency of manifestation of a hereditary disease in individuals who have the dominant or double recessive gene.

Penicillamine A derivative of penicillin used to treat rheumatoid arthritis and heavy metal poisoning.

Penicillin Antibiotic synthesized by various molds, bactericidal to gram positive cocci, spirochaetes and rickettsiae by inhibition of cell wall synthesis.

Penicillinase An enzyme that breaks up molecule of some penicillins.

Penicillium A genus of molds that occasionally produce infection of external ear, skin and respiratory passage.

Penicilloyl-polylysine A substance used to test sensitiveness of a person to penicillins by intradermal skin test or instillation to conjuctival sac.

Penile prosthesis Implantable device in the penis to achieve erection; the device is in form of inflatable plastic cylinders implanted to corpora cavernosa attached to a pump embedded in scrotal pouch. The fluid reservoir to fill the cylinders is implanted behind the rectus.

Penile reflex Contraction of bulbo cavernosus muscle on percussion of dorsum of penis or compression of glans penis.

Penile ring A malleable ring that by preventing venus return from penis helps to maintain erection and delaying orgasm.

Pennifonn Feather shaped.

Pentaerythritol tetranitrate Organic nitrate for angina pectoris.

Pentagastrin Synthetic gastrin to stimulate HCl secretion.

Pentamidine An antimonial used to treat leishmaniasis.

Pentavalent Having valency of five.

Pentazocine An analgesic with strong addictive potential.

Pentobarbital A hypnotic-sedative agent.

Pentolinium Ganglion blocking agent.

Pentosuria Excretion of pentose sugars in urine.

Pentothal sodium Thiopental sodium, used for induction of anesthesia.

Pentoxyphylline Aa vasodilator

Pepsin Proteolytic enzyme of gastric juice which converts proteins into proteoses and peptones.

Pepsinogen The inactive precursor of pepsin found as granules in chief cells of stomach.

Peptic ulcer An ulcer occurring at sites of peptic mucosa, i.e. lower end of esophagus, stomach, first part of duodenum.

Peptide Compound formed by combination of 2 or more amino acids.

Peptidoglycan The material making the cellwall of most microorganisms.

Peptococcus Anaerobic gram positive cocci present in oral cavity, intestine and urinary tract.

Peptone Nitrogenous compounds formed by action of proteolytic enzymes on certain proteins.

Peptostreptococcus Gram positive anaerobic cocci.

Percentile One of 100 equal divisions of a series of items or data.

Perception Process of being aware or being conscious.

Percolate To filter, to strain.

Percolator Apparatus used for extraction of a drug with a liquid solvent

Percussion The use of fingertips to tap the body directly or indirectly to determine position, size and consistency of underlying structure.

Percutaneous Through skin.

Percutaneous ultrasonic lithotriptor Device using ultrasound applied externally to break up kidney stone.

Percutaneous transluminal coronary angioplasty (PCTA) A non-operative balloon dilatation of partially occluded coronary vessels.

Perforation A hole.

Perfusion Supply of an organ/tissue with blood.

Periactin Cyproheptadine hydrochloride, antiserotonin.

Periadenitis Inflammation of tissue surrounding a lymph node.

Perianal Around the anus.

Periarteritis Inflammation of outer coat of an artery.

Periarthritis Inflammation of joint capsule.

Peribronchial Surrounding the bronchus.

Pericardiocentesis Drainage of pericardial sac.

Pericardial rub Friction between the inflamed layers of pericardium.

Pericardiectomy Excision of pericardium.

Pericardiopexy Increasing blood supply to heart by joining pericardium to adjacent tissue.

Pericarditis Inflammation of pericardium often with serofibrinous effusion and rarely constriction.

p. constrictive Pericarditis leading to restriction in ventricular filling with equalisation in diastolic pressure in both ventricles and atria.

Pericardium A bilayer fibroserous sac enclosing heart.

Pericholangitis Inflammation of tissue surrounding bile duct.

Perichondritis Inflamed perichondrium.

Perichondrium Fibrous membrane around the cartilage.

Pericranium Periosteum of skull.

Perikarion Cell body of a neuron.

Perikymata Transverse grooves on surface of enamel of newly erupted anterior teeth

Perimysium Connective tissue sheath around bundle of muscle fiber

Perineoraphy Repair of perineal tear caused during parturition.

Perineotomy Incision into perineum to facilitate delivery as in rigid perineum of primi.

Perinephric Around the kidney.

Perineum The structures occupying the pelvic outlet and constituting pelvic floor.

p. tears of First degree tear involves vaginal mucosa, second degree involves the musculature in addition and in third degree tear the anal sphincter is also torn.

Perineural Around the nerve.

Perineurium Connective tissue sheath around bundle of nerve fibers.

Period The menstruation; the time interval between two events.

p. absolute refractory The period during which any strong stimulus cannot bring about muscle contraction.

p. gestation Period of pregnancy, i.e. 10 lunar months or 280 days measured from onset of last menstrual period.

p. incubation Time from contacting infection till appearance of first symptom.

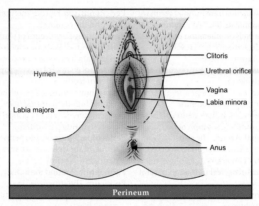

Perineum

p. isoelectric In ECG electrical neutrality or balancing positive and negative charges.

p. latent Time between application of stimulus and onset of contraction.

p. missed Non-occurrence of menstruation at expected time.

p. puerperal The six weeks period immediately following child birth.

p. safe The period during the menstrual cycle during which intercourse cannot lead to conception. It usually includes the first 5 days after stoppage of period and the last 10 days prior to next period.

Periodicity Recurring at more or less regular intervals.

Periodic table The chart depicting chemical elements arranged by their atomic numbers.

Periodontal abscess Abscess formation in gingiva, periodontal pockets.

Periodontal disease Disease of supporting structure of teeth with bleeding gum, loosening of teeth, etc.

Periodontal ligament The fibrous bundles attaching tooth to alveolar bone.

Periodontics The branch of dentistry dealing with study and treatment of periodontal disease.

Periodontitis Inflammatory or degenerative disease of dental periosteum, alveolar bone, cementum and gingiva.

Periodontium The structures that support the teeth and firmly anchor it to alveolar bone.

Periodoscope Pregnancy table for knowing expected date of delivery.

Perionychia Inflammation around a nail.

Perioperative Period immediately before or after an operation.

Perioral Around the mouth.

Periosteitis Inflamed periosteum.

Periosteum A fibrous membrane covering the bone, supporting the blood vessels supplying bone and giving attachment to ligaments and muscles. Its inner cellular layer forms new bone.

Periostotomy Incision of peripsteum.

Periosteophyte New bone formation from periosteum.

Peripheral nervous system Included in this are 12 cranial nerves, 31 spinal nerves, sympathetic and parasympathetic nerves.

Periphlebitis Inflammation of outer coat of vein or tissue around the vein.

Periportal Around the portal vein or its branches.

Periproctitis Inflamed loose areolar tissue around anus and rectum.

Periprostatic Around the prostate.

Perirenal Around the kidney.

Perisplenitis Inflammation of splenic capsule.

Peristalsis Wave like contraction occurring in hollow viscus.

Peristasis A temporary decrease in blood flow in early inflammation.

Peritomy Incision around cornea to treat pannus.

Peritoneal dialysis Removal of toxic metabolic byproducts and some poisons from body by irrigation of peritoneal cavity by dialysate and then draining out the dialysate.

Peritoneopexy Fixation of uterus by way of vagina.

Peritoneoscope An endoscope to visualize abdominal cavity through an incision in the abdominal wall.

Peritoneum A serous membrane reflected over abdominal viscera and lining the abdominal cavity.

Peritonitis Inflamed peritoneum manifesting with board like rigidity of abdomen and aperistalsis, commonly follows rupture of hollow organ, pelvic inflammation, or is primary; can be localized or generalized; acute or chronic, adhesive and aseptic.

Peritrichous Cilia or flagella covering entire surface'of micro organism

Periurethral Around the urethra.

Permeability The quality of being permeable that which can be traversed.

Pernicious anemia Vitamin B_{12} deficient anemia due to antibodies to gastric parietal cells leading to deficient intrinsic factor secretion.

Pernio Swelling of skin due to cold.

Perone Fibula.

Peroneal Concerning fibula.

Peroneal sign In tetany tapping over peroneal nerve causes dorsiflexion and eversion of foot.

Peroral Through the mouth.

Peroxidase An enzyme essential for oxygen transfer, hence important in cellular respiration.

Peroxisome Granules in cell cytoplasm that contain a variety of enzymes.

Perphenazine Antipsychotic agent.

Perseveration Repetition of meaningless words, phrases or answers.

Personality The composition of one's characteristics, behavior, grooming etc.

p. compulsive A type of personality where individual's perfectionism, indecisiveness hampers with social adjustment and interpersonal relationship.

p. extroverted Individual's activities and libido are directed to other individuals or environment.

p. histrionic Personality with self exaggeration, dramatisation, irrational and angry outbursts.

p. introverted Person's activities and libido are directed towards himself.

p. paranoid Undue suspiciousness, mistrust and hypersensitiveness.

p. schizoid Shyness, seclusiveness, eccentricity.

Perspiration Water loss from skin via evaporation of sweat; 1 liter of sweat evaporation removes 580 calories of heat from the body.

p. insensible The evaporation is without prior appearance of moisture on skin.

p. sensible Perspiration that forms moisture on skin.

Perthe's disease Osteochondritis of femoral head due to compromised circulation.

Perturbation Agitated, uneasiness of mind.

Pertussis Acute infectious respiratory disease caused by *B. pertussis, SYN*— whooping cough.

Pertussis immune globulin Globulin derived from patients immunized with pertussis vaccine, used for passive immunization.

Pertussis vaccine Killed pertussis bacilli used for active immunization.

Perversion Deviation from normal accepted path.

p. sexual Abnormal sexual behavior.

Pervert One who has deviated from normal path.

Pervious Capable of being permeated.

Pes Foot.

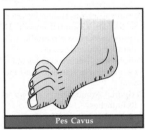
Pes Cavus

p. cavus Increased concavity of foot.

p. equinovalgus Elevation and lateral rotation of heel.

p. equinovarus Elevation and internal rotation of heel.

p. equinus Walking on forefoot, the heel not touching the ground.

Pessary Device inserted into vagina to support pelvic structures like uterus, urethra.

Pessimism A state of mind where one feels dejected, hopeless and gloomy.

Pest Destructive insect.

Pesticide Chemicals used to kill pests.

Pestilence Epidemic of a disease.

Petechiae Hemorrhagic spots on the skin.

Pethidine Meperidine hydrochloride.

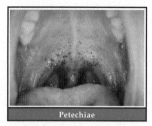
Petechiae

Petit mal Little illness. A form of epilepsy.

Petit's ligament Utero sacral ligament.

Petit's triangle An area on lateral abdominal wall bounded by iliac crest, posterior margin of external oblique and lateral margin of latissimus dorsi.

Petridisk A shallow dish with a cover to hold solid media for culture.

Petrifaction Process of hardening.

Petrositis Inflammation of petrous part of temporal bone.

Peutz-Jegher's syndrome Small intestinal polyposis with hypermelanosis of skin and mucous membrane.

Peyer's patch Lymphoid tissue in small intestine as circular/oval patches in the mucosa-submucosa in the antimesenteric border.

Peyronie's disease Hardening of corpora cavernosa which leads to painful erection and a curved penis.

pH Expresses acidity or alkalinity. pH of 7 is neutral, that above is alkaline and below acidic. Maximum acidity is pH-0 and maximum alkalinity is 14. pH is logarithm of hydrogen ion concentration divided into one

Phacomatosis A group of hereditary diseases manifesting with cutaneous and neurological symptoms. Included in this group are von-Recklinghausen's disease, Hippel-Lindau disease, Sturge-Weber syndrome, tuberous sclerosis and incontinentia pigmenti.

Phage Viruses that can lyse bacteria.

Phage typing A method of identifying particular strains of bacteria that are lysed by only strain specific bacteriophages.

Phagocyte A cell capable of ingesting and digesting cell debris, protozoa, bacteria etc.

Phagocytic index Average number of bacteria ingested by each leukocyte.

Phagocytosis The process of ingestion and digestion of bacteria by phagocytes.

Phagolysosome The body formed when membrane bound phagosome inside a macrophage fuses with lysosome.

Phagomania Abnormal craving for food.

Phagosome A membrane bound vacuole inside a phagocyte containing matters to be digested.

Phakoma Microscopic gray white tumor of retina in tuberous sclerosis.

Phalanx Bones on finger and toes; proximal, middle and distal.

Phalen's test A test for diagnosis of carpal tunnel syndrome when flexon at wrist of fully extended arm causes pain

Phallic Pertaining to penis.

Phalliform Shaped like a penis.

Phalloidin Poisonous peptide from mushroom *Amanita phalloides.*

Phallus Penis.

Phaneromania Abnormal tendency to bite nails, pull or play with hair, beard or moustache.

Phantasy A daydream or disregard for reality.

Phantom An appearance or illusion of body part.

p. limb Following amputation, patient feels as if the limb exists.

p. tumor Muscular contraction or abdominal fat mistaken as tumor.

Pharmaceutics Science of dispensing medicines.

Pharmacodynamics Study of drugs and their action on living organisms.

Pharmacognosy The science of natural drugs and their properties.

Pharmacology The science of drugs, their property and effect.

Pharmacy The practice of compounding and dispensing medicines; a drug store.

Pharyngeal bursa A small blind sac occasionally present in lower portion of pharyngeal tonsils.

Pharyngeal reflex Contraction of pharyngeal musculature following its stimulation by contact.

Pharyngismus Spasm of pharyngeal muscles.

Pharyngitis Inflammation of pharyngeal mucosa.

Pharyngocele Hernia through pharyngeal wall.

Pharyngo conjunctival fever An adenovirus infection.

Pharynx The common gateway in throat for food and air extending from base of skull to 6th cervical vertebra. Nasopharynx is the portion above palate: oropharynx lies between palate and hyoid bone and laryngo-pharynx below the hyoid bone.

Phase A stage of development.

Phenacemide Anticonvulsant agent, rarely used because of serious side effects.

Phenacetin An analgesic and antipyretic agent.

Phenanthrene A coal tar derivative with high carcinogenic potential.

Phenazopyridine Urinary analgesic causing red urine.

Phencyclidine A hallucinogen, also used as anesthetic in veterinary medicine (angel dust).

Phenelzine An antidepressant.

Phenergan Promethazine hydrochloride.

Phenformin An oral hypoglycemic agent, having propensity to cause lactic acidosis.

Phenindione An anticoagulant.

Pheniramine maleate An antihistaminic agent.

Phenmetrazine A sympathomimetic often used to treat obesity.

Phenobarital Phenyl ethyl barbituric acid used as a hypnotic and anticonvulsant.

Phenol A coal tar derivative effective as a bacteriostatic agent (*SYN*—carbolic acid).

Phenology Study of effects of climate on living things.

Phenolphthalein A laxative.

Phenolsulphonphthalein A dye used for renal function test.

Phenomenon A change perceivable by senses.

p. Bell's Rolling of eyeball upward and outward on attempting to close the affected eye in lower motor neurone facial palsy.

Phenothiazine The basic compound used for manufacture of tranquilizers, anthelmintics, dyes and some insecticides.

Phenotype The physical appearance or the sum total of visible traits which characterize the members of a group.

Phenoxyacetic acid A fungicide.

Phenoxy benzamine An alfa-adrenergic blocking agent that causes peripheral vasodilatation.

Phenozygous A developmental anomaly where the skull is much narrower than the face.

Phenprocoumon An anticoagulant.

Phensuximide Anticonvulsant useful for petit mal.

Phentermine Sympathomimetic drug used as anorexic agent.

Phentolamine An alpha adrenergic blocking agent used in diagnosis of pheochromocytoma.

Phenylalanine An essential amino acid.

Phenyl butazone An analgesic anti-inflammatory agent sparingly used for adverse effects on marrow.

Phenylephrine Adrenergic agent used as nasal decongestant.

Phenylethyl alcohol An antibacterial agent used as a preservative.

Phenylhydrazine Used as a test reagent for detecting sugar in urine.

Phenyl ketonuria An autosomal recessive disease where due to defective enzyme system phenylalanine is not converted to tyrosine and there is likelihood of brain damage.

Phenyl mercuric acetate A bacteriostatic agent, also fungicide and herbicide.

Phenyl mercuric nitrate A bacteriostatic agent employed for wound dressing and preservation of IV solutions.

Phenylpyruvic acid A metabolic derivative of phenyl-alanine.

Phenytoin Anticonvulsant drug, also antiarrhythmic.

Pheochromocyte The chromaffin cells of adrenal medulla giving yellowish reaction with chrome salts.

Pheochromocytoma A benign chromaffin cell tumor of adrenal medulla producing adrenaline and noradrenaline.

Pheromone A chemical substance which acts as a means of communication between species of insects through its smell.

Philadelphia chromosome Dislocation of long arm of chromosome 21 to chromosome 9, seen in 90% patients of chronic myelocytic leukemia.

Philtrum The median groove on upper lip.

Phimosis Narrowing of prepucial orifice so that it cannot be retracted over glans penis.

Phlebectomy Surgical resection of vein.

Phlebitis Inflammation of a vein.

Phlebogram A venous pulse tracing.

Phlebography X-ray imaging of the veins by contrast injection.

Phlebolith A concretion in a vein.

Phlebotom Lancent used in incising vein.

Phlebotomus A genus of sandflies, the blood sucking insects transmitting leishmaniasis, oroya fever.

Phlegmasia Inflammation.

p. alba dolens Edema of leg due to thrombophlebitis.

p. malabarica Inflammation with hypertrophy and induration of skin *SYN* — elephantiasis.

Phlegmon Acute inflammation with suppuration of subcutaneous tissue.

Phlyctenula A tiny vesicle or pustule.

Phobia Irrational fear resulting in desire to avoid the feared object / situation.

Phocomelia Congenital malformation where proximal part of a limb is ill developed.

Pholcodine Morphine analog, high addictive potential.

Phonation Production of vocal sounds.

Phonetics Science of pronunciation and speech.

Phono cardiogram Graphic recording of heart sounds.

Phosgene A poisonous gas used in production of pharmaceutical and chemical products.

Phosphatase Enzymes that catalyze hydrolysis of phosphoric acid esters.

p. acid Present in semen, prostatic secretion, osteoclasts and odontoclasts.

p. alkaline Present in developing bone, plasma, and teeth; excreted by liver, increase in obstructive jaundice, bone metastasis and osteomalacia.

Phosphate Salt of phosphoric acid (PO_4). Monosodium and disodium phosphates help to maintain acid-base balance of blood.

p. acid Phosphate in which one or two atoms of hydrogen in phosphoric acid are replaced by a metal.

p. triple Calcium - ammonium and magnesium phosphate.

Phosphaturia Increased excretion of phosphate in urine.

Phosphocreatine An important compound in muscle metabolism.

Phosphofructokinase A glycolytic enzyme.

Phosphorescence The emission of light without heat.

Phosphoric acid Principally used to etch enamel of teeth during restoration work.

Phosphorylase Enzyme catalyzing formation of glucose-l phosphate from glycogen.

Phosphorylation The reaction of phosphate with an organic compound.

Photic epilepsy Convulsion following light stimulation.

Photo dermatitis Skin allergy due to ultraviolet light.

Photocoagulation Light energy used to coagulate tissue proteins as in retinal detachment or diabetic proliferating retinopathy.

Photometer Device for measuring the intensity of light.

Photomicrograph Photograph of an object under microscope.

Photon Unit of energy of light ray.

Photophobia Intolerance to light, a feature of keratitis, uveitis etc.

Photophone Instrument for production of sound by action of light.

Photopsia Subjective feeling of seeing flashes of light as in disease of hind brain (occipital cortex).

Photoptometry Measurement of light perception.

Photoptometer Instrument determining the smallest amount of light required to make an object visible.

Photoreceptor Sensory nerve endings or cells capable of being stimulated by light, e.g. rods and cones.

Photoretinitis Macular burn on exposure to intense light.

Photosensitizer Substance that compounds abnormal reaction of skin to light

Photosynthesis The process by which plants combine water and trapped carbon dioxide to produce carbohydrates.

Phototherapy Therapeutic use of sunlight or artificial blue light to reduce serum bilirubin in newborn.

Phototropism Tendency of plants and some microorganisms to grow towards light.

Phrenic Concerning diaphragm.

Phrenicotomy Severing the phrenic nerve to produce paralysis of diaphragm in order to provide rest to that lung.

Phthirus A genus of blood sucking lice.

Phthisic Concerning pulmonary tuberculosis.

Phycomycosis A fungal disease caused by inhalation of spores.

Phyletic Concerning a race.

Phylogeny Growth and development of a race.

Phylum One of the primary divisions of animal or plant kingdom.

Physiatrist Physician specializing in physical medicine.

Physical Concerning body or material things.

Physical therapy Rehabilitation for restoration of functions and prevention of disability by using exercise, heat, massage, ultraviolet etc.

Physician A doctor practising medicine.

Physicist A specialist in physics.

Physics The science of laws of matter, their properties and various forms of energy.

Physiological Concerning normal body function.

Physiology The branch of science dealing with functions of living organisms.

Physiotherapy Treatment with physical means.

Physostigmine Cholinergic agent, acts by destruction of cholinesterage in nerve ending; used in myasthenia gravis.

Phyton Calcium or magnesium salt of inositol and hexaphosphoric acid; present in cereals.

Phytobezoar An accumulated mass of vegetable matter found in the stomach.

Phytogenesis The origin and development of plants.

Phytohemagglutinin A plant lectin agglutinating red blood cells.

Phytonadione Synthetic vitamin K.

Phytophotodermatitis Dermatitis produced from exposure to certain plants and then to sunlight.

Phytosis Disease caused by vegetable parasite.

Phytotoxin Plant toxin.

Pica Perverted appetite with eating of uneatables like plastic, clay, plaster etc.

Pickwickian syndrome Obesity with hypoventilation.

Pico = 10^{-12}

Picornavirus RNA virus group that includes coxsackie, ECHO and rhinoviruses.

Picrotoxin A CNS stimulant, a shrub derivative not in use now.

Piedra Niodular masses around hair of beard/mustache (white or black) due to a fungus

Pierre-Robin syndrome Small jaw, cleft palate and absent gag reflex.

Piezoelectricity Production of electricity by application of pressure to certain crystals like mica, quartz, etc.

Pigeon breast Sternum projecting forward due to rickets or childhood respiratory obstruction.

Pigeon-breeder's lung A form of hypersensitive pneumonitis due to exposure to excreta of pigeons and parakeets.

Pigeon toed *SYN* — Pes varus; walking with feet turned inward.

Pigment Any organic coloring material in the body.

p. bile Bilirubin and biliverdin, the hemoglobin degradation products in blood secreted in bile, urobilin and bilifuscin excreted in stool and urine.

p. blood Hematin, hemin, methemoglobin and hemosiderin, all derivatives of hemoglobin.

Pigmentophore A cell that carries pigment.

Pile Hemorrhoid.

p. sentinel Thickened anal mucous membrane at the lower end of an anal fissure.

Pili Hairs.

p. annulata Monilethrix or ringed appearance of hairs.

p. incarnati Ingrowing hair.

p. torti Broken and twisted hair.

Pillation Formation and development of hair.

Piliform Hair like.

Pill A medicine presented as a solid mass for swallowing; oral contraceptive.

Pillar An upright support/column.

p's of fornix Downward extension of cerebral hemispheres.

p's of diaphragm Two bundles of muscle fibers extending from lumbar vertebra to the central tendon of diaphragm.

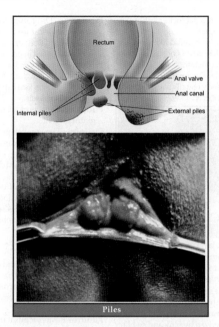

Piles

p's of fauces Folds of mucous membrane between which are situated the tonsils.

Pilobezoar Trichobezoar; hairball concretion in GI tract.

Pilocarpine A cholinergic causing pupillary contraction, used in glaucoma.

Piloerection Standing out of body hairs due to contraction of arrector pili muscles.

Pilojection Introduction of hair into aneurysm (usually intracranial) to promote blood coagulation.

Pilomotor reflex Goose flesh formation when cold is applied to skin or during emotion.

Pilonidal cyst Sacrococcygeal cyst from the entrapped epithelial tissue beneath the skin, a developmental defect.

Pimple A papule or pustule of the skin from blockage of sebaceous glands.

Pindolol A betablocker antihypertensive agent.

Pineal body A gland like structure near splenium of corpus callosum secreting melatonin.

Pinealoma Encapsulated tumor of pineal body usually causing precocious puberty.

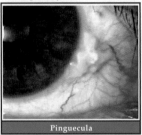
Pinguecula

Pinguecula Yellowish triangular thickening of bulbar conjunctiva adjacent to cornea.

Pinhole pupil Extremely contracted pupil as in opium poisoning and pontine hemorrhage.

Pink disease A disease of infancy characterized by pink and swollen extremities often with arthrosis, a hypersensitive reaction to mercury.

Pinna The auricle or external ear.

Pinocytosis A process by which cells absorb and ingest nutrients.

Pinosome The fluid filled vacuole formed during pinocytosis.

Pinta A nonvenereal skin disease caused by *(Treponema carateum)* and spreading by body contact.

Pinworm Enterobius vermicularis.

Piperazine Drug used for enterobiosis and ascariasis.

Pirenzepine Belladona alkaloid derivative, used in peptic ulcer.

Piriformes syndrome Pain in the hip and bullock down to leg due to sciatic nerve entrapment in piriformis muscle

Piroxicam Nonsteroidal antiinflammatory agent.

Pisiform The smaller pea shaped carpal bone in proximal row of wrist.

Pitch The quality of sound dependent upon frequency.

Pithiatry Treatment of disease by suggestion or persuasion.

Pitressin Vasopressin secreted from posterior pituitary (contains ADH + pressor agent).

Pitting Removal of senesent RBC by spleen.

Pituitary Endocrine gland.of size 1.3 cm. × 1 cm × 0.5 cm at base of brain secreting various hormones like TSH, GH, ACTH, LH, oxytocin and vasopressin.

Pituitrin Posterior pituitary extract.

Pityriasis Skin disease with brany scales.

p. alba Patches of macular scaly lesions, commonly in children.

p. rosea Acute inflammatory skin disease with macular eruption, rose red in color, symmetrical distribution and a clearing center.

p. rubia pilaris Persistent general exfoliative dermatitis.

p. versicolor Superficial fungal infection caused by *Malassezia furfur.*

Placebo An inactive substance, used in controlled studies of drugs.

Placenta The oval structure in pregnant uterus through which fetus derives its nutrition.

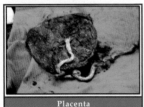
Placenta

p. accreta Placenta whose cotyledons have invaded the uterine musculature so that placental separation after delivery is difficult.

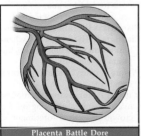
Placenta Battle Dore

p. battle dore Umbilical cord is inserted into margin of placenta.

p. circinate Cup shaped placenta.

p. circumvallate Cup shaped placenta with raised edges.

p. percreta Placental cotyledons invade uterus right up to serosal lining threatening rupture of uterus.

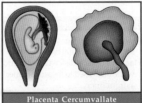
Placenta Cercumvallate

p. previa Placenta implanted to lower uterine segment, often causing painless profuse third trimester bleeding.

p. retained Placenta not expelled even 2 hours after fetal delivery.

p. succenturiate An accessory placenta having vascular connection with main placenta.

p. velamentous Placenta where the umbilical cord is attached to membranes, so that the umbilical vessels enter placenta at its margins.

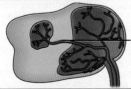
Blood vessel running through the chorion from the placenta to accessory lobe
Placenta Succenturiata

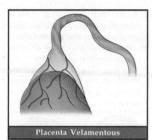

Placenta Velamentous

Placental souffle Auscultatory sound of placental blood flow.

Placido's disk A disk with black and white lines used to measure corneal astigmatism.

Pladaroma Warty growth on eyelid.

Plagiocephaly Irregular closure of cranial sutures resulting in deformed skull.

Plague Disease caused by *Pasteurella pestis*.

p. bubonic Common form of plague with suppurative lymphadenitis.

p. hemorrhagic Rare form of plague with prominent hemorrhagic manifestations particularly into skin.

p. pneumonic Virulent form of plague with extensive involvement of lungs.

Plane A smooth surface; imaginary cut through a body part.

p. Baer's Plane through upper border of zygomatic arches.

p. bite Plane formed by biting surface of teeth.

p. coronal Vertical plane at right angles to sagittal plane so that body is divided into anterior and posterior halves.

p. Hodge's Plane parallel to pelvic inlet passing through second sacral vertebra.

p. median Antero-posterior plane dividing body or organ into two equal parts.

p. sagittal Plane dividing body into equal right and left halves.

Planned parenthood The concept of choosing the time to have children.

Planoconcave An optical lens concave on one side but plane on the other side.

Planoconvex An optical lens convex on one side but plane on the other side.

Planorbis The genus of fresh water snails that serve as intermediate hosts for schistosoma.

Plantar arch The arch of the foot.

Plantaris A slim muscle in the calf.

Plantigrade The type of foot where the entire sole of foot touches the ground while walking.

Plaque A patch on skin or mucous membrane.

p. dental A gummy mesh harboring microorganism growing on the crowns of teeth, a forerunner of dental caries.

Plasma The liquid portion of blood, the medium for transporting nutrients and suspending the corpuscles.

Plasmacyte A plasma cell as found in connective tissue with eccentric nucleus.

Plasmacytoma Myeloma arising from marrow.

Plasma exchange Removal of patient's, plasma with replacement by colloid solution. This removes the immune complexes, excess antibodies or drugs and poisons.

Plasmapheresis Similar to plasma exchange.

Plasmid Extranuclear cell inclusion having genetic function; commonly seen in bacteria and used in DNA cloning and recombinant DNA technology.

Plasmin Fibrinolytic enzyme derived from plasminogen.

Plasmodium A genus of protozoa that includes causative agents of various types of malaria.

Plaster 1. Plaster of Paris used to immobilize a part or make an impression. 2. Medicinal agents formed into a tenaceous mass, e.g. belladona plaster.

Plastic bronchitis Bronchitis with fibrin casts of bronchi.

Plastic surgery Surgery for reconstruction, repair or restoration of body parts.

Plate 1. A flattened part or portion 2. Disk holding culture medium.

p. bite In dentistry used for getting dental impression of bites.

p. epiphyseal The cartilage between diaphysis and epiphysis on which depends the longitudinal growth of bone.

Plateau Elevated and flat area or steady and consistent phase of disease or fever.

Platelet Round or oval disk like cells in blood which help in blood coagulation and hemostasis.

Platelet concentrate Platelets prepared from few units of blood and suspended in plasma.

Platinum A hard heavy silver white metal.

Platybasia A developmental defect where the floor of posterior fossa of skull protrudes upwards often causing hydrocephalus and high cervical cord compression.

Platycephaly Flattening of the skull.

Platysma A thin aponeurotic muscle of neck which on contraction causes wrinkling of skin of neck and depression of jaw.

Platysmal reflex Dilatation of pupil on pinching platysma muscle of neck.

Plegia Suffix meaning paralysis.

Pleocytosis Increased number of lymphocytes in CSF.

Pleomorphism Having many shapes or forms.

Pleoptics A method of eye exercises to train and stimulate amblyopic eye.

Plethora Congestion with fluid.

Plethysmography The method of measuring volume, of blood flow through a part from change in volume.

Pleura A bilayered membrane that encloses the lungs.

Pleural cavity Space between the fibrous parietal pleura and serous visceral pleura.

Pleural effusion Fluid collection in pleural cavity, may be serous, serofibrinous or hemorrhagic.

Pleural fibrosis Thickening of pleura from inflammation, irritation.

Pleurisy Inflammation of pleura; may be primary or secondary, acute or chronic, serous or sero sanguinous.

p. diaphragmatic Inflammation of diaphragmatic pleura causing intense pain under margin of the ribs, hiccough, and often dyspnea.

p. dry Pleurisy where a fibrinous exudate covers the pleural surface causing pain during respiration.

p. encysted Pleurisy with effusion encysted by adhesion.

Pleurodesis Production of adhesion between visceral and parital pleura.

Pleurodynia Sharp pain in intercostal muscles due to fascitis of chest wall.

Pleurolysis Loosening of pleural adhesions.

Plexiform Resembling a network.

Pleximeter The one that receives the percussion.

Plexus A network of nerves, lymphatics or blood vessels.

p. brachial Network of nerves along the neck, axilla and arm.

p. enteric One of the two plexues of nerve fibers and ganglion cells lying in the wall of alimentary canal namely Auerbach's plexus and submucosal Meissner's plexus.

p. pampiniform A network of veins draining the testis in male or ovary in the female.

p. lumbar Network of nerves in the lumbar region.

Plica A fold.

p. circular Transverse folds in small intestine.

p. epiglottic Three folds of mucous membrane lying between the tongue and epiglottis.

p. palmate Mucosal folds in cervical canal.

p. semilunar of colon Transverse mucosal folds in the colon between the sacculations.

Plicate Folded.

Plication The stitching of folds or tucks to reduce the size of an organ.

Ploidy The number of chromosome sets in a cell.

Plombage A method of collapsing the apex of the lung.

Plototoxin A toxic substance present in cat fish.

Plug A mass closing or intending to close a hole.

p. Dittrich's A putrid mass of bacteria and fatty acids crystals in bronchiectasis.

Plumbism Lead poisoning.

Plummer-Vinson syndrome Iron deficiency anemia with dysphagia, achlorohydria, koilonychia and esophageal web, occurring commonly in women.

Pluripotent An embryonic cell having power to differentiate into different kinds of cells.

Plutomania Delusion of richness.

Plutonium A fissile material derived from uranium.

Pneodynamics The dynamics of breathing.

Pneogram Spirogram.

Pneumarthrogram X-ray of joint after air injection.

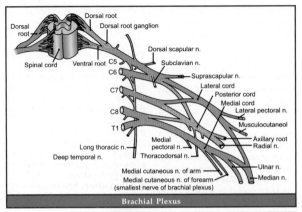

Brachial Plexus

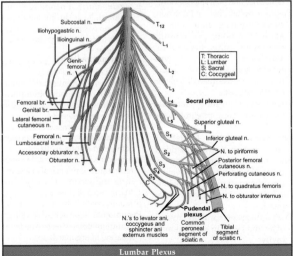

Lumbar Plexus

Pneumatics Branch of physics dealing with properties of gases.

Pneumatization Formation of air-filled cavities especially of mastoid.

Pneumatocele A swelling containing gas or air.

Pneumatosis Presence of air or gas in abnormal location of body.

Pneumaturia Presence of gas in urine due to vesico vaginal fistula.

Pneumococcal vaccine polyvalent A vaccine containing 23 of the known 83 pneumococcal capsular polysaccharides; providing immunity for 3-5 years. The vaccine is particularly useful in patients with sickle cell disease, immunodeficiency and post splenectomy.

Pneumococcus Encapsulated nonspore forming gram positive organism causing pneumonia, meningitis, otitis, mastoiditis, keratitis etc.

Pneumoconiosis Occupational diffuse lung disease due to inhalation of mineral dusts.

Pneumocystis carinii A protozoan parasite causing pneumonia in AIDS patients.

Pneumocystography Cystogram after injection of air into bladder.

Pneumoencephalogram X-ray for subarachnoid cisterns and ventricles of brain after injectin of air into subarachnoid space via lumbar puncture.

Pneumo hemo pericardium Presence of air and blood in the peritoneal cavity.

Pneumohydrothorax Presence of air and fluid in the thoracic cavity.

Pneumo mediastinum Presence of gas in the mediastinum.

Pneumomelanosis Pigmentation of lung as seen in pneumoconiosis.

Pneumonectomy Excision of lung.

Pneumonia Inflammation of lung tissue.

p. alba Pneumonia of newborn due to congenital syphilis.

p. aspiration Pneumonia following aspiration of purulent matter from throat/mouth or gastric content.

p. caseous Pneumonia associated with tuberculosis.

p. interstitial Pneumonia with infiltration of pulmonary interstitium.

p. eosinophilic Pneumonia with eosinophilia as during migration of round worm larva, micro filaria or due to drugs like nitrofurantoin, penicillin.

p. Friedlander's Lobar pneumonia caused by *Klebsiella pneumonae.*

p. giant cell An interstitial pneumonia of childhood with infiltration of lung by multinucleated giant cells, e.g. post measles.

p. hypostatic Pneumonia of aged and debilitated patients due to congestion of one part of lung at all times.

p. atypical Mild pneumonia but with radiological evidence of extensive lung infiltration as caused by *Mycoplasma pneumonae.*

p. woolsorter's Pulmonary anthrax.

Pneumonitis hypersensitive Diffuse granulomatous disease due to inhalation of organic dusts.

Pneumonosis Any noninfective lung disease.

Pneumo peritoneum Presence of air in the peritoneal cavity.

Pneumoradiography Injection of air into a part for X-ray examination.

Pneumorrhachis Presence of gas in the spinal canal.

Pneumothorax Presence of air in pleural cavity.

p. artificial Intentionally induced pneumothorax to cause pulmonary collapse as a treatment option in pulmonary tuberculosis.

p. tension A type of pneumothorax where air enters pleural space with each act of respiration but without an exit leading to high pleural pressure and collapse of lung.

Podagra Gout involving great toe or foot.

Podalic version Rotating the fetus to bring feet to the lower pole.

Podiatrist A specialist in diagnosis, treatment and care of diseases of foot.

Podocyte A special type of epithelial cell lining the glomeruli.

Podology The study of anatomy and physiology of foot.

Podophyllum Preparation from roots of *Podophyllum peltatum* to treat warts.

Poikilocyte Red blood cells of abnormal shape.

Poikiloderma A skin disorder characterized by pigmentation, telangiectasia, purpura, pruritus and atrophy.

Poikilothermy The condition of having same temperature as that of the environment.

Point A minute spot, sharp end of any object.

p. Boa's A tender spot on left of 12th thoracicfs vertebra in patients of gastric ulcer.

p. far Point (20 feet or more) at which normal eye does not use accommodation. The far point is less than 20' in myopia and there is no far point for hypermetropic eye.

p. Lian's A point at junction of outer and middle thirds of a line drawn from umbilicus to anterior superior iliac spine, suitable for paracentesis.

p. McBurney's Point 4-5 cm above the right anterior superior iliac spine on the line joining it to umbilicus, the point of tenderness in appendicitis.

p. Monro Point halfway between left anterior superior iliac spine and the umbilicus.

Poison Any substance which when inhaled, ingested or injected disturbs normal body function.

Poison IVY A climbing vine which on contact produces severe dermatitis.

Poison Oak A climbing vine producing dermatitis similar to ivy.

Poliomyelitis Acute viral disease that causes destruction of anterior horn cells in spinal cord and often cranial nerve nuclei with ensuing palsy.

p. ascending The paralysis begins in lower extremity and then ascends up trunk often to involve respiratory muscles.

p. bulbar Paralysis of cranial nerves and the respiratory center.

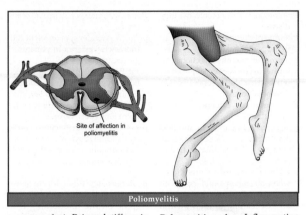

Site of affection in
poliomyelitis

Poliomyelitis

p. non paralytic Pain and stiffness in muscles but no paralysis.

Poliosis Whiteness of hair.

Polio vaccine Available as oral live attenuated vaccine or injectable killed vaccine prepared from types I, II, III polioviruses, given in 3 doses starting at 1½ months of age and then repeated for 2 more doses at 4-6 weeks interval.

Politzer bag Rubber bag used for inflating middle ear.

Pollen The microspores of a seed plant constituting the male gametocyte. Many airborn pollens are allergens.

Pollinosis Nasal congestion due to contact with pollens.

Poltophagy Thorough chewing of food.

Polyandry Having more than one husband.

Polyarteritis nodosa Inflammation of medium and small vessels segmentally with necrosis, an autoimmune disorder.

Polyarthritis Inflammation of more than one joint.

Polyarticular Involving many joints.

Polychondritis Inflammation of several cartilages.

Polychromasia Having many colours.

Polychromatophilia The quality of a cell being stainable with more than one stain.

Polyclinic A clinic catering for many variety of ailments.

Polycystic Having many cysts.

Polycystic ovary An endocrine disorder with anovulation and multiple cysts in the ovaries.

Polycythemia An excess of red blood cells.

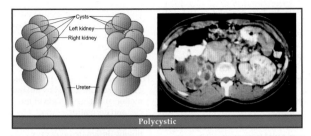

Polycystic

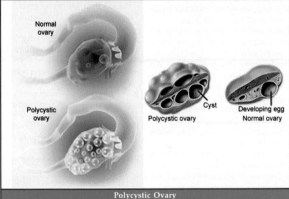

Polycystic Ovary

p. rubra vera A malignant disorder of marrow with increase in RBC mass, WBC and platelets.

Polydactylism Having supernumerary fingers or toes.

Polydipsia Excess thirst.

Polydystrophy Condition of having multiple congenital anomaly of connective tissue.

Polyendocrine deficiency syndrome Hypofunction of many endocrine glands; may be type I or type II; Type I-hypoparathyroidism, adrenal insufficiency, mucocutaneous candidiasis, Type II: IDDM, thyroid deficiency and adrenal insufficiency.

Polyesthesia Abnormal sensation of touch in which single stimulus is felt at two or more places.

Polyethylene A polymer used in production of IV tubing.

Polyethylene glycol Used as ointment base.

Polygamy Practice of having several wives or husbands.

Polygraph Machine that records arterial and venous pulse.

Polyhydramnios Excess of amniotic fluid.

Polymelia Having supernumerary limbs

Polymenorrhea Menses occurring at rapid frequency.

Polymer A synthetic substance made of two or more molecules.

Polymerase An enzyme catalyzing polymerization of nucleosides to form DNA.

Polymerase chain reaction An investigation technique for diagnosis of microbial diseases, genetic diseases by invitro production of numerous copies of DNA from the sample

p choanal a nasal polyp that extends to pharynx

p juvenile benign hamartoma of large bowel.

p laryngeal polyp of vocal cord causing hoarseness of voice

Polymerization The process of changing a simple chemical substance into another of higher molecular weight.

Polymorph A polymorpho nuclear leukocyte.

Polymorphism Appearing in many forms.

Polymyalgia rheumatica A connective tissue disorder of autoimmune nature affecting women with high ESR, weakness of proximal muscles and prompt response to low dose corticosteroids.

Polymyoclonus Muscular contraction proceeding in waveform to involve many muscle groups.

Polymyositis A connective tissue disorder characterized by inflammation and degeneration of muscles and dermatitis.

Polymyxin Aminoglycoside antibiotic designated polymyxin A, B, C, D, E, highly nephrotoxic.

Polyneuropathy Involvement of many peripheral nerves.

p. amyloid Polyneuropathy with thickening of nerves due to amyloid deposits.

p. erythroderma Polyneuropathy of children with skin disorder.

p. porphyric Polyneuropathy of porphyria with pain, paresthesia and often paralysis.

Polyneuro radiculitis Inflammation of nerve roots, peripheral nerves and spinal ganglia.

Polynuclear Having more than one nucleus.

Polynucleotide Nucleic acid composed of one or more nucleotides.

Polyomavirus A papovavirus family causing malignancy in lower animals.

Polyopsia Multiple images seen of the same object.

Polyorchidism Condition of having more than two testicles.

Polyostotic Concerning many bones.

Polyp A tumor with a pedicle.

p. adenomatous Benign polyp from glands.

Polypeptide Union of two or more amino acids.

Polyphagia Frequent and excess eating.

Polypharmacy Concurrent use of multiple drugs

Polyphrasia Talkativeness.

Polyploidy Condition characterized by twice or more number of normal haploid chromosome numbers of gametes.

Polyposis Presence of many polyps.

p. familial Multiple polyps in colon with rectal bleeding and chances of malignant changes.

p. ventriculi Multiple polyps of stomach associated with chronic atrophic gastritis.

Polypotrite Instrument for crushing polyps.

Polyradiculitis Inflammation of several nerve roots.

Polysaccharide Complex sugars which on hydrolysis yield more than 2 molecules of simple sugar.

Polyserositis Inflammation of many serous cavities, e.g. pleural effusion, ascites, pericardial effusion.

Polysinusitis Simultaneous inflammation of many sinuses.

Polystyrene A synthetic resin.

Polythiazide A mercurial thiazide diuretic.

Polyunsaturated Pertains to fatty acids having many carbon atoms joined by double or triple bonds.

Polyuria Excessive passage of urine of low specific gravity.

Polyvalent Substance with combining power of more than two atoms of hydrogen.

Polyvinyl alcohol A water soluble synthetic resin used for preparation of ophthalmic solutions.

Polyvinyl pyrrolidine Povidone.

Pomade A perfumed ointment.

Pompe's disease Glycogen storage disease type II.

Pompholyx Deep seated vesicles of palm and sole associated with contact allergy or fungal infection.

Ponderal index Height in inches/cube root of weight in pounds.

Pontic An artificial tooth set in a bridge.

Pontocaine hydrochloride Topical or spinal anesthetic.

Paples Posterior region of knee.

Popliteal Concerning back of knee.

Popliteus Muscle that flex the knee.

Poppy Any plant of genus papaver; opium is obtained from juice of unripe pods.

Porcine Piglike, obtained from porks.

Pore A small opening.

Pore of Kohn Pores for passage of gas from one alveolus to another, a way to prevent atelectasis

Porencephaly A congenital brain anomaly where ventricles extend up to subarachnoid space.

Porion The midpoint of upper margin of auditory meatus

Pornography Sex stimulating photographs or literature.

Porphobilinogen An intermediate product in heme biosynthesis, often present in urine in patients of porphyria, when exposed to air for long time changes to porphobilin imparting red colour to urine.

Porphyria A group of disorders of porphyrin metabolism.

p. acute intermittent Autosomal dominant trait characterized by abdominal pain, photosensitivity and neurological disturbances.

p. congenital erythropoitic Autosomal recessive trait with hemolysis, splenomegaly and skin reaction.

p. variegate Hepatic porphyria with fragile skin, recurrent episodes of abdominal pain and neuropathy.

Porphyrin Nitrogen containing organic compounds obtained from hemoglobin and chlorophyll.

Porphyrinuria Excess excretion of porphyrin in urine.

Porta Point of entry for nerves and vessels.

Portal circulation The circulation of blood in liver via portal vein and hepatic vein.

Portal hypertension Increased pressure in portal vein due to obstruction to portal blood flow in liver.

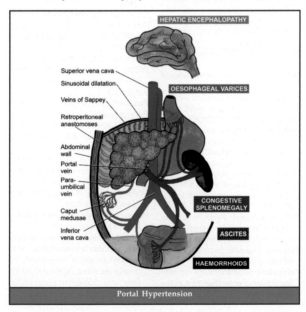

Portal Hypertension

Portal system The portal vein and its branches which drain the abdominal viscera and carry the blood to liver to be drained to inferior vena cava via hepatic vein.

Portal vein The vein formed from union of superior and inferior mesenteric, splenic, gastric and cystic veins.

Portography X-ray of portal vein after injection of contrast.

Portwine mark Superficial purple red birthmark.

Position Manner in which the body of patient is put.

p. Fowler's The position where head end of bed is elevated by 1½ feet and knees are elevated.

p. genucubital Position with patient on knees and elbows.

p. left lateral recumbent Patient lies on left side; right knee and thigh drawn up.

p. lithotomy Patient lies on back with thighs drawn on abdomen and abducted.

p. Trendelenburg Dorsal position with patient supine on a bed tilted to about 45° with head low.

Positive end expiratory pressure A method to prevent collapse of alveoli at end expiration.

Positron Positively charged particle.

Positron emission tomography A method of demonstrating brain image by use of positron emitting radionuclides.

Posology Branch of medicine dealing with dose of medicine.

Possum Device that permits a disabled individual to perform some job by forcefully breathing into master control apparatus.

Post myocardial infarction syndrome Pericardial pain aggravated on breathing, swallowing and change in body position with pericardial friction rubs.

Post polio syndrome Wasting of muscle years after recovery from polio.

Post traumatic stress disorder Re experiencing traumatic event, avoiding stimuli associated with trauma, recurrent arousal, hyper vigilant

Postcibal After meals.

Postclimacteric After menopause.

Postcoital After sexual intercourse.

Post connubial After marriage.

Posterior Situated at back or behind; dorsal.

Posterior drawer sign A test for posterior cruciate ligament tear of knee.

Postterm pregnancy Pregnancy continuing beyond 42 weeks of gestation

Posteroanterior Movement from back to front.

Posteromedial On the back towards midline.

Postfebrile After fever.

Post ganglionic fiber The autonomic nerve fiber passing from ganglia to visceral effector.

Posthaemorrhagic Occurring after a bleeding episode.

Posthumous Occurring after death

Posthetomy Circumcision, removal of foreskin of penis.

Posthitis Inflammation of prepuce.

Postictal Following an attack of epileptic fit.

Postmature Infant born after 42 weeks of gestation.

Postmortem After death.

Postmortem examination Dissection of dead body to determine the cause of death and pathological changes.

Postnatal Occurring after birth.

Postnasal Located behind the nose.

Post palatine Behind the palate.

Postpaludal After an attack of malaria.

Postpartum After child birth.

Postpartum depression Depression occurring in puerperium.

Postpartum hemorrhage Bleeding after childbirth in excess of 500 ml usually due to uterine atony, or cervical laceration.

Postpartum psychosis Psychosis occurring within the six months following childbirth. The symptoms and signs are hallucination, delusion, preoccupation with death etc.

Postprandial After a meal.

Postpubescent Following puberty.

Poststenotic Distal to a stenosed site.

Posttransfusion syndrome Fever, splenomegaly, atypical lymphocytosis that follow blood transfusion.

Postulate Supposition.

Postural Related to posture or body position.

Postural drainage Drainage of secretion from bronchi or pus from a cavity by positioning the patient so that gravity allows free drainage; usually done in bronchiectasis, lung abscess and following any prolonged surgery.

Postural hypotension Severe drop in blood pressure on assuming erect posture.

Posture Attitude or position of body.

Postviral fatigue syndrome Muscle fatigue unrelieved by rest after attack of viral fever.

Potable Water free from impurities and hence fit for drinking.

Potash Potassium carbonate.

p. caustic Potassium hydroxide.

Potassium Mineral element found in combination with other elements in the body. *SYN*— halium.

p. bicarbonate Used to neutralize acid in stomach.

p. chloride Used in IV solutions and as oral preparation to supplement during digoxin and diuretic therapy.

p. citrate Used as alkalizer.

p. iodide Used in expectorant preparations.

p. permanganate Topical astringent and antiseptic, antidote for phosphorus poisoning.

p. tartarate A cathartic.

Potency Strength, power, ability to perform sexual intercourse in case of male.

Potent Powerful, highly effective.

Potentiate To augment or increase the potency.

Potion Liquid medicine.

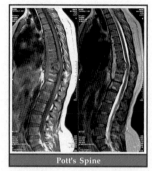
Pott's Spine

Pott's disease Tuberculosis of vertebra.

Pott's fracture Fracture of medial malleolus of tibia with lower end of fibula and outward and backward dislocation of foot.

Pouch Any pocket or sac.

p. Broca's A sac in tissues of labia majora.

p. laryngeal Blind mucosal pouch in the ventral larynx.

p. pharyngeal paired lateral pouches in embryonic pharynx.

p. Rathke's An embryonic outpocketing that forms anterior lobe of pituitary.

p. rectouterine Pocket between anterior rectal wall and posterior uterine wall.

Poultice Counter irritant preparation in the form of plaster.

Poupart's ligament The rolled up lower end of external oblique aponeurosis stretching between anterior superior iliac spine and pubic tubercle. *SYN* — Inguinal ligament.

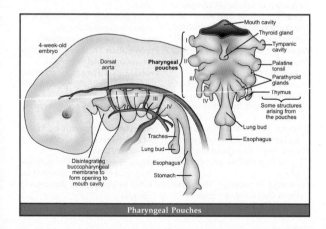
Pharyngeal Pouches

Povidone A synthetic polymer.

Povidone iodine A complex of povidone and iodine used for skin preparation prior to surgery, as vaginal tablets, as lotions and ointments for antiseptic purposes.

Pox Pustular lesion.

Praecox Early.

Praevia Going before in time or place.

Pragmatagnosia Inability to recognize even familiar object.

Pragmatic Pertains to practical aspect of anything.

Pralidoxime A cholinesterase reactivator used in organophosphorus poisoning.

Pramoxime A topical anesthetic.

Prandial Related to meal.

Prausnitz Kustner reaction Intracutaneous transfer of antibody to a healthy person followed by application of suspected allergen to produce wheal and flare. Not recommended now-a-days because of fear of AIDS and viral hepatitis.

Praxiology Study of behavior.

Praxis Planning and execution of co-ordinated movements.

Prazepam Anti-anxiety medicine.

Praziquantel Broad-spectrum antihelminth and antischistosomal drug.

Prazosin Alpha-adrenergic receptor blocker; antihypertensive agent.

Precancerous Any growth or lesion that will probably become cancerous.

Precentral convolution The frontal convolution or motor area.

Precipitate The process of deposition of substances from solutions.

Precipitin An antibody in animal, due to soluble protein antigen.

Precipitin test The formation of precipitate in a solution containing soluble antigen on addition of antibody.

Precocious Development, physical or mental earlier than expected.

Precordium The area of chest overlying the heart.

Precornu Anterior horn of lateral ventricle of brain.

Precursor A substance that precedes another substance, e.g. angiotensinogen is a precursor substance of angiotensin.

Prediabetes The stage or condition prior to development of clinical diabetes.

Predisposing A susceptibility to disease.

Predisposition The potential to develop a certain disease.

Prednisolone A glucocorticoid.

Predormition The state immediately preceding actual sleep.

Preeclampsia Toxemia of pregnancy with albuminuria, hypertension and edema.

Preeruptive Before eruption in exanthema.

Preexcitation Premature excitation of the ventricle by an impulse bypassing A-V node.

Preganglionic fibers Fibers transmiting autonomic impulse from CNS to peripheral autonomic ganglia.

Pregnancy The condition of development of embryo in the uterus.

p. abdominal Development of embryo in the abdominal cavity drawing its blood supply from omentum.

p. ampullar Implantation of ovum in the ampulla of fallopian tube.

p. cornual Pregnancy in one of the horns in a bicornuate uterus.

p. ectopic Condition where ovum develops outside the uterus.

p. molar Pregnancy where ovum degenerates into moles.

Pregnancy test Tests employed to confirm pregnancy by using patient's urine or blood which assess the chorionic gonadotropins. The test is positive beginning 40th day from the last menstrual period. Radioimmunoassay is better and more accurate.

Pregnanediol Progesterone metabolite (end product) in urine.

Pregnanetriol An intermediate metabolite of progesterone.

Pregnenolone A synthetic corticosteroid.

Prehension The primary functions of hand that includes pinching, grasping etc.

Preleukemia Some blood changes that may be forewarners of leukemic process, i.e. unexplained anemia, purpura, mucositis.

Preload In cardiac physiology it is ventricular wall stretch at end diastole.

Premarin Conjugated estrogen.

Premature Before full development.

Premature ejaculation Ejaculation shortly after the onset of sexual excitement.

Premature infant Infant with birth weight below 5 lb or born prior to 37 weeks of gestation.

Premenstrual tension syndrome The syndrome of irritability, anxiety, depression, rage, edema and breast tenderness prior to the onset of menstruation.

Premolar One of the permanent teeth occurring between canine and molar.

Premonition A feeling of an impending event.

Premorbid Prior to onset of disease.

Prenatal diagnosis Diagnosis of developmental defects and diseases while the baby is in utero by use of chemical tests, ultrasound, amnioscopy and amniocentesis.

Preoperative care Care preceding an operation like preparation of operation site, sedation, bowel wash, breathing exercise etc.

Preoptic area The anterior portion of hypothalamus.

Prepatellar bursitis Inflammation of bursa in front of patella *SYN* — housemaid's knee.

Preprandial Before a meal.

Prepubescent Just prior to puberty.

Prepuce The foreskin or skinfold over glans penis.

Prepucial glands Sebaceous glands at corona of penis secreting smegma. *SYN* — Tyson's glands.

Prepyloric Preceding the pylorus of stomach.

Prerenal 1. In front of kidney 2. uremia or any condition occurring prior to defects or changes affecting the kidney.

Presbycusis Sensory neural deafness of old age.

Presbyopia Recession of near point of eye with advancing age due to loss of elasticity of crystalline lens.

Prescribe To advise or indicate medicines/treatment to be taken.

Prescription A written order or direction for using a drug. A prescription consists of four main parts, i.e. superscription, inscription, subcription and signature.

Presenile Premature old age.

Presenium Prior to onset of senility.

Presentation In obstetrics the fetal part presenting at the pelvic inlet; can be breech, vertex, face, brow.

Preservative A chemical additive to drug preparations and foodstuffs that prevents growth of molds and fungi.

Pressure Compression, force exerted on any body tissue, e.g. blood vessel.

p. blood Pressure exerted by moving column of blood against arterial wall.

p. central venous Pressure in the right atrium.

p. end diastolic Pressure in the ventricles at the end of diastole.

p. intracranial Pressure to which CSF is subjected in sub-arachnoid space.

p. intraocular Pressure within the eyeball, maintained by vitreous and aqueous humor, usually 10-20 mm Hg.

p. negative Pressure less than atmospheric pressure.

p. oncotic Osmotic pressure exerted by colloids in a solution.

p. osmotic The force at which solvent like water passes through a semi-permeable membrane separating solutions of different concentrations.

p. wedge Pressure obtained by wedging a fluid filled catheter in a distal branch of pulmonary artery which is equivalent to left atrial pressure.

Pressure palsy Temporary palsy due to pressure on a nerve, e.g. saturday night palsy.

Pressure point Areas where pressure is applied to control bleeding. These points are where the bleeding artery passes over a bone little above the site of bleed, e.g. common carotid artery —2" above clavicle, temporal artery — in front of ear, subclavian artery — behind clavicle, brachial artery — mid arm or just above elbow; radial artery at wrist against radius and ulnar artery at wrist against ulna; femoral artery — compression of artery against femoral head in abduction and external rotation of limb; popliteal artery in popliteal space; anterior tibial artery at ankle in front; and posterior tibial artery behind.

Pressure sore A sore caused by pressure of splint or other appliance or pressure of body on bed at contact points particularly when the skin is insensitive or person is in coma or lies immobile for long time.

Preterm In obstetrics labor occurring before 37th week of gestation.

Pretibial fever A fever of leptospirosis with rash on leg, fever, splenomegaly

Prevalence The number of cases of a disease present in a specified population at a given time.

Preventive medicine The branch of medicine concerned with prevention of mental and physical illness and disease.

Prevertebral In front of vertebra.

Prevesical In front of bladder.

Prezonular Pertains to posterior chamber of eye.

Priapism Painful sustained penile erection without any sexual desire.

Priapitis Inflammation of the penis

Prickle cell A cell with rod shaped processes.

Prickly heat The blockage of sweat pores with escape of sweat to epidermis and formation of itchy tiny vesicles.

Primates An order of vertebrates highly developed in respect to nervous system and brain, e.g. monkey, apes and man.

Primaquine Antimalarial, for radical treatment of *P. vivax.*

Prime Period of greatest health and strength.

Primidone An anticonvulsant.

Primigravida Woman conceiving for first time.

Primipara Woman who has delivered a viable baby.

Primitive Early in point of time.

p. groove The longitudinal depression in the dorsum of the embryonic area.

Prinzmetal's angina Angina of coronary spasm with ST elevation.

Prion A small proteinaceous infectious particle

Prion disease They include kuru, C.J. disease, GSS syndrome, fetal familial insomnia and madcow disease

Prism A transparent solid, three sides of which are parallelograms. Light rays passing through a prism are split into primary colors.

p. maddox Two base together prisms used in testing cyclophoria or torsion of eyeball.

Privacy Right of the patient to revelation of data concerning illness.

Private practice Medical practice not under external policy control other than professional ethics.

Privileged communication Confidential information given by patient to treating doctor which is not to be divulged by the latter.

Proactivator A substance that contains a portion which can be split off and then it is able to activate another substance.

Proantithrombin The substance of plasma which is converted to thrombin by action of heparin.

Probability The ratio that expresses the likelihood of occurrence of specific event important in health statistics.

Proband The initial person with disease who serves as nucleus to study the same disease in his family and subsequent generations.

Probang A device to apply medicines in larynx.

Probanthine Propantheline bromide, an anticholinergic agent.

Probe An instrument for knowing depth and direction of sinus and wound.

Probenecid A benzoic acid derivative, urico suric and delays excretion of penicillin and its derivatives.

Probucol An anti-hyperlipidemic drug.

Procainamide Drug used for ventricular arrhythmia.

Procaine A local anesthetic used in infiltration anesthesia, nerve block, and spinal anesthesia.

Procarbazine A cytotoxic agent used in treatment of lymphomas.

Procedure A way of accomplishing a task to obtain desired result.

Proceious Concave anteriorly.

Procerus muscle A muscle that arises in the skin over the nose and is connected to forehead.

Process A projection or outgrowth of tissue; the steps or method of action.

p. alar Process of cribiform plate of ethmoid articulating with frontal bone.

p. alveolar Inferior border of maxilla or superior border of mandible containing tooth sockets.

p. ciliary About 70 meridional ridges projecting from the corona ciliaris to which suspensory ligament of fens is attached.

p. clinoid The anterior, middle and posterior clinoid processes of sphenoid bone.

p. condyloid The process from mandible articulating with temporal bone.

p. coracoid A beak shaped process extending from neck of scapula.

p. coronoid Sharp projection from semilunar notch of ulna.

p. odontoid Tooth like extension from axis.

Prochlorperazine A phenothiazine derivative for treating nausea and vomiting.

Procidentia Complete prolapse of uterus where it completely protrudes outside the introitus.

Procollagen Precursor of collagen.

Proconvertin Coagulation factor VIII.

Procreate To give birth.

Proctagra Rectal pain.

Proctalgia Pain in and around anus and rectum.

Proctectasia Dilatation of anus and rectum.

Proctenclisis Stricture of anus or rectum.

Proctitis Inflammation of anus and rectum.

Proctoclysis Infusion into rectum and anus.

Proctocolitis Inflammation of rectum and colon.

Proctology Branch of medicine dealing with diseases of rectum, colon and anus.

Proctoptosis Prolapse of anus and rectum.

Proctoscopy Instrument for examination of rectum.

Proctosigmoidoscopy Visual examination of rectum and sigmoid colon by sigmoidoscope.

Procumbent Lying face down.

Procyclidine Antiparkinsonian drug.

Prodromal Initial stage of disease before appearance of distinguished features.

Prodrome A symptom heralding an approaching ailment.

Prodrug Chemicals which exhibit their pharmacologic property after biotransformation in the body.

Proencephalus Brain protruding through a fissure of skull in the infant.

Proenzyme Inactive form of an enzyme.

Proerythroblast The earliest bone marrow precursor of erythrocyte.

Proestrus The period before menstruation.

Profunda Deep seated esp., blood vessel.

Progenitor An ancestor.

Progeny Offspring.

Progeria Premature senility occurring in childhood.

Progestational Concerned with luteal phase of menstrual cycle; action of hormone progesterone.

Progesterone Hormone secreted by placenta, corpus luteum and adrenal cortex; essential for secretory phase of endometrium, mammary growth and development and growth of placenta.

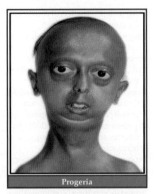

Progeria

Progestin Group of synthetic drugs having progesterone like effect on uterus.

Proglotid A segment of tapeworm containing both male and female reproductive organs.

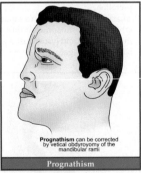

Prognathism can be corrected by vetical obdyroyomy of the mandibular rami

Prognathism

Prognathism Prominent jaws projecting beyond line of face.

Prognosis Prediction of course and outcome of a disease.

Prognosticate To state about outcome of a disease.

Progranulocyte Promyelocyte.

Progressive Advancing as bad to worse.

Progressive muscular atrophy Gradually advancing muscle atrophy due to disease of spinal cord.

Progress notes Notes endorsed by doctors and nurses during course of treatment.

Prohormone Precursor of hormone.

Proinsulin Insulin precursor produced in pancreas.

Projectile vomiting Vomiting where the stomach content is ejected with great force.

Projection A part extending beyond the level of its surrounding; referral of peripheral sensory stimuli to higher centers in CNS for interpretation.

Prokaryote Organism with a single circular chromosome without mitochondria and lysosomes, e.g. bacteria and algae.

Prolabium Central portion of upper lip.

Prolactin Hormone of anterior pituitary that helps in milk production.

Prolapse Falling down of a body part or organ.

p. cord Umbilical cord coming out before fetus.

p. of iris Protrusion of iris through corneal wound.

p. of rectum Protrusion of rectal mucosa through anal orifice.

p. of uterus Downward displacement of uterus.

Proliferate To increase by reproduction of similar forms as to the parent source.

Proliferous cyst Cyst with epithelial lining which proliferates and protrudes from its inner surface.

Prolific Fruitful, reproductive.

Proline An amino acid.

Promazine An antipsychotic agent, often used in obstetrics for sedation and tranquility during labor.

Promegakaryocytes Precursor cell of platelets.

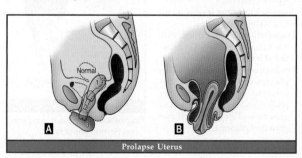

Prolapse Uterus

Prometaphase A stage in mitosis when the nuclear membrane disintegrates and the chromosomes move towards the equatorial plate.

Promethazine An antihistaminic agent.

Promine A tissue extract that promotes growth of certain tumors in mice.

Prominence A projection or eminence.

Promonocyte Precursor of monocyte.

Promontory A projecting surface or part.

p. of sacrum The anterior projecting surface of sacrum.

Promyelocyte A large mononuclear myeloid cell

p. penile A device implanted into penis to assist in erection; consists of inflatable plastic cylinders implanted into corpora cavernosa, a pump embedded in socrotal pouch and the fluid sac in rectus muscle.

Pronation The position of face downwards or palm facing downwards.

Pronator syndrome Syndrome of median nerve entrapment at elbow with paresthesia, thumb weakness, and tenderness in thenar muscles.

Pronephric duct Duct that connects posteriorly to cloaca and to which pronephric tubules are connected.

Pronephric tubules Tubules that open into cranial portion of pronephric duct and communicate with coelom.

Pronephros The earliest and simplest type of excretory organ in vertebrates.

Pronestyl Procainamide hydrochloride.

Pronormoblast An early precursor of redblood cells.

Pronucleus Nucleus of ovum or spermatozoa after fertilization.

Propantheline Anticholinergic agent.

Proparacaine Topical anesthetic.

Properdin A serum protein with some bactericidal property.

Prophase First stage of mitotic cell division.

Prophylaxis Prevention of disease.

Propriolactone A disinfectant used in preparing certain viral and bacterial vaccines.

Propiomazine A sedative agent.

Propionic acid A constituent of sweat.

Propositus Index case or prohand in investigation of hereditary disease.

Propoxycaine hydrochloride Local anesthetic agent.

Propoxyphene hydrochloride Analgesic agent.

Propranolol Betaadrenergic blocking agent used for hypertension, arrhythmias, angina pectoris, portal hypertension etc.

Proprietary medicine Any preparation used in treatment of diseases and has patent and copyright.

Proprioception Knowledge of body position, movement.

Proprioceptor Receptors responsible for body position and equilibrium e.g., muscle spindles, pacinian corpuscles and labyrinthine receptors.

Proptometer Instrument for measuring degree of exophthalmos.

Proptosis Protrusion of eyeball as in exophthalmic goiter, retroorbital mass or cavernous sinus thrombosis.

Propyleneglycol A demulcent agent used as solvent.

Propylhexedrine A sympathomimetic used as inhalation for nasal congestion.

Propyliodone Radiopaque dye used in bronchography.

Propylparaben An antifungal agent used as preservative.

Propylthiouracil Antithyroid drug for hyperthyroidism.

Prosection Dissection for demonstrating anatomic structures.

Prosector One who dissects body for demonstration.

Prosencephalon Embryonic forebrain giving rise to telencephalon and diencephalon.

Prosody The normal rhythm, melody and articulation of speech.

Prosopagnosia Inability to recognise a person from face.

Prosopectasia Abnormal enlargement of face.

Prosoplasia Progressive development of cells to produce cells with higher degree of function.

Prospective study A clinical or epidemiological investigation over a period of time.

Prostacyclin The precursor intermediate of prostaglandins; vasodilator.

Prostaglandin A group of 20 carbon unsaturated fatty acids, metabolites of arachidonic acid, e.g. PGD_2, PGE_2, PGF_2, PGI_2.

Prostatalgia Pain in prostate.

Prostate The musculoglandular organ of the size of $2 \times 4 \times 3$ cm that surrounds neck of urinary bladder and urethra in male.

Prostatic plexus Plexus of nerves and veins that lie in the capsule of prostate.

Prostatic urethra That portion of urethra surrounded by prostate.

Prostatism Symptoms of nocturia, increased frequency and dribbling of any cause.

Prostatitis Inflammation of prostate, whether acute or chronic with aching pain in perineum, urethral discharge often with fever, dysuria, chills and constipation.

Prostatolith A calculus in the prostate.

Prostatosis Any non-inflammatory and non-malignant condition of prostate.

Prosthesis An artificial part or organ.

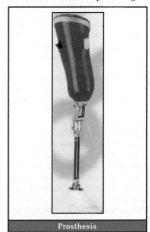

Prosthesis

Prosthetics Branch of surgery dealing with prosthesis.

Prosthodontics Branch of dentistry dealing with construction of artificial appliance for the mouth.

Prostitute Woman who sells herself for sexual exploitation, the major cause of spread of AIDS and other venereal diseases.

Prostration Extreme exhaustion.

Protal Existing before birth, i.e. congenital.

Protamine A simple strongly basic protein used to neutralize excess heparin or to slow down absorption of insulin.

Protanopia Red color blindness.

Protean Variable.

Protease Protein splitting enzyme.

Protein Complex nitrogenous compounds which are essential for growth and development. Basic building block of proteins are amino acids.

Lysine(Lys)

Amino Acids

p. Bence Jones A light chain protein found in urine in patients of myeloma, lymphoma etc.

Protein C A blood protein which on conversion to protein *Ca* inhibits blood coagulation. Its deficiency leads to thrombotic tendency.

Protein calori malnutrition Symptoms complex due to deficiency of protein and calori in small children *SYN*— kwashiorkor.

Protein hydrolysate A solution of amino acids and short chain peptides.

Protein losing enteropathy Excessive protein loss into G.I. tract as in extensive G.I. ulceration or constrictive pericarditis.

Proteinosis Accumulation of excess proteins in tissues.

Proteinuria Loss of protein usually albumin in urine.

p. orthostatic Proteinuria occurring on assuming erect posture but not during recumbency. Hence morning urine is protein free but urine of daytime contains albumin.

Proteolysis Hydrolysis of proteins.

Proteopexy Fixation of proteins within body.

Proteose An intermediate product of proteolysis.

Proteus A genus of enteric bacillus, *P. vulgaris* causes urinary infection while *P. morgagni* in addition causes enteritis: *P. mirabilis* is usually saprophytic.

Prothrombin A blood coagulation factor synthesized in liver which is converted to thrombin.

Prothrombinase An enzyme that catalyzes conversion of prothrombin into thrombin in presence of calcium and platelets.

Prothrombin time The time taken for decalcified plasma to clot on addition of thromboplastin and calcium. Usually employed to evaluate effects of anticoagulants.

Prostiology The science of microorganisms.

Protocol Description of steps to be taken in an experiment.

Protodiastole The first phase of diastole occurring immediately after closure of aortic and pulmonary valves.

Protoduodenum The upper half of duodenum.

Proton A positively charged particle in the atom.

Protoplasm A thick viscous colloid, the physical basis of all living organisms.

Protoporphyrin A tetrapyrole, derivative of hemoglobin.

Protoporphyrinuria Protoporphyrin in urine.

Protozoa Unicellular organism multiplying by binary fission.

Protractor Instrument for removing foreign bodies from wounds.

Protriptyline An anti-depressant.

Protrude To project.

Protuberance A prominent part.

Provitamin Any substance which is converted to vitamin within body, e.g. carotene as precursor of vitamin A.

Prurigo A chronic skin disease with recurrent discrete deep-seated itchy papules usually on extensor surfaces, of unknown etiology.

Pruritus Itching.

p. senilis Pruritus in aged due to degeneration of skin.

p. vulvae Itching around vulva, a feature of diabetes.

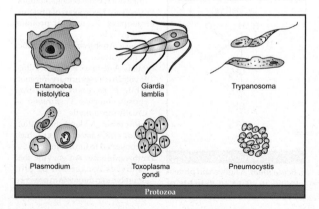

Entamoeba histolytica

Giardia lamblia

Trypanosoma

Plasmodium

Toxoplasma gondi

Pneumocystis

Protozoa

Prussak's space Tiny space in middle ear between sharpnell's membrane laterally and neck of malleus medially.

Prussic acid Hydrocyanic acid, a potent poison.

Psammoma A small tumor of choriod plexus and other areas of brain containing sandlike calcareous particles.

Psammoma bodies Laminated concretions in pineal body.

Psammoma sarcoma Sarcoma with psammoma bodies.

Psammotherapy Use of sandbaths as therapy.

Psammous Sandy-gritty.

Pseudacusis Hearing of false sounds.

Pseudoarthrosis Development of false joint consequent to nonunion of a fracture.

Pseudoacanthosis nigricans Velvety pigmented thickening of flexure surfaces as occurring in obese persons.

Pseudoaneurysm Dilatation of vessel giving impression of aneurysm.

Pseudocele The cavity of septum pellucidum, so called 5th ventricle.

Pseudocoxalgia Osteochondrosis of head of femur.

Pseudocyesis Symptoms of pregnancy like amenorrhea, abdominal enlargement, morning sickness etc., in absence of uterine enlargement as occurring in women who are too keen to have pregnancy.

Pseudocyst A dilatation resembling cyst.

Pseudodementia Social withdrawal but without mental deterioration.

Pseudoedema Puffy skin resembling edema.

Pseudoesthesia A false or imaginary sensation.

Pseudofracture A line of decalcification as seen in osteomalacia.

Pseudogeusia A subjective sensation of taste in absence of any stimulus to taste buds.

Pseudoganglion Local thickening of nerve resembling ganglion.

Pseudogout Joint pain resembling gout but caused by calcium pyrophosphate dihydrate crystals.

Pseudohermaphrodite Individual with sex chromatin and sex organs of one sex but with some of the physical appearance of opposite sex.

p. male Genetically male with a small rudimentary penis and a scrotum without testes resembling labia; usually occurs due to disease of adrenals or feminizing tumors of undescended testis.

p. female A genetically female with large clitoris resembling penis and hypertrophied labia mimicking scrotum.

Pseudohypertrophy Increase in size of tissue but with diminished function.

Pseudohypoparathyroidism Features of hypoparathyroidism due to tissue resistance to parathormone. Features are short stature, cataract, tetany etc.

Pseudojaundice Yellow coloration of skin due to carotinemia.

Pseudomania Pathological lying or a form of psychosis where patient falsely accuses himself for crimes which he has not committed.

Pseudomembrane A false membrane as in diphtheria.

Pseudomenstruation Bleeding from uterus without menstrual changes of endometrium.

Pseudomonas A genus of motile gram negative bacilli some of which produce yellow and blue pigments.

p. aeruginosa Causes urinary tract infection and wound infection.

p. pseudomallei Causes melioidosis.

Pseudomyxoma A peritoneal tumor containing a thick viscid fluid resembling myxoma.

Pseudoneuroma A tumor forming at the end of amputation stump.

Pseudopapilledema Optic neuritis causing swelling of optic nerve head.

Pseudoparesis Hysterical palsy.

Pseudopodium Any temporary outpouching of cell membrane in protozoa for locomotion.

Pseudopolyp Hypertrophied area of mucous membrane resembling polyp.

Pseudo pseudohypoparathyroidism Pseudo hypoparathyroidism without any biochemical changes.

Pseudopsia False perception, visual hallucination.

Pseudosmia Perversion of smell.

Pseudotuberculosis A group of diseases resembling clinically tuberculosis but caused by gram negative organism, *Yersinia pseudotuberculosis.*

Pseudotumor cerebri Benign intracranial hypertension of unknown cause, most patients recover spontaneously.

Pseudoxanthoma elastium Chronic degenerative skin disease with angioid streaks in retina, degeneration of vessel walls.

Psilocybin A hallucinogen obtained from mushrooms.

Psi phenomena Events without explanation, e.g. telepathy.

Psittacosis Fever with pulmonary symptoms caused by *Chlamydia psittaci.*

Psoas A muscle in the loin, inserted to lesser throchanter of femur. It flexes the thigh, adducts and rotates it medially.

Psoas abscess A cold abscess in the sheath of psoas major muscle often noticed above inguinal ligament or near attachment of psoas muscle to femur.

Psoralen Plant derivatives causing phototoxic dermatitis; used in psoriasis and vitiligo.

Psoriasis A chronic itchy disorder of skin marked by lesions on extensor surfaces with silvery yellow white scales. A psoriatic skin produces nearly 2700 cells/cm^2 in comparison to 1250/cm^2 per day in normal person and cell cycle is reduced to 36 hours in comparison to the normal of 311 hours.

p. annularis Ringlike or circular lesion.

p. guttate Small distinct body lesions following streptococcal infection.

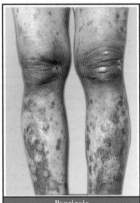

Psoriasis

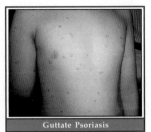

Guttate Psoriasis

Pustular Psoriasis

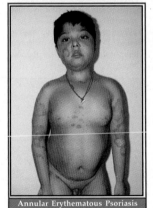

Annular Erythematous Psoriasis

p. numular Disc and plaque lesions on trunk.

p. pustular Small sterile pustules that dry up to form a scab.

Psyche Mind.

Psychedelic Drugs producing visual hallucinations like LSD.

Psychiatry The branch of medicine dealing with diagnosis, treatment and prevention of mental illness.

Psychoanalysis A method of obtaining detailed account of past and present experiences and repressions.

Psychodynamics The scientific study of mental force.

Psychogenesis The origin and development of mind.

Psychogenic Of mental origin.

Psychograph A chart that lists personality traits.

Psychokinesis Impulsive maniacal behavior caused by defective inhibition.

Psycholepsy Sudden alteration of mood.

Psychologist Person trained in methods of psychological analysis, therapy and research.

Psychology Branch of science dealing with mental processes and their influence on behavior.

Psychometry The measurement of psychological variables like intelligence, aptitude, behavior and emotion.

Psychomotor epilepsy Temporal lobe epilepsy.

Psychomotor retardation Generalized slowing of physical and mental reactions.

Psychoneurosis Emotional maladaptation due to unresolved emotional conflicts.

Psychopathy Any mental disease.

Psychopharmacology The science of drugs effecting behavior and emotions.

Psychoplegic Drug reducing excitability.

Psychosexual Pertains to mental and emotional aspects of sexuality.

Psychosexual disorders Disorder of sexual function not due to organic causes e.g., paraphilias, transvestism, pedophilia, etc.

Psychosis An impairment of mental function to the extent of interfering with individual's adaptation to family, society, self care and ordinary demands of life. There is personality disintegration and loss of contact with reality; hallucinations and delusions.

p. alcoholic Psychosis in chronic alcoholism.

p. depressive Psychosis characterized by excessive depression, melancholia.

p. manic depressive Alternating periods of mania and depression.

p. organic Psychosis resulting from any CNS pathology.

p. situational Psychosis due to excessive stress.

Psychosomatic Pertains to body and mind, i.e. a disease producing physical symptoms due to some disturbance in emotional state.

Psychotherapy A method of treating disease by mental means like suggestion, hypnotism rather than physical means.

Psychrophobia Abnormal aversion or sensitiveness to cold.

Psyllium seeds Used as mild laxative.

Pterion Point of suture of frontal temporal, parietal and sphenoid bones

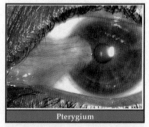
Pterygium

Pterygium Triangular thickening of bulbar conjunctiva with apex towards pupil.

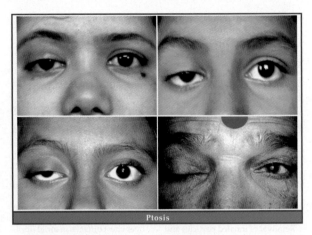

Ptosis

Pterygoid Wing shaped.

Pterygoid process Downward projection from sphenoid bone at junction of body and greater wings.

Ptomaine A nitrogenous putrefactive product from bacterial action on proteins.

Ptosis Drooping of an organ or eyelid.

Ptylagogue Agent that stimulates secretion of saliva.

Piyalin A salivary enzyme that hydrolyzes starch and glycogen to maltose and glucose.

Ptyalism Excessive secretion of saliva.

Ptyalography X-ray of salivary glands and ducts.

Puberty The period of sexual maturity between 13-15 years in boys and 9-16 years in girl, probably related to decrease in secretion of pineal gland.

p. precocious Onset of puberty earlier than normal.

Pubescence Puberty.

Pubic hair Hair in pubic region, appearing on sexual maturity.

Pudenda External genitalia especially of female.

Puerile Concerning puerperium.

Puerperal sepsis Infection of genital tract in the puerperium.

Puerperium Period of six weeks following childbirth.

Pulmometer Spirometer; device to measure lung capacity.

Pulmometry Determination of lung capacity.

Pulmonary alveolar proteinosis Eosinophilic material deposition in alveoli causing dyspnea.

Pulmonary arterial webs Web like deformities in pulmonary angiogram at the site of previous thromboembolism.

Pulmonary artery wedge pressure Pressure at the capillary end of pulmonary arterial system usually below 16 mm Hg, is equal to mean left atrial pressure and left ventricular end diastolic pressure.

Pulmonary function tests Tests done to measure functional ability of lungs, e.g. total lung capacity, vital capacity, peak flow rate, gas exchange.

Pulmonary insufficiency Failure of pulmonary valve to close completely during diastole.

Pulmonary mucociliary clearance Removal of inhaled particles and sputum from bronchial tree by ciliary action of bronchial mucosa.

Pulmonary stenosis Narrowing of pulmonary valves.

Pulmonary valve The valve between right ventricle and pulmonary artery, has three cusps 2 posterior and one anterior.

Pulmonary veins 4 set of veins draining the lungs into left atrium.

Pulp Soft vascular portion of the center of tooth; the soft part of fruit.

Pulp amputation Removal of exposed pulp.

Pulp capping Covering and protecting the exposed or infected pulp by metal cap thus allowing it to heal and be protected by formation of secondary dentin.

Pulpectomy Extirpation of dental pulp.

Pulpitis Inflammation of pulp.

Pulsate To throb, or beat.

Pulsation The rhythmic beat

Pulse The waveform of blood passing through an artery as a consequence to cardiac contraction.

p. alternating Pulse with weak and strong beats.

p. anacrotic Pulse with a secondary wave on ascending limb.

p. bigeminal Pulse where every third beat is irregular.

p. collapsing Pulse striking the finger with force but then abruptly subsiding.

p. corrigans Bounding and forceful pulse of aortic regurgitation.

p. deficit Pulse rate counted from wrist and cardiac rate auscultated over chest differ as in atrial fibrillation.

p. paradoxical Pulse disappearing at the end of inspiration as in pericardia! tamponade.

p. thready Barely perceptible pulse.

p. waterhammer Sudden jerky pulse with immediate collapse.

Pulse generator The component of cardiac pacemakers that provides electrical discharge.

Pulseless disease Aortoarteritis causing absence of brachial and radial pulse.

Pulse pressure Difference between systolic and diastolic pressure. Pulse pressure above 50 and below 30 are considered abnormal.

Pulverization To crush any hard substance into powder form.

Punchdrunk Boxers with repeated head trauma leading to multiple scars and intellectual deterioration and Parkinsonian features.

Punched out Small clearly defined hole like appearance.

Punctate Pinpoint punctures or depressions.

Punctate rash Minute rash.

Puncture To make a hole, or wound by a sharp pointed instrument.

p. cisternal Puncture of cerebro-medullary cisterns through sub-occipital space to obtain CSF.

p. lumbar Puncture of subarachnoid space between L 3-L4 vertebrae to obtain CSF for analysis, or to do myelogram.

p. sternal Aspiration of bone-marrow from sternum.

Pupil The opening at the center of iris.

p. Argyl Robertson Pupil that reacts to accommodation but with loss of light reflex.

p. Hutchinson's One side dilatation of pupil with contraction on other side due to intracranial space occupying lesion.

p. pinpoint Excessively constricted pupil in opium poisoning, myopias and in pontine hemorrhage.

Pupillary reflex Constriction of pupil upon stimulation of retina by light

Pupilometer Instrument for measuring diameter of pupil.

Purgative Drug stimulating bowel movement.

Purge To evacuate the bowel.

Purine End products of nucleoprotein digestion consisting of adenine, guanine and uric acid.

Purine free diet Diet devoid of meat, liver, kidney, poultry, fish, condiments, alcohol, sweets, pastries, fried foods.

Purine low diet Diet that excludes foods like meat, fish, fowl, spinach, lentils, mushrooms, peas, aspargus.

Purkinje Anatomist and physiologist.

p. cells Large neurons that have dendrites extending from cortex to deep white matter.

p. fibers A type of muscle fibers which conduct electrical impulse to ventricular muscle.

p. network Fibrous network of large muscle cells beneath the endocardium.

p. phenomenon The maximum pupillary movement while dark adaptation occurs in green rather than yellow light.

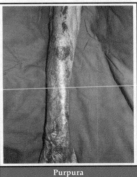
Purpura

Purpura Hemorrhages into skin, mucous membrane first appearing as red, then purple and finally brownish yellow before disappearing; can be allergic to food, drugs, micro organisms, and idiopathic as well as due to other causes like thrombocytopenia and vasculitis.

Purpurin An acid dye used to stain nuclei, a red pigment often present in urine.

Purulent Containing pus, suppurative.

Puruloid Like pus.

Pus Liquid product of inflammation containing albuminous substances, leukocytes and organisms. Blue or green pus is due to infection by pseudomonas group and fetid pus is due to growth of anaerobes.

Puscells Dead and degenerated leukocytes.

Pustule Small elevated skin lesion containing pus, may be flat, round or umbilicated.

Putrefaction Decomposition of protein with production of malodorous and toxic products like ptomaines, mercaptans, hydrogen sulphide, caused by bacteria and fungi. Decomposition occurring spontaneously in sterile tissue is called autolysis.

Putrefy To undergo putrefaction.

Putrescence Decay, rottenness.

Putrescine A poisonous polyamine formed by bacterial action on arginine.

Pyarthrosis Pus in a joint.

Pycnemia Thickening of blood.

Pycno Dense or thick (Pykno).

Pyelectasia Dilatation of renal pelvis.

Pyelocystitis Inflammation of renal pelvis and bladder.

Pyelogram X-ray of ureter and renal pelvis.

Pyelolithotomy Operation to remove stone from renal pelvis.

Pyelonephritis Inflammation of kidney substance and pelvis, in 85% caused by *E. coli*.

Pyemia Presence of pus forming organisms in blood, a form of septicemia, causing metastatic abscess.

Pygmy A very small person or dwarf.

Pygodidymus Conjoined twins with fusion of chest and head but free abdomen and limbs.

Pyknocyte A form of spiculated red cell.

Pyknodysostosis A form of osteopetrosis, but without hematologic and neurologic abnormalities.

Pyknosis Shrinking of cell through degeneration and becoming thick.

Pylephlebitis Inflamed portal veins.

Pylethrombosis Occlusion of portal vein.

Pylon A temporary artificial leg.

Pyloric antrum First part of pylorus leading into pyloric canal.

Piloric canal The short narrow lowermost portion of stomach entering into duodenum.

Pyloric stenosis Narrowing of pyloric orifice due to peptic ulcer or post pyloric duodenal ulcer or congenital hyperplasia of pyloric circular muscles.

Pylorodiosis Dilatation of pylorus.

Pyloroplasty Surgical enlargement of the opening of pylorus.

Pylorospasm Contraction of pyloric orifice secondary to ulcer in pyloric antrum or duodenum.

Pylorotomy Incision into pyloric submucosa to relieve hypertrophic stenosis.

Pylorus The lower orifice of stomach which opens intermittently to allow partly digested food to enter into duodenum.

Pyocele Any cavity distended with pus.

Pyoderma Purulent lesions in skin.

p. gangrenosum Pyoderma of skin associated with ulcerative colitis or any chronic wasting disease.

Pyogenic Pus producing.

Pyometra Pus in the uterus.

Pyovarium Pus in the ovary.

Pyopneumopericardium Pus and air in pericardial cavity.

Pyopneumothorax Pus and gas present in pleural cavity.

Pyorrhea A discharge of purulent matter.

p. alveolaris A periodontal inflammatory disease with resorption of alveolar bone, and loosening of teeth.

Pyoureter Pus in the ureter.

Pyramid An object whose three triangular sides meet at an apex.

p. of medulla A pair of elongated prominences on the anterior surface of medulla oblongata representing descending corticospinal tract.

p. of tympanum The space in middle ear cavity through which passes stapedius muscle.

p. renal Cone shaped structures making the medulla of the kidney, the apex that projects as renal papilla into the renal sinus.

Pyramidal tract One of the three descending tracts (lateral, ventricular, andventrolateral) of the spinal cord whose fibers are axons of giant Betz cells of motor cortex.

Pyrantel pamoate Drug used in helminthiasis especially ascariasis and enterobiasis.

Pyrazinamide Bactericidal antitubercular drug, very effective in killing intracellular slowly growing bacilli.

Pyrethrum Compounds having antipeduculosis property and insecticidal.

Pyrexia Fever.

Pyrexin A substance isolated from inflammatory exudate that produces fever.

Pyridium Urinary antiseptic and soothing agent.

Pyridostigmine An anti-cholinesterase drug used in myasthenia.

Pyridoxal -5 phosphate A derivative of pyridoxine acting as a coenzyme.

Pyridoxamine One of the vitamin B_6 group.

Pyridoxine Vitamin B_6 that includes pyridoxal and pyridoxamine.

Pyriform Shaped like a pear.

Pyrilamine maleate Antihistaminic agent.

Pyrimethamine Antimalarial agent (Daraprim).

Pyrimidine Nitrogenous compound containing uracil, cytosine and thymine.

Pyrogen Agent that produces fever.

Pyrophosphatase An enzyme that catalyzes splitting of phosphoric groups.

Pyrophosphate Any salt of phosphoric acid.

Pyrosis Burning in epigastrium and lower chest *SYN* – heart burn.

Pyrrobutamine phosphate An antihistaminic agent.

Pyrrole A heterocyclic substance acting as a building block for hemoglobin and others.

Pyrrolidine Substance obtained from pyrole or tobacco.

Pyruvate Ester of pyruvic acid.

Pyruvic acid An intermediate product in metabolism of carbohydrates and fats. Its blood level increases in thiamine deficiency.

Pyrvinium pamoate A drug for pinworms.

Pyuria Pus in the urine.

Q

Q Symbol for long arm of a chromosome

Q angle A angle formed by a line from anterior superior iliac spine through center of patella and a line from tibial tubercle through the patella normal is 15°.

Q fever Acute infectious disease caused by *Coxiella burnetti*, a rickettsial organism, characterized by fever, sweating, myalgia.

QT segment In ECG the period from beginning of Q wave to the end of T wave.

Quack Person who pretends to have knowledge and skill of medicine.

Quadrangular Having 4 angles.

Quadrangular lobe A region on superior surface of each cerebellar hemisphere.

Quadrangular membrane Upper portion of elastic membrane of larynx extending from aryepiglottic folds above to the level of ventricular folds below.

Quadrantanopia Diminished vision or blindness in one quadrant of visual field.

Quadrate Square like.

Quadrate lobe A small lobe of liver on the visceral surface lying in contact with pylorus and duodenum.

Quadriceps Four headed muscle of thigh consisting of rectus femoris, vastus lateralis, vastus medialis, and vastus intermedius.

Quadriceps reflex Extension of leg following contraction of quadriceps muscle.

Quadrigeminal Having four equal parts.

Quadriplegia Paralysis of all four extremities and the trunk usually due to injury to spinal cord above Cs segment. Lesion above Cs causes death due to diaphragmatic palsy.

Quadruped Four footed animal.

Quadruplet Giving birth to 4 children at a time.

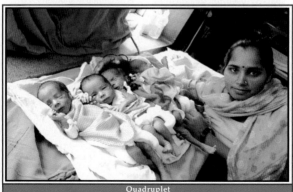

Quadruplet

Quantum A definite amount.

Quarantine The period of isolation when one is exposed to infectious disease which is the longest incubation period of disease.

Quartan Occurring every fourth day.

Quartz Silicon dioxide.

Queckenstedt's test Rise in cerebrospinal fluid pressure on compression of jugular veins of neck. A failure in rise of pressure means spinal subarachnoid block.

Quervain's disease Chronic tenosynovitis of abductor pollicis longus and extensor pollicis brevis.

Quickening Feeling of first movements of fetus in utero usually between 18-20 weeks of pregnancy.

Quick lime Calcium oxide.

Quick's test A liver function test for measuring hippuric acid after a dose of sodium benzoate.

Quinacrine hydrochloride An agent sparsely used for treatment of malaria and often *Giardialamblia*.

Quincke's disease Giant urticaria.

Quincke's pulse Capillary pulsation in finger nails, a sign of aortic incompetence.

Quinethazone A diuretic.

Quingestanol A progestational agent.

Quinghasu A plant product for resistant malaria.

Quinidine sulfate Anti-arrhythmic agent from cinchona bark.

Quinine An antimalarial alkaloid from cinchona bark used orally as sulfate, bisulfate and hydrochloride and parenterally as dihydrochloride. Quinine tannate is tasteless, best for giving to young children, used for falciparum malaria.

Quinoline An amine from coaltar whose salts are used as analgesic, antipyretic and in amebiasis.

Qinolone A class of compounds whose well known derivatives are norfloxacin, ciprofloxacin, pfloxacin and ofloaxacin.

Quinsy Peritonsillar abscess.

Quintan Occurring every fifth day.

Quintuplet Birth of 5 children at same time to a mother.

Quotidian Occurring daily.

Quotient Number of times a number is contained in another.

q. intelligence. Division of one's mental age by actual age,

q. respiratory Division of amount of CO_2 in expired air by the oxygen. Normal value is 0.9.

q. wave The downward defection before R wave in ECG. Prominent Q waves indicate myocardial necrosis.

R

Rabid One having rabies.

Rabies An acute infectious CNS disease with fatal outcome; transmitted to humans by bite of rabid animals like dogs, foxes and cats. Bats, foxes and raccoons serve as reservoir of infection.

Rabies immune globulin Antibodies against rabies isolated from plasma of those immunized with rabies vaccine. It is used for imparting passive immunity.

Raccon sign Periorbital ecchymosis in patients of basilar skull fracture

Race A distinct ethnic group who originated from a common ancestor, or a taxonomic classification of individuals within the same species who exhibit distinct genetic characteristics.

Racemase An enzyme that helps in production of an optically active compound.

Rachial Concerning spine.

Rachialgia Pain in the spine.

Rachi graph Device for outlining the spinal curvature.

Rochilysis Mechanical treatment of scoliosis by traction and pressure.

Rachiometer Device for measuring curvature of spine.

Rachischisis Spina bifida.

Rachitis Rickets.

Rachitism Propensity for rickets.

Rachitome Instrument for opening spinal canal.

Radial reflex Flexon of forearm on percussion on lower end of radius.

Radiant Transmitted by radiation; coming out from a common center.

Radiation The process by which energy is propagated through space or matter. Ionizing radiation is used for therapeutic and diagnostic purposes.

r. auditory Fibers fanning out from medial geniculate body of thalamus to auditory cortex.

r. electromagnetic Rays travelling at speed of light (186000 miles/sec) exhibiting both electrical and magnetic properties.

r. optic The fibers extending from lateral geniculate body of thalamus to visual cortex.

r. ultraviolet Radiant energy from 2900-3900 AU.

r. visible Visible spectrum of light: Violet (3900-4550 AU); blue (4550-4920 AU); green (4920-5770 AU); yellow (5770-5970 AU); orange (5970-6220 AU) and red (6220-7700 AU).

Radiation absorbed dose The quantity of ionizing radiation absorbed by any material per unit mass measured as ergs per gram.

Radiation injury Injury to cells by ionizing radiation which can lead to cell death or malignancy.

Radiation carcinoma Squamous cell carcinoma of skin attributed to radiation injury.

Radiation protection Preventive measures against radiation like shielding of source, keeping appropriate distance, use of protective clothing, dosimeter, lead appron and limiting the dose and duration of exposure.

Radiation sickness Acute nausea and vomiting following therapeutic radiation. Prolonged exposure may lead to sterility, carcinogenesis, leukemia and bone marrow aplasia.

Radical A group of atoms acting as single unit.

r. free A molecule containing an odd number of electrons and an open bond, hence highly reactive to cause myocardial injury.

Radical treatment Treatment, medical or surgical aimed at providing absolute cure.

Radicle Rootlet.

Radiculitis Inflammation of spinal nerve roots.

Radiculomyelopathy Any disease involving spinal cord and nerve roots.

Radiculopathy Disease of nerve roots.

Radioactive Capable of emitting radiant energy.

Radioactive decay The decrease in number of radioactive atoms in a substance with passage of time.

Radioactive patient A patient who was treated with radioactive substance or was accidentally contaminated with radioactive material and hence remains radioactive to be a source of radiation injury to family and friends.

Radioactivity The ability of a substance to emit rays or particles (alpha, beta or gamma) from its nucleus.

Radio allergo sorbent test A test to measure the quantities of IgE.

Radio autograph Photograph of tissue section to show distribution of radioactive substances.

Radiobiology Branch of biology dealing with effects of ionizing radiation on living organisms.

Radiochroism The ability of substances to absorb radioactive rays.

Radiocinematography Simultaneous recording of images during fluoroscopy.

Radiocystitis Inflammation of bladder following X-ray exposure.

Radiode The metal container for radium.

Radiodermatitis Inflammation of skin on exposure to X-ray or radioactive elements.

Radioimmunoassay A method for determining concentration of substances particularly protein bound hormones to the range of picograms.

Radioimmunodiffusion Study of antigen-antibody interaction by use of radioisotope labelled antigens or antibodies diffused through a gel.

Radioimmunoelectrophoresis Electrophoresis involving use of radioisotope labelled antigens or antibody.

Radioiodine Radioactive isotope of iodine[131] used in diagnosis of thyroid disorders.

Radioisotope A radioactive form of an element.

Radiologist A doctor practising the art of diagnosis and treatment by use of radiant energy.

Radiolucency The property of being partly or fully permeable to radiant energy.

Radiolucent Permitting the X-rays to pass through.

Radiometer Equipment for measuring the intensity of radiation.

Radiomimetic Imitating the biological effects of radiation, e.g. alkylating agents.

Radionecrosis Tissue destruction on exposure to radiant energy.

Radionuclide Atom that disintegrates by emission of electromagnetic radiation.

Radiopaque Impermeable to X-ray or other form of radiation.

Radiopelvimetry Measurement of pelvis by use of X-rays.

Radiopharmaceuticals Radioactive chemicals or their combination with carriers. Used for determining size and function of body organs.

Radioprotective drugs Drugs protecting against lethal effects of ionizing radiation.

Radio resistant Tumors that cannot be destroyed by radiation, and hence are radio resistant.

Radiotelemetry Transmission of data via radio from a patient to a remote monitor for analysis.

Radiotherapist Doctor trained in therapeutic use of radiant energy.

Radiotherapy The treatment of disease by application of X-rays, radium, ultraviolet or other forms of radiations.

Radium A radioactive and fluorescent metallic element with half life of 1622 years.

Radium needles Metallic needle shaped containers which contain radium and are inserted to tissue to destroy malignant growths.

Radon A radioactive gaseous element resulting from disintegration of radium. It occurs in nature and is estimated to cause 5-10% of lung cancers occurring in general population.

Raffinose A trisaccharide which on hydrolysis yields fructose and melibiose.

Ragsorter's disease Pulmonary anthrax in rag sorters.

Raillietina A genus of tapeworm whose species demerariensis infests humans in S. America.

Raimiste's phenomenon In hemiplegia resistance to hip abduction or adduction in the noninvolved extremity evokes same response in involved limb.

Rale Abnormal sound heard during auscultation of chest produced by passage of air through diseased bronchi, (means both rhonchi and crepitation); can be dry or moist, coarse, crackling, bubbling, clicking, amphoric, sibilant and sonorous.

Ramus A branch or division of a forked structure.

Rancid Disagreeable smell or taste from decomposition of fatty substances.

Random controlled trial An experimental study for testing the effectiveness of a drug or treatment regime in which subjects are divided at random into two groups: experimental and control.

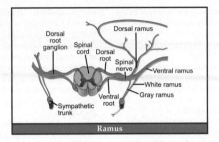

Ramus

Randomization *SYN*—double blind technique; a method used to assign subjects into treatment or non-treatment group by procedures like tossing a coin or use of numbers.

Random sample The selection of samples from population where each individual in the group has same opportunity of being selected.

Ranitidine H_2 receptor blocker, used in peptic ulcer.

Ranula A blue cystic swelling in mouth under the tongue due to obstruction of sublingual or submandibular ducts.

Ranviers' nodes Constriction in myelin sheath of nerve fibers at regular intervals.

Rape Intercourse, homosexual or heterosexual, against consent or with consent which is obtained by force. The age of victim for consent varies from countries to countries. In India it is 16 years.

Raphania A spasmodic disease caused by ingestion of seeds of white radish.

Raphe A ridge, crease or point of joining of two halves of a part.

r. abdominal Linea alba.

r. penis A median ridge on the dorsum of penis continuous with raphe on scrotum.

r. tongue A median groove on the dorsum of tongue.

r. perineal A ridge or raphe in the midline of perineum.

Rapport A relationship of mutual trust.

Rarefaction Decreased density, e.g. of bone due to mineral loss.

Rash Any eruption of skin usually associated with communicable disease.

r. butterfly Skin rash on cheeks and over the bridge of nose as seen in systemic lupus erythematosus.

r. diaper Skin inflammation in diaper areas in infants.

r. drug Rash due to drugs like ampicillin, sulphas, iodides and bromides.

r. macular Flat rash not protruding above the skin surface.

r. mulbery Dusky rash in typhus fever.

r. nettle Smooth, elevated itchy rash *SYN*—urticaria.

Rasion Grating of drugs by use of a file.

Rasura The process of scraping, filing or shaving.

Rat A rodent of genus rattus that serve as reservoirs of many infections and infestations, e.g. ratbite fever.

Ratbite fever Fever, bodyache and joint pain caused by *Streptobacillus moniliformis* and *Spirillum minus* transmitted by bite of rat.

Rate The frequency of occurrence of an event expressed with respect to time or some other standard.

r. birth The number of live births per 1000 in a given population per year.

r. case fatality The ratio of the number of deaths caused by a disease to the total number of people who contracted the disease.

r. death The number of deaths in a year per a specified population.

r. glomerular filtration Rate of filtrate formation in glomeruli of the kidneys; normal 120 ml/min.

r. heart The number of heart beats per minute.

Rathke's pouch A depression in the embryo giving origin to anterior lobe of pituitary.

Ratio Relationship between two substances.

r. albumin globulin Ratio of albumin to globulin in blood; usually 1.3:1 or 1.4:1.

r. arm In chromosome the ratio of long arm to short arm.

r. lecithin-sphingomyelin The ratio of lecithin to sphingomyelin in amniotic fluid, an indicator of fetal maturity, usually at term.

r. Odd's In epidemiological and case control studies a relative measure of disease occurrence.

r. therapeutic A ratio of effective therapeutic dose to minimum lethal dose.

Ration Fixed food and drink per day/month.

Rational Logical.

Rationale The reasoning for course of action.

Rationalization In psychology, a justification for an unreasonable or illogical act or idea to make it appear reasonable.

Rattle A gurgling sound.

r. death The crepitant rale heard due to fluid accumulation in trachea in a dying person.

Rattle snake A poisonous snake that produces a characteristic rattle.

Raucous Hoarse or harsh.

Rauwolfia The dried roots of *Rauwolfia serpentina* from which are extracted the potent hypotensive agents like reserpine.

Rave Irrational talk, as in delirium.

Ray Any narrow beam of light, the line of propagation of any radiant energy.

r. alpha The less penetrative rays composed of positively charged particles of helium having powerful fluorescent, photographic and ionizing properties.

r. beta Negatively charged electrons of disintegrating radio active elements.

r. cosmic Electromagnetic radiation of short wavelength and high penetrance coming from sources in outerspace.

r. delta Highly penetrating waves of radioactive substances.

r. gamma High velocity and penetrating rays coming from nucleus of radioactive elements with wavelength of 1.4 to 0.00 1AU.

r.s. heat Visible rays from 3900 to 7700 AU and infrared rays from 7700 to 1400 AU.

r. medullary In the kidney, slender processes composed of straight tubules projecting into renal pyramids.

Raynaud's disease Intermittent pallor and cyanosis of digits on exposure to cold in females due to abnormal vascular response.

React To respond to stimulus; to participate in chemical reaction.

Reaction Response of an organism to a stimulus.

r. anaphylactic A hypersensitive reaction with vasomotor collapse, laryngo-tracheobronchial spasm to allergens usually mediated by IgE.

r. conversion Hysterical neurosis.

r. dissociative A sudden temporary alteration in the normal functions of consciousness even forgetting self identity.

r. leukemoid Appearance of few blasts with high leukocytes count in some nonleukemic conditions.

r. Quellong Swelling of capsules of bacteria when mixed with their specific antisera, e.g. pneumococcus.

r. transfusion Agglutination and hemolysis of donor's or recipient's blood following mismatched transfusion.

Reaction time The time interval between application of stimulus and response to it.

Reactive depression Depression following situations like bereavement, financial loss, slander etc.

Reading lip Interpretation of ones speech from movement of his lips.

Read only memory The part of computer's memory that contains permanent instructions in contrast to random access memory which holds only a temporary memory (program).

Reagent A substance that reacts in a chemical reaction to detect presence of another substance.

Reagin IgE antibody.

Reamer Instrument of dentists for enlargement of root canal.

Reanimate To revive, resuscitate.

Rebound phenomenon When a limb or part is moved against resistance and the resistance is suddenly withdrawn, the limb moves abruptly in the direction of effort, a feature of cerebellar disease.

Recall Recapitulation.

Recepjaculum chyli Inferior pear shaped expanded portion of lower end of thoracic duct in abdomen.

Receptor In pharmacology, a cell component that combines with a drug or hormone to alter the function of the cell.

r. adrenergic Consists of alpha and beta adrenergic receptors: Alpha receptors cause vasoconstriction where as betareceptor stimulation causes tachycardia, vasodilatation and bronchodilatation. Beta receptors can be beta$_1$ and beta$_2$ the former being in smooth muscles of bronchi and the latter in heart.

r. cholinergic Sites in nerve synapses or effector cells that respond to acetylcholine.

r. of proprioception Muscle or tendon spindles which serve for kinesthetic or position sense.

r. sensory Sensory nerve endings which once stimulated give rise to afferent sensory impulse, e.g. 1. Stretch receptors—muscle spindles and Golgi tendon apparatus 2. temperature—Krause's end bulbs for cold and Ruffini's corpuscles for warmth 3. touch—Merkle's disc, Meissner's corpuscles.

Recess A small depression or indentation.

r. cochlear A small hollow between the two limbs of vestibular crest of the ear that accommodates the beginning of cochlear duct.

r. epitympanic *SYN*—attic. The middle ear cavity that lies above the level of tympanic membrane and contains head of malleus and short limb of incus.

r. infundibular A small projection of third ventricle extending into infundibular stalk of hypophysis.

r. omental These are three pocket like extensions of omental bursa extending towards caudate lobe of liver, hilum of spleen and into greater omentum.

r. pharyngeal *SYN*—fossa of Rosenmuller. The recess in the lateral wall of nasopharynx lying above and behind the opening of auditory tube.

r. piriform A deep fossa in the lower pharynx bounded laterally by thyroid cartilage and medially by cricoid and arytenoid cartilages. It is the common site for lodgement of foreign bodies.

Recession In dentistry, the atrophy of gingival tissue leading to exposure of the roots.

Recessive gene Gene that does not express itself in presence of its dominant allele.

Recidivism Habitual criminality; repetition of criminal act.

Recidivity Tendency to relapse or to return to a former position/condition.

Recipe A medicine formula.

Recipient One who receives, e.g. blood kidney, heart-lungs, etc.

Reciprocal Mutual, complementary.

Recklinghausen German pathologist.

R's canal Rootlets of lymphatics.

R's disease Multiple neurofibromata of nerve sheath, arising from cranial and spinal nerve roots and peripheral nerves.

R's tumor Adenoleio myofibroma on the wall of fallopian tube or posterior uterine wall.

Recline To lie down; to be in recumbent position.

Reclus' disease Multiple benign cystic growth in the breast.

Recombinant DNA Insertion of DNA segment from one organism into DNA of another organism.

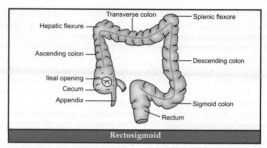

Recombination In genetics, the joining together of gene combinations
in the offspring that were not
present in the parents.

Recon In genetics, the smallest unit
that can enter into recombination.

Recover To regain lost health after
the illness.

Recovery The process of becoming
well after illhealth.

Recovery room The room where
patients are kept to recover from
effects of anesthesia after the surgery.

Recrudescence Relapse or return of
symptoms after a remission.

Recruitment 1. In audiology, an increase in the perceived intensity of
sound out of proportion to the actual increase in the sound level,
failure of recruitment indicates
lesion. 2. Increase in the intensity
of a reflex by activation of greater
number of motor neurones by a
reflex action even though strength
of stimulus remains unchanged, e.g.
patellar reflex augmented by clasp-
ing/pulling the hands apart.

Rectal crisis Rectal pain and tenesmus in CNS disorders.

Rectal reflex Desire to defecate
when rectum is filled with stool.

Rectified Made pure or set right.

Rectifier In electricity, a device for
transforming alternating current
into direct current.

Rectocele Prolapse of posterior
vaginal wall along with anterior
wall of rectum.

Rectoclysis Slow introduction of
fluid into rectum.

Rectopexy Surgical fixation of rectum.

Rectosigmoid Upper portion of rectum and adjoining sigmoid colon.

Rectourethral Concerning rectum
and urethra.

Rectouterine Concerning rectum
and uterus.

Rectovaginal Concerning rectum
and vagina.

Rectovesical Concerning rectum and
bladder.

Rectum The lower 5" of large intestine, responsible for initiation of
defecation reflex through S_1-S_2-S_3
sacral segments of spinal cord.

Rectus muscle 1. The short muscles of eye. 2. Two long midline muscles of abdominal wall stretching from pubic bone to ensiform cartilage and 5th, 6th and seventh ribs.

Recumbent Lying down.

Recuperation To recover, restoration to normal health.

Recurrence Return of symptoms after a period of quiescence or relapse.

Recurrent Returning at intervals.

Red A primary colour.

r. congo Amyloid material treated with congo red produces green fluorescence in polarized light.

r. cresol A pH indicator; yellow in pH 7.4 and red in pH exceeding 9.

r. methyl A pH indicator; red when pH 4.4 and yellow at pH 6.2.

r. scarlet An azo dye used for staining tissues for microscopic examination.

Red cross Internationally recognized sign of medical installation or a medical personnel bearing impunity against attack in war.

Redia A stage in life-cycle of trematode following sporocyst which develop into infecting cercaria.

Red nucleus Gray matter in the tegmentum of midbrain.

Redox Combined form to indicate oxidation reduction reaction.

Reduce 1. To restore to normal apposition as in fracture 2. In chemistry a type of reaction in which a substance gains electrons.

Reducing agent A substance that loses electrons easily, e.g. hydrogen sulfide, sulphur dioxide.

Reductase An enzyme accelerating the process of reduction in a chemical reaction.

Reduction division Cell division occurring in gametogenesis so that the chromosome number is reduced to half.

Redundant Superfluous, more than necessary.

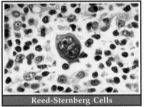
Reed-Sternberg Cells

Reed-Sternberg cells Giant connective tissue cells with large nuclei (owl-eye), characteristic of Hodgkin's disease.

Reentry In electrophysiology of heart, a mechanism to explain tachyarrhythmias where a stimulus passing down the conduction system is blocked in one pathway but travels down in an alternative pathway and again ascends up in previously blocked pathway to give rise to a circus movement.

Reference man A concept employed in nutritional investigation and surveys where a man weighing 70 kg, of 22 years of age engaged in light physical activity consumes 2800 kca l/day.

Reference woman Woman of around 22 years of age weighing 58 kg and consuming 2000 kcal/day.

Referred pain Pain felt at a point remote from point of origin due to similar segmental inervation.

Reflection 1. The condition of being turned back on itself, e.g. peritoneum 2. In psychology mental consideration of something already considered.

Reflex Involuntary instantaneous response to a stimulus; usually purposeful and adaptive. In a simple reflex the reflex circuit consists of a sensory receptor, afferent neuron, reflex center in brain or spinal cord, efferent neurone supplying the organ (muscle or gland).

r. Babinski Flexion of great toe and fanning out of other toes on stroking the lateral aspect of sole of foot in healthy persons.

r. Bainbridge Acceleration of heart rate with ventricular distention.

r. cat eye The yellow pupillary reflex of children due to retinoblastoma.

r. crossed extension Extension of opposite extremity on painful stimulation of skin over other extremity.

r. grasp Grasping reaction of finger on stimulation of hollow of palm, its presence in adults is evidence of diffuse cerebral disease, e.g. G.P.I, dementia etc.

r. Hoffman's Flickering of tip of nail of index finger; produces flexion of

phallanges in thumb and other fingers, an evidence of pyramidal tract lesion (upper motor palsy).

r. hung up Abnormal slowness of relaxation phase of deep tendon reflex, e.g. hung up ankle jerk in hypothyroidism.

r. light Contraction of pupil on focussing a bright light on it.

r. mass A condition following complete trans-section of cord where a weak stimulus brings about widespread responses (muscle contraction, defecation, urination, etc.), due to release from inhibition of higher cortical centers.

r. Mayer's Downward pressure on index finger causes apposition and adduction of thumb, flexion at metacarpo phallangeal joint and extension at interphallangeal joint.

r. Mendel-Bekhtena Plantar flexion of toes on percussion of the dorsum of foot.

r. monosynaptic Reflex involving only two neurones, i.e. afferent and efferent.

r. neck righting Turning of the body in the direction of head rotation in supine infants elicited between 4 months to 2 years of age.

r. nociceptive Reflex obtained by painful stimulus.

r. palm-chin Scratching of thenar eminence producing contraction of lower lip on same side.

r. parachute Extension of arms, hands and fingers when the infant is suspended in prone position and dropped a short distance to a soft surface. Asymmetrical response indicates motor abnormality in children above 9 months of age.

r. rooting Stroking the cheek of the infant causes turning of mouth towards the stimulus. It is present upto 7th month of age.

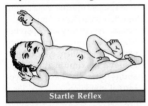

Startle Reflex

r. startle Reflex reaction in a newborn child in step once to a sudden unexpected stimulus such as loud noise or sudden change in position.

r. stepping Leg movements simulating walking when the infant is held erect, inclined forward with sole of feet touching a flat surface. The reflex is present at birth and is gone by 6 weeks of age.

r. tonic neck In the infant forcibly turning the head causes extension of extremities on the side to which head is turned with flexion of extremities on the other side.

Reflex arc The neural pathway or circuit between the point of stimulation and the responding organ.

Reflex center An area in the brain or spinal cord where afferent input initiates impulses in the efferent pathway.

Reflux Regurgitation or backward flow.

Refraction The change in the direction of light rays while passing from one medium to another medium of a different density.

r. errors of pathological condition where parallel rays of light are not

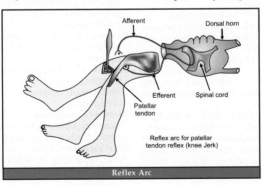

Reflex arc for patellar tendon reflex (knee Jerk)

Reflex Arc

brought to focus on retina because of defect in refractive media, i.e. cornea and lens.

Refractive power The degree to which a transparent object deflects a ray of light from its straight path.

Refractometer Instrument for measuring refractive power.

Refractometry Measurement of refractive power of lenses.

Refractory period Period of relaxation of a muscle during which excitation is not possible.

Refrigerant Agent producing cooling.

Refrigeration Cooling.

Refsum disease A hereditary disorder of phytanic acid metabolism manifesting with ataxia, neuropathy, visual disturbances (night blindness) and heart disease.

Regel Menstruation.

Regeneration Regrowth, repair.

Regimen A systematic plan of therapy.

Region A body part or area.

Regression Return to a former state.

Regulation The state of being controlled.

Regurgitation Backward flow.

r. aortic Backflow of blood from aorta to left ventricle during diastole due to incompetent aortic valve.

r. duodenal Reflux of duodenal secretions and bile into stomach.

r. mitral Backflow of blood from left ventricle into left atrium during ventricular systole due to incompetent mitral valve.

r. pulmonary Backflow of blood from pulmonary artery into right ventricle.

r. tricuspid Regurgitation of blood from right ventricle into right atrium.

Rehabilitation The processes of treatment and education for a disabled patient to achieve maximum function and independent living.

r. cardiac A combination of psychological support, progressive exercise and patient education to achieve maximum functional ability after one has had myocardial infarction.

Rehydration Restoration of body hydration or water balance.

Reichert's cartilage The second branchial arch in embryo giving rise to stapes, styloid process, stylohyoid ligament, etc.

Reid's baseline Line drawn from lower margin of orbit to center of external auditory canal to center of occipital bone.

Reimplantation Replacement of a part from where it was taken out, e.g. tooth, finger, ear.

Reinfection A second infection by the same organism.

Reinforcement Augmentation or strengthening

Reissner's membrane The thin membrane separating the cochlear canal from the scale vestibule.

Reiter's syndrome A symptom complex consisting of urethritis, arthritis and conjunctivitis commonly occurring in young men with a preceding history of gastro-intestinal upset.

Rejection Destruction of trans-planted tissue/organ due to host immune response. Rejection can be hyperacute, acute or chronic.

Relapse Reappearance of symptoms after apparent cure.

Relapsing fever Infectious disease caused by *B. recurrentis*.

Relative risk In epidemiological studies it is the ratio of incidence rate of a disease in the exposed group to that in the unexposed group.

Relax To diminish anxiety, tension, nervousness.

Relaxant An agent decreasing tension, tone of a muscle.

Relaxin A polypeptide hormone secreted by corpus luteum of ovary during pregnancy that inhibits uterine contraction.

Relieve To provide relief.

Remak's ganglion A group of nerve cells in the coronary sinus near its entry into right atrium.

Remedy Cure.

Remission Abatement in severity of symptoms.

Remittent fever Fever alternately increasing and decreasing but not touching the normalcy.

Remodelling The reshaping or reconstructing of a part or area.

Renal failure Failure of kidneys to perform excretory and metabolic functions resulting in anuria/metabolic changes.

Renal transplant Surgical implantation of donor kidney to replace a diseased host kidney.

Renal tubular acidosis A group of 4 disorders in which bicarbonate loss in urine is increased with reabsorption of more chloride and resulting acidosis

Reniform Shaped like a kidney.

Renin An enzyme secreted by juxtaglomerular apparatus of kidneys that converts angiotensinogen to angiotensin.

Renin substrate Alpha-2 globulin.

Rennin An enzyme present in gastric juice of animals that coagulates milk.

Renography X-ray of kidneys.

Renshaw cells Small cells with short axons connecting motor nerve axons with each other and thereby inhibit motor neurons.

Reovirus A class of viruses found in the intestinal and respiratory tract of healthy humans.

Repellent An agent that repels insects, ticks and mites, e.g. dimethy-pthalate.

Reperfusion injury Reinstitution of blood flow to previously ischaemic zone may cause washout of toxic cellular products with arrhythmia

Repletion Complete fullness or satisfied.

Replication The process of doubling of tissue, cell, genetic material.

Repolarization Restoration of basal electrical status in muscle or nerve fiber after excitation.

Reposition Restoration of an organ or tissue to its original position.

Repositor Instrument for reposition.

Reproduction The process by which plants and animals give rise to off-springs.

r. asexual Reproduction by fission or budding without involvement of sex cells.

Repulsion Act of driving back or use of force to cause separation.

Res ispa liquitor The thing speaks for itself e.g. inadvertent removal of a healthy part/organ or leaving a sponge or forceps in patient's body.

Research Scientific and diligent study, investigation and experi-mentation to establish facts and intelligently analyze them to derive conclusion.

Resect To cut out, e.g. a part of intes-tine in gangrene of bowel.

Resection Partial excision.

r. wedge Resection of a piece of tissue in form of a wedge as in polycystic ovary.

Resectoscope Instrument for resec-tion of prostate through urethra.

Reserpine Derivative from plant Rauwolfia acting as a hypotensive agent.

Reserve That which is held back for future use.

r. alkali Alkali content of body available for neutralization of acid.

r. cardiac The ability of heart to increase cardiac output during strenuous physical work.

Reserve air Additional amount of air that can be expelled from lungs over the normal quantity.

Reservoir Any human being, animal or insect in which an infecting agent lives, multiplies and reproduces for transmission to susceptible host.

Resident A doctor under training after internship.

Residual Relates to that left as a residue.

Residual urine Urine left in bladder after urination; commonly it is less than 50 ml.

Residue-free diet Diet free of cel-lulose or roughage.

Resilience The property of coming back to original shape after stretch is released.

Resin 1. Some natural substances ob-tained as exudation from plants. 2. A class of solids or soft organic compounds that includes most polymers like polyethylene, polys-tyrene and polyvinyl.

r. ionexchange Ionizable synthetic substances either anionic or cationic, used to remove acid or basic ions from solutions.

Resistance 1. Power of resisting 2. In psychology, the force which prevents repressed thoughts from entering conscious mind from the unconscious 3. The power of body to withstand infection.

Resistance transfer factor A genetic factor in bacteria that control resistance to drugs.

Resolution 1. The subsidence of infla-mmation and return to normalcy, 2. The ability of a ultrasonic transducer system to show fine details of organ scanned.

Resolve To return to normal after pathological process subsides.

Resonance The musical quality elicited on percussing an air containing cavity.

r. vocal The vibrations of voice transmitted to ears during auscultation. It is increased in consolidation, and over cavities in communication with bronchus.

Resorb To absorb again or to undergo resorption.

Resorbent An agent that promotes absorption of blood and exudates.

Resorcinol A mild antiseptic, keratolytic and fungicidal agent.

Resorption Act of removal by absorption, e.g. callus following bone fracture, root of deciduous tooth, blood from hematoma.

Respiration The act of breathing for interchange of gases, i.e. O_2 and CO_2.

r. abdominal Use of diaphragm and abdominal muscles for respiration as in rib fracture, pleurisy.

r. paradoxical A condition seen in paralysis of diaphragm whereby the affected side diaphragm moves up during, inspiration and moves down during expiration.

r. Cheyne-Stokes Abnormal bizarre breathing with periods of apnea followed by gradually increasing depth of respiration followed by a slow decline to end in apnea; seen in diencephalic dysfunction.

r. kussmaul's Deep gasping respiration of diabetic ketoacidosis.

r. thoracic Respiration performed entirely by expansion of chest as in peritonitis, diaphragmatic inflammation.

Respiratory center The centers in medulla oblongata controlling the act of respiration. Consists of an inspiratory center in rostral half of reticular formation overlying olivary nuclei, an expiratory center dorsal to it and a pneumotaxic center in the pons.

Respirator An apparatus which rhythmically inflates and deflates the lungs; either pressure cycled or volume cycled.

Respiratory distress syndrome Dyspnea in newborn due to deficient pulmonary surfactant, causing atelectasis, commonly seen in prematures *SYN*—hyaline membrane disease.

Respiratory failure Inability of lungs to perform ventilatory function with PaO_2 of ≤ 60 mm Hg and $PCO_2 \geq 50$ mm Hg.

Respiratory quotient The relationship between CO_2 produced and oxygen consumed.

Respiratory syncytial virus A virus that induces formation of syncytial masses in infected cell cultures; causes acute respiratory disease in children.

Response The reaction like that of muscle or gland following a stimulus.

r. anamnestic The rapid production of an antibody response after injection of an antigen.

r. inflammatory Dilatation of blood vessels with exudation of plasma proteins and accumulation of leukocytes following injury.

r. triple Three phases of vasomotor response following skin injury, i.e. red reaction, flare or spreading of flush and wheal.

Restiform Rope like.

Restiform body Inferior cerebellar peduncle on lateral border of 4th ventricle.

Resting potential The potential difference existing between inside and outside of a cell membrane while the cell is at rest.

Restitution Return to a former status.

Restless leg Irrepressible ache in the legs of unknown etiology compelling the patient to move the legs to bring some relief.

Restoration Return of anything to its previous state; in dentistry material or device that restores or replaces a tooth.

Restraint Preventing or restricting from any action.

Resuscitation Revival after apparent death.

Retardation Slowing down, delayed mental or physical response.

Retch To make an involuntary attempt to vomit.

Rete A network of vessels and nerves.

r. testes A network of tubules in mediastinum testis that receives sperms from seminiferous tubules. From rete testis efferent ducts convey sperm to epididymis.

Retention 1. Keeping within body of substances like urine, stool. 2. holding back.

Retention cyst Cyst caused by retention of secretion in a gland due to closure of the duct.

Retention enema Enema retained in colon to provide medication or nutrition.

Reticular In the form of a network.

Reticular activating system The system essential in maintaining wakefulness. It consists of reticular formation, hypothalamus and medial thalamus.

Reticular cells Phagocytic cells present in bone marrow and lymph nodes, constitute the reticular tissue.

Reticular formation The group of cells and fibers forming a diffuse network in brainstem and connecting to the ascending and descending tracts around. Responsible for wakefulness and sleep.

Reticular layer Connective tissue layer in deeper portion of dermis beneath the papillary layer.

Reticulation Formation of a network.

Reticulin A proteinacious substance in the connective tissue.

Reticulocyte Immediate precursor of mature RBC, contains a network of granules or filaments, constitute 1% of circulating RBC.

Reticulocytosis Raised number of reticulocytes in peripheral blood indicating active erythropoisis; occurs after hematinics in treatment of anemia, following bleeding episode.

Reticuloendothelial cell A phagocytic cell of reticuloendothelial system.

Reticuloendothelial system The phagocytic cell system of body capable of ingesting paniculate matter like bacteria, colloid particles. It includes macrophages, (both fixed and wandering), reticular cells, Kuffer cells of liver and spleen, microglia of CNS, adventitial cells of blood vessels and dust cells of lungs.

Reticuloendotheliosis Hyperplasia of reticuloendothelium.

Reticuloid Resembling reticulosis.

Reticuloma Tumor composed of reticuloendothelial cells.

Reticulosarcoma A malignant tumor composed of large monocytic cells originating from reticuloendothelial system.

Reticulosis Reticulocytosis, a fatal lymphoma, often familial, with hepatosplenomegaly, lymphadenopathy, anemia and granulocytopenia.

Retina The innermost light sensitive layer of eye extending from optic disk to margin of pupil. The various layers of retina from without inward are: pigment epithelium, rods and cones, external limiting membrane, external nuclear layer, external plexiform layer, internal nuclear layer, internal plexiform layer, layer of ganglion cells, layer of nerve fibers, internal limiting membrane.

r. detachment Complete or partial separation of retina from choroid following trauma, choroidal hemorrhage or tumors.

Retinaculum A band or membrane holding any organ or part in its place.

r. extensor, of ankle Both superior and inferior on dorsum of foot.

r. flexor of ankle Extends from medial malleolus to the medial tubercle of calcaneus:

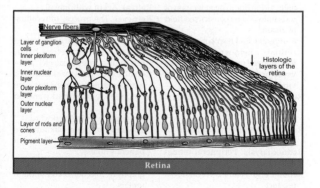

Retina

r. extensor of wrist An oblique band on dorsal aspect that contains six separate compartments for extensor tendons.

r. flexor of wrist Extends from trapezium to pisiform bones.

r. of hip joint Three bands along neck of femur continuous with capsule of hip joint.

Retinene Orange—yellow carotenoid pigment formed by action of light on rhodopsin.

Retinitis Inflammation of retina.

r. actinic Retinitis following exposure to intense light.

r. circinate Retinitis where there is a circle of white spots around macula.

r. diabetic Retinitis of long standing diabetes characterized by microaneurysm, waxy exudates and hemorrhages.

r. pigmentosa A degenerative condition, usually hereditary, beginning in childhood with pigmentary changes. Manifests with defective night vision due to degeneration of rods followed by constricted field of vision.

r. proliferans End result of recurrent retinal hemorrhage with vascularized masses of connective tissue projecting from retina into vitreous.

Retinoblastoma Malignant glioma of retina giving yellow reflex (cat's eye reflex).

Retinochoroiditis Inflammation of retina and choroid.

Retinodialysis Peripheral retinal detachment.

Retinoic acid Vitamin A breakdown product.

Retinoid Resembling a resin.

Retinol A form of vitamin A.

Retinopathy Any disorder of retina; may be arteriosclerotic, diabetic, hypertensive, syphilitic etc.

Retinopexy Refixation of detached retina

Retinoschisis A splitting of retina into two layers with cyst formation in between

Retinoscopy A method of determining refractive power of the eyes.

Retinosis Non-inflammatory degeneration of retina.

Retort Long necked glass vessel used in distillation.

Retractile Capable of being drawn back.

Retraction Shortening, state of being drawn back.

Retraction ring A ridge of uterus separating upper contractile segment from lower dilating segment.

Retractor Instrument for holding back a tissue.

Retreat Act of withdrawal.

Retrieval The process of recalling past memory.

Retro Situated behind or backward in position, e.g. retro-ocular, retrobulbar, retrocecal, etc.

Retroflexed Bent backwards, a retroflexed uterus is the state where uterine body is bent backwards on cervix.

Retrograde Moving backward.

Retrograde amnesia Memory loss for events just preceding the time of patient's illness.

Retrograde pyelography Pyelography by injection of dye through ureters.

Retrograde ejaculation Semen discharge into bladder rather than through urethral meatus as in diabetic neuropathy.

Retrolental fibroplasia Bilateral retinal vessel occlusion followed by fibrous proliferation often involving the vitreous in premature newborns exposed to high concentration of oxygen.

Retroperitoneal fibrosis Fibrotic tissue growth in retroperitoneal space often compressing ureters, vena cava and aorta, a sequel to mathysergide treatment of migraine, *SYN—* Ormond's syndrome.

Retroposition Backward displacement of an organ.

Retropulsion Moving backward involuntarily as in Parkinson's disease.

Retrospective study A study where patient's records are analyzed after they have experienced the disease.

Retroversion of uterus Backward tilting of entire uterus including cervix so that the latter points towards symphysis pubis.

Retroviruses A group of viruses containing reverse transcriptase, e.g. RNA containing tumor viruses causing leukemia, lymphoma, in lower animals and AIDS infection in human.

Rett's syndrome A multiple deficit developmental disorder with decline in motor and cognitive function.

Retzius Swedish anatomist,

R. *lines* Concentric lines in transverse section of tooth enamel.

R. *space* Space between bladder and symphysis pubis containing fat and a plexus of veins.

R. *veins* Veins communicating mesenteric veins and inferior vena cava.

Revascularization Restoration of blood flow to a part.

Reverberation 1. Repeated echoing of a sound. 2. In neurology the process by which a single applied impulse causes continuous discharge of impulses from collaterals of the neurones.

Reye syndrome A syndrome characterized by encephalopathy, and hepatic failure in children in consequence to viral infection, aspirin use.

Rhabdomyolysis A disease wilh destruction of muscle cells, common sequence to snake venom.

Rhabdomyoma Benign tumor of striated muscle.

Rhabdomyosarcoma Malignant tumor of striated muscle.

Rhabdovirus Rod shaped RNA virus, e.g. Rabies virus.

Rhachischisis Congenital cleft in spinal canal.

Rhaphe A ridge.

Rh. blood group A blood group antigen on human RBCs, in common with rhesus monkeys. A Rh -ve mother if bears a Rh +ve fetus, Rh antibodies produced in mother may cross the placenta to destroy the fetal RBCs.

Rheology Study of deformation and flow of materials.

Rheostosis A form of osteitis occurring in streaks in long bones.

Rheumatic fever A systemic illness that follows streptococcal sore throat manifesting with carditis. fleeting polyarthritis, chorea, erythema marginatum, subcutaneous nodules, etc. believed to be an autoimmune phenomenon.

Rheumatism A generic term to denote inflammation of muscle, joint pain.

r. palindromic A disease of unknown etiology manifesting with joint pain, joint swelling lasting from few hours to days with periods of complete normalcy.

r. soft tissue Pain around a joint not related to any joint pathology, e.g. bursitis, tendinitis, perichondritis, Tietz syndrome etc.

Rheumatoid Resembling rheumatism.

Rheumatoid arthritis Bilaterally symmetrical polyarthritis involving the fingers and toes with bony erosion, joint deformity and involvement of great vessels, vertebra etc.

Rheumatoid factor An IgM autoantibody present in upto 75% of

Rheumatoid Arthritis

patients suffering from rheumatoid arthritis.

Rheumatology Branch of medicine dealing with rheumatic diseases.

Rh immune globulin Anti Rh gammaglobulin, usually given to Rh -ve mothers within 72 hours of giving birth to a Rh +ve baby or following abortion.

Rhinecephalon The part of brain concerned with reception and integration of olfactory impulses.

Rhinitis Inflammation of nasal mucosa, can be allergic, atrophic (rusting and bad odor), hyperplastic, etc.

Rhinocleisis Nasal obstruction.

Rhinolalia Nasal quality of voice.

Rhinologist A specialist dealing with diseases of nose.

Rhinomiosis Reduction in size of nose by surgery.

Rhinophyma Hypertrophy of tissue over the nose with congestion and retention of sebum.

Rhinoplasty Plastic surgery of nose.

Rhinorrhea Thin watery nasal discharge.

Rhinoscleroma An infective disease of nose caused by *Klebsiella rhinoscleromatis* manifesting with hard nodular growth often spreading to lower respiratory tract.

Rhinosalpingitis Inflammation of nasal mucosa and eustachian tube.

Rhinoscopy Examination of nasal passage.

Rhinosporidiosis A fungal disease caused by *Rhinosporidium seberi* characterized by growth of pedunculated polyps in nose, larynx and genital tracts.

Rhinovirus A subgroup of picorna virus causing common cold.

Rhitidectomy Removal of wrinkles by plastic surgery.

Rhitodosis Wrinkling of cornea, a feature of approaching death.

Rhizo Root.

Rhizoid Root like.

Rhizometic Concerning hip and shoulder joints.

Rhizotomy Section of nerve roots.

Rhodopsin The purple pigment of rods responsible for vision in dimlight.

Rhombencephalon A primary division of embryonic brain giving rise to brainstem and cerebellum.

Rhomboid An oblique parallelogram.

Rhoncus Rattling sound resembling snoring; pleural = rhonchi.

Rhubarb Extract from root and stem of plant used as cathartic and astringent.

Rhythm Regularity of occurrence of an action or movement or impulse.

r. alpha In EEG a rhythm of 8-12 per second.

r. beta Rhythm frequency of 15-30 per second in EEG, predominantly in frontomotor leads.

r. cicardian The recurrence of biological activities every 24 hours not being influenced by environment.

r. delta A slow EEG rhythm of 4 or less per second with relatively high voltage, usually recorded over tumor or hematoma.

r. ectopic Impulse originating outside SA node.

r. escape An impulse originating from a site other than SA node when the latter fails to initiate the impulse.

r. gallop Three heart sounds heard (S_1 S_2 S_3) in sequence in each cardiac contraction resembling gallop of horse.

r. gamma In EEG 50/second rhythm.

r. idioventricular Impulse originating from bundle of His or myocardium in consequence to complete A-V block.

r. theta An EEG rhythm of 4-7 cycles/sec.

r. tic-tac A rhythm where S_1, and S_2 are of same quality usually in cardiac distress or in fetus.

Rhytidectomy Plastic surgery for wrinkles.

Rhytidosis Wrinkling of cornea.

Rib One of the 12 pairs of narrow curved bones of chest wall connecting sternum to vertebra.

r. cervical A super numerary rib arising from 7th cervical vertebra and often causing thoracic inlet syndrome by compression of lower cord of brachial plexus.

Riboflavin Yellow-orange crystalline powder of B complex group functioning as coenzyme in cellular oxidation; Richly found in milk and milk products, green leafy vegetables, fish and meat; deficiency causes glossitis, seborrhea, cheilosis and corneal vascularization.

Ribonuclease An enzyme that breaks down RNA.

Ribonucleic acid (RNA). RNA differs from DNA in that its sugar is ribose and the pyrimidine compound it contains is uracil rather than thymine. RNA is principal constituent of cytoplasm and of certain viruses. Messenger RNA carries the transcription code for specific amino acid sequences from DNA to cytoplasmic reticulum for protein synthesis. Transfer RNA carries the amino acid groups to the ribosomes for incorporation into proteins.

Ribose A pentose sugar present in RNA and riboflavin.

Ribosome A constituent of cell cytoplasm that receives genetic information and translates them into synthesis of proteins.

Ricin A white highly toxic protein of castor beans.

Ricinoleic acid An unsaturated, fatty acid with a strong laxative action, principally found in castor oil.

Rickets A vitamin D deficiency disease in children where mineralization of newly formed osteoid tissue is defective. The child is restless with aches and pains, hepatosplenomegaly, delayed dentition, soft skull bones with proneness to skeletal deformilies like kyphoscoliosis, bow leg, pigeon chest.

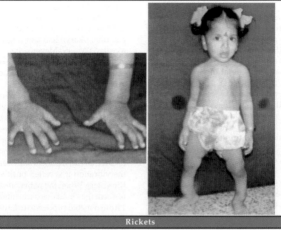

Rickets

r. renal Rickets in chronic renal failure primarily due to inadequate formation of active vitamin D_3 and accompanying acidosis causing bone dissolution.

r. vitamin D resistant Defects of renal tubular function causing excessive renal calcium and phosphorus loss so that the accompanying ricket responds poorly to vitamin D.

Rickettsia Microscopic organism in between viruses and bacteria causing typhus fever, Q fever, rockymountain spotted fever; transmitted by arthropods.

Rickettsial pox A self limited acute, febrile disease caused by *Rickettsia akari*.

Rider's bone Bone formation in adductor longus muscle of thigh in horse riders.

Ridge Long projecting surface or crest

r. alveolar The bony process on maxilla or mandible containing tooth sockets.

r. dental Elevation on crown of tooth.

r. epicondylar Two ridges on humerus for muscular attachment.

r. genital Ridge in developing embryo giving rise to gonads.

r. gluteal Ridge on upper femur for attachment of gluteus maximus muscle.

r. pronator Ridge on front surface of ulna for attachment of pronator quadratus.

r. pterygoid Ridge on greater wing of sphenoid bone.

r. supracondylar Ridges on lower end of humerus.

Riedel's lobe A tongue shaped process of liver.

Rifampin An antibiotic from streptomyces, used in treatment of mycobacterial diseases (leprosy, tuberculosis) and meningitis prophylaxis.

Right handedness Proneness of a person to dominantly use the right hand.

Rigidity Stiffness; one who resists all changes.

r. cerebellar Stiffness of body parts from disease of middle lobe of cerebellum.

r. clasp knife Rigidity seen in pyramidal disease where flexion of a limb causes increased resistance of extensors but if flexion is continued, there is a sudden giving way.

r. cogwheel Jerky resistance felt while stretching a hypertonic muscle.

r. decerebrate Sustained contraction of extensor muscles from lesion of brainstem.

Rigor Paroxysmal chill.

Rima A fissure or crack.

r. glottidis An elongated slit between the vocal folds.

r. vestibuli Space between the vocal folds.

Rimiterol A beta$_2$ agonist for use in bronchial asthma.

Rimantadine An analog of amantadine, the antiviral agent.

Ring Band around circular opening, circular form.

r. abdominal Apertures in abdominal wall, often producing herniations, e.g. inguinal, femoral, etc.

r. Bandl's Retraction ring of uterus.

r. lymphoid Lymphoid tissue in a ring fashion in pharynx consisting of palatine, pharyngeal and lingual tonsils *SYN*—Waldeyer's ring.

Ringworm Dermatomycosis caused by trichophyton and microsporum group of fungi.

Rhine test Tuning fork test for testing bone and air conduction. The base of vibrating tuning fork is held in contact with the mastoid process till vibrations are no longer heard by the patient, then it is held close to external ear. If patient still hears the vibration it is called positive Rinne test. When the patient does not hear the vibrations once shifted 1 from mastoid process to external ear, air conduction is tested first by placing the vibrating fork in front of external ear until the sound is no longer heard, then the stem of the fork is placed on mastoid. If vibration is still heard it is called negative Rinne test. All normal persons are Rinne positive and those with defective air conduction are Rinne negative.

Ripening 1. Softening and dilatation of cervix during labor 2. maturation of cataract.

Risk-benefit analysis In medicare the analysis of risk and benefit from a procedure discussed between patient, doctor and relations.

Risk factor Factors that predispose a person to development of a disease, e.g. hypertension, diabetes, hyperlipidemia, cigarette smoking, etc. are high risk factors for developing coronary artery disease.

Risorius The muscle arising over massetor and inserted to corners of the mouth.

Ristocetin An antibiotic obtained from cultures of *Nocardia lurida.*

Risus Laughter.

r. sardonicus A peculiar grin as in tetanus due to spasm of facial muscles.

Ritodrine-Beta$_2$ agonist for use in bronchial asthma.

Ritualistic surgery Surgery without scientific justification performed in primitive societies.

Robert's pelvis Transverse contraction of pelvis due to osteoarthritis of sacroiliac joints

Rocking A technique to increase muscle tone in hypotonic muscles through vestibular stimulation.

Rocky-mountain spotted fever A tick born typhus with fever, rash and myalgia caused by Rickettsia rickettssi.

Rodent Mammals like mice, rats and squirrel.

Rodenticide Chemicals that kill rodents.

Rodent ulcer Basal cell carcinoma commonly occurring on upper face with destruction of underlying tissue and bone.

Roentgen German physicist who discovered roentgen rays, (X-rays) and won noble prize in 1901.

Rokitansky's disease Acute yellow atrophy of liver.

Rolando's fissure Fissure between parietal and frontal lobes.

Romberg's sign Inability to stand still with the eyes closed and feet drawn together in patients of sensory ataxia.

Root canal The pulp cavity in root of a tooth.

Rorschach test Psychological test consisting of 10 inkblot designs. Interpretation hints at personality disorder.

Rosacea A disease of unknown etiology manifesting with papules, pustules and hyperplasia of sebaceous glands principally affecting face.

Rosary Resembling a string of beads.

r. rachitic Swollen costochondral junctions in rickets.

Rose Bengal Iodine 131 along with ^{131}I rose Bengal used for liver scanning.

Rosenmuller's body A rudimentary structure in mesosalpinx homologous to head of epididymis in male.

Rosenmuller's sign Fine tremor of closed eyelids in hyperparathyroidism

Roseola Rose colored rash.

r. infantum Non-infectious rose colored'rash appearing in infants with splenomegaly, high fever.

Rosette Something resembling a rose.

Ross bodies Copper color round bodies with dark granules seen in blood and tissue fluids of syphilis.

Rossolimo's reflex Plantar flexion of second to fifth toes in response to percussion on plantar surface of toes.

Rostellum A fleshy protrusion on anterior end of scolex of tapeworm bearing spines or hooks.

Rostral Towards cephalic end of body.

Rostrum Any hooked or beaked structure.

Rotavirus Virus causing epidemic and sporadic enteritis.

Roth spots Small white spot on retina close to optic disk in acute infective endocarditis.

Rotoxamine tartarate An antihistaminic drug.

Rotor syndrome A form of conjugated hyperbilirubinemia inherited as autosomal recessive.

Roughage Fibers in cereals, fruits and vegetable, essential for patients of diabetes and those with constipation but inadvisable for patients of colitis.

Round ligament Round cord like structures passing from uterus in the broad ligament and then through the inguinal canal to end in soft tissues of labia majora.

Rub The sound of friction of one roughened surface moving on another, e.g. pleural rub, pericardial rub.

Rubefacient Agents causing redness of skin by vasodilatation, e.g. liniments of turpentine.

Rubella Acute infectious disease of viral origin causing rash, cervical and post auricular lymphadenopathy, in first trimester can cause fetal anomalies and in pubertal girls can cause oophoritis.

Rubeola *SYN*—measles.

Rubeosis iridis Vascularization of anterior surface of iris with retinal vein thrombophlebitis often responsible for hemorrhagic glaucoma in diabetics.

Rubidium A soft silvery metal that bursts into flames spontaneously in air.

Rubin's test Carbon dioxide/air uterine insufflation to test tubal patency.

Rubor Redness caused by inflammation. The other three classical signs of inflammation are calor.(heat) dolor (pain) and tumor (swelling).

Rubrospinal The descending tract from rednucleus of midbrain to gray matter of spinal cord.

Rudiment 1. Remnant of a part which was functional in earlier stage of development or in ancestors, 2. undeveloped.

Ruffini's corpuscles Encapsulated sensory nerve endings of skin to mediate sensation of warmth.

Ruga A fold of mucous membrane, e.g. of stomach or vagina.

Ruggeri's reflex Rise in pulse rate on convergence of eyes on a near object.

Rugose, rugous Having many wrinkles or creases.

Rugosity Condition of having wrinkles or being folded.

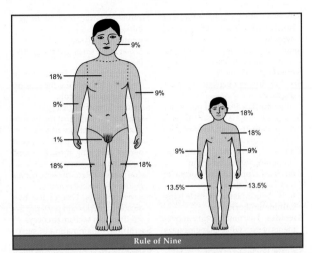

Rule of Nine

Rule of nine Formula for estimating percentage of body surface area, where head represents 9%, front and back of trunk 18% each, each lower extremity 18%, each upper extremity 9% and perineum 1%.

Rum fits Convulsion occurring within 48 hours following abstinence in habitual drinkers.

Rumination 1. Regurgitation of previously swallowed food. 2. Obsessional preoccupation with thoughts.

Rump Gluteal region or buttocks.

Rumpl's symptom In neurasthenia, rise in pulse rate on pressure over a painful spot.

Rupia A thick cutaneous syphilitic erruption often with extensive ul-ceration.

Rupture Breaking apart of any organ or tissue, e.g. of amniotic membrane, uterus, intestines fall-opian tubes.

Rush The first spell of pleasure produced by a narcotic drug.

Russel bodies Small spherical hyaline bodies in cancerous and simple inflammatory growths.

Russian bath Steam bath followed by friction and plunge in cold water.

Rutin A crystalline glucoside derived from buckwheat closely related to hesperidin, used in hemostatic preparations.

Rye A cereal used for food and beverages.

Rytidosis Wrinkling of cornea preceding death.

S

Saber sin Convex prominent anterior border of tibia in congenital syphilis.

Sabin vaccine Oral polio vaccine containing inactivated polio virus.

Sabulous Sandy, gritty.

Sac A cavity or pouch often containing fluid.

s. alveolar The terminal part of air passage consisting of alveoli connected to respiratory bronchiole by alveolar duct.

s. hernial Peritoneal protrusion containing herniated organ.

s. lacrimal Upper dilated portion of nasolacrimal duct.

s. yolk A rudimentary vesicle lying within the chorion sac.

Saccades Fast involuntary movements of eyes while changing gaze from one point to another.

Saccate Enclosed in a sac.

Saccharide A group of carbohydrates including mono, di, tri, and polysaccharides.

Saccharase An enzyme catalyzing breakdown of disaccharides to monosaccharides.

Saccharic acid A dibasic acid produced by action of nitric acid on dextrose.

Saccharin A coal tar product, 300-500 times sweeter than sugar, used as artificial sweetener.

Saccharolytic Capable of splitting up sugar.

Saccharomycosis A disease due to yeasts.

Saccharose Sucrose, or cane sugar.

Saccular Resembling a sac.

Sacculation Group of sacs or formed into group of sacs.

Saccule A small sac.

s. laryngeal A small diverticulum of larynx.

s. vestibular The smaller sac in vestibule that contains the sensory area—macula sacculi.

Sacculus Singular of saccule.

Sacralization Fusion of the sacrum and the 5th lumbar vertebra.

Sacral nerves The 5 pairs of mixed nerves emerging through sacral foramina.

Sacral plexus Plexus of sacral nerves giving rise to sciatic nerve.

Sacrococcygeus One of the two muscles, anterior and posterior extending from sacrum to coccyx.

Sacroiliitis Inflammation of sacroiliac joint.

Sacrospinalis A large muscle lying on either side of vertebral column consists of iliocostalis and longissimus.

Sacrovertebral angle Angle formed between base of sacrum and fifth lumbar vertebra.

Sacrum The triangular bone of buttock lying in between the two iliac bones forming sacroiliac joints. Male sacrum is narrower and more curved.

Saddle A seat for horse riders.

Saddle area The areas of buttocks coming in contact with the saddle during horse riding.

Saddle joint A joint where the articulating surfaces are convex and concave.

Saddle nose A depressed nasal bridge, due to congenital absence of bony or cartilaginous support or destructive disease like leprosy and syphilis.

Sadism Sexual pleasure from inflicting physical or mental torture on others.

Sadist One who practises sadism.

Sadness Feeling of dejection or melancholy.

Safelight Dark room lights whose wavelength does not hamper undeveloped X-ray film.

Safflower oil It has high content of linoleic acid but low saturated fatty acids

S. botryoids A sarcoma of uterus of infant and children

Sagittal Anteroposterior direction.

Sagittal plane The plane that divides body into left and right halves.

Sagittal sinus The superior longitudinal sinus.

Sagittal suture Suture between two parietal bones.

Sago A starch preparation; when taken as food, leaves little residue.

Saint Vitus, dance Sydenham's chorea.

Salam spasm Infantile epilepsy with nodding of head due to spasm of sternocleidomastoids.

Salbutamol Beta$_2$ agonist bronchodilator.

Salacious Lustful.

Salicylate Salt of salicylic acid, Methyl salicylate is a counter irritant whereas sodium salicylate is analgesic and antipyretic.

Salicylic acid A phenol derivative used for making aspirin and used as keratolytic and antifungal agent.

Saline Solution of salt or salty; can be hypertonic > 0.9% or hypotonic < 0.85% concentration.

Saline enema 1 teaspoon of salt dissolved in a pint of water to which is added magnesium sulfate (epsum salt) to induce catharsis.

Saliva Colourless, odorless, weakly alkaline secretion of salivary glands. Contains ptyalin, maltase and lysozymes. Daily secretion is upto 1500 ml.

Salivant Agents that stimulate flow of saliva.

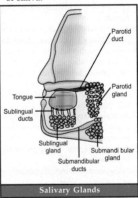

Salivary Glands

Salivary glands The parotid, sublingual and submandibular paired glands and the unpaired palatal, buccal, lingual glands secreting saliva.

Salk vaccine Formalin inactivated poliomyelitis vaccine for intramuscular use.

Salmefamol Beta$_2$ adrenergic stimulant

Salmonellosis Infection with salmonella group of organism producing typhoid fever, gastroenteritis and septicemia.

Salmonpatch Salmon colored areas of cornea in syphilitic keratitis.

Salpingectomy Surgical removal of fallopian tubes.

Salpingitis Inflammation of fallopian tubes usually due to gonococci, tuberculosis, strepto and staphylococci.

Salpingography Imaging of fallopian tubes by injection of radioopaque dye in investigation of infertility.

Salpingolysis Surgical procedure to free the fallopian tubes of adhesions.

Salpingo-oophorectomy Excision of ovary and fallopian tube.

Salpingo-oophoritis Inflammation of fallopian tube and ovary.

Salpingopexy Surgical fixation of fallopian tube.

Salpingoplasty *SYN*—tuboplasty; plastic surgery of fallopian tube to promote fertility.

Salpingorrhaphy Ligation of fallopian tube.

Salpingostomy Surgical opening up of a fallopian tube.

Salpingotomy Incision on a fallopian tube.

Salpinx The fallopian or eustachian tube.

Salsalal Salicyl-salicylic acid.

Salt 1. Sodium chloride 2. A chemical compound formed from action of an acid with a base.

s. bile Salt of glycocolic and taurocolic acids present in bile, help in absorption of fat.

s. iodized Salt containing 1 part of sodium or potassium iodide per 10, 000 parts of sodium chloride for iodine deficiency.

s. smelling Aromatized ammonium carbonate.

Saltatory Dancing or leaping movement.

Saltatory conduction Nerve conduction where impulse skips from node to node.

Salt free diet Diet containing < 500 mg salt/day.

Salubrious Good for health, wholesome.

Saluresis Excretion of salt in urine.

Salutary Promoting health.

Salvarsan Arsenic salt previously used for syphilis.

Sample A portion of population or any substance that is representative of entire population or that substance.

s. biased In epidemiology, a sample of a group of which each member did not have an equal opportunity of being selected in the sample.

Sampling The process of selecting portion or part to represent the whole.

Sanatorium A place or establishment for promotion of good-health or treatment of chronic ailments, e.g. tuberculosis.

Sand Fine particles from disintegration of rock.

s. auditory Calcareous concretions in inner ear.

s. pineal Calcium deposit near base of pineal gland.

Sandflies Flies belonging to genus phlebotomus transmitting sandfly fever, oroya fever and various forms of leishmaniasis.

Sandfly fever An arbovirus disease mimicking influenza but without respiratory symptoms, transmitted by sandflies.

Sandhoff's disease A gangliosidosis where enzymes hexosaminidase A and B are absent.

Sane Mentally sound.

Sanfilippo's disease A form of mucopolysaccharidosis with mental retardation, dwarfism, hepatosplenomegaly and skeletal defects.

Sanguine Pertains to blood, cheerful.

Sanguinous Bloody.

Sanies Wound discharge which is thin, fetid and green.

Sanitary Clean; conditions conducive to good health.

Sanitary napkin Perineal pad used during menstruation.

Sanitation Establishment of conditions favorable to health.

Sap Any fluid essential for life.

Saphenous nerve A deep branch of femoral nerve supplying innerside of foot and leg.

Saphenous veins The long saphenous vein extends from foot to saphenous opening in upper thigh whereas short saphenous vein runs up behind lateral malleolus to join popliteal vein.

Saponification 1. Conversion into soap, i.e. hydrolysis of fat by an alkali yielding glycerol and salts of fatty acid 2. In chemistry hydrolysis of an ester into corresponding alcohol and acid.

Saponin Some plant glycosides that produce gastroenteritis.

Saporific Imparting taste or flavor.

Saprogen Any microorganism causing or produced by putrefaction.

Saprophyte Organisms living on decaying or dead organic matter.

Saralasin Converting enzyme inhibitor for hypertension.

Sarcoblast Embryonic cell that develops into a muscle cell.

Sarcocele A fleshy tumor of testicle.

Sarcoid 1. Resembling flesh 2. Small tuber like lesion characteristic of sarcoidosis.

Sarcoidosis A granulomatous disease of unknown etiology affecting lungs, lymph nodes, skin, eyes, small bones of hand and feet.

Sarcolemma A thin membrane surrounding each striated muscle fiber.

Sarcoma Cancer of connective tissue like muscle and bone.

s. chondro Sarcoma composed of cartilages.

s. Ewing's A fusiform swelling of long bones containing round endothelial cells.

s. kaposi's A skin sarcoma in AIDS victims.

s. osteogenic Sarcoma in metaphysis of long bones containing variously shaped cells.

s. reticulum cells A form of malignant lymphoma.

Sarcomere That portion of a striated muscle fibril lying between two adjacent dark lines.

Sarcoplasm The cytoplasm inside muscle cells.

Sarcoptes A genus of Acarina that includes mites: e.g. *Sarcoptes scabiei* causing scabies.

Sarcosporidia A protozoa which is parasitic in muscles of higher vertebrates

Sarcous Concerning flesh or muscle

Sartorius The thin longest muscle of body in the thigh acting as weak knee flexor.

Satellite A small structure attached to a larger one.

Satiety Feeling satisfied with food.

Saturated compound Any compound with all its carbon bonds saturated.

Saturation A state in which all of a substance, that can be dissolved in a solution. Adding more of the substance will not increase its concentration.

Saturday Night palsy Paralysis of radial nerve in alcoholics from its compression against the chair.

Saturnine gout Gout like symptoms produced by lead poisoning.

Satyriasis Uncontrollable or excessive sexual urge in males.

Saucerization Surgical creation of a shallow area in tissue.

Sauna An enclosure where a person is exposed to high temperature and humidity for brief period and then he is given cold bath; a process to relieve aches and pains, loosen stiff joints and loose weight.

Savory Appetizing taste or odor.

Saxifragant Dissolving or breaking of bladder stones.

Saxitoxin A toxin of marine life like mussels, clams and plankton; lethal if inhaled or consumed by CNS depression

S. botryoids A sarcoma of uterus of infant and children

Scab Crust formed on a wound, pustule or ulcer.

Scabicide Agents effective against scabies organism, i.e. *Sarcoptes scabiei.*

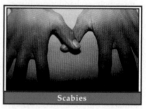
Scabies

Scabies A mite borne contagious skin disease characterized by papule, vesicle, pustule, with intense itching.

Scala One of the three spiral passages of cochlea: the scala media, scala tympani and scala vestibuli.

Scald Burn caused by moist heat or hot vapors.

Scalded skin syndrome Staphylococcal necrotizing skin infection.

Scale Thin dry exfoliation from upper layers of skin, maximum in psoriasis, eczema, seborrhea sicca etc.

Scalenotomy Division of scalenus muscle to contain apical tuberculosis of lungs.

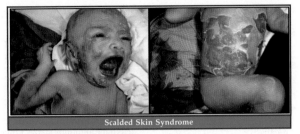
Scalded Skin Syndrome

Scalenus Scalenus anterior, medius and posterior muscles originating from transverse processes of C_3-C_6 vertebra and inserted to Ist and 2nd ribs.

Scalenus syndrome Thoracic inlet syndrome due to compression of brachial plexus and subclavian artery manifesting with pain, paresthesia in upper limb with atrophy of small muscles of hand.

Scaler An instrument used for removing dental calculus.

Scaling Removal of calculus from teeth.

Scalp The hairy portion of head, consisting from out to inwards: skin, dense subcutaneous tissue, occipitofrontalis muscle with the galea aponeurotica, and periosteum.

Scalpel A straight surgical knife with a convex edge.

Scalp tourniquet Tourniquet applied to scalp during IV administration of anti-neoplastic drugs to prevent alopecia.

Scanning electron microscope An electron microscope that provides three dimensional views of an object.

Scanning speech A symptom of cerebellar disease where words are pronounced by syllables, slowly and hesitantly.

Scaphoid Boat shaped.

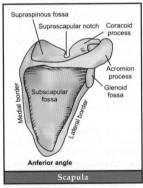

Supraspinous fossa
Suprascapular notch
Coracoid process
Acromion process
Glenoid fossa
Medial border
Subscapular fossa
Lateral border
Anterior angle
Scapula

Scapula The flat triangular bone at the back of shoulder articulating with clavicle and humerus.

s winged Paralysis of serratus anterior or trapezius causing prominence of medial border of scapula.

Scapular reflex Muscular contraction on percussion between scapulae.

Scapulohumeral reflex Reflex in which the upper arm is abducted and rotated outward when medial border of scapula is percussed.

Scar Healing of wound or injury leaving a mark on skin or internal organs.

Scarlatina Scarlet fever.

Scarlatiniform Resembling scarlet fever or its rash.

Scarlet fever A streptococcal infection characterized by sore throat, strawberry tongue, rose colored rash and fever.

Scarpa's fascia Deep layer of superficial abdominal fascia.

Scarpa's triangle Triangular space bounded laterally by inner edge of sartorius, above by inguinal ligament and medially by adductor longus.

Scatology Scientific study and analysis of fecal material or interest in obscene literature.

Scatoma Mass of dry hard stool in colon resembling a tumor.

Scatter Diffusion of X-rays after striking an object.

Scatter radiation X-rays changing direction because of collision with matter.

Scattergram Display of data on a paper where each value is indicated by a symbol and the individual symbols are not connected by a line.

Scavenger cell A phagocytic cell like macrophage that removes tissue debris.

Schaffer's reflex Dorsiflexion of toes and flexion of foot on pinching tendo-Achilles.

Schatzki ring A mucosal web like ring at the squamocolumnar junction of lower esophagus often causing dysphagia.

Shicks test Skin test in diphtheria to determine immunity status. 1 ml. of diphtheria toxin is injected intradermally and result is read after 72 hours. Presence of immunity is indicated by absence of any erythema and inflammation at point of injection.

Schilder's disease *SYN* — adrenoleukodystrophy, manifesting with diffuse cerebral demyelination and adrenal atrophy.

Schiller's test A test to demonstrate superficial cancer cervix. Iodine is applied on the cervix. As the cancer cells do not contain glycogen, they fail to stain with iodine.

Schilling test A test using radioactive B_{12} for assessment of vitamin B_{12} absorption and diagnosis of intrinsic factor deficiency as in pernicious anemia.

Schistocyte Fragmented red blood cells of various shapes and irregular surfaces.

Schistosoma A genus of blood flukes living in blood vessels of internal organs and discharging eggs through urine and feces.

s. *haematobium* The schistosoma inhabit in vesical plexus and discharge egg in urine; produce hematuria, cystitis and bladder wall calcification.

s. japonicum Adults live in branches of superior mesenteric vein and produce dysentery.

s. mansoni Adults live in branches of inferior mesenteric veins.

Schistosomiasis Infestation with the blood flukes, the schistosoma.

Schizencephaly Deformed fetus with a longitudinal cleft in the skull.

Schizogony Asexual reproduction by binary fission as in case of malarial parasite.

Schizoid Resembling schizophrenia.

Schizoid personality disorder A personality cult with difficult interpersonal relationship, and a limited range of emotional experience and expression; the cold, lonely, aloof personality.

Schizont A stage in life-cycle of sporozoa when it reproduces asexually to 12-24 merozoites inside RBC.

Schizophrenia A form of psychosis with disorder of thinking, affect and behavior. Patients have delusions and hallucinations with loss of self-identity.

s. catatonic Patients have catatonic stupor or mutism, catatonic rigidity, catatonic posturing etc.

s. paranoid Patient has delusions of persecution, jealousy.

Schlemm's Canal Canaliculi or spaces at sclerocorneal junction of eye in anterior chamber for drainage of aqueous.

Schmorl's nodes Herniation of nucleus pulposus into vertebral body producing X-ray density.

Schonlein's disease Allergic or anaphylactoid purpura in response to serum sickness, sensitiveness to drugs or most often idiopathic.

Schuffner's dots Minute granules present within RBC infected by *Plasmodium vivax.*

Schultze's bundle Fasciculus cuneatus of spinal cord.

Schwabach's test A test of hearing using 5 tuning forks, each of different tone.

Schwann cell Cells of ectodermal origin, form neurilemma.

Schwannoma Benign tumor of Schwann cells.

Sciatic Pertains to hip or ischium.

Sciatica Pain along the course of sciatic nerve from back of thigh along lateral border of leg to little toe usually due to disk prolapse at L_5-S_1.

Sciatic nerve The largest nerve in body (L_{4-5} $S_{1,2,3}$) passing from pelvis through greater sciatic foramen down the back of the thigh where it divides into tibial and peroneal nerves. Its lesion cause paralysis of hamstrings, peroneal and calf muscles and toe extensors.

Science Branch of knowledge utilizing systematic study and intelligent analysis to understand, explain, quantitate and predict the phenomena of life and natural laws.

Scintillascope Device for viewing the effect of ionizing radiation, alfa particles on a fluorescent screen.

Scintillation The emissions coming from radioactive substances.

Scintiphotography Photography of scintillations emitted by radioactive substances injected into body.

Scintiscan The scintiphotography record to indicate the differential accumulation of a substance in various parts of body.

Scintiscanner The machine performing scintiscan.

Schirrhus Hard cancerous overgrowth of fibrous tissue.

Scission To divide, split or cut.

Scissor gait Crossing of the legs while walking as in cerebral diplegia.

Scissor leg Contraction of thigh adductor causing the legs to have abnormal tendency to cross to the otherside.

Scissors A cutting instrument with two opposing blades with handles held together by a pin.

Sclera The outer tough white fibrous tissue of eyeball extending from optic nerve to corneal margin.

s. blue Abnormally thin sclera with visible choroid as in osteogenesis imperfecta.

Scleredema A benign self-limited skin disease characterized by edema and induration of skin.

Sclerema Hardening of the skin.

Scleriasis Hardening of the eyelid.

Scleritis Inflammation of sclera, can be anterior (adjacent to cornea), posterior or annular (in ring fashion around cornea).

Sclerodactyly Hardening of skin of fingers and toes.

Scleroderma A chronic disease of unknown etiology causing sclerosis of skin, esophageal dysmotility, pulmonary fibrosis, etc. The skin is tough, taut, hard and leather bound.

Scleroma Circumscribed indurated area of granulation tissue in skin or mucous membrane.

Scleromalacia Softening of sclera as in late rheumatoid arthritis.

Sclerophthalmia A congenital condition where opacity of sclera advances over the cornea.

Scleroproteins A group of insoluble proteins found in cartilage, hair, nails and skeletal tissue.

Sclerosent Any substance that produces sclerosis.

Sclerosis Hardening or induration of a tissue due to excessive growth of fibrous tissue, a feature of degeneration.

s. amyotrophic lateral A form of motor neurone disease which results in atrophy of anterior horn cells and the pyramidal tracts.

s. multiple A slowly progressive disease of central nervous system marked by widespread demyelination producing visual disturbances, sensory motor deficit, and cerebellar symptoms.

Sclerotherapy Use of sclerosing agents for hemorrhoids and bleeding varices.

Sclerosing agents Urea, alcohol, polydachonol tetradecyl sulphate.

Sclerothrix Brittleness of hair.

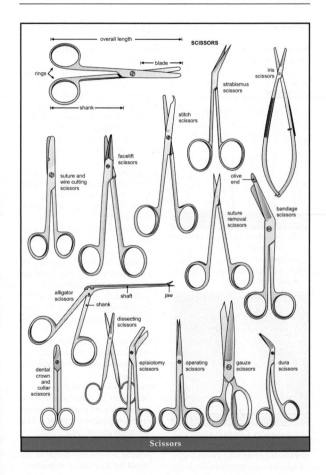

SCISSORS

overall length

rings

blade

shank

strabismus scissors

iris scissors

stitch scissors

facelift scissors

suture and wire cutting scissors

olive end

suture removal scissors

bandage scissors

alligator scissors

shaft

jaw

shank

dissecting scissors

dental crown and collar scissors

episiotomy scissors

operating scissors

gauze scissors

dura scissors

Scissors

Sclerotome Knife used for incision of sclera.

Scolex The head of tapeworm possessing hooks, suckers or grooves for attachment.

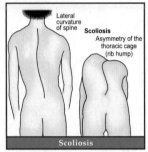

Scoliosis

Scoliosis Lateral curvature of spine; the abnormal curve and the compensatory curve in opposite direction; can be congenital, myopathic, ocular, paralytic, etc.

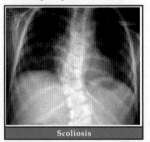

Scoliosis

Scoliosometry Determination of degree of spinal curvature.

Scombroid poisoning Poisoning by histamine like toxin present in the undercooked fish of suborder scombroidea.

Scoop Spoon shaped surgical instrument.

Scopalamine A plant alkaloid producing smooth muscle relaxation and twilight sleep.

Scopophilia Sexual pleasure obtained from seeing nude and obscene picture.

Scorbutic Concerning scurvy.

Score A rating or grade as compared to standard.

s. Apgar A scoring system for evaluation of neurological maturity of newborn from pulse, respiration, reflexes, skin color, grimace etc.

Scorpion sting Symptoms from scorpion bite resembling spider bite or of strychnine poisoning. The venom contains neurotoxin, hemolysins and agglutinins. Stings are fatal to children below 3 years. As the venom is heat labile emersion of part bitten in hot water for 30-90 minutes neutralizes the toxin.

Scoto Pertains to darkness.

Scotochromogen Microorganisms that produce color when grown in darkness.

Scotoma Dark or blind areas in visual field, can be annular, arcuate, central (around point of fixation), centrocecal (covering point of fixation to blindspot), peripheral.

s. scintillating An irregular outline around a luminous patch in the visual field as seen in migraine.

Scotometer Device for detecting and measuring scotoma in visual field.

Scotopic vision Dark adaptation.

Scotopsin The protein portion of rods of retina that combines with retinol to form visual purple, i.e. rhodopsin.

Scratch test An allergy test where the allergen is placed over a skin scratch. In sensitive persons wheal develops within 15 minutes.

Screen 1. A flat surface for projecting slides or movies or visualizing X-ray films. 2. To make fluoroscopic examination 3. To thoroughly examine and investigate a person for a disease 4. Materials used to protect the body parts from ionizing radiation/X-rays.

s. Bjerrum One meter square surface which is viewed from one meter to chart blind spot, scotoma and extent of visual field.

Scribner shunt Arteriovenous shunt made of polypropylene for facilitating hemodialysis.

Scrofula Tubercular cervical lymphadenopathy.

Scrofuloderma Tubercular skin ulcer or sinus.

Scrotal reflex Contraction of scrotal muscle (dartos) on stroking the perineum.

Scrotum The double cavity male pouch containing testicles and epididymis, composed of layers of skin, non-striated dartos muscle, cremasteric, infundibular and spermatic fascia, cremasteric muscle and tunica vaginalis.

Scrubbing Thorough washing of hands and finger nails before performing any surgical procedure.

Scrub typhus Typhus fever caused by *Rickettsia tsutsugamushi* transmitted by mites.

Scum The floating impurities in surface of a culture.

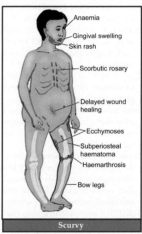

Scurvy

Scurvy Vitamin C or ascorbic acid deficiency manifest with bleeding spongy gums, subperiosteal hemorrhage, muscle pain and induration, loosening of teeth and poor wound healing.

s. infantile SYN — Barlow's disease, results from prolonged use of milk (milk is deficient in vitamin C) without vitamin C supplementation, manifest with anemia, pseudoparalysis, bony tenderness and often epiphyseal fracture.

Scybala Hard rounded masses of fecal matter.

Sea-sickness Akin to motion sickness with giddiness, nausea, vomiting and headache while travelling in ship.

Seasonal affective disorder Mental depression especially in winter.

Seatle foot Artificial foot developed in Seatle (USA) that has a spring back quality making it feel like a real foot.

Seat worm *SYN* — pinworm, *Enterobius vermicularis* causing perianal itching.

Sebaceous cyst Sebum filled cyst of sebaceous gland with a black head, may need complete extirpation rather than drainage.

Sebaceous gland Holocrine glands (secretion arising from complete disintegration of cells) in the skin that open into hair follicle and secrete oily substance, the sebum.

Sebolith Concretion in a sebaceous gland.

Seborrhea A functional disease of sebaceous glands marked by increased secretion of altered quality sebum. Commonly affects scalp (dandruf), face and trunk.

s. sicca Seborrhea with gray brown or yellow scale and crust.

Sebum A fatty secretion from sebaceous gland, that from the ear is called cerumen and from pepuce is called smegma.

Secobarbitol Short acting barbiturate used for its hypnotic effect.

Secondary areola Pigmentation around nipple during pregnancy.

Secondary hemorrhage Hemorrhage occurring after 48 hours of injury or operation commonly due to sepsis.

Secondary intention Healing by formation of granulation tissue that fills the gap between torn or incised edges.

Secretin A hormone secreted from duodenum that stimulates secretion of pepsinogen and inhibits secretion of acid by stomach.

Secretion Substances produced or the process of glandular secretion.

s. apocrine A process by which the secreting cell breaks off to extrude the secretion, e.g. milk production.

s. holocrine The process where the entire cell and its contents are extruded, e.g. sebum.

s. merocrine The process where the cell remains intact and discharges its secretion through cell membrane.

Secretogogue Agent that stimulates secretion.

Secretomotor Nerve fibers that promote glandular secretion.

Sectarian Medical practice based on unscientific practice.

Section Process of cutting or dividing.

s. cesarean Delivery of fetus by incision of uterus.

s. frozen Freezing of a cut section of tissue followed by microscopic examination.

s. sagittal Section cut parallel to the median plane of body.

Sector The area within a circle between two radii and the arc.

Sectorial Having cutting edges like teeth.

Sedative Agent that soothes, quietens or brings tranquility.

Sedentary Work with minimal physical exertion.

Sediment The substance settling at the bottom of a liquid.

Sedimentation rate A test to determine the speed at which RBCs settle down when suspended in a test tube. The speed depends upon the size of RBC aggregate which is further dependent upon fibrinogen content of blood. Fibrinogen is an acute phase reactant and is increased in infection, inflammation of any etiology. ESR is reduced in polycythemia, congenital cyanotic heart disease and microcytic hypochromic anemia. Normal ESR is 10-15 mm/hr. in male and slightly higher in female.

Segment A portion.

Segmentation Division into similar parts; division of fertilized egg into many smaller cells.

Segregation Separation.

Seiditz powder Effervescent cathartic composed of tartaric acid, sodium — potassium tartarate and sodium bicarbonate.

Seizure A sudden attack of pain, disease or certain symptoms like convulsion, epilepsy.

Seldinger technique A method of introducing a catheter into a vein or artery. The vessel is punctured with a needle that contains a wire. The needle is removed and the catheter is then advanced over the wire, the latter being finally withdrawn.

Selenium sulfide Drug used in treatment of tinea versicolor and dandruff.

Self-limited A disease which without treatment pursues a definite course within a limited time.

Sella turcica The concavity on superior surface of body of sphenoid that holds the pituitary gland.

Selzer water Naturally occurring water with high CO_2 and mineral content.

Semantics The field of language concerning meaning.

Semeigraphy Description of signs and symptoms of disease.

Semen Thick viscid fishy odor discharge per male urethra during sexual climax. It contains the sperms 60-150 million/ml. 80% are motile and normal in morphology. Semen is alkaline without any leukocytes, volume per ejaculation is 2-5 ml.

Seminuria Passage of semen in urine.

Semi Prefix meaning half.

Semicircular Half of a circle.

s. canals The superior, inferior and posterior structures of inner ear for maintenance of body posture.

Semicoma Mild degree of impaired consciousness.

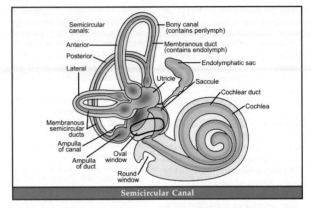

Semicircular canals:
- Anterior
- Posterior
- Lateral

Bony canal (contains perilymph)
Membranous duct (contains endolymph)
Endolymphatic sac
Utricle
Saccule
Cochlear duct
Cochlea
Membranous semicircular ducts
Ampulla of canal
Ampulla of duct
Oval window
Round window

Semicircular Canal

Semilunar Shaped like a crescent.

s. cartilage The medial lateral, fibro cartilages of knee between tibia and femur.

Semilunar valves The pulmonary and aortic valves.

Semimembranosus A large muscle at inner and back portion of thigh, a knee flexor.

Seminal vesicle Two sac like structures close to prostate in the male giving rise to ductus deference. Act to store semen and secrete a thick viscus fluid that forms part of semen.

Seminiferous tubule Tubules in testes forming and conducting semen.

Semitendinosus Fusiform muscle of posterior and inner part of thigh.

Senescence The process of growing old or period of old age.

Sengstaken — Blackmore tube A three lumened tube used to stop bleeding from esophageal varices.

Senility Pertains to old age and its changes, physical and mental.

Senna Leaves of a plant, used as cathartic.

Sennosides Anthraquinone glucosides present in senna, used as cathartic.

Sensation Feeling or awarness.

Sense 1. The general faculty responsible for perceiving the outside world 2. To perceive 3. Normal power of understanding.

s. proprioception Appreciation of body position from sensory input from skin and joints.

s. stereognosis Judgement of size, shape and weight of an object through fingers.

Sensible 1. Reasonable 2. Can be perceived by senses.

Sensitive 1. Able to feel a sensation 2. Abnormal response to substances like drugs and foreign proteins.

Sensitivity 1. The term is employed in relation to accuracy of diagnostic tests/observations. It is the proportion of people who truely have a specific disease as identified by the test 2. Susceptibility of bacteria to antimicrobials.

Sensitization Making a person susceptible to a substance by its repeated injection.

Sensitizer A substance that makes the susceptible individual react to same or another irritant.

Sensorium The sensory apparatus of body or consciousness.

Sensory area The post central gyrus of cerebral cortex responsible for analysis of somatosensory input.

Sensory integration Skill and performance required in the development and coordination of sensory input and motor output.

Sensory nerve A nerve conveying afferent impulses to brain.

Sensualism State of emotions dominating one's actions.

Sensuous Affecting senses or susceptible to influence through the senses.

Sentiment Mental feeling or opinion, an emotional attitude towards an object.

Sentinel node Cancer metastasis into supraclavicular nodes.

Separator Any device or instrument used for separating two substances, e.g. cell separators.

Sepsis A pathological state due to bacterial multiplication and toxin production.

s. puerperal Infection of genital passage resulting from childbirth. Common infecting agents are strepto, staphylo *and Escherichia coli.*

Septa Partition.

Septate Having a partition or wall.

Septic Infected

Septicemia Multiplication of pathogenic bacteria in peripheral blood producing toximia, disseminated cellulitis, lymphangitis etc.

Septic fever Fever due to presence of pathogenic organisms or their products in blood, producing shaking chills with abrupt rise in temperature and sweating.

Septometer Instrument used for measuring bacterial contamination of air.

Septoplasty Plastic surgery on nasal septum for deviated nasal septum.

Septostomy balloon atrial (Raskind procedure) where interatrial opening is widened by balloon to reduce RV load in some congenital heart diseases.

Septum A partition wall dividing two cavities, e.g. interatrial, inter ventricular, atrioventricular, nasal septum, rectovaginal.

s. pellucidum A thin triangular sheet of nervous tissue forming the medial wall of the lateral ventricles.

s. primum The embryonic septum dividing the two atria in a developing heart.

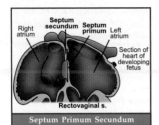

Septum Primum Secundum

Septulet Seven children in one pregnancy.

Sequela The final outcome of a disease with or without treatment.

Sequestration Formation of sequestrum.

s. *pulmonary* A nonfunctioning area of the lung receiving blood from systemic circulation.

Sequestrum The necrotic bone separated from adjacent healthy bone in osteomyelitis.

Serendipity Finding some thing by chance

Series In row or chain, form of arrangement.

s. *aliphatic* Chemical compounds with open chain carbon atoms.

s. *aromatic* Organic compounds possessing benzene ring.

s. *erythrocytic* Immature precursor cell series in bone marrow that develop to mature erythrocyte.

s. *granulocytic* Immature cell series of bone marrow developing into mature granular white blood cells.

Serine protease inhibitor Compounds that inhibit platelet aggregation and blood coagulation.

Serodiagnosis Diagnosis from tests involving patient's serum.

Seroepidemiology Epidemiological study of a disease by investigating for presence of diagnostic characteristic in the serum.

Serology The scientific study of serum.

Seroma A localized collection of serum resembling a tumor, commonly after stitching of operational wounds.

Seronegative Negative serological tests.

Seropositive Positive serological tests.

Serosa A serous membrane like pleura, pericardium and peritoneum.

Serosanguinous Discharge containing serum and blood.

Serositis Inflammation of serous membrane.

Serotherapy Treatment of disease by injection of serum containing antibodies thereby conferring passive immunity.

Serotonin 5 hydroxy tryptamine present in platelets, mastcells, argentaffin cells of carcinoid tumors. A potent vasoconstrictor incriminated in migraine.

Serotonin reuptake inhibitor compounds that inhibit serotonin reuptake at nerve ending increasing its availability; used to treat depression.

Serotype A classification of microorganisms based on antigenic structure of cell.

Serous cavity Cavity lined by serous membrane like pleural, pericardial and peritoneal cavities.

Serpiginous Creeper like course.

Serrate Tooth like, notched.

Serratia Gram negative rod of enterobacteriaceae family.

S. marcescens causes septicemia and pulmonary disease

Serratus A muscle arising or inserted by a series of tooth like processes.

Sertoli's cells Supporting cells in the seminiferous tubules that nourish the spermatids.

Serum The straw coloured fluid after blood coagulates.

Serum glutamo oxaloacetic trans-aminase (SGOT) *SYN* — aspartate transaminase (AST). An intra-cellular enzyme present in muscle, liver and brain. Its serum level is increased in necrosis of above tissues.

Serum glutamopyruvic trans-aminase (SGPT) *SYN* — Alanine amino transferase (ALT) Like SGOT, this enzyme is also present in muscle, liver and brain tissue and its level increases in necrosis of above tissues.

Serum sickness A type III hypersensitivity immune response following injection of animal sera (antitoxins) with arthritis, lymphadenopathy and spleno-megaly.

Sesamoid Resembling a grain sesame.

s. cartilage Cartilage plates present between lateral nasal and greater alar cartilages of nose.

Severe combined immune deficiency (SCID) Deficient cell mediated and humoral immunity with infection by bacteria and fungi

Sever's disease Apophysitis of calcaneus in adolescents

Sewer gas Methane and hydrogen sulphide produced in sewage, may be used as fuel.

Sex The distinctive characteristics that separate living beings and plants into males and females.

s. chromosomal Sex differentiation based on xx (female) or xy (male) chromosome pattern.

s. morphological Sex determined from external genitalia.

s. nuclear Sex determination from presence or absence of sex chro-matin in body cells.

Sex chromatin *SYN* — Barr body. It represents the inactivated 'x' chromosome in female somatic cells (Lyon hypothesis).

Sex chromosome The x and y chromosomes which determine the sex of an individual.

Sex-linked A character controlled by genes on sex chromosome.

Sextuplet Six children in one preg-nancy.

Sexual dysfunction Sexual dissatis-faction due to defective arousal, or-gasm, pain or penetration.

Sexual maturity rating The order and extent of development of sexual chacteristics.

Sexually transmitted diseases (STD) Diseases acquired during sexual intercourse with partner. They include syphilis, gonorrhea, lymphogranuloma venereum, granuloma inguinale, chancroid, acquired immunodeficiency syndrome, genital herpes and warts, viral hepatitis B, chlamydia urethritis etc.

Sexual reflex Erection and ejaculation and ejaculation from sexual stimulation (whether direct or indirect) irrespective one is asleep or awake.

Sezary cells An atypical mononuclear cell containing mucopoly saccharide filled cytoplasmic vacuoles.

Sezary syndrome Exfoliative skin disease characterized by infiltration of skin by sezary cells; a variant of mycosis fungoides.

Shakes Shivering or tremulousness.

Shaking palsy Parkinson's disease.

Shaman A traditional healer who while in a trance, uses spirits to cure diseases.

Shagreen patch Thick granular grayish green skin of tuberous sclerosis.

Shear A force applied parallel to the planes of an object but opposite in direction to existing force.

Sheath A connective tissue covering. *s. axon* Myelin sheath or neurilemma.

s. carotid Enclosure of carotid artery, vagus nerve and internal jugular vein by cervical fascia.

s. dural Covering of optic nerve.

s. lamellar Connective tissue covering a bundle of nerve fibers.

s. myelin Layers of lipid and protein forming a semifluid covering of nerves, an extension of plasma membrane of Schwann cells.

s. synovial Double walled tube like bursa enclosing the tendon of hands and feet.

Shedding Casting off surface layer of epidermis.

Sheehan's syndrome Hypopituitarism secondary to pituitary infarction following post-partum hemorrhage and shock.

Sheep cell agglutination test (SCAT) A test for rheumatoid factor when sheep erythrocytes sensitized with rabbit anti sheep RBC immunoglobulin are agglutinated by patient's serum containing rheumatoid factor.

Sheet Linen.

s. draw Folded linen placed under a patient which can be withdrawn without lifting the patient.

Shellen chart A chart for testing visual acuity using letters that subtend an angle of 5°.

Shenton's line A radiographic line used to determine the relationship of head of femur to acetabulum.

Shield A protective device.

Shigella Non motile gram negative bacilli causing bacillary dysentery and alimentary disturbances, e.g. S. *boydii, S. dysenteriae, S. flexneri, S. sonnei.*

Shigellosis Disease produced by shigella.

Shin Anterior edge of tibia.

Shingles *SYN* — Herpes zoster producing painful vesicles along course of a nerve.

Shirodhkar operation Placement of purse-string suture around cervix to prevent premature delivery in incompetent cervix.

Shiver Involuntary muscle contraction during cold, fear or at onset of some fevers.

Shock A state of poor tissue perfusion due to deficient circulating blood volume, pump failure or sudden fear, anaphylaxis, overwhelming infection, drugs, toxins.

s. anaphylactic Shock following injection of foreign substances to a sensitized patient.

s. cardiogenic Shock due to pump failure following myocardial infarction or electrical disturbances.

s. endotoxic Shock from endotoxins of gram negative bacteria.

s. Insulin Shock due to insulin induced hypoglycemia.

s. spinal Acute flaccid paralysis with loss of all sensations and reflexes following complete transection of spinal cord.

Shohl's solution Solution of citric acid and sodium citrate used for acidosis.

Short bowel syndrome Poor absorption of nutrients following resection of sizeable length of small intestine.

Shortsightedness *SYN*—myopia. A condition where parallel rays are brought to focus in front of retina.

Shot A subcutaneous injection.

Shoulder The junction of upper arm with collar bone and scapula.

s. dislocation Slipping of humeral head from glenoid cavity of scapula.

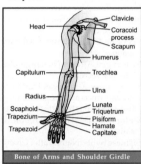

Bone of Arms and Shoulder Girdle

Show Blood mixed thick mucoid discharge from vagina during first stage of labor.

Sharpnell's membrane The triangular portion of tympanic membrane lying above the malleolar fold. *SYN*- pars flaccida.

Shred Thin strand of mucus.

Shrink To reduce in size.

Shudder Convulsive tremor from fear, aversion.

Shunt Diversion of flow.

s. arteriovenous Congenital abnormal arteriovenous communication or the one done for hemodialysis.

s. left to right Passage of blood from left side of heart to right side chambers as in VSD, ASD, PDA.

s. right to left Reverse of above occurring in Fallot tetralogy, transposition of great vessels, single ventricle, DORV and Eisenmenger syndrome.

Shy-Drager syndrome Chronic orthothostatic hypotension due to primary autonomic failure.

Sialism Excessive salivary secretion.

Sialoadenitis Inflammation of salivary gland.

Sialocele Cyst or tumor of salivary gland.

Sialogogue An agent that promotes salivary secretion.

Sialography X-ray examination of salivary ducts and the gland by die injection through the duct opening.

Sialoporia Deficient secretion of saliva.

Siamese twins (Named after Chang and Eng joined Chinese twins born in Siam), cogenitally joined twins.

Sib A blood relative, brother or sister.

Sibilant Hissing or whistling sound.

Sibilismus A hissing sound.

Sibling Children of same parent.

Siccus Dry.

Sick Not well, ill.

Sickle cell Crescent shaped RBC

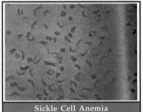
Sickle Cell Anemia

Sickle cell anemia A form of congenital hemolytic anemia where there is abnormal hemoglobin (Hbs) resulting in sideling during splenic hypoxic conditioning.

Sickle cell crisis Capillary plugging by sickle cells causing joint pain, abdominal pain, renal pain, etc. due to infarction.

Sickling Tendency of RBC to assume sickle shape.

Sickness Illness.

s. *motion* Nausea and vomiting experienced during motion by road, air or water.

s. *morning* Nausea and vomiting of early pregnancy.

s. *mountain* Nausea, anorexia, insomnia and dyspnea of high altitude due to oxygen lack.

s. *sleeping* 1. Trypanosomiasis involving CNS (Chaga's disease), transmitted by tsetsefly. 2. Encephalitis lethargica.

s. *serum* Joint pain, fever, lymphadenopathy following injection of serum.

Sick-sinus syndrome SA node dysfunction manifesting as excessive bradycardia, brief periods of sinus arrest or tachy-brady syndrome.

Side effect Undesirable effects of a drug.

Sideroblast Ferritin containing normoblast in bone marrow that constitute 20-90% of bone marrow normoblasts. The ferritin gives prussian blue reaction indicating presence of ionized iron.

Siderocyte RBC containing iron in any form other than hemoglobin.

Siderophil A cell having affinity for iron.

Siderosis A form of pneumoconiosis due to inhalation of iron dusts/fumes.

Siderosome A reticulocyte with iron containing granules.

Sieve A mesh with uniform sized pores.

Sigh A deep inspiration followed by a slow but loud expiration.

Sight Vision.

Sigmoid Shaped like capital greek letter sigma.

Sigmoid flexure Lower part of sigmoid colon shaped like S.

Sigmoido proctostomy Artificial communication of sigmoid flexure with colon.

Sigmoidoscope Tubular instrument for examination of rectum and sigmoid colon.

Sigmoidoscopy Examination of rectosigmoid by sigmoidoscope.

Sigmoido sigmoidostomy Artificial creation of communication between two segments of colon.

Sign Any objective evidence or manifestation of disease.

Silastic Silicone material which are usually inert and hence compatible with body and used in reconstructive surgery.

Silent Mute.

Silent period Period in a tendon reflex immediately following muscle contraction when another neural impulse entering the reflex center cannot excite efferent motor neurone.

Silent angina Angina pectoris without subjective symptoms like precordial pain.

Silica Silicon dioxide.

Silicate A salt of silicic acid.

Silicon A non-metallic element constituting 25% of earth's crust.

Silicone A group of polymeric organic compounds used in adhesives, lubricants and prosthesis.

Silicosis A form of pneumoconiosis resulting from inhalation of silica (quartz) dusts producing nodules, fibrosis and often emphysema.

Silo-filler's disease Hypersensitive pneumonitis in workers working in silos caused by nitric acid and nitrogen dioxide that are produced by fermenting organic matter.

Silver White malleable metal used for astringent and antiseptic effect.

s. amalgam Alloy of silver within or copper used as a dental restorative material.

s. halide The coating on radiographic films which when exposed to radiant energy forms the image.

s. sulfadiazine Used for topical application on burn.

Silver-fork deformity Malunited Colle's fracture resembling back of the fork.

Silver nitrate A germicide and local astringent used for throat cauterization; causes grayish discoloration of mucous membranes.

Silvester's method A method of artificial respiration where patient lies on back with arms raised to the sides of head, then brought down and pressed against the chest.

Simethicone Dimethyl polysiloxanes, an antifoaming agent used to treat intestinal gas.

Simian crease A single tranverse crease on palm as in monkeys. Its presence may signify Down's syndrome, rubella syndrome, Turner's syndrome, Klinefelter's syndrome.

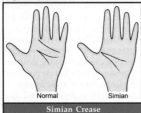

Simian Crease

Similimum A therapeutic concept in homeopathy where a medicine produces symptoms similar to that of the disease for which it is prescribed.

Simmond's disease Hypopituitarism due to pituitary atrophy.

Simmon's position An exaggerated lithotomy position with elevation of buttock and abduction of thighs, employed for operation of vagina.

Simulation Imitation, pretention.

Simulator Any device that creates a situation similar to one that might be encountered, a technique useful in teaching in flying practice, engine testing.

Simulium A genus of insects that includes black flies, *S. damnosum*, serves as intermediate host of *Onchocerca volvulus*.

Sinciput Front and upper part of head.

Sinemet Combination of levodopa and carbidopa.

Sineguan Doxepin hydrochloride, an antidepressant.

Singer's node A swelling between arytenoid cartilages in singers.

Sinister Evil, wickedness; in anatomy left or present on left side of body.

Sinistral Showing preference for left sided organs like left hand, eye or foot in certain actions.

Sinistrality Left handedness.

Sinistrous Awkward, clumsy, unskilled; opposite to dextrous.

Sinoatrial node Node at entry of superior vena cava into right atrium, the pacemaker of heart.

Sinogram X-ray of sinus after radiopaque dye injection.

Sinuous Winding, wavy, tortuous.

Sinus A cavity within bone, dilated venous channel, a cavity with small opening.

s. cavernous The intracranial sinus extending from sphenoidal fissure to the apex of the petrous portion of temporal bone.

s. circular A venous sinus around pituitary body communicating on each side with the cavernous sinus.

s. coronary The vein in the atrioventricular groove of heart draining into right atrium.

s. dermal A congenital sinus tract connecting spinal canal with exterior.

s. frontal An irregular asymmetrical cavity in frontal bone.

s. inferior petrosal A large venous sinus along lower margin of petrous part of temporal bone draining into cavernous sinus.

s. *lateral* One of the two venous sinuses inside brain draining into jugular vein.

s. *marginal* A large venous sinus around the margin of placenta; around white pulp of spleen.

s. *maxillary* Cavity in the maxilla communicating with middle meatus of nose. Both maxillary sinuses are usually symmetrical.

s. *of valsalva* Dilatation of aorta opposite the semilunar valve.

s. *renal* The area of the kidney comprised of renal pelvis, renal calices, vessels and nerves.

s. *sigmoid* Continuation of transverse sinus along posterior border of petrous part of temporal bone to the jugular foramen to continue as jugular vein.

s. *superior sagittal* A straight sinus along upper border of falx cerebri from the crista galli to the internal occipital protuberance where it joins transverse sinus, the left or right.

s. *transverse* The sinus uniting both inferior petrosal sinuses.

s. *urogenital* The common receptacle of the genital and urinary ducts.

Sinus arrhythmia Rise and fall in heart rate in inspiration and expiration respectively; usually innocuous.

Sinusitis Inflammation of paranasal sinuses, the maxillary, frontal, ethmoidal and sphenoidal with headache, fever and chills. A consequence to chronic allergic rhinitis, deviated nasal septum, or nasal polyp.

Sinusoid A large blood channel with reticuloendothelial lining found in liver, spleen, adrenal and bone marrow.

Sinus rhythm The normal cardiac rhythm originating from SA node.

Siphon A tube bent at an angle with two unequal parts for transfering liquids from one container to another.

Sipple syndrome Multiple endocrine neoplasia type III.

Siriasis Sunstroke.

Site Position or location.

Sitophobia Abnormal psychic aversion for particular food.

Sitosterols A mixture of saturated sterols that increase fecal elimination of cholesterol and therefore used as lipid lowering agent.

Sitting height In anthropometry a vertical height taken from the table on which patient is sitting to the vertex.

Situs A position.

s. *inversus* An anomaly where visceral positions are reversed.

Situational crisis In psychiatry any brief transient period of psychological stress.

Sitz bath Emersion of patient's buttocks and perineal region in hot water.

Sixth cranial nerve Abducent nerve that supplies the external rectus.

Sjögren's syndrome A combination of rheumatoid arthritis with xerostomia, keratoconjunctivitis sicca and parotid enlargement.

Sjögren-Larson syndrome Mental ratardation, ichthyosis, spastic diplegia, inherited as an autosomal recessive trait.

Skater's gait Flexion and extension of trunk while walking in patients with advanced Huntington's chorea akin to that of skaters.

Skatole A nitrogenous decomposed product of protein formed from tryptophan with bad odor.

Skeletal muscle A muscle attached to bone and involved in body movements.

Skeletal survey X-ray of entire skeleton to detect any metastasis or disease.

Skeletal traction Traction applied directly to bone through inserted pins and needles.

Skeletization Wasting of soft parts leaving only the skeleton.

Skeleton The bony framework supporting and protecting the viscera. It consists of 206 bones, 80 axial and 126 appendicular.

Skene's glands Paraurethral glands opening to the floor of terminal urethra. Constantly involved in gonococcal infection.

Skew Asymmetrical, to slant.

Skew deviation A condition where one eyeball is deviated upward and outward, the other being inward and downward.

Skin The integument covering the body. It is the largest organ system consisting of epidermis and dermis. The layers of epidermis are stratum corneum, statum luciderm, stratum granulosum, stratum basale.

Skin clip An alternative to sutures to close the skin wound.

Skin fold thickness Measuring thickness of subcutaneous fat over triceps, in upper abdomen and in subscapular region to assess the nutritional status.

Skoda's resonance Tympanic resonance above the line of fluid in pleural effusion or above consolidation in pneumonia

Sleep The periodic state of rest in which there is diminution of consciousness and relative inactivity.

Sleep apnoea Cessation of breathing for atleast 10 sec occurring 30 or more times during 7 hours sleep recording.

Sleep paralysis Transient paralysis with spontaneous recovery occurring while falling asleep or on awakening.

Sleeping sickness African trypanosomiasis, encephalitis lethargica.

Sleep spindle In electro encephalography, the bursts of about 14 per second waves occurring during sleep.

Slide A piece of glass on which specimens are examined under microscope.

Sliding flap A simple flap that is rotated on a broad base to fill an adjacent defect.

Sliding hernia A variety of indirect irreducible inguinal hernia in which a section of viscus forms one wall of the sac.

Sling A bandage usually slung from neck to support the arm.

s. clove-hitch Sling made as follows: A close hitch is placed at the center of a roller bandage. Its ends are

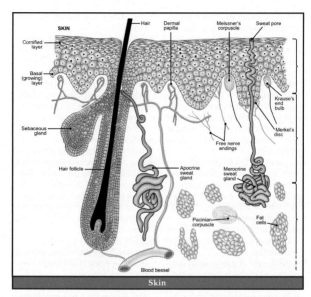

Skin

carried over shoulder and tied beside neck with a square knot.

s. counterbalanced A rehabilitation device that suspends arm by way of an overhead frame and pulley with weight system.

s. open Sling made by placing the point of a triangular cloth at the tip of elbow and bringing the two ends around back of neck and tied.

Slipped disk Herniated intervertebral disk.

Slipped epiphysis Displacement of upper femoral epiphysis, common to children.

Slit A narrow opening.

Slit lamp An instrument consisting of a light source providing a narrow beam of high intensity light and a microscope for better visualization of anterior segment of eye.

Slough A mass of necrotic tissue, to cast off a mass of necrotic tissue.

Slow reacting substance of anaphylaxis A chemical substance (leukotriene) produced by mast cell degranulation in allergic conditions. It causes smooth muscle contraction, e.g. bronchospasm.

Slow virus infection Virus infection manifesting after long latency period, e.g. kuru.

Sludge Any solid, semisolid or liquid waste arising from municipal, commercial or industrial waste water treatment; gall bladder sludge.

Slurry A thin watery mixture.

Small pox Synonym variola, a viral exanthema with papulo-vesicular lesions on skin and constitutional symptoms.

Smegma The thick odorous secretion from Tyson's glands under prepuce and under labia minora.

Smellies forceps Obstetric forcep for delivery of aftercoming head in breech presentation.

Smellies scissors Special scissors with external cutting edges for fetal craniotomy.

Smelling salt A preparation containing ammonium carbonate and stronger ammonia water scented with aromatic substances.

Smelter's chills Zinc poisoning.

Smith-Hodge pessary A retroversion pessary.

Smith-Hemil-Optiz syndrome Small stature, mental retardation, crypto-orchidism, and failure to thrive.

Smith fracture Fracture of lower end of radius with forward displacement of lower segment.

Smith-Piterson nail A special nail that on crosssection has three flanges, used for stabilization of fracture neck of femur.

Smog Dense fog combined with smoke.

Smokeless tobacco Tobacco used for chewing or as snuff. They irritate oral mucosa and increase the risk of oral cancer.

Smoker's cancer Cancer of lip, throat or lungs caused by tobacco smoke.

Smoking passive Exposure to tobacco smoke of smokers around (involuntary smoking)

Snudging A speech defect where difficult consonants are omitted.

Snake A reptile possessing scales but no limbs, external ears and eyelids.

Snake venom A secretion of posterior superior labial glands of poisonous snake containing neurotoxin, hemolysins, cytolysins and hemocoagulins.

Snap A sharp cracking sound.

s. opening A high pitched sound heard during opening of diseased valves, e.g. mitral stenosis.

Snapping hip Presence of an abnormal tendinous band on gluteus maximus muscle which slips to produce a snap during certain hip movements.

Snapping jaw An audible and palpable snap on closing and opening of mouth due to displaced meniscus of temporomandibular joint.

Snapping knee An audible snapping sound on sudden extension of knee caused by slipping of biceps femoris tendon or displaced menisci.

Snare An instrument with a wire loop to remove polyps, tonsils and small growths with a pedicle.

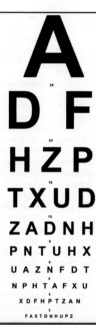

Snellen Chart

Sneeze A sudden spasmodic expiration through nose.

Snell chart A chart for testing visual acuity using letters that subtend an angle of 5°.

Snore The noise produced while breathing through mouth during sleep.

Snout reflex A variant of sucking reflex in which sharp tapping of mid upper lip results in exaggerated contraction of the lips, positive in infants and in diffuse brain disease.

Snuff Powdered form of tobacco inhaled through nose.

Snuff box anatomical Triangular area at the base of thumb. Tenderness in this area indicates scaphoid fracture.

Soap A salt of one or more higher fatty acids with an alkali or metal.

Soluble soaps are detergents and are prepared from alkali metals sodium and potassium.

Soap liniment A solution of soap and camphor in alcohol and water. Used as a stimulant and rubefacient.

Sociology Study of human social behaviour and the origin, institutions and functions of human groups and societies.

Sociopathy The condition of being antisocial.

Socket A hollow in a joint or bone.

s. alveolar The bony space occupied by tooth and periodontal ligament.

Soda Salts of sodium.

s. baking Sodium bicarbonate.

s. caustic Sodium hydroxide.

s. lime Mixture of calcium hydroxide and sodium hydroxide used to absorb carbon dioxide.

Soda water A solution of carbon dioxide under pressure.

Soda ash Commercial sodium carbonate.

Sodium Light, silvery white alkali metal which violently decomposes water forming sodium hydroxide and hydrogen.

s. acetate Systemic and urinary alkalizer.

s. alginate A food additive.

s. benzoate A food preservative.

s. bicarbonate Used IV to treat acidosis.

s. carbonate Washing soda.

s. chloride Table salt; 0.9% solution is osmotically compatible with blood.

s. lactate In one sixth or on fourth molar solution used IV to correct acidosis.

s. monofluoro phosphate For topical application on teeth to prevent caries.

s. morrhuate A sclerosing agent used to obliterate varices.

s. nitrite Antidote for cyanide poisoning.

s. nitroprusside A powerful vaso-dilator.

s. polystyrene sulphonate Cation exchange resin used to lower body potassium.

s. propionate Possesses antifungal action.

s. salicylate Analgesic and an tipyretic.

s. thiosulphate Antidote for cyanide poisoning.

Soft palate The posterior portion of roof of mouth.

Soft sore Venereal ulcer caused by Ducrey's bacillus.

Soleus The flat broad muscle at back of calf of leg.

Solitary Single or lonely.

Solubility Capable of being dissolved.

Solute The substance that is dissolved in a solution.

Solution A homogeneous mixture of solid, liquid or gaseous substance in a liquid from which the dissolved substance can be recovered by crystallization or other physical process.

Solution aqueous Solution containing water as the solvent.

s. buffer Solution of weak acid and its salt solvent for maintaining constant pH.

s. hypertonic Solution with greater osmotic pressure than that of body fluids.

s. hypotonic Solution with osmotic pressure less than that of body fluids.

s. isotonic Solution with similar osmotic pressure as that of body fluids.

s. Ringer's Solution containing chlorides of sodium, calcium and potassium.

Solvent A liquid that dissolves another substance.

Soma The body as distinct from mind.

Somatesthesia The consciousness of the body.

Somatic Pertains to body, the non-reproductive cells, skeletal muscles.

Somatist One who believes that mental disorders have an organic basis.

Somatization Expression of emotional conflicts as bodily ailment.

Somatoform disorders A group of disorders in which there are symptoms of a disease but no objective evidence to explain the symptoms.

Somatomedin Insulin like growth factors derived from liver (Somatomedin C and A) that stimulate growth under influence of growth hormone.

Somatopagus Twins with merged body.

Somatostatin A hypothalamic hormone that inhibits release of somatotropin, insulin, and gastrin.

Somatotropin Growth hormone.

Somnambulism Sleep walking, the performance of any fairly complex act while in a sleep like state or trance.

Somniferous Promoting sleep.

Somniloquism Talking during sleep.

Somnolence Sleepiness.

Somogyi phenomenon In diabetes mellitus, rebound hyperglycemia following an attack of hypoglycemia that triggers release of counter regulatory hormones. Reduction in dose of insulin helps to control the hyperglycemia by abolishing hypoglycemia.

Sonogram Ultrasonography record.

Sonolucent Condition of not reflecting the ultrasound wave back to the source.

Sonorous rale Low pitched rale caused by mucous secretion in bronchus.

Sophistication In medicine, the adulteration.

Soporific A drug producing sleep, narcotic.

Sorbefacient Agent promoting absorption.

Sorbitol A crystalline alcohol used as sweetening agent.

Sordes Foul brown crusts about the lips in some fever.

Sore Painful lesion of skin or mucous membrane.

s. bed Gangrene of skin due to pressure.

s. canker A sore on the mucous membrane of mouth.

s . cold Herpes simplex on the lips.

s. Delhi Cutaneous leishmaniasis.

s. soft SYN — Chanchroid.

Sororiation Growth of breasts during puberty.

Sotalol Betaadrenergic blocking agent used as antihypertensive agent, antiarrhythmic too.

Souffle A bruit, soft blowing sound.

s. uterine Blood flow within uterine arteries producing the sound.

Sound Auditory sensation produced by vibrations, noise, measured in decibels.

s. bronchial Pattern of breath sound over consolidation.

s. bronchovesicular A mixture of bronchial and vesicular sound.

s. ejection High pitched clicking sound heard during systole.

s. Korotkoff's Sounds heard over an artery during blood pressure measurement.

s. succussion Splashing sound heard over a cavity filled with fluid.

s. tubular Breath sound heard over trachea and large bronchi.

Southern blot An analytical method in DNA analysis

Space dead In respiratory physiology, the area from nose to bronchioles which do not take part in exchange of oxygen and carbon dioxide.

s. epidural Space between the dura mater and vertebral periosteum.

s. subarachnoid Space between the pia mater and the arachnoid containing CSF.

s. of Fontana Spaces at the angle of iris allowing passage of aqueous humor from anterior chamber to the canal of Schlemm.

s. Tenon's Lymph spaces between sclera and Tenon's capsule.

Space medicine Branch of medicine dealing with pathological and physiological problems encountered by humans in the space.

Sparge To introduce gas or air into liquid.

Spargosis 1. Swelling of skin as in elephantiasis. 2. Distention of lactating breast with milk.

Spasm Sudden involuntary muscle contraction, can be clonic (alternate contraction and relaxation) or tonic (sustained contraction).

Spasmophilia A tendency towards spasm and convulsion as in rickets.

Spastic colon A motility disorder of colon with lower abdominal pain and alternating constipation and diarrhea.

Spasticity Increased muscle tone with muscular stiffness as in upper motor neurone lesions.

Spatial Pertaining to space.

Spatula Flat instrument for mixing or spreading semisolids.

Specific-gravity Weight of a substance compared with equal volume of water. Specific gravity of water is taken as 1000.

Spectinomycin Injectable antibiotic used for gonorrhea.

Spectrometer An instrument to measure wavelength based on the principle of prism or diffraction grating.

Spectrophotometry Estimation of depth of colour by using spectrophotometer.

Spectroscope An instrument for separating radiant energy into its component frequencies or wavelengths.

Spectrum The series of components or images obtained when a beam of electromagnetic wave is dispersed and the constituent waves are arranged according to their frequencies or wavelengths.

s. invisible Spectral portion below the red (infra red) or above violet (ultraviolet) which is invisible to the eyes lying below 3900 angstrom units and above 7700 angstrom units.

s. visible Colors from red to violet with wavelengths of 3900-7700 AU.

Speculum Instrument for examination of canals, e.g. ear speculum, vaginal speculum.

Speech Expression of thoughts by spoken words or sound symbols.

s. atoxic Defective speech due to muscular incoordination as in cerebellar ataxia.

s. esophageal Speech produced by modulation of air expelled from esophagus in laryngectomised patients.

s. scanning Speech with pauses in between syllables.

s. staccato Slow and labored speech wilh each syllable being pronounced separately.

Spermatic cord The cord suspending the testis and is composed of vas deferens, spermatic arteries, veins and lymphatics.

Spermatic vein The vein draining the testis. The left vein drains into left renal vein while the right vein empties into inferior vena cava.

Spermatid A precursor cell of spermatozoon derived from secondary spermatocyte.

Spermatin A mucilaginous substance present in semen.

Spermatocele A cystic tumor of epididymis.

Spermatocyte The cell arising from spermatogonium that forms the spermatids.

Spermatogenesis The process of formation of mature spermatozoa, i.e. spermatogonium-primary spermatocyte-secondary spermatocyte-spermatid-motile functional spermatozoa.

Spermatorrhea Involuntary loss of semen without orgasm.

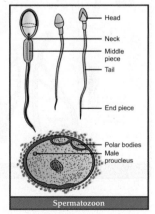

Spermatozoon

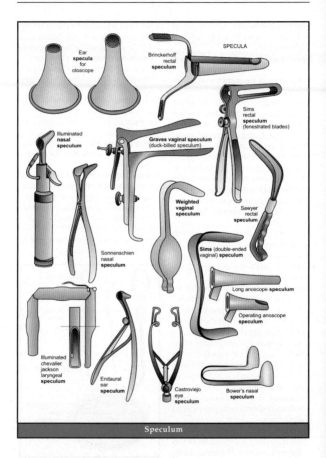

SPECULA

Ear specula for otoscope

Brinckerhoff rectal **speculum**

Sims rectal **speculum** (fenestrated blades)

Illuminated **nasal speculum**

Graves vaginal speculum (duck-billed speculum)

Sawyer rectal **speculum**

Weighted vaginal speculum

Sonnenschien nasal **speculum**

Sims (double-ended vaginal) **speculum**

Long anoscope **speculum**

Operating anoscope **speculum**

Illuminated chevalier jackson laryngeal **speculum**

Endaural ear **speculum**

Castroviejo eye **speculum**

Bower's nasal **speculum**

Speculum

Spermatozoon The mature male germ cell formed within the seminiferous tubules of testis, freely mobile resembling a tadpole.

Spermaturia Semen passed with urine.

Spermicide Agent that kills spermatozoa.

Sphenoid Wedge shaped.

Sphenoid bone Large bone placed at base of skull between the parietal and temporal bones laterally, occipital bone behind and ethmoid in front.

Sphenoiditis Inflammation of sphenoidal sinus cells.

Sphenoid spine Downward projection from the posterior extremity of greater wing of sphenoid, giving attachment to sphenomandibular ligament.

Sphenosis Condition in which fetus becomes wedged in the pelvis.

Sphere Globe like structure.

Spherocyte Erythrocyte assuming globular shape.

Spherocytosis A form of congenital hemolytic anemia characterized by hemolysis, anemia, splenomegaly and jaundice with increased red cell fragility.

Spherule A very small sphere; the structure present in tissues infected with *Coccidiodes imitis,* each spherule containing hundreds of endospores.

Sphincter Circular muscle fibers that close an orifice when contracted, e.g. anal sphincter, lower esophageal sphincter, pyloric sphincter and sphincter of Oddi.

Sphingolipid Lipid containing sphingosine bases.

Sphingolipidosis Hereditary disease with defective metabolism of sphingolipids. Included in this group are Tay-Sachs disease, Fabry's disease, Kuf's disease, Krabbe's disease and Nieman-Pick disease.

Sphingomyelins Phosphorus containing sphingolipids principally

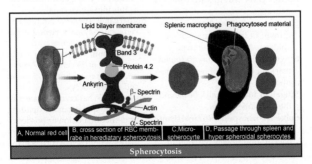

Spherocytosis

found in nervous tissue. They are derived from choline phosphate and a ceramide.

Sphygmo Pulse.

Sphygmobolometer Device that measures force of pulse.

Sphygmograph Instrument for recording shape and force of pulse wave.

Sphygmoid Resembling the pulse.

Sphygmomanometer Instrument for indirect measurement of arterial blood pressure, can be aneroid or mercurial.

Spica A reverse spiral bandage, the turn of which crosses like letter V.

Spicule Small needle shaped.

Spider black widow Black female spider with four pairs of legs and poison fangs. Its bite causes excruciating abdominal pain and ascending motor palsy.

Spider finger Abnormally long phallanges of hand.

Spider cells Branching cells in neuroglia.

Spider nevus Branched capillary growth in the skin resembling a spider as in cirrhosis of liver.

Spigelian line Line on abdomen marking the edge of rectus abdominis.

Spigelian lobe A small lobe behind the right lobe of liver.

Spike The main peak, or a rapid sharp wave appearing suddenly in the background slow wave rhythm.

Spill Overflow.

s. cellular Dissemination of cells through lymphatic or hematogenous route as in metastasis.

s. radioactive Leaking of radioactive material.

Spillway The contour of teeth allowing food to escape from the cusps during mastication.

Spina The spine.

s. bifida Congenital nonunion between the laminae of vertebra.

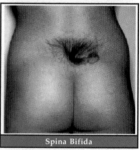
Spina Bifida

Spinal anesthesia Anesthesia produced by injection of anesthetic agents into spinal canal.

Spinal canal The canal bounded by vertebral body and vertebral arches that contains the spinal cord.

Spinal column The vertebral column consisting of 33 vertebra: 7 cervical, 12 thoracic, 5 lumbar, 5 sacral and 4 in the coccyx.

Spinal cord The nervous tissue contained in spinal canal extending from medulla to lower border of first lumbar vertebra. The gray matter within spinal cord is in the form of H.

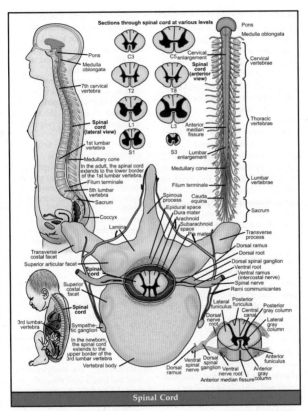

Spinal Cord

Spinal curvature Curvature of spine which is often physiological like cervical and lumbar lordosis and thoracic kyphosis.

Spinal fluid Cerebrospinal fluid lying in the central canal and around the spinal cord within the subarachnoid space.

Spinal nerves 31 pairs of nerves arising from spinal cord; 8 cervical, 12 thoracic, 5 lumbar 5 sacral and coccygeal. Each nerve has a ventral efferent motor root and an afferent dorsal sensory root. Each nerve has white and gray rami communicant which pass to the ganglia of sympathetic trunk.

Spinal shock Complete arcflexic flaccid palsy following complete transection of spinal cord.

Spindle A fusiform shaped body.

s. muscle Specialized nerve tissue in voluntary muscles involved in stretch and myotatic reflex.

s. neuromuscular A complex sensory nerve ending enclosed within a capsule and supplied by an afferent nerve fiber to mediate proprioceptive sensations and reflex.

s. neurotendinous SYN—organ of Golgi, the proprioceptive nerve ending in the tendon.

Spine A sharp process from a bone.

Spinnbarkeit Evaluation of elasticity of cervical mucus for determining time of ovulation.

s.cell RBC with spikes due to membrane deformity as seen in alcoholic cirrhosis

Spinobulbar Concerning the spinal cord and medulla oblongata.

Spiral Coiling around a center like the thread of screw.

s. lamina A thin bony plane of inner ear dividing the cochlear canal into upper scala vestibuli and lower scala tympani.

s. organ of Corti The sensory endorgan containing hair cells that act as receptors for sound.

Spirillium minus A flagellated aerobic bacteria in blood of rats causing rat bite fever.

Spirochaeta A genus of slender spiral motile microorganism causing diseases like syphilis, pinta, yaws.

Spirogram A record made by a spirograph depicting respiratory movements.

Spirograph Graphic record of respiratory movements.

Spiroma Multiple, benign, cystic epithelioma of the sweat glands.

Spirometer An apparatus for measuring the air capacity of the lungs.

Spironolactone Aldosterone antagonist that excretes sodium but conserves potassium, useful in cirrhotics.

Spissated Thickened.

Spit To expectorate.

Spittle Sputum, which is expectorated.

Spitz-Holter valve Used to drain hydrocephalus.

Splanchnic Pertains to viscera.

s. nerves Three nerves from thoracic sympathetic ganglia distributed to viscera.

Splanchnology The study of structure and function of viscera.

Spleen A lymphoid vascular organ in left hypochondrium at the tail of pancreas, consisting of red and white pulp, functions as erythropoietic organ in embryo, and filtrates bacteria, senescent red blood cells, inclusion bodies from the blood.

Splenectomy Surgical removal of spleen.

Splenadenoma Enlargement of spleen caused by hyperplasia of its red pulp.

Splenic flexure Junction of transverse colon with descending colon.

Spleniform Resembling the spleen.

Splenitis Inflammation of the spleen, acute or chronic, hypertrophic or suppurative.

Splenium of corpus callosum The thickened posterior end of corpus callosum.

Splenius A flat muscle in upper back on either side.

Splenoportal Pertaining to spleen and portal vein.

Splenoportogram Radiographic picture of spleen and portal vein after injection of radiopaque material into spleen.

Splenorenal shunt Anastomosis of splenic vein to renal vein as in portal hypertension.

Splenorrhagia Bleeding from ruptured spleen.

Splenorrhaphy Suturing of any splenic wound.

Splint An appliance used for protection, fixation or union of injured part, can be movable or immovable.

s. *Agnew's* Splint used for fracture of patella and metacarpus.

s. *anchor* Splint for fractured jaw.

s. *Balkan* Splint for continuous extension in fracture of femur.

s. *Bond's* Splint used for fracture of lower end of radius.

s. *Cabot's* Metal splint for immobilization of lower limb.

s. *Denis Browne* Splint used for correction of talipes equinovarus.

s. *Dupuytren's* Splint used to prevent eversion in Pott's fracture.

s. *dynamic* Splint that assists in movements initiated by patient.

s. *Fox's* Splint used in fracture of clavicle.

s. *Gordon's* Splint for Colle's fracture.

s. *Thomas* A long wire splint with a proximal ring that fits into upper thigh, used for fracture femur.

Splinter A sharp piece of material piercing the body.

Splinter hemorrhage Small linear bleeding under the nail as in subacute bacterial endocarditis.

Splinting Fixation of injured part with a splint.

Split Division or fissure.

Split tongue Bifid tongue.

Spondylos Vertebra.

Spondylitis Inflammation of vertebra.

Spondylolisthesis Forward subluxation of lower lumbar vertebra on sacral vertebra.

Spondylosis Degenerative disease of vertebra and the inter vertebral disk with new bone formation at vertebral margins and facet joint arthropathy.

Spondylotherapy Spinal manipulation in treatment of disease.

Sponge An absorbent pad made up of cotton and gauze to absorb fluids and blood, used in wound dressing.

s. *gelatin* Spongy substance of gelatin used to stop internal bleeding.

Spongiform Having appearance or quality of a sponge.

Spongioblast The precursor cell of astrocytes and ependymal cells that develop from neural tube.

Spongioblastoma A glioma arising from spongioblasts.

Spongiocyte A neuroglial cell.

Spontaneous fracture Fracture of a osteoporotic bone.

Spoon nail Concave nail of iron deficiency anemia.

Sporadic Occurring occasionally.

Spore An asexual reproductive unit of plants, some protozoa and bacteria.

Sporoblast Structure within the oocyst of certain protozoa.

Sporocyst A reproductive cell containing spores.

Sporogony Reproduction by development of spores.

Sporothrix A genus of fungi.

Sportrichosis A chronic granulomatous fungal infection involving skin and lymph nodes with abscess formation, nodularity and ulceration.

Sporozoa A subdivision of protozoa that includes plasmodia, toxoplasma and isospora.

Sports medicine Application of medical knowledge for treatment and prevention of sports injuries and improvement of training methods.

Sporulalion Production of spores.

Spot A small area distinguishable from surrounding area.

s. *blind* The optic disk containing opaque optic nerve fibers.

s. *cherry-red* Red spot in retina in Tay-Sach's disease.

s. *Koplik* Bluish white spots on oral mucous membrane before appearance of rash of measles.

s. *Mongolian* Blue or mulbery coloured spots in sacral region present at birth that disappear later.

Spotted fever Name for eruptive fevers like typhus, and other rickettsial fevers.

Spotting Appearance of blood tinged discharge from vagina in between periods or at onset of labor.

Sprain Trauma to the ligamentous capsular support of a joint with tearing of fibers and haemorrhage.

Sprain fracture Separation of a tendon or ligament from its bony insertion site taking along with it a piece of bone.

Spray A jet of fine medicated vapor.

Spring conjunctivitis Conjunctivitis occurring in each spring.

Spring ligament Calcaneoscaphoid ligament in the sole of foot.

Sprue Intestinal malabsorption disorder often due to dietary factors, folic acid deficiency producing bulky, frothy, offensive stool.

Spur A sharp bony outgrowth.

s. *calcaneal* An exostosis from calcaneus.

Spurious False, adulterated.

Sputum Material expelled by coughing containing bronchial secretions, alveolar collections.

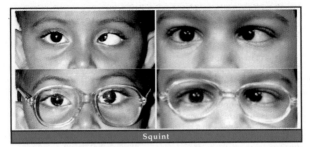

Squint

s. numular Round coin shaped flat forms of sputum sinking in water as seen in bronchiectasis.

Squalene An unsaturated carbohydrate present in vegetable oils, precursor of cholesterol.

Squamous Scale like.

Squamous bone Upper anterior portion of temporal bone.

Squamous cell Flat scaly epithelial cell.

Square knot Double knot in which ends and standing parts are together and parallel to each other.

Squatting Sitting on ones haunches and heels.

Squill Obsolete expectorant and diuretic.

Squint An abnormality where visual axes do not converge on a single point.

Stab Piercing with a sharp pointed instrument.

Staccato speech Jerky pronunciation with separation of each syllable and word by pauses.

Stachyose A nonabsorbable carbohydrate present in beans; hence causing flatulence.

Staging The process of classifying tumors with respect to their degree of differentiation, response to therapy and prognosis.

Stain A dye used to colour objects for microscopic examination.

s. acid Stain where the colour bearing ion is anion, i.e. eosin.

s. acid-fast Staining for mycobacteria which retain carbolfuschin even when washed with acid-alcohol.

s. basic Stain where colour bearing ion is cation, e.g. methylene blue.

s. dental Staining of enamel or denture due to tea, coffee or tobacco or inhalation of metals like copper (green) manganese (black), iron (brown).

s. Giemsa Stain containing azur II-eosin.

Stalk An elongated structure that attaches or supports an organ.

s. infundibular Stalk connecting diencephalon with pituitary.

Stamina Strength, endurance.

Stammering Speech disorder with hesitation, mispronunciation, made worse by anxiety and fear.

Standard deviation In statistics, it is the square root of variance.

Standard error A measure of variability; the difference between means of two samples.

Standstill Cessation of activity.

Stannosis Exposure to an inorganic dust (finoxide) but without pulmonary symptoms

Stannous fluoride A fluoride compound in toothpaste that prevents dental caries.

Stanolone Anabolic steroid.

Stanazolol Anabolic steroid, used for muscle building.

Stapedectomy Excision of stapes as in otosclerosis.

Stapedius A small muscle in the middle ear attached to stapes.

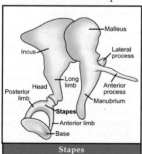

Stapes

Stapes Ossicle in middle ear whose foot plate fits into oval window.

Staphyle Uvula, the fleshy mass hanging from soft palate.

Staphylococcus Gram positive cocci appearing as bunch of grapes. Cause boils, carbuncles, internal abscess, food poisoning, toxic shock syndrome and scalded skin syndrome.

Staphyloderma Cutaneous infection with staphylococci.

Staphyloma Protrusion of sclera or cornea.

Staphylopharyngeus Muscle of soft palate whose contraction narrows the fauces and occludes the nasopharynx.

Staphyloplasty Plastic surgery of uvula or soft palate.

Staphylorrhaphy Suture of cleft palate.

Staphylotoxin Toxins produced by staphylococci, e.g. the enterotoxin, hemotoxin, dermo necrotic toxin, etc.

Staple food Any principal food item of a community supplying more than 25% of calori and eaten regularly.

Stapling Fastening of incised wounds by metal staples.

Starch A plant polysaccharide of high molecular weight which on absorption is reduced to simple sugars to provide energy. Starch is converted to sugar when some fruits ripen while peas and corn change sugar into starch as their seeds develop.

Stare Fixed gaze at any object.

Starling's law Starling law of heart depicts that the force of contraction of heart muscle is directly related to length of muscle fiber at beginning of contraction.

Starvation Food deprivation.

Stasis Stagnation in the flow.

State A condition.

Static electricity Electricity produced by friction.

Stationary Fixed.

Statistics The systematic collection, organization and analysis of data and their interpretation.

Statoconia Minute beats of calcium adhering to the hair cells of macule and utricle responsible for maintenance of posture. *SYN*—statolith.

Stature Height of body in standing position.

Status A state or condition.

s. asthmaticus Persistent and intractable asthma. SYN — acute severe asthma.

s. epilepticus Recurrent convulsive episodes without regain of consciousness in between.

s. sternuens Continuous sneezing.

s. vermcosus Warty appearance of surface of brain due to defective development of cerebral gyri.

Steapsin SYN — Lipase, the pancreatic lipolytic enzyme.

Stearate Salt of stearic acid.

Stearic acid A fatty acid mainly found in animal fats.

Stearin Ester of stearic acid and glycerine.

Stearrhea Excessive secretion of sebum.

Steatadenoma Tumor of sebaceous glands.

Steatitis Inflammation of adipose tissue

Steatocele Fatty tumor within the scrotum.

Steatorrhea Fatty diarrhea of pancreatic enzyme deficiency; increased secretion of sebaceous glands.

Stein-Leventhal syndrome Polycystic ovary syndrome with amenorrhea and infertility.

Stein man's pin A metal pin inserted into bone for application of traction.

Stelazin Trifluoperazine hydrochloride.

Stellate Star shaped.

s. fracture Fracture with radiating fracture lines from center of trauma.

s. ganglion A sympathetic ganglion formed by fusion of inferior cervical and first thoracic ganglions.

s. veins Venous plexus beneath capsule of kidney.

Stellwag's sign Widening of palpebral fissure with infrequent blinking, a feature of Graves' disease.

Stem Stalk like structure.

Stem cell The cell which is initial precursor of specific differentiated red blood cells.

Stenosis Constriction or narrowing.

Stensen's duct Parotid duct.

Stensen's foramina Foramina in hard palate transmitting anterior branches of descending palatine vessels.

Stent Any material used to hold tissue in place, provide support for graft, to keep a passage open, e.g. prostatic stent, esophageal stent and coronary stents.

Stephanion Point of intersection of superior temporal ridge and coronal suture.

Steppage gait High stepping gait of foot drop as in anterior tibial nerve palsy.

Stercobilin A brown pigment derived from bile that imparts the color to feces.

Stercolith A fecal concretion.

Stercus Feces.

Stereoanesthesia Inability to recognize objects by feeling their form.

Stereochemistry Chemistry dealing with atoms in their space relationship.

Stereognosis Ability to recognize objects by touch.

Stereoisomerism Compounds having same number of atoms but in differing arrangement, e.g. dextrose and levulose.

Stereo-orthopter A mirror reflecting device for treatment of squint.

Stereophotography Photography that gives depth, i.e. three dimensional picture.

Stereoscope Instrument that gives three dimensional view of objects seen by combining images of two pictures.

Stereotaxis A method of precisely locating areas of brain concerned with a particular function by moving a probe or electrode along coordinates for measured distances from certain external landmarks.

Stereotypy Persistent repetition of words, posture or activity.

Sterile Free from living micro-organism; unable to procreate.

Sterility The state of being free from living microorganisms; state of being sterile.

Sterilization The process of destroying all microorganisms either by heat, chemical or ionizing radiation.

Sterilizer Appliance used for achieving sterilization.

Sternal puncture Removal of bone marrow for examination by pressing wide bore needle into sternum.

Sternocleidomastoid Muscle arising from sternum and clavicle, attached to the mastoid, helps in rotation of the head.

Sternohyoid Muscle attached to medial end of clavicle and sternum and the hyoid bone.

Sternum The narrow fat bone in the midline of thorax in front.

Steroid Any organic compound containing cyclopentano perhydrinophenanthrine ring.

Steroidogenesis Production of steroid hormones.

Sterols Group of substances related to fats. They are alcohols with CPPP nucleus.

Stertorous Snoring sound.

Stethograph Device to measure chest movements in respiration.

Stethoscope Instrument used to appreciate internal body sounds, i.e. respiratory, cardiovascular and intestinal.

Stevens-Johnson syndrome Erythema multiforme.

Stibium Antimony.

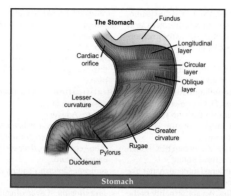

Stibophen Trivalent antimony compound used in treatment of schistosomiasis.

Stiffman syndrome A disease of unknown etiology manifesting with muscle stiffness that limits voluntary movements.

Stigma Any mark, spot on the skin, the spot on ovarian surface where graffian follicle ruptures.

Still birth Birth of dead fetus.

Still's disease Juvenile rheumatoid arthritis with prominent visceral involvement.

Stimulant Agent that increases functional activity.

Stimulus Any agent or factor that brings changes in living tissue, e.g. muscular contraction, secretion from gland, initiating an impulse.

Sting Punctured wound made by an insect.

Stippling Spotted appearance.

Stitch To unite skin or flesh; suture material; sharp spasmodic pain.

Stock culture Permanent culture of a microorganism reinforced from time to time by fresh media.

Stockinet Tubular woven elastic material to place uniform pressure around a body part.

Stock The original individual or tribe from which others have descended.

Stoke A unit of viscosity.

Stokes-Adam's syndrome Feeling of light headedness and becoming unconscious due to poor blood supply to brain as in complete heart block.

Stokes' law Paralysis of a muscle lying adjacent to inflamed serous or mucous membrane.

Stoma A mouth or opening.

Stomach The most dilated saclike portion of alimentary tract in between esophagus and duodenum, secretes hydrochloric acid and pepsinogen, destroys the microorganisms and subserves as a reservoir.

Stomachic Medicine that stimulates actions of stomach.

Stomatitis Inflammation of mouth.

s. *aphthous* Development of minute tiny painful ulcers on mucosa of mouth and tongue due to avitaminosis.

Stomatocyte A swollen RBC with a slit like central pallor

Stone Hardened mineral matter like gallstone, kidney stone.

Strabismus An abnormality of the eyes in which optic axes do not meet at the desired point due to incoordinate action of extraocular muscles.

s. *concomitant* Strabismus in which both eyes move freely but retain unnatural relationship to each other.

s. *paralytic* Extraocular muscle palsy where secondary deviation is greater than primary.

Strabometer Instrument for measuring degree of strabismus.

Strachan syndrome The neurological syndrome of amblyopia, painful neuropathy and dermatitis in under nourished and alcoholics

Strain Excessive use of a muscle or joint; to pass through a filter, to make great effort as in affecting bowel movement; a stock of bacteria.

Strait A narrow passage.

Strangle To choke or suffocate.

Strangury Painful and interrupted urination.

Strap A band to hold parts together.

Strapping Substance used to bind things together or hold dressings place.

Stratification The process of arraning in layers.

Stratum A layer.

s. *basale* Innermost layer of epidermis and other stratified squamous epithelium, deepest layer of endometrium.

s. *corneum* Outermost horny layer of epidermis.

s. *granulosum* Layer of cells containing deeply staining granules of keratohyalin in the epidermis next to stratum basale.

s. *spinosum* Prickle cell layer so called because of prominent intercellular attachment.

s. *spinosum* Middle layer of decidua.

Strawberry tongue Red papillated tongue.

Streak A line or stripe.

Streptobacillus Bacilli found in chains.

Streptococcus Gram positive cocci occurring in chains differentiated into alpha, beta and gamma types based on their reaction on agar plates. Those of alpha type *(St. viridans)* produce a greenish coloration about colonies and partially nemolyze the blood; those of beta type *(St. pyogenes)* form a clear zone about colonies and completely hemolyze the blood, gamma type *(St. faecalis)* are non-hemolytic and produce grayish discoloration about the colonies.

St. pneumoniae Gram positive spherical capsulated cocci causing lobar pneumonia, otitis media.

St. pyogenes Hemolytic streptococci producing rheumatic fever, scarlet fever, puerperal sepsis.

St. viridans Organism producing endocarditis.

Streptokinase Catalytic enzyme produced by hemolytic streptococci. It activates blood fibrinolytic system, used for dissolution of coronary thrombus.

Streptodornase Enzyme secreted by hemolytic streptococci which along with streptokinase is used for enzymatic debridement of infected tissue.

Streptolysin Hemolysin (O and S) produced by *Streptococcus pyogens*.

Streptomyces A genus of aerobic nonacid fast nonfragmenting organisms with branching filaments occupying a position between bacteria and fungi. They serve as source of antibiotics.

Streptomycin Aminoglycoside antibiotic from *Streptomyces griseus* used for pulmonary tuberculosis and gram positive cocci.

Streptozocin Antineoplastic drug, used in pancreatic cancer.

Stress Any stimulus that tends to disrupt body homeostasis to cause disease/disability.

Stress fracture Hairline fracture often only visible 3-4 weeks after undue muscle stress as in runners.

Stress test Method of evaluating cardiovascular fitness by exercise on treadmill or bicycle ergometer or after drugs (dipyridamole, dobutamine).

Stress ulcer Peptic ulcer caused by excessive stress as in burn, head trauma.

Stretch To lengthen.

Stretcher A litter or carriage for patients.

Stretch receptor Proprioceptors in muscle or tendon that are stimulated by stretch or pull.

Stretch reflex Contraction of a muscle as a result of pull exerted on its tendon.

Stria A line or band differing in color and texture from surrounding tissue.

s. of Retzius Benign incremental lines seen periodically in calcified enamel of teeth.

Striatal epilepsy A form of epilepsy characterized by tonic seizure of arm and leg due to disease of corpus striatum.

Striated Stripped as striated muscles.

Striated arteries Branches of middle cerebral arteries supplying basal nuclei of brain.

Striated muscles Skeletal muscles consisting of fibers marked by cross striations.

Striatum The caudate and lentiform nuclei of brain taken together.

Stricture Narrowing or constriction.

Stridor High pitched respiratory sound resembling blowing wind due to obstruction in air passage.

Stridulous Characterized by stridor.

Stringent Rigorous, strict.

Strio nigral Tract arising from putamen and caudate nucleus and ending in substantia nigra.

Strobila Adult form of tapeworm.

Stroboscope A device by which moving object may appear to be at rest; a rapid motion may appear to be slowed.

Stroke 1. A sharp blow 2. Sudden neurological deficit with or without unconsciousness due to cerebral thrombosis, hemorrhage or embolism.

Stroke volume Amount of blood ejected from ventricle during systole.

Stroma Supporting framework of an organ including its connective tissue, vessels and nerves.

Stromatosis Presence of mesenchyma like tissue throughout the endometrium of uterus.

Strongyloides stercoralis A round worm that inhabits human intestine and its motile larvae are passed in stool.

Strontium Radioactive isotope fall out from atomic explosions, principally stored in bone.

Struma Enlarged thyroid gland.

s. *ovarii* Form of ovarian teratoma composed of thyroid follicles filled with colloid.

Strumpell's sign Dorsiflexion of foot when thigh is flexed on abdomen.

Struvite Crystals of magnesium ammonium phosphate.

Strychnine A poisonous alkaloid from plant nux vomica, a potent CNS stimulant.

Stuart-Prower factor Factor x of blood coagulation *SYN* — thrombokinase.

Stupe Counter irritant for topical use.

Stupor A state of lessened responsiveness.

Sturge-Weber syndrome A form of neurocutaneous dysplasia with facial naevus, intracranial railroad calcification, angiomas of leptomeninges and choroid, epileptic seizures, and mental retardation.

Stuttering Speech defect with stumbling and spasmodic repetition of same syllable.

Stye Inflammation of glands of Zeis and Moll at the edge of the lid. Internal stye involve meiobomian or tarsal glands.

Stylet A thin probe.

Styloglossus Muscle connecting tongue and styloid process that helps to retract and raise the tongue.

Styloid process Pointed process of temporal bone, distal end of radius.

Stylopharyngeus Muscle that elevates and opens up the pharynx.

Stylus A probe or slender wire for stiffening or clearing a canal or catheter.

Styptic Anything that stops bleeding by contracting blood vessels or by astringent action.

Sub Under, beneath, less in quantity.

Subacromial Under the acromial process.

Subacute A course of disease in between acute and chronic.

Subacute myelo-optic neuropathy Neurological disease characterized by sensory motor disturbances, impaired vision, abdominal pain and ataxia occurring as a toxicity of chinoquinol (iodochlorhydroxyquin).

Subacute sclerosing panencephalitis A cerebral degenerative disease with decreasing mental function, and myoclonic jerks and rigidity. Probably related to chronic measle virus infection of CNS.

Subatomic Less than the size of an atom.

Subclavian Under the clavicle or collar bone.

Subclavian artery Left subclavian is a direct branch of aortic arch while right subclavian is a branch of innominate artery; gives rise to vertebral arteries and terminates as brachial vessels supplying the arm.

Subclavian steal syndrome Shunting of blood away from cerebral circulation via vertebral artery to subclavian when subclavian is occluded at its origin. Exercise of involved arm then produces dizziness due to cerebral anoxia.

Subclavian triangle Triangle shaped part of neck formed by clavicle and the omohyoid and sternomastoid muscles.

Subclavius A tiny muscle from first rib to under surface of clavicle.

Subclinical Pertains to period before the appearance of typical symptoms.

Subcortical Area beneath the cerebral cortex.

Subcutaneous Beneath the skin.

Subdural space Space between dura and arachnoid.

Suberosis Hypersensitive pneumonitis in workers exposed to cork.

Subfamily In taxonomy between family and a tribe.

Subjective Concerned with the individual or perceived by individual himself but not by examiner.

Sublimate A solid or condensed substance obtained by heating a solid material which passes to vapor phase and then back to solid phase.

Sublimis Near the surface.

Sublingual Beneath the tongue.

Sublingual gland Salivary gland situated at the floor of mouth.

Subluxation A partial or incomplete dislocation.

Submandibular gland Salivary gland about the size of wallnut that lies in digastric triangle beneath the mandible. Its main duct (Wharton's duct) opens by side of frenulum linguae.

Submerge To dip in water.

Submucosa Connective tissue layer below the mucosa con–taining vessels and nerves.

Submucous resection Resection of cartilaginous tissue below the mucosa for correction of deviated nasal septum.

Subphrenic Below the diaphragm.

Subscription That part of prescription containing directions for compounding ingradients.

Subsidence Gradual disappearance of symptoms of disease.

Subsistence Minimum or barely needed essentials for life.

Substance PA 11 amino acid peptide acting as neurotransmitter in pain fiber system.

Substantia Matter.

s. *nigra* Black substance (pigmented cells) in crux cerebri.

Substituent One part of a molecule substituted with another atom.

Substitute Something used in place of another.

Substitutive therapy Treatment of a particular inflammation by exciting a nonspecific inflammation.

Subthalamic nucleus An elliptical mass of gray matter lying in ventral thalamus above the cerebral peduncle and rostral to substantia nigra.

Subtle Very fine or delicate; causing injury without attracting attention.

Subtilin Antibiotic biosynthesized by Bacillus subtilis.

Subtraction A method of removing overlying shadows in radiography.

Succedaneum Something which can be used as a substitute.

Succenturiate Acting as a substitute.

Succinylcholine A neuromuscular blocking agent used as muscle relaxant during anesthesia.

Succus A juice or fluid secretion.

Succussion Shaking up a person to detect fluid in body cavity from presence of splashing sound.

Suck To draw fluid into mouth.

Suckle Breast feed.

Sucralfate Drug used in peptic ulcer.

Sucrase Enzyme present in intestinal juice which splits cane sugar into glucose and fructose.

Sucrose A disaccharose which is broken down into glucose and fructose.

Suction The act of sucking, e.g. suction abortion, suction biopsy.

Sudafed Pseudoephedrine hydrochloride.

Sudamen Noninflammatory lesion of sweat gland due to retention of sweat forming whitish vesicles.

Sudan Biological stain for fat.

Sudanophilic Staining easily with sudan stain.

Sudation Excessive perspiration or sweating.

Sudek's atrophy Acute atrophy of bone at the site of injury.

Sudor Secretion from sweat glands.

Sudoresis Profuse sweating.

Sufentanil An opioid analgesic.

Suffocation Feeling choked.

Suffusion Spreading or extravassation of body fluid or blood; pouring of water on body as a treatment method.

Sugar Sweet tasting carbohydrate either monosaccharose or disaccharose.

s. *beet* Sucrose.

s. *brain* Galactose.

s. *cane* Sucrose.

s. *grape* Glucose.

s. *liver* Glycogen.

s. *milk* Lactose.

s. *muscle* Inositol, but not a true sugar.

s. *wood* Xylose.

Suggestion Imparting an idea indirectly or the psychological process of having an individual accept an idea without hesitation.

Suicide Voluntarily bringing an end to one's own life.

Suit An outer garment.

Sulcal artery A small branch of anterior spinal artery.

Sulcus A furrow, groove, depression.

s. calcarine A horizontal fissure on the medial surface of occipital lobe of brain.

s. central Fissure dividing frontal and parietal lobes.

Sulfacetamide A sulfonamide for ophthalmic use particularly in trachoma.

Sulfadiazine An absorbable sulfa which penetrates well into brain, hence was previously used in meningococcal meningitis, now chiefly used in rheumatic fever prophylaxis.

Sulfadoxine Sulfa used in malaria.

Sulfamerazine A derivative of sulfadiazine.

Sulfamethizole Sulfa for urinary tract infection.

Sulfamethoxazole Sulfa usually combined with trimethoprim for broad spectrum action and complimentary bactericidal effect.

Sulfanilamide A formerly used coaltar product for infections.

Sulfapyridine Sulfonamide used in the treatment of dermatitis herpetiformis.

Sulfasalazine Poorly absorbable sulfa used in treatment of ulcerative colitis.

Sulfatase An enzyme that hydrolyzes sulfuric acid esters.

Sulfathiazole A rapidly absorbable sulfa.

Sulfatide Any cerebroside with a sulfate radical esterified to galactose.

Sulfhemoglobin A form of greenish hemoglobin formed by action of hydrogen sulfide on blood, causes cyanosis if in excess.

Sulfinpyrazone Antigout agent.

Sulfonamide Amides of sulfanilic acid, derived from their parent compound sulfanilamide. They are bacteriostatic.

Sulfisoxazole Sulfa used in urinary tract infection.

Sulfoxone sodium A drug for treatment of leprosy and dermatitis herpetiformis.

Sulfur Yellow inflammable element.

s. dioxide A bactericide and disinfectant

s. precipitated A keratolytic agent.

s. sublimated A scabicide and keratolytic agent.

Sulfuric acid 10% solution used as an astringent and for gastric hypoacidity.

Sulindac Non-steroidal antiinflammatory drug.

Sulpiride Agent used in peptic ulcer.

Summation Cummulative action or stimuli.

Sunburn Solar keratitis due to ultraviolet (290-320 nm).

Sunscreen Agents like PABA used for protection against solar dermatitis.

Sunscreen protective factor index The ratio of the amount of exposure needed to produce minimal erythema response with the sunscreen in place divided by amount of exposure required to produce the same reaction without the sunscreen.

Sunstroke Hyperpyrexia with cessation of sweating, headache and stupor due to failure of heat regulating mechanism.

Super antigen An antigen that simultaneously activates large number of T cell e.g. exotoxin of streptococci

Super ego The portion of personality associated with ethics, self-criticism, and moral standards of community, usually developed in childhood.

Superfecundation The fertilization of two or more ova ovulated more or less simultaneously by two or more coital acts, not necessarily involving the same male.

Superfetation Fertilization of two ova in the same uterus at different menstrual periods within a short interval.

Superinfection A new infection caused by a different organism from that which caused initial infection.

Superior Situated above or higher.

Superjacent Immediately above.

Supernatant The clear liquid remaining at top as the heavy particles settle down below.

Supernumerary In excess of regular number, e.g. supernumerary teeth and supernumerary breast.

Superoxide A highly reactive form of oxygen (oxygen with single electron) produced during phagocytosis and bacterial digestion by neutrophils, lipid metabolism.

Superoxide dismutage Enzyme that destroys superoxide, being tried in myocardial infarction.

Superscription The beginning of prescription marked by letter Rx meaning "you take".

Superstructure Any visible part external to the main structure.

Supination Turning the palm or foot upward, lying on the back.

Supinator Muscle causing supination of forearm.

Suppository A substance in the form of semisolid introduced into the vagina or rectum serving as vehicle for medicine.

Suppurate To form or generate pus.

Suppuration The process of pus formation.

Supra Meaning above, beyond.

Suprachoroid lamina Superficial layer of choroid consisting of transparent layers.

Supraclavicular fossa Depression on either side of neck above the clavicle.

Supraglottic Situated above the glottis.

Suprahyoid muscles The digastric, geniohyoid, myohyoid and stylohyoid muscles.

Suprameatal triangle Triangular space bordered by posterior wall of external auditory meatus and the posterior root of zygomatic process of temporal bone.

Supraorbital notch A notch in the superior margin of orbit for transmitting supraorbital vessels and nerves.

Suprapubic cystostomy Surgical opening of urinary bladder from an approach above the symphysis pubis.

Suprapubic reflex Deviation of linea alba towards the stroked side of abdomen above inguinal ligament.

Suprarenal Gland lying superior and medial to kidney secreting adrenaline and noradrenaline.

Suprasellar Above the sella turcica.

Supratentorial Located above the tentorium.

Supratrochlear Above the trochlea of humerus.

Sura Calf or calf muscles.

Suramin A urea derivative used in treatment of trypanosomiasis.

Surfactant An agent that lowers surface tension.

s. pulmonary A phospholipid in nature that controls the surface tension of air-liquid emulsion in the alveoli. Its absence causes hyaline membrane disease and respiratory distress in infants.

Surgery Branch of medical science dealing with operative procedures for diagnosis or treatment of diseases, and deformities.

s. maxilofacial A branch of dental surgery.

s. plastic Deals with repair and restoration of defective/missing parts for functional improvement or cosmetic appearance.

Surgical dressing Sterile gauze or other material for wound dressing.

Surgical neck Constricted part of shaft of humerus below the tuberosities, the common site for fracture.

Surrogate Someone or something replacing another.

Surrogate mother Mother who bears a child for another couple. She is impregnated with the fertilized ovum from that couple.

Surveillance The monitoring of some programme.

Susceptible More prone to disease, suggestion; easily influenced or impressed.

Suscitate To stimulate or reactivate.

Suspensory bandage A sling/bag for support of testicles.

Sustentaculum Supporting structure.

Suture 1. The line of bony union as in skull bones 2. to unite by stitching 3. the thread, wire or other material used to stitch body parts together.

s. absorbable Sterile strand from mammalian collagen.

s. basilar Suture between the occipital bone and the sphenoid bone.

s. catgut Suture made from sheep's small intestine.

s. cobbler's Suture having needles at each end.

s. continuous Wound closure by means of one continuous thread.

s. coronal Suture between the frontal and parietal bones.

s. lamboid Suture between parietal bones and superior border of occipital bones.

s. non-absorbable Suture materials like silk, silkworm gut, horse hair, synthetic material and wire.

s. purse string Suture around the periphery of a circular opening which when drawn taught closes the opening.

s. sagittal Suture between the parietal bones.

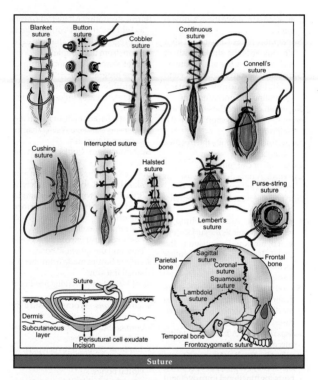

Suture

s. *silkworm gut* Type of suture that causes little irritation, friction and is less pliable and does not twist or curl.

s. *mattress* An interrupted suture where the needle pierces both flaps of wound and then reenters to emerge at the same side of insertion and then tied. Particularly useful in holding together thick fragile tissues.

Suxamethonium A muscle relaxant used during anesthesia *SYN* – Succinyl choline.

Swab Cotton or gauze on end of a slender stick used for cleaning wounds, applying medicines or obtaining secretion for bacteriological culture.

Swallowing The act that enables passage of food or drink from mouth along esophagus into the stomach.

Swan-Ganz catheter A soft flexible catheter with a balloon at its tip. The balloon helps to guide the catheter into pulmonary artery. The balloon is inflated in distal pulmonary artery and the pressure is recorded which is pulmonary wedge pressure equivalent to left atrial pressure.

Swan-neck *deformity* Deformity of hand in rheumatoid arthritis with hyperextension of proximal interphalangeal joints due to tight interossei. Swan-neck deformity of renal tubules is a feature of adult Fanconi syndrome.

Sweat A salty aqueous slightly turbid fluid secreted by sweat glands.

Sweat gland Simple coiled tubular glands present all over body surface except in glans penis and inner surface of prepuce. The glands lie in dermis and the duct passes through epidermis to open outside. Most sweat glands are merocrine but those of axilla, labia majora and perianal region are apocrine.

Sweet's syndrome Dense dermal invasion with mature neutrophils causing raised painful plaques; of unknown cause

Swelling Enlargement mostly localized.

s. calabar Swelling in filaria loa loa.

s. cloudy Tissue degeneration marked by cloudy appearance and appearance of tiny albuminoid granules within the cells.

Swimmer's itch Itchy eruptions on skin due to swim in water containing cercariae of schistosomes.

Sycophant Flatterer, praiser of persons in command of wealth or influence.

Sycosis Chronic inflammation of hair follicle.

s. barbae Sycosis of beard with papulopustular eruptions.

Sydenham's chorea Involuntary purposeless repetitive movements of distal parts as a remote manifestation of rheumatic fever.

Sylvian fissure The fissure separating temporal lobe from frontal and parietal lobes.

Symbiosis Living in perfect harmony in case of two organisms, a state beneficial to both.

Symblepharon Adhesion of lids to eyeball.

Syme's amputation Amputation just above ankle joint with removal of malleoli.

Sympathectomy Surgical excision of part of sympathetic system; either nerve, ganglia or plexus.

Sympathomimetic Producing effect similar to stimulation of sympathetic nerves.

Symphysiotomy Section of symphysis pubis to increase capacity of contracted pelvis to facilitate child birth.

Symphysis Fibrocartilaginous union of bones.

Symptom Subjective description or manifestation of disease.

Synapse The point of junction between two adjacent neurones.

Synarthrosis A type of joint where skeletal elements are joined by a continuous intervening cartilage, fibrous tissue or bone. Hence movement is limited or absent and joint cavity is lacking, e.g. *SYN* — chondrosis, suture joints.

Synchysis Degenerative condition of vitreous.

Syncope Transient loss of consciousness due to inadequate blood supply to brain.

s. cardiac Syncope of cardiac origin as in Stokes-Adam's attack, tachycardia, tight aortic stenosis, HOCM.

s. carotid sinus Hypersensitive carotid sinus being stimulated by neck movement or tight collar producing bradycardia and syncope.

s. vasovagal Syncope occurring due to abrupt fall in blood pressure due to fall in peripheral resistance and hence reduced venous return.

Syncytiotrophoblast Outer layer of chorionic villi.

Syncytium A mass of cytoplasm with numerous nuclei but no division into separate cells.

Synchondrosis A joint in which the surfaces are connected by plate of cartilage.

Syndactylism Fusion of two or more fingers or toes.

Syndectomy Excision of a circular strip of conjunctiva around the cornea to relieve pannus.

Syndesis The state of being bound together, surgical fixation or ankylosis of joint.

Syndesmectomy Excision of a section of ligament.

Syndesmitis Inflammation of a ligament; inflammation of conjunctiva.

Syndesmology Study of ligaments, joints, their movements and disorders.

Syndesmopexy Joining of two ligaments or fixation of a ligament at a new place for correction of dislocation.

Syndesmophyte A bony bridge between adjacent vertebrae or bony outgrowth from a ligament.

Syndesmosis A form of articulation where bones are united by cartilages.

Syndrome A group of signs and symptoms that provide a framework of reference to investigate as they characterize a definite lesion or pathology.

s. adrenogenital Syndrome characterized by early puberty, over masculization, hirsutism, etc. due to excess production of adrenocortical hormones.

s. dumping Palpitation, diarrhea sweating and syncope occurring, after food intake in patients of partial gastrectomy due to rapid emptying of food into jejunum.

s. Frohlich's Obesity, genital atrophy, due to hypothalamic pituitary lesions.

s. Gradenigo's Infection of petrous temporal bone causing 6th nerve paralysis as in otitis media.

s. Horner's Ptosis, myosis, enophthalmos, and lack of sweating on affected side of face due to paralysis of cervical sympathetic.

s. Korsakoff's A form of psychosis in chronic alcoholism with disorientation, loss of recent memory, confabulation, insomnia and hallucinations.

s. Marfan's A connective tissue disorder with long arm span, spider finger, lax ligaments, dislocation of lens, high arched palate, aortic root dilation and, mitral valve prolapse.

s. Weber's A form of crossed paralysis caused by a lesion in the upper border of pons involving cerebral peduncle and oculomotor nucleus. Hence there is third nerve palsy on one side with spastic hemiplegia on the opposite side.

Synechia Adhesion of iris to lens and cornea.

s. annular Iris is adherent to lens throughout entire pupillary margin.

s. anterior Adhesion of iris to cornea.

s. posterior Adhesion of iris to lens capsule.

Synergetic Working together in cooperation, e.g. muscle groups.

Synergism Harmonious action of two agents to produce an effect greater than that produced by either agents singly.

Synergist A muscle acting in cooperation with another.

Synergy Coordinated action of two or more agents.

Synesthesia 1. A subjective sensation of a sense other than the one being stimulated, e.g. hearing of a sound to producing a sensation of smell 2. A sensation experienced in one part of body following stimulation of another part.

Synagmus laryngeus A nematode a inhabiting respiratory tract of birds and mammals often accidentally infecting man.

Syngamy Union of gametes in fertilization.

Syngeneic Individuals or cells without tissue incompatibility.

Synkaryon A nucleus resulting from fusion of two pronuclei.

Synkinesis An involuntary movement of one part occurring simultaneously with reflex or voluntary movement of another part.

Synonym Having the same or similar meaning.

Synopsia Congenital fusion of the eyes.

Synopsis A summary; general review.

Synorchidism Partial or complete fusion of two testicles within scrotum or abdomen.

Synoptophore Apparatus for diagnosis and treatment of squint.

Synosteotomy Dissection of joints.

Synostosis Union of separate bones by osseous tissue.

Synovectomy Excision of synovial membrane.

Synovia A colourless viscid lubricating fluid in the joint cavity, bursae and tendon sheaths.

Synovial cyst Accumulation of synovia in a bursa.

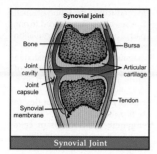

Synovial Joint

Synovial folds Smooth folds of synovial membrane inside joint cavity.

Synovial villi Slender avascular processes on the surface of synovial membrane.

Synovioma A tumor of synovial membrane.

s. dendritic Synovitis with villous growths.

s. dry Synovitis without effusion.

s. serous Synovitis with copious nonpurulent effusion.

Syntasis Stretching.

Syntaxis Articulation between two bones.

Synthesis Union of elements to produce new compounds.

Synthetase An enzyme that acts as a catalyst to unite two molecules.

Syntonic A personality with cool temperament, normal emotional responsiveness.

Syntropy Turning or pointing in same direction.

Syphilis Chronic venereal disease involving all tissues in body caused by *Treponema pallidum,* the spirochaete.

s. cardiovascular Syphilis with aortic aneurysm, root dilatation and aortic incompetence.

s. congenital Syphilis transmitted from mother to fetus in the womb with stigmatas at birth or infancy like choroidoretinitis, sabre tibia, Hutchinson's teeth, craniotabes etc.

s. latent Syphilis where symptoms are absent but disease is transmissible and serum tests are positive.

s. meningovascular A form of neurosyphilis due to involvement of meninges and the cerebral blood vessels.

Syphilitic macules Small red nonitchy eruptions all over the body in secondary syphilis.

Syringe Instrument for injecting fluids or wash out purpose.

Syringomyelia A chronic progressive disorder with formation of cavities with surrounding gliosis in the spinal cord.

Syringomyelocele A form of spina bifida in which the projecting syrinx communicates with central canal of spinal cord.

Syrinx Eustachian tube; pathological cavity within spinal cord, a fistula.

Syrup Concentrated sugar in water.

System A group of cells/organs that perform a particular function.

s. haversian Architectural unit of bone consisting of haversian canal with alternate layers of matrix and cell, the haversian lamellae.

s. *reticuloendothelial* The phago-cytic system of body excluding leukocytes, e.g. macrophages histiocytes, Kuffer's cells of liver, microglia of brain, and reticular cells of lymphatic system.

Systemic circulation Blood flow from left ventricle to aorta and to arteries and return to heart via the superior and inferior vena cava.

Systole The period of myocardial contraction, usually of 0.3 seconds in a heart beat.

Systolic pressure Maximum blood pressure during cardiac contraction.

T

Tabacosis Chronic tobacco poisoning or pneumoconiosis from inhalation of tobacco dust.

Tabes Chronic progressive wasting disease.

t. dorsalis Degeneration of posterior column of spinal cord in syphilis.

t. mesenterica Tuberculosis abdomen leading to malabsorption of nutrients.

Tabetic crises Paroxysms of pain occurring during course of tabes dorsalis.

Tablespoon A rough measure equivalent to 15 ml.

Taboo Setting apart of thing as sacred, thus forbidden for general use.

Taboparaesis Tabes dorsalis associated with general paralysis.

Tabular bone A flat bone composed of an outer and an inner table of compact bone with cancellous or diploe between them.

Tache A coloured spot or macule on skin.

Tachogram A graphic tracing of rate of blood flow.

Tachyarrhythmia Abnormally rapid heart rate with or without irregularity.

t. atrioventricular reentrant occurs due to presence of two conducting pathways – av node the normal one and an abnormal slowly conducting one.

t. nodal results from increased rhythmicity of av node over SA node

t paroxysmal atrial results from atrial hyper excitation

t paroxysmal supraventricular tachycardia focus in proximal to his bundle bifurcation

Tachycardia bradycardia syndrome – sick sinus syndrome, a defect in sinus node impulse generation or conduction

Tachycardia Rapid heart rate; can be atrial, nodal, ectopic, ventricular or sinus depending upon the site of origin of the impulse.

Tachymeter Instrument for estimating the speed of anything in motion.

Tachyphrasia Rapidity of speech.

Tachysterol One of the isomers of ergosterol.

Tactile Perceptible to touch.

Tactile discrimination The ability to localize two points of touch on skin surface as two discrete sensations.

Tactile disk Tiny expanded end of a sensory nerve fiber found in the epidermis or root sheath of hair.

Tactile localization Ability to accurately identify the site of tactile stimulation (touch, pain or pressure).

Tactometer Instrument for determining acuity of tactile sensitiveness.

Taenia A genus of parasitic, elongated ribbon like worms, the body being segmented.

t. saginata Tapeworm whose larvae live in flesh of cattle and adult worms (15 to 20 feet long) in human intestine. Men acquire the infestation by eating undercooked beef.

t. solium Tapeworm whose larval stage is in pigs and adult worms in human intestine. The disease is acquired by eating undercooked pork containing cysticercus cellulosae.

Taenia coli Three bands in large intestine into which muscular fibers are collected.

Tag A small polyp or growth; a label.

Tag skin Small outgrowth of skin.

Tagging Incorporating radioactive isotope into chemical compounds to trace the metabolism.

Takayasu arteritis Aortic branch occlusion of unknown origin, often involving ophthalmic artery.

Talc Hydrous magnesium silicate, used as dusting powder.

Talipes Congenital non-traumatic abnormal deviation of foot.

t. calcaneus The heel alone touches the ground.

t. equinus The person walks on the toes; can be varus or valgus depending on whether the heel is turned inward or outward.

Talus The ankle bone articulating with tibia fibula above and calcaneus and navicular bone below.

Talwin Pentazocine, an opioid analgesic.

Tam Horsfall protein A mucoprotein secreted from renal tubules.

Tamoxifen Antiestrogen drug used in adjuvant therapy of breast cancer.

Tampon A roll of pack made of various absorbent substances used to absorb body secretions or arrest hemorrhage, e.g. menstrual tampon.

Tamponade Pathologic compression of an organ or part.

t. balloon Used to arrest variceal bleed.

t. cardiac Increased pericardial pressure due to pericardial bleed or excess fluid causing compression of heart to the extent of compromising its function.

Tangier disease A syndrome of HDL deficiency first discovered in Tangier island. Symptoms and signs include polyneuropathy, lymphadenopathy, coffee, orange tonsils, hepatosplenomegaly.

Tannin An acid substance found in tea and an astringent, topical hemostatic and antidote for various poisons.

Tantrum Bad temper or anger.

Tapeinocephaly A flattened skull with vertical index less than 72.

Tapetum Fibers from corpus callosum forming roof and lateral walls of inferior and posterior horns of lateral ventricle.

Tapeworm Parasitic worms belonging to class cestoda having a scolex with hooks and suckers and a series of proglottids.

t. beef Taenia saginata.

t. broad Diphylobothrium latum.

t. dog Dipylidium caninum.

t. dwarf Hymenolepis nana.

t. pork Taenia solium.

Tapia syndrome Paralysis of pharynx, larynx and atrophy of tongue due to paralysis of tenth and twelfth cranial nerves.

Tapping Removal of fluid from cavity, percussion in massage.

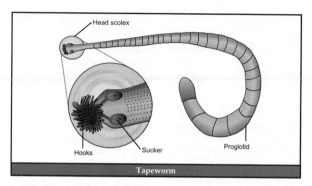

Tapeworm

Tar Thick brown to black liquid obtained from distillation of carbonaceous matter.

Taractan Chlorprothixene, an antidepressant.

Tarantula a venomous spider

Tardieu's spot Subpleural spots of ecchymosis following death by strangulation.

Tardive Tending to be late.

Target cell An abnormal erythrocyte which when stained shows a central and peripheral rim of hemoglobin with intermediate unstained area resembling a target.

Tarnier's sign A sign of impending abortion; the disappearance of angle between upper and lower uterine segments of uterus.

Tarnish Discoloration.

Tarsal glands Branched sebaceous alveolar glands in the eyelids. *SYN* — meiobomian glands.

Tarsal tunnel In the ankle, the bony fibrous passage for the posterior tibial vessels, nerves and flexor tendons.

Tarsal tunnel syndrome Weakness of plantar flexion of toes and numbness of sole of foot due to compression of tibial nerve in the tarsal tunnel.

Tarsitis Inflammation of margin of eyelid; inflammation of tarsal bones (the seven bones of ankle).

Tarso Flat of the foot, or edge of the eyelid.

Tarsomalacia Softening of tarsal cartilages of eyes.

Tarsorrhaphy The procedure of suturing the edges of upper and lower eyelids for purpose of reducing width of palpebral fissure.

Tarsus The ankle with its seven constituent bones, i.e. talus, calcaneus, cuboid, navicular and the three cuneiform bones.

Tartrazin A pyrazole aniline dye used to colour foods, cloth and drugs.

Taste A sensation produced by stimulation of taste buds by sweet, sour, bitter and salty substances.

Taste buds Sensory end organs located on surface of tongue, on soft palate that mediate the sensation of taste.

Tattooing Production of permanent colors on the skin by introducing vegetable and mineral pigments.

Taurocholic acid Bile acid that yields taurine and cholic acid on hydrolysis.

Taussing Bing syndrome A congenital deformity of heart in which aorta arisen from RV and pulmonary artery from both ventricles with presence of VSD

Taxis The response of an organism to its environment.

Taxonomy Laws and principles of classification of animals and plants.

Tay-Sachs disease Autosomal recessive form of gangliosidosis (lipid storage disease) manifesting with mental retardation, blindness, cherry red spot in macula, etc., due to deficiency of hexosaminidase. A leading to accumulation of sphingolipid in CNS.

T cells Thymus derived lymphocytes consisting of helper inducer cells (T_4), killer T cells and suppressor T cells.

Tea black Tea made from the leaves that have been fermented before they are dried.

Tea green Tea made by heating the leaves in open trays.

Tear A watery saline solution secreted by lacrimal glands that lubricates the eyeball and eyelids.

Teaspoon Measure equivalent to 5 ml.

Teat The nipple of mammary gland.

Teatulation The development of nipple like elevation.

Technetium 99M An isomer of technetium that emits gamma rays with a half-life of 6 hours, used for vascular imaging.

Technology The scientific knowledge and its practical application.

Tectocephaly Boat shaped head.

Tectospinal tract A descending tract from tectum of midbrain to spinal cord.

Tectum Structure resembling a roof; dorsal midbrain consisting of superior and inferior colliculi.

Teenage Age bracket of 13-19 years.

Teeth Hard bony projections from jaw helping in mastication.

t. deciduous Milk teeth which are shed and replaced by permanent teeth.

t. Hutchinson's Notched upper central incisors and peg-shaped lateral incisors.

t. wisdom The third molar of permanent dentition, last to erupt.

Tegmen A structure that covers a part.

Tegmentum The dorsal portion of midbrain containing red nucleus, and oculomotor nuclei.

Tegument The skin covering of body.

Teichoic acid A polymer focused on some bacterial cell wall.

Teichopsia Zigzag lines bounding a luminous object in visual field as in migraine.

Tela Any web like structure.

Telalgia *SYN* — referred pain, i.e. pain felt at a distance from its stimulus.

Telangiectasia Dilatation of group of capillaries to form elevated dark red wart like spots.

Telangioma Tumor made of dilated capillaries and arterioles.

Telangion Terminal arteriole.

Tele canthus Increased distance between inner canthi.

Teleceptor A sense organ responding to stimuli arising from some distance from body like eyes and ears.

Telediagnosis Diagnosis based on data transmitted electronically to the doctor.

Telemetry Transmission of data to a distant place by electronic means.

Telencephalon The embryonic forebrain that develops into olfactory lobes, cerebral cortex and corpora striate.

Teleneurite The branching end of an axon.

Teleology The belief that everything in nature is directed towards some final purpose.

Teleopsia A visual perceptive disorder where objects appear to have excess depth or close objects appear to be away.

Telepaque Iopanoic acid.

Telepathy Communication of one's thought and mental process to another at a distance.

Teleradiography Radiography with radiation source at about 2 meters away from body.

Telogen Resting stage of hair growth.

Telophase The final stage of mitosis.

Temazepam A benzodiazepine, anxiolytic.

Temper State of one's mood, disposition and mind.

Temperament The combination of intellectual, emotional and physical characteristic of an individual.

Temperate Moderate.

Temperature The degree of intensity of heat.

t. ambient Temperature of surrounding.

t. inverse A state where morning body temperature is higher than evening body temperature.

t. normal Oral temperature of 98.6°F(37°C).

t. rectal More accurate than oral or axillary temperature. It is about 1°F higher than oral temperature, whereas axillary temperature is 1°F lower than oral temperature.

Temper tantrums Spells of uncontrollable anger especially in children.

Template A pattern, form or mold used as a guide in duplicating, e.g. in preparation of denture.

Temple Forehead, the portion lying in front of ear and above the zygomatic arch.

Temporal Related to or limited in time.

Temporalis The muscle in temporal fossa inserted into coronoid process of mandible, a muscle of mastication.

Temporal fossa The fossa above ear that contains temporalis muscle.

Temporal lobe Lobe of cerebrum concerned with olfaction.

Tenacious Adhesive, sticky.

Tenacity Condition of being tough, stubborn.

Tenaculum Sharp hook like instrument.

Tenalgia Pain in the tendon.

Tenderness Sensitive to pain on pressure.

t. rebound Intensification of pain during release of pressure, a feature of peritonitis.

Tenderizer Preparations containing proteolytic enzymes like papain to make the meat more tender.

Tendinitis Inflammation of a tendon.

Tendinitis rotator cuff Especially supra spinatus tendon is involved following injury or over use.

Tendinous synovitis Inflammation of tendon's synovial sheath.

Tendon Fibrous connective tissue attaching a muscle to bone.

t. Achilles The thickest and strongest tendon of gastrocnemius muscle attached to calcaneus.

t. central Central portion of diaphragm consisting of a flat aponeurosis into which the muscle fiber of diaphragm are inserted.

t. superior of Lockwood Portion of fibrous ring from which superior oblique muscle of eye originates.

Tendon spindle Fusiform nerve ending in a tendon.

Tendovaginitis Inflammation of tendon and its sheath.

Tenesmus Ineffectual painful effort in bladder and bowel evacuation.

Teniposide Antineoplastic agents of podophylotoxin group.

Tennis elbow Pain over lateral epicondyle of humerus at the site of attachment of extensor tendons.

Tenon's capsule Connective tissue covering of eyeball.

Tenon's space Space between the posterior surface of eyeball and Tenon's capsule.

Tenosynovectomy Excision of tendon sheath.

Tenosynovitis Inflammation of tendon sheath.

Tenotome Instrument for cutting tendon.

Tenotomy Surgical section of a tendon.

Tensilon Edrophonium chloride.

Tension Expansive force that stretches; a state of mental strain.

t. premenstrual Nervous instability, irritability, headache and depression occurring few days before menstruation.

Tension headache Headache caused by sustained contraction of muscles of head and neck.

Tension suture Suture used to reduce pull of the edges of wound.

Tensor Any muscle that makes a part tense.

Tensor vali palatini A muscle of soft palate arising from cartilaginous medial end of auditory tube and inserted into palatal aponeurosis.

Tentacle A slender projection of invertebrates used for tactile purposes or feeding.

Tentative Provisional.

Tenth cranial nerve Vagus nerve supplying heart, lungs, abdominal viscera, esophagus etc.

Tentorial notch An arched cavity formed by anterior and inner border of tentorium cerebelli.

Tentorial pressure cone The herniation of uncus of temporal lobe and midbrain through tentorial notch due to raised intracranial pressure.

Tentorium cerebelli The process of dura mater between cerebrum and cerebellum supporting the occipital lobes.

Tepanil Diethylpropion hydrochloride.

Tepid Lukewarm.

Teratoblastoma A tumor containing embryonic tissue.

Teratocarcinoma Carcinoma developing from epithelial element of a teratoma.

Teratogen Any substance capable of disrupting fetal growth and producing fetal malformation.

Teratology Scientific study of teratogens and their mode of action.

Teras A severely malformed fetus.

Teratoma Congenital tumor containing one or more of three embryonic germ layers.

Teratosis Deformed fetus.

Terbutaline Synthetic sympathomimetic amine used as bronchodilator.

Terconazole A ketoconazole derivative, antifungal agent.

Teres Round and smooth.

Terfenadine H_1 receptor blocker, antiallergic agent.

Terminal Pertains to end or placed at the end.

Terminal arteriole Arteriole without any branches which ends in capillaries.

Terminal illness Illness from which recovery is impossible, hence death is imminent.

Terminology Nomenclature, a system of technical terms used in arts, science and trade.

Terpene A hydrocarbon used as an expectorant.

Terracing Suturing in several rows through thick tissues in wound closure.

Terramycin Oxytetracycline, synthesized by *Streptomyces rimosus*, effective against bacteria, rickettsia and chlamydia.

Terror Great fear.

Tertian Occurring every third day as in malaria.

Tertiary Third in order.

Tertiary care A level of medicare.

Tertiary syphilis Third and most advanced stage of syphilis with general dissemination.

Tesla A measure of magnetic strength, one tesla equalis 1 weber per square meter

Testis The male reproductive gland located in scrotum about 4 cm long and 2 cm wide.

Testmeal A meal of definite quality and quantity given for analysis of stomach function.

Testosterone An androgenic hormone secreted by Leydig cells of testes.

Test Examination, chemical reaction

t. acetic acid test to detect albumin in urine

t. acetone to urine is added nitroprusside and strong ammonia; appearance of magenta ring indicates presence of acetone

t. coin – for detection of pneumothorax

t. creatine clearance best indicator of renal function, normal is 95-135ml/min.

t. finger nose a test of cerebellar function.

t. guaic acid a test for occult blood in feces

t. limulus amebocyte lysate a test to detect bacterial endotoxin and pyrogens in samples

t. liver function tests for liver cell function like AST, ALT, bilirubin, gamma GTT

t. McMurray a test for torn meniscus in knee

t. ninhydrin a test to detect sympathetic response after healing of nerve injury as indicated by sweat.

t nonstress an external electronic monitoring procedure for accessing fetal well being

t. Schiller a test for cervical cancer. Painting with iodine causes glycogen containing normal cells to take iodine colour and those cells without glycogen paint white/yellow

t. shake test of fetal lung maturity. Amniotic fluid is diluted with NS, mixed with 95% ethyl alcohol and shaked for 30 sec. appearance of foamy bubbles indicates spresence of surfactant

t. sickling red cells placed in oxygen free condition will sickle if contain HbS.

t. thematic appreciation a projective test for insight into subjects personality

t. tourniquet a test for capillary fragility.

Test tube baby A baby born to a mother whose ovum was removed, fertilized outside her body and implanted in her uterus.

Tetanolysin A hemolytic component of the toxin produced by *Clostridium tetani.*

Tetanospasmin The toxin of *Clostridium tetani* responsible for spasm.

Tetanus An acute infectious disease caused by anaerobe *Clostridium tetani* manifesting with painful tonic-clonic spasm of voluntary muscles.

t. anticus Form of tetanus with forward bowing of body.

t. ascending Tetanus in which muscle spasm occurs first in the lower part of body to spread upward to involve muscles of head and neck.

t. neonatorum Tetanus in neonates following umbilical sepsis.

Tetanus antitoxin Serum containing antibody against tetanus obtained from immunized horses or humans.

Tetanus toxoid Modified tetanus toxin capable of promoting active immunity.

Tetany A state of increased neuro-muscular excitability caused by

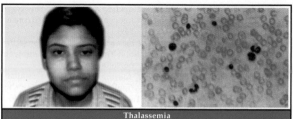
Thalassemia

decreased serum ionized calcium or phosphorus and in alkalosis.

Tetracaine Local anesthetic used topically.

Tetrachlorelhylene A clear colorless bitter liquid used as anthelmintic, potentially hepatotoxic.

Tetracycline A broad spectrum antibiotic.

Tetrad A group of four things.

Tetradactyly Having four digits on a hand or foot.

Tetrahydrocanabinol Principal active component of *Canabis indica.*

Tetrahydrozoline A vasoconstrictor used in ophthalmic and nasal drops.

Tetraiodothyronine One of the principal hormones secreted by thyroid *SYN*— thyroxine (T_4).

Tetralogy A combination of four symptoms or elements.

t. of Fallot Congenital heart disease with infundibular pulmonary stenosis, right ventricular hypertrophy, over-riding aorta, and high ventricular septal defect.

Tetramisole Anthelmintic.

Tetraparesis Paresis of all four limbs.

Tetraplegia *SYN* — quadriplegia.

Thalamic nuclei The anterior, lateral, medial and posterior thalamic nuclei.

Thalamic syndrome Severe sharp boring and burning pain caused by vascular lesions of thalamus.

Thalamotomy Destruction of thalamus by several means to treat psychosis or intractable pain.

Thalamus Large ovoid masses of gray matter on either side of third ventricle, serving as gateway for all sensory projections to brain.

Thalassemia A group of congenital hemolytic anemia due to impaired synthesis of hemoglobin polypeptide chains, alpha or beta.

t. major The homozygous form of deficient beta chain synthesis manifesting with severe microcytic anemia, splenomegaly, jaundice, gall stones, leg ulcers and thickened cranial bones.

t. minor Heterozygous state for alpha or beta chain production with mild microcytic hypochromic anemia and raised Hb A_2.

Thalidomide Alfa glutarimide previously used as sedative but now only used in lepra reaction; causes severe birth defects if given to pregnant mothers.

Thallium A metallic element used as rodenticide.

Thanatology The science of death.

Thanatophobia Morbid fear of death.

Tharatophoric dwarfism dwarfism caused by generalized failure of endochondral bone formation.

Thayer-marten medium medium used for growth of N. gonorrhoea.

Theaism Chronic poisoning from excessive intake of tea.

Thebaine An alkaloid present in opium.

Thebesian valve An endocardial fold at entrance of coronary sinus into right atrium.

Thebesian vein Small veins draining blood from myocardium directly into heart chambers.

Theca A sheath.

Thecitis Inflammation of sheath of tendon.

Thecoma A benign tumor of ovary.

Thecomatosis Increased connective tissue in the ovary.

Thelalgia Pain in the nipples of breast.

Thelarche The beginning of breast development during puberty.

Thelothism Nipple erection by contraction of its smooth muscles.

Thenar Palm of hand or sole of foot; fleshy eminence at base of thumb.

Thenar muscles Abductor and flexor muscles of thumb.

Theobromine A smooth muscle dilator, used as a mild stimulant and diuretic.

Theomania Religious insanity.

Theophylline A plant product and bronchodilator.

t. ethylenediamine Aminophylline.

Theorem A proposition proved by logic or argument.

Theory An assumption based on certain evidence or certain observations but lacking scientific proof.

Therapeutic A curative.

t. abortion Termination of pregnancy that disrupts mother's physical or mental health (as a sequence of rape) or is likely to produce a physically or mentally handicapped child.

t. index The ratio of toxic dose of a substance to its therapeutic dose; an index of safety of the drug.

Therapeutics The branch of medical science dealing with treatment of disease.

Therapist Practitioner of some kind of therapy.

Therapy The means employed to effect a cure or manage a disease.

t. collapse Production of pneumothorax to effect pulmonary collapse as a method of treatment of non healing cavitary pulmonary tuberculosis.

t. electroconvulsive Passing of electric current in the convulsive dose to treat psychosis or suicidal depression.

t. photodynamic Method of treating cancer by using light absorbing chemicals that are selectively retained by malignant cells.

t. physical Use of physical agents such as massage, heat, hydration, electricity, exercise in the treatment of disease.

t. replacement Therapeutic use of medicine as substitute for natural body substances, e.g. thyroid hormone, insulin.

Thermalgesia Pain caused by heat.

Thermanalgesia Insensitiveness to heat.

Thermesthesia Capability to perceive heat and cold.

Thermic Pertains to heat.

Thermistor An apparatus for determining small changes in temperature.

Thermobiosis Ability to withstand high temperature.

Thermocoagulation Coagulation or destruction of tissue by passage of high frequency current.

Thermocouple Device for measuring slight temperature changes.

Thermodilution A technique for determination of cardiac output from injection of cold saline into blood stream and measuring the temperature change downstream.

Thermogenesis Production of body heat.

Thermography A technique to study blood flow into limbs and to detect breast cancer.

Thermoluminescent dosimeter A monitoring device that stores energy of ionizing radiation. When heated it emits light proportional to the amount of radiation to which it has been exposed, used by radiographers and those working near radiation source.

Thermometer Instrument for recording temperature.

Thermometry Measurement of temperature.

Thermophilic Thriving best in environment of raised temperature.

Thermophylic Resistance to destruction by heat.

Thermoregulation Heat regulation.

Thermoregulatory center Hypothalamic center that regulates heat production and heat loss.

Thermostasis Maintenance of body temperature.

Thermostat A device that automatically regulates temperature.

Thiabendazole Anthelmintic used for strongyloidiasis and cutaneous larva migrans.

Thiamine Vitamin B_1 present in wheat germ, rice water, animal and plant foods. Acts as a coenzyme in carboxylation of pyruvic acid. Deficiency produces beriberi.

Thiersch's graft Partial thickness skin graft.

Thiamine

Thimerosal An organic mercurial antiseptic used topically and as a preservative.

Thio Prefix meaning sulfur.

Thioguanine An antimetabolite and immunosuppressant.

Thiopental sodium An ultrashort acting barbiturate used for inducing surgical anesthesia.

Thioridazine Antipsychotic agent.

Thiotepa An alkylating agent, antineoplastic drug.

Thiothixene An antipsychotic drug.

Thiouracil Antithyroid agent.

Thiourea Antithyroid drug.

Third degree burn Burn involving entire thickness of skin and deeper structures.

Third degree heart block Complete heart block.

Third heart sound Heart sound occurring at the end of rapid ventricular filling.

Thirst Desire for water or the sensation arising out of lack of body fluids.

Thoma's splint A splint with a proximal ring with two long steel rods used to place traction on the leg in long axis.

Thomsen's disease Myotonia congenita.

Thompson test In Achiles rupture squeezing of calf does not cause plantar flaxion of foot.

Thoracentesis Puncture of chestwall to drain out pleural fluids.

Thoracic cage The bony structure surrounding the chest.

Thoracic duct The main lymphatic duct of body arising at cisterna chyli, ascending up to join left subclavian vein near its junction with left internal jugular vein.

Thoracic outlet syndrome Brachial neuritis and vascular/vasomotor disturbance in upper limb due to compression by cervical rib/ scalenus anterior.

Thoracocentesis Drainage of thoracic cavity through needle puncture.

Thoracometer Instrument for measuring chest expansion.

Thoracoplasty Partial resection of ribs to induce collapse of underlying lung as in lung abscess, or empyema.

Thoracoscopy Endoscopic examination of pleural cavity.

Thoracostomy Surgical resection of chest wall for drainage.

Thorax The part of the body between diaphragm below and base of the neck above.

t. barrel shaped Rounded chest as in emphysema.

t. Peyrot's Obliquely oval chest as in large pleural effusion.

Thorel's bundle A muscle bundle joining SA node and AV node.

Thorium Radioactive metallic substance.

Thoron A radioactive isotope of radon.

Threadworm *Enterobius vermicularis.*

Threonine Alpha amino beta hydroxybutyric acid an essential amino acid.

Threshold 1. Point at which physiological response is produced

2. A measure of sensitivity of an organ or function.

Threshold dose Minimum dose that will be effective.

Thrill A palpable murmur.

Thrix Hair.

Throat The pharynx and the fauces.

Throbbing Pulsatile.

Throe A severe spasm or pain.

Thrombasthenia A platelet disorder with prolonged bleeding time, and abnormal clot retraction.

Thrombectomy Excision of a thrombus.

Thrombin An enzyme derived from prothrombin by action of thromboplastin.

Thromboangitis Inflammation of blood vessel with thrombus formation.

t. obliterans Chronic occlusive vascular disease common to cigarette smokers commonly affecting the feet with propensity for gangrene formation. *SYN* — Buerger's disease.

Thromboclasis Lysis of thrombus.

Thrombocythemia Absolute increase in platelet count.

Thrombocytopenia Decrease below normal in number of platelets. ($\leq$ 50,000 cmm)

Thrombocytosis Increase in number of platelets. ($\geq$ 400,000 cmm)

Thromboembolism A detached thrombus causing occlusion of a vessel.

Thrombogenesis The process of formation of blood clot.

Thrombokinase Factor 'x' or Stuart factor.

Thrombolysis Dissolution of blood clot.

Thrombophlebitis Inflammation of vein with thrombus formation.

Thromboplastin The coagulation factor III present in most tissues which accelerates clot formation by converting prothrombin to thrombin.

Thrombosis The formation or existence of thrombus or clot within the vessel.

Thrombus A blood clot.

t. hyaline Thrombus with a glassy appearance.

t. parietal or mural Thrombus attached to wall of a vessel or heart.

Thrush Infection caused by *Candida albicans* in mouth and throat with formation of white patches and ulcers.

Thrust The sudden move forward.

Thumb The short thick first finger on radial side of hand having two phallanges in place of three.

Thymectomy Surgical removal of thymus.

Thymine A base present in DNA.

Thymocyte A lymphocyte that migrates from bone marrow to thymus where it matures and is released to blood as T lymphocyte.

Thymoma Tumor from epithelial tissue of thymus.

Thymopoietin A substance produced by thymus gland that helps in differentiation of thymocytes.

Thymus The capsulated bilobed organ in anterior mediastinum which is essential for immune function of body.

Thyroepiglottic muscle Muscle arising from inner surface of thyroid cartilage and inserted into epiglottis. Acts to depress the epiglottis.

Thyroglobulin Iodine containing protein secreted by thyroid gland and stored within the colloid.

Thyroglossal duct A duct which in the embryo connects the thyroid diverticulum with the tongue.

Thyroid cartilage The V shaped principal cartilage of larynx, known as Adam's apple.

Thyroidectomy Excision of thyroid gland, usually done in hyperthyroidism.

Thyroid function tests A group of tests done to assess the level of functioning of thyroid gland. They include thyroid radio-iodine uptake studies, estimation of T_3, T_4 and TSH.

Thyroid gland The bilobed gland joined by isthmus located at the base of the neck, secreting T_3 and T_4.

Thyroiditis Inflammation of thyroid gland.

t. giant cell Thyroiditis characterized by presence of giant cells, round cell infiltration, fibrosis and destruction of the follicles.

t. Hashimoto's A form of autoimmune thyroiditis common to women. There is thyromegaly and hypothyroidism.

Thyroid stimulating hormone (TSH) Hormone secreted by anterior pituitary which stimulates thyroid to secrete T_3 and T_4.

Thyroid storm A complication of thyrotoxicosis precipitated by infection, surgery; manifests with high fever, restlessness and congestive failure.

Thyromegaly Enlarged thyroid gland.

Thyroprivia Hypothyroid state.

Thyroptosis Downward displacement of thyroid.

Thyrotoxic Pertains to hyperactivity of thyroid gland.

Thyrotoxicosis Hyperfunctioning of thyroid gland with tachycardia, fine tremor, anxiety, nervousness, diarrhea etc.

Thyrotropic Agent that stimulates thyroid gland.

Thyrotropin Thyroid stimulating hormone.

Thyroxine Tetra-iodo-thyronine, the principal hormone of thyroid gland.

Tibia The inner larger bone in the leg.

t. saber Gummatous periosteitis of tibia with increased outward curvature.

Tic A sudden involuntary muscle contraction.

t. douloureux Lightening pain along the branches of trigeminal nerve due to degeneration or pressure on the nerve.

Ticarcillin A semi synthetic penicillin effective against pseudomonas.

Tick A group of blood sucking acarids; can be hard tick or soft tick; transmit typhus group of fevers, Q fever, Lyme's disease, babesiosis, bereliosis, tularemia etc.

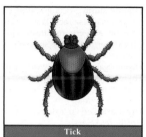
Tick

Tickling Gentle stimulation of sensitive surface and the reflex thereof.

Tidal Periodically rising and falling.

Tietze syndrome Sternal costochondritis of unknown etiology, often requiring injection procaine and steroids locally.

Tincture An alcoholic extraction of animal or vegetable substance.

Tinea Fungus infection.

t. capitis Fungal infection of head.

t. corporis Fungal infections of body with scaly eruptions and clearing center.

t. cruris Fungal infection of genital area.

t. nigra Superficial fungal infection of palm with pigmented non-itchy nonscaly macules.

t. nodosa Sheath like nodular masses in hair of heard, moustache making hairs brittle.

t. pedis Fungal infection of foot (*SYN*— athlete's foot).

t. profunda Fungal skin nodules and plaques which may ulcerate.

t. versicolor Yellow or fawn colored skin patches due to *Malassezia furfur*.

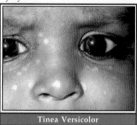
Tinea Versicolor

Tinel's sign Tingling sensation on pressing or tapping a damaged or degenerating nerve.

Tingle Pricking or stinging sensation.

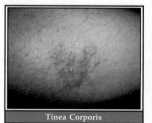
Tinea Corporis

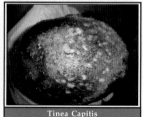
Tinea Capitis

Tinidazole An imidazole used in amebiasis.

Tinnitus Ringing sensation in the ear.

Tissue A group or collection of similar cells performing a particular function.

t. adipose Tissue containing densely packed fat cells.

t. areolar Loose connective tissue forming interstitial tissue of most organs.

t. epithelial The cells are arranged in continuous sheets in several layers, e.g. epidermis of skin, glandular tissue lining of tubes, canals and ducts.

t. granulation Newly formed vascular and cellular tissue produced in the early stages of wound healing.

t. lymphoid A collection of developing and mature lymphocytes within supporting network of connective tissue, e.g. adenoids, tonsils, Peyer's patches.

t. osseous Connective tissue with intercellular matrix impregnated with calcium and phosphorus.

t. reticular A form of connective tissue with delicate fibers.

Tissue macrophage A large wandering branched cell with single nucleus capable of ingesting particulate matter.

Tissue plasminogen activator (TPA) A thrombolytic agent that is clot specific, acting on plasminogen causing breakdown of fibrin.

Tetanium dioxide Used in solutions for protection against sunburn.

Titilation Sensation produced by tickling.

Titration 1. Determination of quantity of antibody in the serum, 2. Estimation of the concentration of chemical solution by adding known amount of standard reagent.

Titubation Unsteadiness of posture, swaying of trunk and head while sitting, staggering gait.

TNM classification Method of calssifying malignant tumors based on local characteristics of the tumor, involvement of lymph nodes and distant metastasis.

Toad skin Excessive dryness, wrinkling and scaling of skin as in vitamin A deficiency (phrynoderma).

Tobacco Dried leaves of the plant *Nicotiana tobacum* containing nicotine, picoline, pyridine, collidin, etc. Tobacco chewing is related to oropharyngeal cancer and tobacco smoking to lung cancer, hypertension, heart attack, vasoocclusive disease, etc.

Tobramycin Aminoglycoside antibiotic.

Tocainide A lidocaine analog, antiarrhythmic drug used for VT.

Tocodynamometer Device for estimating force of uterine contraction *SYN* — tocometer.

Tocograph Device for recording force of uterine contraction.

Tocology Science of parturition.

Tocolysis Suppression of uterine contraction.

Tocopherol Compounds with vitamin E activity.

Toilet Wound cleaning.

Toilet training Teachings for a child to achieve control over urination and defecation.

Tolazamide An oral hypoglycemic agent.

Tolazoline An alfa adrenergic blocking agent used for causing peripheral vasodilatation as in chilblain.

Tolbutamide An oral hypoglycemic agent.

Tolerance Progressive decrease in the effectiveness of a drug.

Tolfenamic acid A fenamate anti-inflammatory drug.

Tolnaftate Synthetic antifungal agent used topically.

Tomography A method of X-ray that shows details of image of structures at a particular plane of tissue by blurring images of structures in all other planes.

Tone 1. A state of partial contraction of muscle. 2. normal tension in arterial wall.

Tongue A fleshy leafy organ lying in floor of mouth. Helps in mastication, deglutition, speech production and taste.

t. black hairy Tongue with brown fur like area on its surface composed of pigmented filiform papillae resulting from antibiotic therapy.

t. fissured Tongue with deep furrows on its epithelium often due to syphilis.

t. furred Tongue coated with a layer of white fur as seen in most fevers.

t. geographic Tongue with white raised areas of heaped up epithelium with surrounding atrophy.

t. magenta Magenta colored tongue in riboflavin deficiency.

t. parrot A dry shrivelled tongue as seen in typhus.

t. scrotal Furrowed and fissured tongue.

t. smooth A tongue with atrophy of papillae as in anemia and malnutrition.

t. strawberry A bright red tongue with prominent papillae as in scarlet fever.

Tongue tie Congenital shortness of frenum linguae with poor protrusion, difficulty in articulation and sucking.

Tonicity Property of possessing tone.

Tonography The recording of changes in intraocular pressure.

Tonometer Instrument for measuring intraocular pressure.

Tonometry Measurement of intraocular tension.

Tonsil 1. A mass of lymphatic tissue located in the fauces, 2. Two rounded masses projecting from inferior surface of cerebellum. 3. Lymphatic tissue near the opening of eustachian tube into pharynx.

Tonsillar fossa Depression between the glossopalatine and pharyngopalatine arches accommodating the tonsils.

Tonsillar ring Ring of lymphoid tissue encircling the pharynx, e.g. palatine and lingual tonsils and the adenoids.

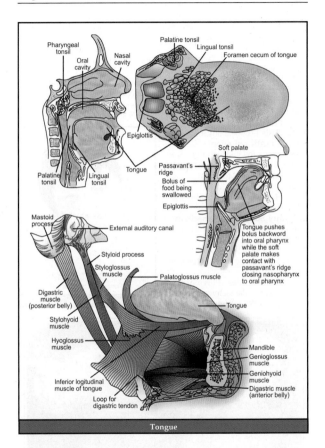

Tongue

Tonsillar sinus Space between the plica triangularis and anterior surface of tonsils.

Tonsillectomy Surgical removal of the tonsils.

Tonsillitis Inflammation of tonsils. *t. follicular* Tonsillitis principally affecting the crypts.

Tooth The hard structure in the jaw for mastication.

Topagnosis Loss of ability to localize site of tactile sensation.

Tophaceous Related to tophus.

Tophus Deposits of sodium biurate in tissue adjacent to a joint.

Topical Local.

Torpent Medicine that modifies irritation.

Torpidity Sluggishness, inactivity.

Torque A force producing rotary motion.

Torr The pressure of 1/760 of standard atmospheric pressure or simply 1mm of Hg.

Torsade-de-pointes Polymorphic rapid ventricular tachycardia with changing QRS configuration.

Torsion Rotation of the vertical meridians of eye; rotation of tooth along its long axis.

Tort A wrong or unlawful action.

Torticollis Spasmodic contraction of neck muscles causing head to tilt to one side and chin pointing to other side.

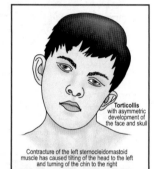

Torticollis with asymmetric development of the face and skull

Contracture of the left sternocleidomastoid muscle has caused tilting of the head to the left and turning of the chin to the right

Torticollis

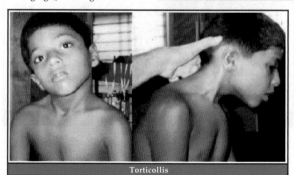

Torticollis

t. ocular Inequality of vision or squint causing torticollis.

Tortuous Having many bends or twists and turns.

Torture Infliction of mental or physical pain.

Torula Former name for cryptococcus, a form of yeast.

Toruloma The nodular lesions of cryptococcosis.

Torulopsis glabrata A yeast closely related to candida, causing serious illness in immunocompromised patients.

Torus A swelling or elevation.

Total hip replacement Replacement of acetabulum and head of femur by metallic or silicone prosthesis in the treatment of advanced disabling hip disease.

Total parenteral nutrition (TPN) Provision of total electrolyte, protein, calorie, vitamin and mineral need via intravenous route.

Totipotent A cell capable of dividing into a large variety of cells.

Touch Tactile sense or perceive from palpation.

Tourette's syndrome A disease with involuntary purposeless movement, ticks, grunts and barks.

Tournay's sign Dilatation of pupil on strong lateral fixation.

Tourniquet Any item used to exert pressure over an artery to stop bleeding.

t. rotating A technique of applying tourniquets to three extremities in rotation to reduce venous return to heart as in pulmonary edema.

Tourniquet test Test for determining capillary fragility from their ability to withstand pressure.

Touton cells Giant multinucleated cells found in lesions of xanthomatosis.

Toxemia Circulation of toxins throughout the body producing symptoms like fever, diarrhea, vomiting, hypotension, flushing tachycardia etc.

t. of pregnancy A series of changes occurring in pregnancy leading to hypertension, proteinuria, convulsion and intrauterine growth retardation.

Toxic allergic syndrome A disease caused by ingestion of adulterated rapeseed oil with aniline producing respiratory distress, eosinophilia, hepatosplenomegaly, etc.

Toxicology Branch of science dealing with toxic substances, their detection, pharmacological action, selection of suitable antidotes, treatment and prevention of their symptoms.

Toxicosis A diseased condition resulting from poisoning.

Toxic shock syndrome Fever, diffuse macular erythematous rash, syncope due to toxins produced by *Staphylococcus aureus*.

Toxiferous Containing a poison.

Toxigenic Producing toxins or poisons.

Toxigenicity The virulence of a toxin producing pathogenic organism.

Toxin A poisonous substance of animal or plant origin.

Toxocariasis Infection with nematode *T. canis* or *T. cati*.

Toxoid A toxin without toxicity but with intact antigenicity so that when injected can produce antibodies.

Toxolysin Substance capable of destroying toxin.

Toxoplasma A form of protozoa, e.g. *T. gondii* causing toxoplasmosis.

Toxoplasmosis A disease due to infection with *Toxoplasma gondii* manifest with pneumonitis, hepatitis, encephalitis (in the severe form) or mild fever and malaise in mild form. In congenital form the newborn may have encephalopathy, jaundice, anemia, hepatosplenomegaly and generalized lymphadenopathy.

Trabecula Fibrous cord of connective tissue extending into an organ from its capsule or wall.

Trabecula carnae The interlacing muscular columns projecting from inner surface of ventricles of the heart.

Trabeculae lienis Fibromuscular bands which pass into the spleen from the capsule.

Trabeculoplasty A drainage surgery of trabecular meshwork in glaucoma

t. ascending white fibers in spinal cord carrying nerve impulses towards brain

t. descending fibers in spinal cord that carry impulse from brain to spinal centers

t. dorsolateral in spinal cord, tract superficial to the tip of dorsal horn, the fibers of pain and temperature

t. ilitibial a thickned part of fascia lata extending from lateral condyle of tibia to iliac crest

t. olfactory extends from olfactory bulb to anterior perforated substance

t. optic fibers of optic nerve beyond optic chiasma, most of which terminate in lateral geniculate body of thalamus

t. pyramidal one of the three descending tracts (lateral, ventrolateral and ventral) arising from Betz cells the motor area of brain

t. rubrospinal tracts from red nucleus of midbrain to spinal cord

t. uveal includes iris, choroid and ciliary body.

Trace 1. Very small quantity. 2. A visible mark or sign.

Trace elements Organic elements normally present in minute quantity but very essential for plant or animal life.

Tracer An isotope which due to its unique physical properties, can be detected in extremely minute quantity, and hence is used to trace the chemical behavior of natural element; used in absorption and excretion studies for identifying intermediary products of metabolism and determination of distribution of various substances in the body. Commonly used tracers are ^{14}C and ^{131}I.

Trachea The round cartilaginous air tube extending from larynx to bronchi (6th cervical to 5th dorsal vertebra).

Trachealis Smooth muscle fibers extending between the ends of

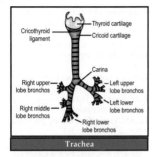

Cricothyroid ligament — Thyroid cartilage — Cricoid cartilage

Carina

Right upper lobe bronchos — Left upper lobe bronchos

Right middle lobe bronchos — Left lower lobe bronchos

Right lower lobe bronchos

Trachea

tracheal rings whose contraction narrows the lumen.

Tracheal ring C-shaped fibrous rings of trachea.

Tracheal tug The downward tugging movement of larynx in thoracic aortic aneurysm.

Tracheitis Inflammation of trachea.

Trachelectomy Amputation of uterine cervix.

Trachelitis Inflammation of cervix.

Trachelology Scientific study of neck, its diseases and injuries.

Trachelorraphy Repair of torn cervix.

Tracheobronchomegaly Congenital enlargement of trachea and bronchi.

Tracheocele Protrusion of tracheal mucous membrane through its wall.

Tracheomalacia Softening of cartilaginous framework of trachea.

Tracheostomy Surgical opening up of trachea to put an airway to facilitate respiration in laryngeal obstruction or a condition requiring prolonged respiratory assistance.

Trachitis Inflammation of trachea.

Trachoma A form of chronic follicular conjunctivitis caused by *Chlamydia trachomatis*.

Trachyphonia Roughness of voice.

Tracing A graphic record of some events like respiration, electrical activity of heart and brain.

Tract 1. A pathway 2. Bundle of nerve fibers within spinal cord or brain acting as an anatomical and functional unit.

Traction The act of drawing or pulling.

t. axis Traction in line with the long axis of the part.

t. aneurysm An aneurysm due to traction on artery, e.g. traction on aorta by an incompletely atrophied ductus.

t. diverticulum A circumscribed sacculation usually of the esophagus due to pull of adhesions.

t. headache Pain arising from traction on intracranial structures by tumors, hematoma, abscess, etc.

Tract of Schuz Periventricular tract.

Tractotomy Surgical section of a tract in CNS, e.g. for pain relief.

Tragion An anthropometric point on tragus of ear.

Tragus Cartilaginous projection in front of external auditory meatus.

Training 1. An organized system of instruction 2. Systematic exercise for physical development or some specialized aim.

Trait A characteristic or property of an individual.

Tramazoline An adrenergic agent.

Trance The state of hypnosis resembling sleep or a state of being mentally out of touch with the environment.

Tranexamic acid An antifibrinolytic drug 10 times potent than aminocaproic acid; used to decrease bleeding.

Tranquilizer A drug reducing mental tension and anxiety without interfering with normal mental activity.

Transaminase An enzyme that catalyzes transamination, i.e. transfer of amino group of an amino acid to a ketoacid.

t. glutamic-oxaloacetic **(SGOT)** Highest concentration in heart muscle and liver; hence raised in myocardial infarction and hepatitis.

t. glutamic-pyruvic Highest concentration in liver. Injury to hepatic cells liberates the enzyme to blood stream.

Transanimation Resuscitation by mouth to mouth respiration.

Transatrial Procedure done through or across the atrium.

Transcortin A corticosteroid binding globulin.

Transcriptase A polymerase that transcripts by converting a DNA base sequence into its complementary RNA base sequence.

Transcription The DNA directed synthesis of messenger RNA.

Transcutaneous nerve stimulation (TNS) Application of mild electrical stimulation to skin electrodes placed over a painful area to block transmission of pain sensation into CNS.

Transducer Device that converts one form of energy into another, e.g. ultrasonic transducers that convert sound energy to electrical energy.

Transection Cutting across the long axis.

Transfer factor A factor present in antigen sensitized lymphocytes.

Transferrin Iron transporting globulin in plasma.

Transfixion The act of piercing through and through.

Transfixion sutures A method of closing a wound by the use of suture which is placed through both wound edges in a figure of eight fashion.

Transformation Change of shape or form, in oncology the change of one tissue into another; a type of mutation occurring in bacteria.

Transfusion Injection of blood, blood products or IV solutions into vein.

t. exchange Transfusion of blood and withdrawal of blood at same time until blood volume is entirely replaced as in hemolytic disease of newborn.

Transfusion reaction A variety of reactions including fever, chill, hemolysis, jaundice, shock and anaphylaxis occurring during transfusion.

Transgrow A special medium for culture of *N. gonorrhea.*

Transient ischaemic attack (TIA) Symptoms of neurological deficit lasting for few hours without residual damage due to transient interference with blood supply to brain.

Transillumination Inspection of a cavity or organ by passing a light through its wall, e.g. examination of paranasal sinus by means of a light placed across mouth; examination of hydrocele contents in scrotum and examination of brain in hydrocephalus in infants.

Transition Passing from one state or position to another.

Translation Protein synthesis under direction of RNA.

Translocation The displacement of part or whole of chromosome to another.

Translucent Permitting a partial transmission of light; somewhat transparent

Transmethylation Transfer of a methyl group from a donor to a receptor compound. Methionine and choline serve as donors of methyl group.

Transmigration A wandering across or through as that of ovum or leukocytes across the capillary wall.

Transmissible Capable of being transmitted from one person to another; communicable, infectious.

Transmission Transfer of anything; like disease or hereditary characteristics.

t. mechanical Passive transfer of causative agent of disease, especially by arthropods, e.g., fly borne diseases.

t. placental Transmission of disease from mother to fetus via the placenta.

t. synaptic The mechanism by which an impulse in one neurone gives rise to impulse in another neurone.

t. transovarian Transmission of a diseased agent to offspring from mother from infection of ovary of latter as in ticks and mites.

Transmural Across a wall, e.g. myocardial infarction involving full thickness of wall in a given area.

Transparent Permitting passage of light rays without obstruction.

Transpeptidase An enzyme that catalyzes the transfer of a peptide from one compound to another.

Transplant To transfer tissue or organ from one part to another.

Transplantation The operation of transplanting an organ or tissue from one person to another, e.g. heart, lung, kidney, liver and bone marrow.

t. heteroplastic Transplantation of a part from one individual to another of the same or closely related species.

t. heterotopic Transplantation in which transplant is placed in a different location in host than it had in donor.

Transport Movement or transfer of substances in biological system; transport may be active, passive or carrier mediated.

Transposition A change in position of an organ or viscera usually to opposite side.

Transposition of great vessels A congenital cardiac anomaly where aorta arises from right ventricle and pulmonary artery from left ventricle.

Trans-sexual An individual who has overwhelming desire or feels psychically to be of opposite sex or has got his external sex changed by surgery.

Transthyretin A serum prealbumin that transports thyroxin.

t. multidrug resistant MDR TB is on rise and bacilli are resistant to many first line drugs.

Transudate A fluid that passes through the capillary wall.

Transudation Oozing of fluid through the membrane.

Transurethral An operation performed through urethra, e.g. transurethral prostatectomy.

Transversalis A structure occurring at right angles to the long axis of body.

Transversalis fascia The thin membrane lying between the transversus abdominis muscle and the peritoneum.

Transverse arrest In obstetrics, arrest of transverse axis of descending fetal head in maternal pelvis.

Transverse mesocolon The transverse portion of mesentery connecting transverse colon with posterior abdominal wall.

Transverse myelitis Inflammation of spinal cord involving entire cord substance at a particular level, usually of unknown etiology.

Transverse sinus A sinus of dura mater running from internal occipital protuberance along attached margin of tentorium cerebelli to reach jugular foramen.

Transvestism Dressing or masquerading in the clothing of opposite

sex to be accepted as a member of opposite sex.

Tranta's dots Chalky concretions of the conjunctiva around the limbus associated with vernal conjunctivitis.

Tranylcypromine An antidepressant of MAO inhibitor group.

Trapezium The first bone of the second row of carpal bones.

Trapezius The muscle arising from occipital bone, nuchal ligament and the spines of thoracic vertebra and inserted into clavicle, acromion and spine of scapula.

Trapezoid ligament The lateral portion of coraco clavicular ligament.

Trauma A physical injury or wound caused by external force or violence.

t. psychic A painful emotional experience.

Traumatology The branch of surgery dealing with wounds and their care.

Tray A flat surface with raised edges.

t. impression In dentistry U shaped receptacle to carry impression material and support it in contact with teeth.

Tranyl cypromine Monoamine oxidase inhibitor antidepressant.

Treacher Collin's syndrome Mandibulofacial dysostosis.

Treatment Any specific procedure employed for amelioration of a disease or pathological condition.

t. empiric Treatment based on observation and experience rather than having a scientific basis.

t. expectant Relief of symptoms that arise during an illness but treatment not directed at specific cause of illness.

t. palliative Symptomatic treatment rather than a cure.

Trechoic acid A polymer found on some bacterial cell wall

Trematoda A class of flatworms commonly known as flukes.

Tremble Involuntary shaking or quivering.

Tremograph A device for recording tremors.

Tremor Involuntary movement resulting from alternate contraction of opposing muscle groups.

t. action Tremor when voluntary motion is attempted.

t. alcoholic Visible tremor in alcoholics.

t. cerebellar Intention tremor of 3-5 Hz frequency seen in cerebellar disease.

t. essential Benign tremor usually of head, chin, outstretched hands, 8-10 cycles per second, made worse by anxiety and action, usually familial.

t. flapping Coarse tremor with momentary loss of tone in muscle groups followed by return of tone *SYN* — asterixis, seen in hepatic encephalopathy.

t. parkinsonian A rest tremor which is suppressed briefly during voluntary activity, usually pill rolling type.

t. physiologic Tremor occurring in normal persons during anger, anxiety, fatigue and hypoglycemia.

Tremulous Trembling or shaking.

Trench fever The disease caused by *Rickettsia quintana,* transmitted by body louse.

Trench foot A condition skin to frost bite due to keeping of feet in wet socks and shoes for prolonged period.

Trench mouth Painful pseudomembranous ulceration of mucous membrane of mouth.

Trend The tendency to proceed in a certain direction.

Trendelenburg position Position in which patient's head is low and the legs are on an elevated and incline position.

Trephine A cylindrical saw for cutting circular piece of bone out of skull.

Trepidant Marked by tremor.

Trepidation Fear, anxiety, trembling motion.

Treponema A genus of spirochetes causing infections in man, e.g. syphilis *(T. pallidium)* pinta *(T. carateum),* frambesia *(T. pertenue).*

Treponea Condition of being able to breathe easily when in a certain position.

Tretinoin Transretinoic acid used topically for acne.

Triacetin Antifungal agent used topically.

Triad Any three things having or denoting something in common.

Triage The screening and classification of sick, wounded or injured during war or disaster to assign priority for medical and nursing attention.

Triamcinolone Synthetic gluco-corticoid used for skin conditions.

Triamterene A potassium sparing diuretic.

Triangle An area formed by three angles and three sides.

t. anal Triangle formed by ischial tuberosities and tip of coccyx.

t. anterior of neck Space bounded by midline of neck, anterior border of sternocleidomastoid and lower border of mandible.

t. digastric Space bounded by mandible, stylohyoid muscle and anterior belly of digastric muscle.

t. femoral Triangle on inner part of thigh bounded by inguinal ligament above and satorius and adductor longus muscles below.

t. Hesselbach's The area in the lower anterior abdominal wall bounded by inguinal ligament below, the edge of the rectus muscle medially and the deep epigastric artery laterally.

t. of Petit The space above the hip bone between the exterior oblique muscle, the latissimus dorsi and the interior oblique muscle.

t. posterior cervical The triangular area bounded by upper border of clavicle, the posterior border of sternocleidomastoid and the anterior border of trapezius muscle.

t. urogenital Triangle with the base formed by a line between the two ischial tuberosities and the apex at symphysis pubis.

Triangular bandage A bandage folded diagonally.

Triangular ligament The ligaments left and right connecting right and left lobes of liver with corresponding portions of diaphragm.

Triatoma A genus of blood sucking bugs, one variety of it transmits *Trypanosoma cruzi*, causative agent of Chaga's disease.

Triazolam Benzodiazepine anxiolytic.

Tribadism A condition where women attempt to imitate heterosexual intercourse with each other.

Tribasic Composed of three replaceable hydrogen atoms.

Tribasilar synostosis Condition resulting from fusion of occipital, sphenoid and temporal bones leading to arrested cerebral development and mental deficiency.

Tribe A taxonomic division between genus and family.

Tribromoethanol An anesthetic agent.

Tricarboxylic acid cycle The metabolic cycle of pyruvic acid breakdown for production of energy; the terminal pathway whereby fats, carbohydrates and proteins are utilized.

Triceps A muscle arising by three heads.

Triceps reflex Extension of forearm on tapping the triceps tendon while the elbow is flexed.

Trichiasis Inwardly directed eye lashes that rub against cornea.

Trichinella A genus of nematode. *Trichinella spiralis* of this genus causes trichinosis from ingestion of undercooked pork containing the cyst.

Trichinellosis Disease caused by *Trichinella spiralis* SYN — trichinosis. Symptoms are swelling of face, firm, tender swollen muscles, fever and eosinophilia.

Trichion The anthropometric point where midsagittal plane of head intersects the hairline.

Trichitis Inflammation of hair bulbs.

Trichloracetic acid The caustic agent used for cauterization of warts, condylomata and hyperplastic tissue.

Trichlorethylene Inhalational anesthetic that supplements nitrous oxide.

Tricho bezoar A hair ball in the stomach.

Trichogen An agent stimulating hair growth.

Trichokryptomania Abnormal desire to break off hair by finger nail.

Trichoma Matted and encrusted state of hair.

Trichology Study of hair, its growth and care.

Trichomatosis Entangled matted hair due to fungal disease.

Trichome A hair or other appendage of skin.

Trichomonal Resembling Trichomonas.

Trichomonas Genus of flagellated protozoa.

T. hominis Intestinal flagellate causing diarrhea and bacillary dysentery like disease.

T. vaginalis Flagellate inhabiting vagina causing profuse white watery often blood stained discharge and intense itching.

Trichomycosis Any fungal disease of hair.

Trichophagia The habit of hair eating.

Trichophytobezoar A hair ball found in the stomach along with vegetable fiber and other debris.

Trichophyton Parasitic fungus living on skin or its appendages.

Trichorrhexis Splitting of hair.

Trichosis Any disease of hair or its abnormal growth.

Trichosporon A genus of fungi growing on hair.

Trichotilomania Unnatural impulse to pull out one's own hair.

Trichotomy Division into three parts.

Trichotoxin A toxin that destroys ciliated epithelial cells.

Trichromatic Able to differentiate three primary colors, which means normal color vision.

Trichuriasis Infestation with *Trichuris trichura*.

Trichuris trichura A nematode that inhabits large intestine and causes diarrhea and abdominal pain.

Tricitrates oral solution Solution of sodium citrate, potassium citrate and citric acid.

Triclophos sodium A sedative-hypnotic preparation.

Tricuspid Having three cusps, e.g. tricuspid valve, tricuspid tooth.

Tricuspid atresia Congenital atresia of tricuspid valve with cyanosis and clubbing.

Tricuspid valve Right atrioventricular valve.

Trident Having three prongs.

Tridihexethyl chloride An anticholinergic agent.

Triencephalus A deformed fetus lacking organs for sight, smell and hearing.

Triethylenemelamine One member of nitrogen mustard group of antineoplastic agent.

Triethylenethiophosphoramide An alkylating agent used in cancer chemotherapy. *SYN*— thiotepa.

Trifluoperazine An antipsychotic agent (Espazine).

Triflu promazine Anti-psychotic agent used mainly for nausea and vomiting (Siquil).

Trifluridine Antiviral agent.

Trifurcation Division into three branches.

Trigeminal nerve The fifth cranial nerve, the sensory-motor nerve dividing into 1. ophthalmic (supplies upper part of face, nasal mucosa, cornea and conjunctiva). 2. maxillary (supplies gums and teeth of upper jaw, upper lip and orbit) and 3. mandibular supplying muscles of mastication, gum and teeth of lower jaw.

Trigeminal neuralgia Neuralgic pain (burning and tingling) in distribution of trigeminal nerve due to any lesion of Gasserian ganglion or compression of its large sensory root by an aberrant artery and often idiopathic.

Trigeminal pulse Pulse where every third beat is an extrasystole.

Trigger To initiate with suddenness. An event or impulse that initiates other events or actions.

Trigger finger A state when finger flexion or extension is accomplished with a jerk due to tenosynovitis.

Trigger zone Any area of hyper excitability in the body which when stimulated precipitates a specific response, e.g. epileptic fit or an attack of neuralgia.

Triglyceride Combination of glycerol with three different fatty acids.

Trigone A triangular area at the base of bladder i.e., between the two openings of ureter and internal urinary meatus.

Trigone olfactory A small triangular eminence at the root of olfactory peduncle.

Tigonitis Inflammation of mucous membrane of the trigone of bladder.

Trihexyphenidyl hydrochloride An anticholinergic drug used in parkinsonism.

Triidothyronine T_3, the active form of thyroid hormone.

Trikates A mixture of potassium acetate, potassium bicarbonate and potassium citrate.

Trilabe A three pronged forcep for removing foreign body from bladder.

Trilaminar Three layered.

Trilobate Having three lobes.

Trilocular Having three compartments.

Triology A series of three events.

Trimeprazine tartarate Antipyretic agent.

Trimester A block of 3 months.

Trimethadione An anticonvulsant.

Trimethaphan Ganglion blocking agent used for treatment of hypertension.

Trimethobenzamide An antiemetic drug.

Trimethoprim Antibacterial agent used for urinary tract infection; when combined with sulfamethoxazole causes sequential block in enzyme synthesis within a wide range of bacteria.

Triethylene Cyclopropane, the general anesthetic agent.

Trimipramine Tricyclic antidepressant.

Trimmer Instrument used to cut and shape things like gingiva, dental plaster.

Trimorphous Having three different forms like larva, pupa and adults as in insects.

Trinitroglycerol Nitroglycerin, the vasodilator.

Trinitrophenol *SYN* — Picric acid, reagent.

Trinitrotoluene *SYN* — TNT, an explosive.

Triorchidism Having 3 testes.

Triose A monosaccharide with 3 carbon atoms.

Trioxsalen Agent that induces repigmentation, hence used in vitiligo.

Trip Hallucinatory experience produced by various drugs.

Tripelenamine citrate An antihistaminic agent.

Tripier's amputation Amputation of foot with part of calcaneus.

Tripotassium dicitrato bismuthate Bismuth compound used in peptic ulcer.

Triple response The three basic response of skin to injury like redness, flare and wheal.

Triplet Three children in one pregnancy.

Triploidy Having three supports or legs.

Tripod Having three sets of chromosomes.

Tripolidine hydrochloride An antihistaminic drug.

Triquetrum Three cornered or triangular, e.g. cuneiform bone.

Triradiate Radiating in three directions.

Trismus Tonic spasm of jaw muscles as in tetanus.

Trisomy Having three homologous chromosomes instead of two.

T13 Trisomy of chromosome 13 manifest with hypertelorism, low set ears, mental retardation and death during infancy.

T18 Same as above.

T21 Down syndrome with simian crease, sloping forehead, epicanthic folds, Brush field's spots, flat nose and mental retardation.

Trisulfapyrimidines A combination of sulfamerazine, sulfa methazine and sulfadiazine.

Tritanopia Blue blindness.

Tritium Heavier form of hydrogen.

Trituration The act of making a substance into powdered form.

Trivalent Combining with or replacing three hydrogen atoms.

Trocar The instrument which is contained within the cannula for removal of fluid from body cavity.

Trochanter Bony processes.

t. greater Outward projection at upper end of femur below its neck.

t. fesser Conical tuberosity at the inner and posterior surface of upper end of femur at the junction of shaft and neck.

Troche Solid cylindrical form containing medicine. *SYN*—Lozenge.

Trochlea 1. The smooth articular surface of bone upon which glides another bone 2. A structure having the function of pulley.

Trochlear fovea A depression in the orbital plate of frontal bone for attachment of the cartilaginous pulley of superior oblique muscle.

Trochlear nerve The fourth cranial nerve emerging from dorsal surface of midbrain and supplying superior oblique muscle.

Trombicula A genus of mite that may serve as vectors for various diseases.

Tromethamine *SYN* — THAM. A systemic alkalizer used in lactic acidosis.

Trophic Relating to nutrition of a part particularly when denervated.

Trophoblast The outermost layer of developing embryo consisting of inner cytotrophoblast and outer syntrophoblast that comes in contact with uterine endometrium.

Trophocyte The supporting cells of Sertoli which nourish the developing spermatozoa.

Trophology The science of nutrition.

Trophozoite The active mobile feeding state of protozoa.

Tropia Deviation of eyes away from visual axis: esotropia means inward; exotropia outward; hypertropia upward and hypotropia downward.

Tropicamide An anticholinergic drug used for producing mydriasis as 2% lotion.

Tropin When suffixed indicates stimulating effect especially of a hormone on target tissue.

Tropism Involuntary response of an organism like turning towards or away from a stimulus.

Tropomyosin A muscle protein involved in the formation of cross bridges during muscle contraction.

Troponin A muscle protein that attaches to actin and myosin. It binds to calcium and inhibits actin-myosin cross bridge formation.

Trousseau's sign Muscle spasm or tetany induced by pressure on the nerve, indicative of latent tetany.

True conjugate The distance from posterior surface of symphysis pubis to sacral promontory (11 cm.)

Trunk The main stem of lymphatic, nerve or blood vessel. The middle portion of body without head and limbs.

Truss Device to occlude hernial orifica.

Trypanosoma A genus of flagellate protozoa found in blood, e.g. *T cruzi* causing Chaga's disease and *T. rodesiense* causing African sleeping sickness.

Tryparsamide An arsenic compound used in sleeping sickness.

Trypsin Proteolytic enzyme formed by action of enterokinase on pancreatic trypsinogen.

Trypsinogen Inactive form of trypsin found in pancreatic juice.

Tryptophan An essential amino acid, the precursor of serotonin.

Tsetse fly Blood sucking fly of genus glossina, transmitter of trypanosomiasis.

Tsutsugamushi fever Scrub typhus.

t. tube A tube placed in common bile duct after cholecystectomy for bile drainage and cholangiography.

Tuaminoheptane A sympathomimetic used topically in nasal drops.

Tube A long hollow cylindrical structure.

t. endotracheal A tube usually with an inflatable cuff put into trachea for airway during anesthesia.

t. nasogastric Rubber tube passed into stomach for aspiration/decompression of stomach.

t. Segstaken-Blackmore Three passaged nasogastric tube for treating bleeding esophageal varices.

t. stomach A wide bore tube for stomach wash in poisoning.

Tubectomy Surgical removal of a part or whole of fallopian tube.

Tuber A swelling or enlargement.

Tuber cinereum A part of base of hypothalamus connected to posterior lobe of pituitary by an infundibulum.

Tubercle 1. A small rounded elevation on bone or skin 2. tubercular granuloma.

t. adductor The bony tubercle on femur serving for attachment of tendon of adductor magnus.

t. dental A small elevation on crown of tooth representing thickened enamel or accessory cusp.

t. deltoid Tubercle on clavicle for attachment of deltoid muscle.

t. genital The embryonic structure which becomes penis or clitoris.

t. miliary Tubercle resembling millet seed, as in tuberculosis.

Tuberculin A preparation from human tubercle bacilli, used for diagnostic test of previous exposure to tubercular infection.

Tuberculin test A test to know if a patient has been exposed to tubercle bacilli in the past 5 or 10 TU is injected intradermally and induration is measured after 72 hours. When induration exceeds 10×10 mm the test is termed positive.

Tuberculoma A tuberculous abscess.

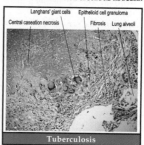
Tuberculosis

Tuberculosis An infectious disease caused by *Mycobacterium tuberculosis* having propensity to infect lungs, bone, GU tract, meninges and the GI tract.

Tuberosity An elevated bony process, e.g. ischial tuberosity.

Tuberous sclerosis A neurocutaneous disorder with adenoma sebaceum, seizure, mental retardation, periventricular nodules.

Tubocurarine A skeletal muscle relaxant used during anesthesia and in convulsive states and to treat black-widow spider bite.

Tubo-ovarian Relates to fallopian tube and the ovary.

Tuboplasty Plastic surgery or repair of fallopian tubes in order to restore fertility.

Tubotympanal Relates to tympanic membrane and the eustachian tube.

Tubule A small tube.

t. collecting Tubules having transport function in renal medulla.

t. convoluted The constituent parts of a nephron of kidney.

t. dentinal Very small canals in the dentine.

t. seminiferous Very small tubules in testis in which the spermatozoa develop and leave the testis to enter the epididymis.

Tubulin A protein present in the microtubules of cell.

Tubulodermoid A dermoid tumor in the persistent remnant tubular structure.

Tuft A small coiled mass or cluster.

Tugging Drag or pull, e.g. tracheal tug, the sign of aortic aneurysm.

Tularemia A plague like illness caused by *Francisella tularensis*, transmitted to man by bite of infected tick or direct contact with infected animal. (Tulare : a place in California).

Tumefacient Producing a swelling.

Tumescence Swelling.

Tumor A swelling or enlargement.

t. carotid body Benign tumor arising from carotid body.

t. connective tissue e.g., lipoma, fibroma and sarcomas.

t. desmoid Tumor of fibrous connective tissue.

t. Ewing's Malignant round cell tumor of bone.

t. giant cell Locally malignant tumor of bone consisting of multinucleated cells surrounded by cellular spindle cell stroma.

t. granulosa cell Tumor arising from granulosa cells of ovary secreting estrogen.

t. islet cells Insulin secreting tumors from islet cells of Langerhans in pancreas.

t. Krukenberg's Tumor of ovary from transperitoneal metastasis of GI tract malignancy.

Tumor angiogenesis factor A protein factor present in all cancerous tissue which stimulates capillary growth.

Tumoricidal Having killing effect on tumor cells.

Tumor markers Certain substances present in blood that indicate possible presence of malignancy, e.g. carcinoembryonic antigen in tumors of colon, lungs and breast; alfa fetoprotein in hepatoma, acid, phosphatase in prostatic malignancy.

Tumor necrosis factor A lymphokine produced by macrophages.

Tumor viruses Viruses causing malignant neoplasms, e.g. EB virus

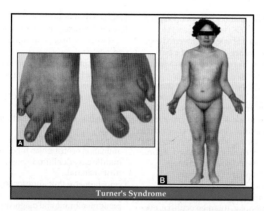

Turner's Syndrome

linked to Burkitt's lymphoma; HSV$_2$ in cancer cervix, AIDS virus in Kaposi sarcoma.

Tunga A genus of fleas.

Tungsten A metallic element used in X-ray tube.

Tunica A covering.

t. adventia The outer fibrous coat of blood vessels.

t. intima The innermost layer of endothelial cells and the basement membrane including the internal elastic lamina of blood vessels.

t. media The middle layer in the wall of a blood vessel containing circular smooth muscle and elastic fibers.

t. serosa The mesothelial lining of the pleura, peritoneum and pericardium.

t. vaginalis The serous membrane surrounding the testes.

Tuning fork A vibrating metallic instrument for testing hearing and sensation of vibration.

Tunnel A narrow channel.

t. carpal The fibro-osseous canal in the wrist through which pass the flexor tendons and the median nerve.

t. tarsal The osteofibrous canal bounded by flexor retinaculum and tarsal bones giving way to posterior tibial vessels, tibial nerve and flexor tendons.

Tunnel vision 1. Severe constriction of visual field as in chronic glaucoma 2. A condition in hysterics where the field of vision remains the same irrespective of the distance from the visual screen.

Turbid Cloudy.

Turbidity The quality of not having transparency of liquid due to contamination or suspended particles.

Turbinate Shaped like inverted cone.

Turgescence Swelling of a part.

Turgor Normal tension in a tissue, swelling.

Turner's syndrome 45 (XO) chromosomal pattern in girls manifested with amenorrhea, infertility, short stature and poor sexual maturation.

Turpentine A pine plant derivative containing mixture of terpenes and other hydrocarbon used in liniments and counter irritants.

Turricephaly Oxycephaly.

Tussis Cough.

Tutamen Tissue with protective action, e.g. tutamen oculi, i.e. eyebrows, eyelashes, etc.

t. wave The positive or negative wave representing repolarisation of heart muscle in electrocardiogram.

Twig A final branch of a nerve or vessel.

Twilight sleep A state of partial anesthesia where perception of pain is greatly reduced.

Twin Two fetuses developing within uterus, in one pregnancy.

t. dizygotic Twins developed from two separate ova.

t. monozygotic Twins developing from a single fertilized ovum; hence have identical genetic makeup, are of same sex, have common placenta and one chorion sac.

t. Siamese Symmetrically united twins.

Twinge A sudden pain.

Twitch Sudden spasmodic muscle contraction.

Tylosis Formation of a callus.

Tyloxapol A detergent used to reduce viscosity of bronchopulmonary secretions.

Tympanic membrane Membrane at the junction middle ear and external ear.

Tympanites Intestinal distention with gas.

Tympanitis Inflammation of middle ear.

Tympanography Radiographic examination of eustachian tubes and middle ear after introducing contrast material.

Tympanometry Procedure for objective evaluation of mobility of tympanic membrane and diagnosis of middle ear diseases.

Tympanoplasty Surgical procedure for middle ear disease or reconstruction.

Tympanum The middle ear or tympanic cavity.

Tympany 1. Abdominal distension with gas 2. Tympanic resonance on percussion.

Typhlectomy Excision of cecum.

Typhlitis Inflammation of cecum.

Typhlodicliditis Inflammation of ileocecal valve.

Typhlology Study of blindness and its causes.

Typhlomegaly Abnormally large cecum.

Typhlopexy Suturing of movable cecum to anterior abdominal wall.

Typhloureterostomy Implantation of ureters into cecum.

Typhoid Resembling typhus.

Typhoid fever Acute infectious fever with inflamed Peyer's patches and mesenteric glands, enlarged spleen and continuous fever; caused by *Salmonella typhi.*

Typhoid vaccine Vaccine containing killed *Salmonella typhi.*

Typhus A group of acute infectious fevers with severe headache, prostration, maculopapular rash, and some neurologic involvement caused by Rickettsia organisms.

t. epidemic Caused by *R. prowazekii,* transmitted by body louse.

t. endemic Caused by *R. mooseri,* transmitted by rat flea.

t. scrub Caused by *R. tsutsugamushi,* transmitted by mites.

Typing Identification of types, e.g. 1. Bacteriophage typing, i.e. determination of bacterial species by bacteriophages. 2. Tissue typing, i.e. testing for histocompatibility of tissues to be used in transplant or graft.

Tyramine An intermediate product during conversion of tyrosine to epinephrine, found in cheese, beer, yeast, beans, wine and chicken liver.

Tyroid Cheesy or caseous.

Tyrosinage An enzyme that converts tyrosine into melanin.

Tyrosine An amino acid serving as precursor for epinephrine, thyroxine and melanin.

Tyrosinemia Increased tyrosine concentration in blood due to deficiency of enzyme tyrosine aminotransferase manifested with mental retardation, keratitis, dermatitis, etc.

Tyrothricin Antibacterial agent.

Tyrrell's fascia Ill defined fascia behind prostate.

Tyson's glands Modified sebaceous glands in prepuce secreting smegma.

Tzanck test Examination of tissue from base of an intact bulla to demonstrate degenerative changes as in pemphigus.

Tzank cell A degenerated cell from keratin layer of skin, seen in pemphigus.

U

Ubiquinone Coenzyme Q, important for intracellular respiration.

Ulalgia Gum pain.

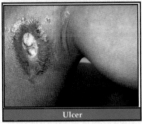
Ulcer

Ulcer Discontinuity in the skin or mucous membrane with sloughing.

u. Curling Stress induced peptic ulcer as in post burn or cerebrovascular accident patient.

u. decubitus Ischemic necrosis and tissue ulceration over bony prominence in bedridden patients.

u. Huner's Painful slowly healing ulcer in urinary bladder.

u. rodent Deeply infiltrating ulcer with undermined edges as in basal cell carcinoma.

u. serpiginous A creeping ulcer that heals in one part but extends to another.

Ulitis Inflammation of gums.

Ulna The inner and larger bone of forearm.

Ulotomy Incision of gums; resection of scar tissue to relieve tension.

Ultrafiltration A filtration process that separates colloidal particles from the suspending liquid.

Ultrasonic Sound frequency above 20,000 cycles per second, not audible to human ear.

Ultrasonography Use of ultrasound to image body organs.

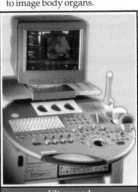
Ultrasound

Ultrasound Sound frequency in the range of 20,000 to 10^9 cycles per second, employed to image body organs and for therapeutic purposes, (ultrasonic ablation/stone dissolution).

Ultrastructure Structure of tissue as visible only under electron microscope but not to normal eye.

Ultraviolet rays Light rays in the spectrum of 3900-1800 angstroms.

Umbilical cord The cord consisting two arteries and one vein embedded in Wharton's jelly attaching fetus to placenta.

Umbilication Formation at the apex of a vesicle or pustule a depression (e.g. in smallpox), any depression resembling the navel.

Umbilicus The navel or depression in the center of abdomen.

Umbo Projecting center of a round surface.

Umbrella filter A filter placed in a vein to prevent passage of emboli as in prevention of pulmonary infarction in deep vein thrombosis.

Uncal herniation Transtentorial herniation of uncus.

Unciform Shaped like a hook.

Unciform fasciculus The bundle of fibers connecting frontal lobes with temporal lobes (uncinate fasciculus).

Unciform process Anterior end of hippocampal gyrus.

Uncinate Hook shaped.

Uncinate bundle of Russel Fibers from cerebellum passing into vestibular nuclei via superior cerebellar peduncle.

Uncinate fits Periodic episodes of olfactory and gustatory hallucinations usually disagreeable or loss of taste and smell.

Uncinate gyrus Rostral portion of hippocampal gyrus.

Unconditioned reflex Natural reflex which is independent of previous experience or training.

Unconscious Lacking awareness of surrounding.

Uncus Hooked anterior end of hippocampal gyrus.

Underweight Weight more than 10% less than the ideal weight for height and age.

Undine A small glass or metal flask for irrigation of eyes.

Undecylenic acid A fungistatic 11-carbon acid.

Undine curse Sleep apnea.

Undulation Continuous wave like motion or pulsation.

Ungual Resembling nails.

Unguentum Ointment.

Unguis A finger or toe nail.

u. incarnatus Ingrowing nail.

Uniceps Having a single head.

Unicorn Having a single horn or cornu as in uterus.

Unicuspid Having a single cusp, e.g. tooth or valve.

Unilateral Affecting or occurring at one side.

Uninucleated Having a single nucleus.

Uniocular Pertains to one eye.

Union Meeting of two or more things at one point.

Uniparous Giving birth to one offspring at a time.

Unipolar Having a single process, e.g. unipolar neurone.

Unit A standard of measurement.

u. angstrom Wave length of 1/10,000,000 of a millimeter.

u. motor A neurone and the muscle cells innervated by it.

u. mouse Least amount of estrogen that brings characteristic change in mouse vaginal epithelium.

u. todd The reciprocal of the highest dilution that inhibits hemolysis as in measurement of antistreptolysin O titre in rheumatic fever.

Univalent Capable of combining with or replacing one atom of hydrogen.

Universal antidote Two parts of activated charcoal, one part magnesium oxide and one part tannic acid used in poisoning by unknown agents by oral route.

Universal donor A person of blood group 'O' Rh -ve.

Universal recipient A person of blood group AB, Rh positive. Unmedullated A nerve without myelin sheath. *SYN* – unmyelinated.

Unna's paste 15% Zinc oxide in glycogelatin base.

Unsaturated Not combined to the full extent or capable of dissolving or absorbing more.

Uptake Absorption of nutrient or radioactive material.

Urachus A fibrous cord extending from apex of bladder to umbilicus. Often urachus remains patent resulting in an umbilical urinary fistula.

Uracil A pyrimidine base of ribonucleic acids.

Uranium A radioactive element

Uranorrhaphy Operation for closure of cleft palate.

Urate A salt of uric acid.

Urea The diamide of carbonic acid derived from ammonia by deamination representing 80-90% of total urinary nitrogen.

Urea cycle The metabolic process of urea formation from metabolism of nitrogen containing foods.

Urea frost Deposits of urea particle on skin in patients of advanced uremia.

Urea plasma A microorganism is sexually transmitted and causes urogenital infection in both partners.

Urease An enzyme that breaks down urea into ammonia and carbon dioxide.

Uremia A complex biochemical abnormality in kidney failure, characterized by azotemia, acidosis, anemia and many systemic symptoms.

u. prerenal Uremia occurring not primarily due to kidney disease but due to fluid loss.

Ureter 28-34 cm fibromuscular tubes conveying urine from kidney to urinary bladder.

Ureterocele Dilatation of ureter near its opening into bladder.

Urodialysis Rupture of ureter.

Ureteroenterostomy Establishment of communication between ureter and intestine.

Ureteroileostomy Anastomosis of ureter into a segment of small intestine.

Ureterolith A stone in ureter.

Ureteropyeloplasty Plastic surgery of pelvis of kidney and ureter.

Ureterovesicostomy Reimplantation of ureters into bladder.

Urethane Compound with diuretic, hypnotic and cytostatic properties, often used in leukemia.

Urethra The canal extending from bladder neck to exterior for discharge of urine.

Urethrismus Irritation or spasm of urethra.

Urethritis Inflammation of urethra.

u. anterior Inflammation of anterior portion of urethra (portion anterior to triangular ligament).

u. gonococcal Gonococcal infection of urethra.

u. nonspecific Chlamydial urethritis.

u. posterior Urethritis involving prostatic and membranous urethra.

Urethroplasty Repair of urethra as in stricture.

Urethroscope An instrument for visualization of interior of urethra.

Urethrostenosis Stricture urethra.

Urethrotomy Incision into urethra as a part of operation for stricture.

Uric acid An end product of purine metabolism responsible for clinical manifestations of gout.

Uricase An enzyme present in most mammals excluding man that breaks uric acid into allantoin and carbon dioxide.

Uricemia Excess uric acid in blood.

Uricocholia Uric acid in bile.

Uricosuria Excessive excretion of uric acid in urine.

Uricosuric Agents that potentiate excretion of uric acid in urine.

Uridrosis Excess of urea in sweat.

Uridine A nucleoside of ribonucleic acids, consisting of uracil and D ribose.

Uriesthesis Normal desire to void urine.

Urinary pigments Urochrome, urosilin, uroerythrin and hematoporphyrin.

Urinary sediment Deposits in urine like bacteria, phosphates, uric acid, calcium oxalate/phosphate/carbonate etc.

Urination The act of voiding urine.

Urine The fluid excreted by kidneys with a specific gravity of 1005-1030, acidic in reaction and amber colored; 24 hour urine contains nearly 75 grams of solids, i.e. 25% as urea, 25% as chloride, 25% as sulfates.

Uriniferous Carrying urine.

Uriniparous Producing urine.

Urinoma A cyst containing urine.

Urinometer Device for measuring specific gravity of urine.

Urobilin A brown pigment formed by oxidation of urobilinogen, a breakdown product of bilirubin.

Urobilinogen A colourless degradation product of bilirubin formed by action of intestinal bacteria.

Urobilinuria Excess of urobilin in the urine.

Urocele Swelling of scrotum with urine.

Urochrome A yellow pigment in urine derived from urobilin.

Uroclepsia Involuntary passage of urine without knowledge.

Urocyanin A blue pigment in urine in certain diseases like scarlet fever.

Urodynamics Study of bladder function both neural and muscular.

Urodynia Painful urination.

Uroerythrin A red pigment found in urine.

Uroflavin A fluorescent compound present in persons taking riboflavin.

Urofuscin A red-brown pigment in urine of patients of porphyria.

Urogastrone A polypeptide present in urine that inhibits gastric acid secretion.

Urogenital diaphragm The sheet of tissue stretching across the pubic arch, formed by deep transverse perineal and sphincter urethrae muscles. *SYN* — triangular ligament.

Urography X-ray study of urinary tract after introduction of radiopaque dye. Can be ascending type: dye is injected into bladder or descending type: the dye is given IV. and is excreted by the kidneys.

Urokinase An enzyme obtained from human urine used for coronary, pulmonary and peripheral thrombolysis.

Urolithiasis Formation of calculi in urinary tract and the associated symptoms thereof.

Urology The branch of medicine concerned with diseases of urinary tract.

Uroporphyrin A red pigment present in urine and feces in porphyria.

Urorosein A red colored pigment in urine.

Uroxanthin A yellow pigment in urine.

Urticaria Eruption of itchy wheals on skin.

u. bullosa Eruption of fluid filled vesicles under the epidermis.

u. cold induced urticaria.

u. hemorrhagica Urticarial lesions filled with blood.

u. pigmentosa Brown itchy eruptions of mastocytosis.

u. solaris Urticaria on exposure to sunlight.

Usher's syndrome Congenital deafness and retinitis pigmentosa progressing to complete blindness.

Uta Infection with *Leishmania braziliensis* causing nasopharyngeal and mucocutaneous lesions.

Uterine souffle The sound of blood flow in uterine vessels in gravid uterus.

Uterine subinvolution Failure of uterus to return to its normal size after child birth.

Uterus The womb, the seat of embryo's embedment and growth; a hollow muscular pelvic organ.

Utricle 1. One of two sacs of the membranous labyrinth in the bony vestibule of inner ear, communicating with semicircular ducts, sacculus and "endolymphatic duct 2. Any small sac.

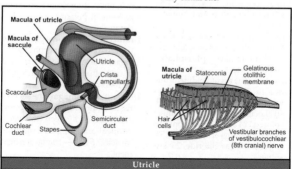

Utricle

u. of prostate A small blind pouch of urethra extending into substance of prostate, a remnant of embryonic mullerian duct.

Uvea The vascular pigmented coat of the eye lying beneath the sclera and consisting of iris, ciliary body, choroid.

Uveitis Inflammation of uvea or any part of it.

u. anterior Inflammation of iris and ciliary body.

u. posterior Choroiditis.

Uveoparotitis Inflammation of uvea and parotid glands as in sarcoidosis.

Uviometer An instrument for measuring the intensity of ultraviolet light.

Uvula A small fleshy structure hanging from soft palate.

u. of vermis A small triangular elevation on the vermis of cerebellum.

Uvulitis Inflammation of uvula.

Uvulopalatopharyagoplasty Plastic surgery of orpharynx to remove redundant tissue to ease breathing in snoring and sleep apnoea

Uvuloptosis A lax pendulous soft palate.

Uvulotome Instrument for performing uvulotomy.

U-wave A low amplitude positive wave that follows T wave in ECG. U-wave inversion indicates coronary artery disease.

V

Vaccination Inoculation with a vaccine to achieve resistance against infectious disease.

Vaccine A suspension of live attenuated/killed infectious agent or its products/parts for achieving immunity against that infectious agent.

v. BCG Bacillus Calmettee-Guerin, a preparation of dried live-culture of mycobacterium tuberculosis whose virulence has been reduced by repeated cultures on glycerinated ox bile.

v. DPT A preparation of diphtheria and tetanus toxoid and killed pertussis organisms given intramuscularly.

v. hepatitis B Vaccine containing recombinant viral capsular antigen of hepatitis B virus.

v. human diploid cell An inactivated rabies virus vaccine prepared in human diploid cell tissue culture.

v. Influenza A polyvalent vaccine containing inactivated antigenic variants of the virus for rendering immunity in chronically ill and aged.

v. measles A live attenuated virus vaccine.

v. mumps A live attenuated virus vaccine.

v. pneumococcal A polyvalent vaccine effective against 23 strains of pneumococci, given to children under 2 years of age and to those who have undergone splenectomy.

v. polio Oral poliovaccine containing 3 types of live attenuated (v. Sabin) or inactivated viruses (v. Salk).

v. typhoid usually given during need and to troops

v. varicella given against chickenpox at 12-18 month

v. yellow fever given to travelers entering endemic areas

Vaccinia Cowpox, the vesicopustular disease of cattles.

Vacuole A clear space in the protoplasm.

Vacuum Empty space.

Vacuum extractor A device with a suction cup which is placed on fetal head for applying traction during delivery.

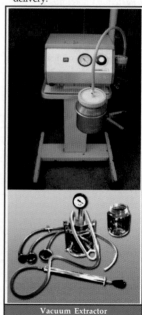

Vacuum Extractor

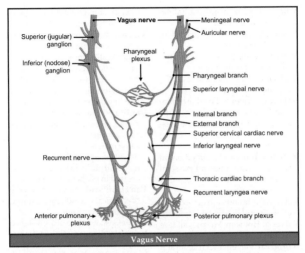

Vagus Nerve

Vacuum aspiration A method of termination of pregnancy by applying suction to a catheter placed in uterine cavity.

Vagabond's disease Body louse infection causing itching and skin discoloration.

Vagal tone Cardiac inhibitory effect by vagus.

Vagina The musculo membranous passage between the cervix and vulva.

Vaginal bulb Small erectile tissue on each side of vestibule.

Vaginal hysterectomy Surgical removal of uterus through vagina.

Vaginal vibrator A vibrator placed in vagina for erotic stimulation.

Vaginismus Painful spasm of vagina often preventing coitus; may be idiopathic, following trauma, vaginitis or psychological aversion to coitus.

Vaginitis Inflammation vagina causing purulent malodorous discharge, itching, pain in perineum, and during coitus and painful micturition.

v. atrophic Atrophy of vagina in postmenopausal women with reduced introitus and dryness.

v. Trichomonial Vaginitis due to Trichomonas causing red frothy discharge with fishy odor.

Vaginosis bacterial Caused by *Gardenerella vaginalis* with characterstic clue cells.

Valgus Bent outward e.g. talipes valgus, caxa valgus.

Valine An amino acid essential for growth of infants.

Vallate papilla Present on posterior dorsal surface of tongue.

Vallecula Depression or crevice

Valproic acid Anticonvulsant.

Valsalva maneuver Forcible expiration against closed glottis, nose, and mouth; used to increase pressure within middle ear to correct retracted ear drum.

Valsalva sinuses The dilatations in the root of aorta behind the semi lunar cusps where the coronary arteries originate.

Valve Membranous structures that allow flow of fluid in one direction.

Valves of Houston Mucosal folds of rectum.

v. ileocecal Valve between ileum and large intestine (cecum) composed of two membranous folds.

v. thebesian Valves at the entrance of coronary sinus into right atrium.

Valvoplasty Dilatation of valve.

Valvotomy Incision into a valve to dilate it.

Valvulae conniventes Circular membranous folds in the lumen of small intestine that retard the passage of food thereby promoting absorption of nutrients. *SYN*—plica circularis.

Van Buren's disease Thick indurated corpora cavernosa *SYN*— Peyronie's disease.

Vancomycin hydrochloride Antibiotic given IV 1-2 gm daily, specific for resistant staphylococcal infection.

Van den Berg's test Blood test for detection of bilirubin.

Vander Wall's forces The weak forces of attraction between the nuclei of atoms. These forces do not exist on the basis of ionic attraction, hydrogen bonding or sharing of electrons

Vanilla Obtained from tropical orchid, an aromatic substance used for flavoring.

Vanilyl mandelic acid (VMA) Metabolite of epinephrine and nor epinephrine in urine, amount increased in pheochromocytoma.

Van't Hoff's rule Doubling of speed of chemical reaction for each 10°C rise in temperature.

Vapor Gaseous state of a substance.

Vaguiz's disease Polycythemia vera.

Variance In statistics, the square of standard derviation.

Variant Having some different characteristic from the original.

Varicella Chickenpox, the viral disease with polymorphic maculo-vesico-pustular eruptions.

v. gangrenosa Varicella where necrosis occurs around the vesicles resulting in ulcerations.

Varicella-Zoster immune globulin An immunoglobulin isolated from human volunteers with high antibody titer against varicella-zoster virus.

Varicocele Dilated pampiniform plexus in the spermatic cord, commonly on left side, feeling like a bag of worms.

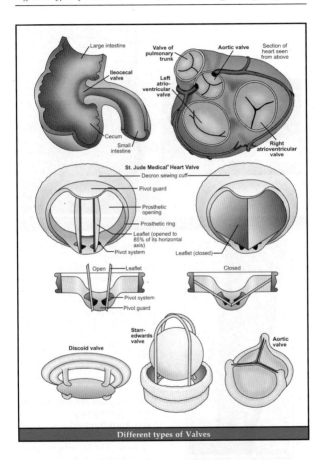

Different types of Valves

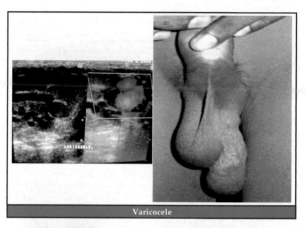

Varicocele

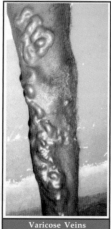

Varicose Veins

Varicose Means distended, tortuous and knotted.

Varicose veins Dilated tortuous veins as developing in legs due to venous incompetence or the development of esophageal varices in portal hypertension.

Varicosity The condition of varicose.

Variola *SYN*—smallpox, the vesico-pustular generalized eruptive viral disease that has disappeared from the globe for past two decades.

Varioloid Resembling smallpox.

Varix Dilatation of a vein, artery or lymphatic channel.

Varus Turned inward.

Vas A duct.

v. deferens The 18" long excretory duct of testis transporting sperm to urethra.

Vasa Pleural of vas.

v. afferentia Lymphatic vessels entering a lymph node.

v. brevia Branches of splenic artery running to greater curvature of stomach.

v. efferentia Lymphatic vessels leaving a lymph node.

v. recta 1. Straight collecting tubules of kidney 2. Tubules that become straight prior to entering the mediastinum testis.

v. vasorum The tiny blood vessels supplying the fibromuscular coats of arteries and larger veins.

Vascularization Growth of new blood vessels in a structure.

Vascular ring A form of congenital anomaly where an arterial ring surrounds trachea and esophagus often causing compression.

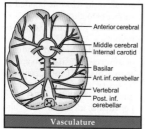

Vasculature

Vasculature The arrangement and interrelationship of blood vessels.

Vasculitis Inflammation of blood or lymph vessels.

Vasculopathy Any disease of blood vessels.

Vasectomy Removal of a segment of vas deferens bilaterally to induce male sterility.

Vasoactive intestinal polypeptide (VIP) A peptide of GI tract that inhibits gastric acid secretion but promotes intestinal secretion, excess secretion causing diarrhea.

Vasoconstriction Spasm or temporary narrowing of blood vessels.

Vasodepressor An agent that depresses circulation, i.e. lowers blood pressure by dilating blood vessels.

Vasodilator Agent causing relaxation of blood vessels.

Vasomotor Pertains to or regulating the contraction and relaxation of blood vessels.

v. epilepsy Epilepsy manifesting with vasomotor phenomena like pallor, urticaria, pruritus, skin discolouration.

v. headache Histamine cephalgia.

v. paralysis Paralysis of vasomotor mechanism with resultant atony and dilatation of blood vessels.

Vasopressin A posterior pituitary hormone having antidiuretic, and vasopressor effect (causes coronary spasm, hence not used to raise blood pressure).

Vasopressor Agent bringing about contraction of blood vessels.

Vasospasm Spasm of blood vessels.

Vasotripsy Stopping bleeding crushing an artery by forceps.

Vasovagal syncope Sudden fainting due to hypotension caused by emotional stress, pain or trauma.

Vasovasostomy Rejoining of torn vas deferens of testis.

Vasovesiculitis Inflammation of vas deferens and seminal vesicle.

Vastus Large or great; one of the three muscles of thigh.

V. Bjork Shiely An artificial synthetic valve previously placed at mitral position

Vector 1. A carrier or disease transmitting living organism like arthropod or insect 2. A force having a magnitude and direction.

v. biological An animal vector in which the infective organism multiplies or develops prior to becoming infective to humans.

v. mechanical A vector in which growth and development of organism does not occur.

Vectorcardiography Analysis of direction and magnitude of electrical forces of cardiac contraction by a continuous series of loops (Vectors), especially useful in diagnosing infarction in the presence of left bundle branch block.

Vecuronium Neuromuscular blocking agent.

Vegan A strict vegetarian who even abstains from milk and milk products.

Vegetate 1. To lead a passive existence either mentally or physically 2. Luxuriant growth.

Vegetation Wart like luxuriant growth from heart valves; consisting of fibrin mesh with enmeshed blood cells.

Vegetative Quiscent, passive.

Vehicle A therapeutically inactive substance that carries the active ingredient.

Vein Vessel carrying unsaturated blood towards the heart except for pulmonary veins that carry saturated oxygenated blood to left atrium.

Velamentous Expanding like a veil or sheet.

Velamentum Membranous covering.

Vellus The fine hair left on the body after the lanugo hairs disappear in the newborn.

Velpean's bandage A special form of roller bandage incorporating shoulder, arm and forearm.

Venal comitantes Two or more veins accompanying an artery.

Veneer In dentistry, materials like acrylic resin which is bonded to surface of tooth.

Venereal Resulting from sexual intercourse.

Venereal collar Mottled condition of skin of neck often seen in syphilis.

Venereal disease Disease acquired by sexual intercourse. It includes gonorrhea, syphilis, AIDS, viral hepatitis B, trichomoniasis, chlamydia infection, granuloma inguinale and lymphogranuloma venereum (LGV).

Venereal wart Moist reddish elevations on genitals and anus.

Venereology The branch of medical science dealing with diagnosis and treatment of venereal disease.

Venesection Surgical incision into a vein for draining out blood or introducing blood/colloids.

Venipuncture Puncture of a vein for drawing out blood or introducing any substance.

Venogram X-ray of the vein by introduction of contrast material.

Venom Poisonous secretion expelled by some animals, reptiles.

v. snake The poisonous secretion of labial glands of snake containing neurocytolysins, hemolysins, hemocoagulants.

Venomous Poisonous.

Venooclusive Pertains to obstruction of veins, e.g. venoocclusive disease of liver.

Venoperitoneostomy Surgically inserting the cut end of long saphenous vein into peritoneal cavity to drain ascitic fluid.

Venostasis Stasis or stagnation of blood within vein, often artificially achieved by putting ligature to reduce pulmonary edema in congestive failure.

Venous artery An artery carrying venous blood, e.g. pulmonary artery.

Venous hum A continuous murmur heard on veins of neck.

Venous return Amount of blood returning to atria.

Venous sinus A channel that carries venous blood, e.g. dural venous sinus.

Vent An opening in any cavity.

Ventilation Circulation of fresh air in lung alveoli.

v. continuous positive pressure Mechanical method of artificial ventilation where the respirator delivers air to the lungs under a continuous positive pressure.

v. intermittent positive pressure The respirator delivers air under positive pressure to initiate inspiration but expiration is passive.

Ventilation coefficient The amount of air that must be respired for each liter of oxygen to be absorbed.

Ventouse Cup shaped.

Ventral Anterior or front side or lower or underneath.

Ventral hernia Hernia through anterior abdominal wall.

Ventricle A small cavity or pouch, e.g. in the heart and in the brain.

v. third The median cavity of brain bounded by thalamus and hypothalamus on either side, anteriorly by optic chiasm; communicating with lateral ventricles and fourth ventricle.

v. fourth The CSF containing cavity at base of brain extending between upper end of spinal canal and cerebral aqueduct. Its roof is formed by cerebellum and floor by rhomboid fossa.

v. lateral The ventricle in each cerebral hemisphere with triangular shaped body, inferior and posterior horns; communicating with their ventricle by interventricular, foramen.

v. of larynx The space between true and false vocal cords.

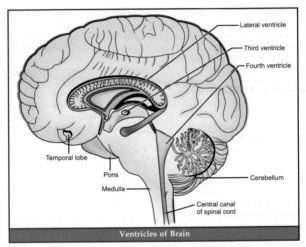

Ventricles of Brain

v. of Morgagni The recess in lateral wall of larynx between vestibular and vocal folds.

Ventricular escape Temporary assumption of pacemaker function by the ventricles either due to complete AV block or sinus standstill.

Ventricular folds The false vocal cords or folds of mucous membrane parallel or above true vocal cords.

Ventricular septal defect A congenital defect in the interventricular septum of heart leading to passage of blood from left ventricle into right ventricle.

Ventriculitis Inflammation of ependymal lining of cerebral ventricles.

Ventriculoatriostomy Establishment of communication between cerebral ventricle and right atrium by placement of a shunt to treat hydrocephalus.

Ventriculocisternostomy Establishing communication between cerebral ventricle and cisterna magna.

Ventriculography Visualization of size and shape of cerebral ventricles by air injection or visualization of size shape and contraction of ventricles of heart after contrast injection.

Ventriculostomy Establishing communication between third ventricle and cisterna interpeduncularis to treat hydrocephalus.

Ventrosuspension Fixation of displaced uterus to anterior abdominal wall.

Venturi mask A mask for controlled administration of O_2.

Venule A tiny vein continuous with capillary.

Verapamil Calcium channel blocker; antiarrhythmic agent.

Verbigeration Repetition of meaningless words.

Verge An edge or margin, e.g. anal verge, i.e. the transitional area between smooth perianal area and the hairy skin.

Vermicidal Capable of destroying intestinal worms or parasites.

Vermicular Resembling a worm, e.g. vermicular movement.

Vermiform Shaped like a worm

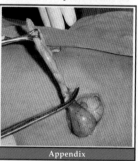

Appendix

Vermiform appendix The long narrow worm shaped tube arising from cecum closed at the distal end.

Vermifuge Agents that expel intestinal worms.

Vermilion border The junction between the skin and oral mucous membrane at the lips.

Vermin Small insects and animals.

Vermis A worm, median lobe of cerebellum between the lateral lobes.

Vernet's syndrome Paralysis of 9th, 10th and llth cranial nerves due to injury to jugular foramen.

Vernix caseosa A sebaceous deposit covering the fetus, abundant on creases and flexor surfaces, consisting of sebaceous secretion, lanugo and exfoliated skin.

Verruca *SYN* — wart.

v. acuminate Reddish moist wart around genitalia and anus.

v. filiformis A small thread like growth on the neck and eyelids.

v. vulgaris Warts on back of hand and fingers.

Verucous Wart like.

Versicolor Having many colours or change in colors.

Version Change in position of fetus within uterus.

v. bipolar A combination of both external and internal manipulation to bring a change in fetal position.

v. cephalic Turning of the fetus so that head becomes the presenting part.

v. external Version of fetus with both hands placed on abdomen.

v. internal Version of fetus with one hand placed inside vagina.

v. podalic Version by holding feet of the fetus to make the presenting part breech.

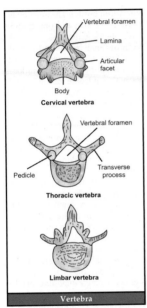

Cervical vertebra

- Vertebral foramen
- Lamina
- Articular facet
- Body

Thoracic vertebra

- Vertebral foramen
- Pedicle
- Transverse process

Limbar vertebra

Vertebra

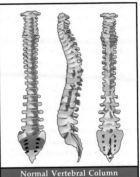

Normal Vertebral Column

Vertex The top portion of head.

Vertical Perpendicular to the horizontal plane, upright.

Vertiginous Afflicted with vertigo.

Vertigo The sensation of moving around in space (subjective vertigo) or experiencing the surrounding objects moving around oneself (objective vertigo).

V. benign positional paroxysmal postioned vertigo with nystagmus on particular head positions

V. epidemic likely to be due to vestibular neuronitis

V. peripheral occurring due to a cause outside brainstem

V. vestibular caused by malfunction of vestibular apparatus.

Verumontanum An elevation on the floor or the prostatic urethra where seminal ducts open.

Vesalius A small opening in base of skull transmitting an emissary vein.

Vertebra One of the 33 bony segments making up the spinal column, consisting of 7 cervical, 12 thoracic (dorsal), 5 lumbar, 5 sacral and 4 coccygeal.

Vertebral canal The cavity within spinal column containing the spinal cord.

Vertebral pedicle The portion of bone projecting backward from each side of body of vertebra and connecting the lamina with body.

Vertebrate Those having a vertebral column.

Vesica A bladder.

Vesical Shaped like a bladder.

Vesical reflex Desire to urinate once bladder is distended.

Vesicant Agent that produces blisters.

Vesicle Elevated skin lesions containing serous fluid.

v. optic Hollow outgrowths from lateral aspects of embryonic brain giving rise to retina and optic nerves.

v. seminal Membranous sacculated tubes at the base of bladder acting as reservoir of semen.

Vesicopustule A vesicle in which pus has formed.

Vesicostomy Surgical opening into bladder.

Vesico uterine pouch Extension of peritoneal cavity downwards between bladder and uterus.

Vesicovaginal Concerning urinary bladder and vagina.

Vesiculation Formation of vesicles.

Vesiculectomy Partial or complete excision of seminal vesicle.

Vesiculitis Inflammation of seminal vesicle.

Vesiculogram X-ray of seminal vesicles.

Vesiculo tympanic Having both vesicular and tympanic qualities.

Vespidal Family of wasps.

Vessel A duct or canal to carry fluids.

Vestibular apparatus The anatomical parts including saccule, utricle, semicircular canals, vestibular nerve and nuclei, concerned with body equilibrium.

Vestibular area A triangular area lateral to sulcus limitans, beneath which lie the terminal nuclei of vestibular nerve.

Vestibular bulbs Two sacculated collection of veins lying on either side of vagina homologous to male corpus spongiosum.

Vestibular nerve The main division of eighth cranial nerve, arising from vestibular ganglion and concerned with body equilibrium.

Vestibule Small cavity or space at the beginning of a canal.

v. of ear The middle part of inner ear containing utricle and saccule.

v. of vagina An almond shaped space between the lines of attachment of the labia minora surrounded anteriorly by clitoris, posteriorly by fourchette. The structures opening into this space are urethra, vagina and the ducts of Bartholin's glands.

Vestibuloplasty Plastic surgery of vestibule of mouth.

Vestige A small incompletely developed structure.

Veterinary Pertains to animal diseases and their treatment.

Viability Ability to live or capable of living, e.g. a fetus reaching 24 weeks gestation or 500 gms of weight can live outside uterus.

Vial A small glass bottle for medicines and chemicals.

Vibrator Device that produces vibration or shaking.

Vibratory sense The ability to perceive vibrations or that transmitted through skin and bone from a vibrating tuning fork.

Vibrio A genus of comma shaped motile gram-negative, bacilli e.g. *V. cholerae,* the organism causing cholera.

Vibrometer 1. A device that produces rapid vibrations of tympanic membrane, a form of massage to treat deafness. 2. Device used to measure vibratory sensation threshold, useful in judging clinical status of peripheral neuropathy.

Vicarious Acting as alternative or substitute.

Vicarious menstruation Blood loss during menstruation at sites other than vagina like nose, breast.

Vidarabine Antiviral agent effective against herpes simplex and zoster.

Vidian artery Artery passing through pterygoid canal.

Vidian canal A canal in the medial pterygoid plate of sphenoid bone for passage of vidian vessels and nerve.

Vidian nerve A branch from sphenopalatine ganglion.

Vigil Wakefulness.

Vigilant Being attentive, watchful and alert.

Vigor Force or strength of body and mind.

Villaret's syndrome A lesion of posterior retroparotid space causing ipsilateral palsy of 9th, 10th, 11th and 12th cranial nerves.

Villiferous Having villi or tuft of hair.

Villus Short slender filamentous processes found on some membranous surfaces.

v. arachnoid Protrusion of arachnoid into dural venous sinus.

v. chorionic Tiny branching processes on surface of chorion that become vascular and form placenta.

v. intestinal The projecting structures into lumen of small intestine that help to absorb fluid and nutrients.

Vinblastine An extract from plant vinca rosea having cytotoxic properties.

Vincent's angina Acute necrotising gingivitis.

Vincristine sulfate A cytotoxic agent extracted from plant vinca rosea.

Vindesine Vinca alkaloid, antineoplastic agent.

Vinegar A weak solution of acetic acid.

Vinyl chloride A chemical often causing lung malignancy.

Violaceous Violet, said of a discoloration of skin.

Violent Great force, fierceness.

Viomycin Antibiotic produced by *Streptomyces griseus,* used in tuberculosis.

Viper A venomous snake of the family viperidae.

Vipoma An islet cell tumor of pancreas that causes watery diarrhea, hypokalemia and achlorhydria.

Viraginity A woman who thinks herself to be male even through she is not .

Virchow cell Lepra cell.

Virchow's node Supraclavicular lymph node.

Virchow-Robin space Perivascular spaces.

Virchow's angle The angle formed by joining the nasofrontal suture and the most prominent point on superior alveolar process with the line joining the same point and superior border of external auditory meatus.

Viremia Presence of viruses in blood stream.

Virgin Woman who has had no sexual intercourse; uncontaminated, fresh.

Virginity The state of being virgin.

Viricide Destructive to viruses.

Virile reflex Contraction of bulbocavernosus muscle on percussing dorsum of penis or compressing the glans penis.

Virilism Appearance of male secondary sexual characteristics in female.

Virility Sexual potency in male; state of possessing masculine qualities.

Virilization Masculine changes in female like appearance of moustache and beard, atrophy of breast, enlarged clitoris, male voice and male type baldness.

Virion A complete virus particle.

Viroids Small naked virus genome without a dormant phase.

Virulence Degree of pathogenicity.

Virulent Highly infectious.

Virus Minute submicroscopic organisms with a central core of DNA or RNA and a capsid but no cell wall. They utilize the cell metabolic processes for their nutrition and replication.

v. cytomegalic (CMV) A member of the herpes virus group transmitted transplacentally from mother to

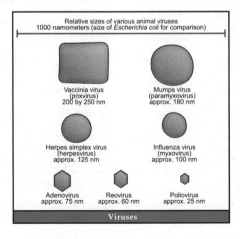

Relative sizes of various animal viruses
1000 namometers (size of *Escherichia coli* for comparison)

Vaccinia virus (poxvirus) 200 by 250 nm

Mumps virus (paramyxovirus) approx. 180 nm

Herpes simplex virus (herpesvirus) approx. 125 nm

Influenza virus (myxovirus) approx. 100 nm

Adenovirus approx. 75 nm

Reovirus approx. 60 nm

Poliovirus approx. 25 nm

Viruses

fetus with mental retardation and hepatosplenomegaly in the newborn.

v. entero cytopathogenic human orphan (ECHO) Virus responsible for epidemic pleurodynia, meningoencephalitis, myocarditis etc.

v. immunodeficiency The RNA virus containing reverse trancrytase that confers it capacity to change the antigenicity indefinitely and hence the difficulty in producing a successful vaccine. It causes the dreaded disease AIDS for which there is no cure.

v. respiratory syncytial The virus causing lower respiratory infection in infancy and childhood and that produces large syncytial masses in cell cultures.

Viscera Internal body organs.

Visceral skeleton The pelvis, ribs, and sternum enclosing pelvic and thoracic viscera.

Visceromotor Conveying motor impulses to viscera.

Visceroptosis Downward displacement of a viscus.

Viscid Sticky, adhering, gummy.

Viscosimeter Device for estimating viscosity of fluid.

Viscosity 1. The state of being sticky or gummy. 2. Resistance of a fluid medium to changeability due to existing intermolecular force.

Vision Act of seeing external objects; sense by which light and color are perceived,

v. binocular Vision produced by fusion of the images in brain perceived by each eye.

v. central Vision resulting from rays falling on fovea centralis.

v. dichromatic A form of defective colour vision in which only two primary colours are perceived.

v. multiple Seeing of one object as many.

v. peripheral Vision resulting from rays falling on peripheral parts of retina.

Visual acuity A measure of the resolving power of eye. A normal person is able to read letters at a distance of 20 feet that subtend angle of 5°.

Visual evoked response A test to know about integrity of visual pathway. While the patient watches a pattern projected on screen, the wave form is recorded and from its latency and amplitude site of delay can be pinpointed.

Visuognosis The recognition and appreciation of what is seen.

Vital capacity The quantity of air that can be expelled following deep inspiration.

Vitality The state of being alive, vigor.

Vital signs The traditional signs of life: like pulse, blood pressure, respiration, urination.

Vital statistics Statistics relating to birth, death, marriage, sickness etc.

Vitamin Micronutrients essential for metabolism, growth and development.

Vitamin A Fat soluble vitamin derived from carotenes (alpha, beta and gamma) in food, responsible for growth, development and integrity of epithelial tissues, and functioning of Rhods, the visual sensory cells that contain visual purple for dim vision.

Vitamin B1 Thiamine, an essential coenzyme for decarboxylation of pyruvate to acetyl coenzyme.

Vitamin B2 Riboflavin; constituent of flavoproteins responsible for tissue oxidation.

Vitamin B6 Pyridoxine, a coenzyme for over 60 different enzyme systems, required for heme synthesis and neuro excitability.

Vitamin B12 Cyanocobalamin, essential for cytoplasmic maturation of red cells and intactness of neurones.

Vitamin C Ascorbic acid, a factor essential for integrity of intercellular cement in many tissues, especially capillaries.

Vitamin D One of several vitamins (D_2, D_3, D_4, D_5) that have antirachitic property. Vitamin D_2 (calciferol) D_3 (irradiated 7 dihydro cholesterol), D_4 irradiated 22 dihydro ergosterol, D_5 (irradiated dehydro sitosterol), all are essential for calcium and phosphorus metabolism.

Vitamin E Tachysterol, (alpha tocopherol), which prevents oxidation of polyunsaturated fatty acids in cell membranes.

Vitamin K Naphtha quinone derivative that helps in synthesis of prothrombin in liver.

Vitellin An egg yolk protein containing lecithin.

Vitelline duct The duct connecting yolk sac with the embryonic gut.

Vitelline veins Two veins carrying blood from yolk sac.

Vitellus The yolk of an ovum.

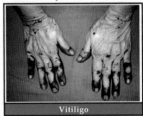
Vitiligo

Vitiligo A skin depigmentory disorder of unknown etiology.

v. capitis Depigmentation scalp skin and the hairs.

Vitrectomy Removal of vitreous.

Vitreous Transparent jelly like mass that fills the posterior chamber, enclosed by hyaloid membrane.

Viviparous Giving birth to young alive offspring rather than larvae or embryo.

Vocal cord Two thin mucous folds in larynx enclosing vocal ligaments responsible for production of sound.

Vocal fremitus Palpable vibration on chest wall while patient speaks.

Vocal ligament A strong band of elastic tissue lying within vocal cord.

Vocal muscle The inner portion of thyroarytenoid muscle which lies in contact with vocal ligament.

Vocal process The part of arytenoid cartilage to which are attached the vocal cords.

Voice Sound produced in human beings by vibration of vocal cords.

Void To evacuate bladder and bowel.

Volar Relates to palm of hand and sole of foot.

Volatile Easily evaporable.

Vole A mouse like rodent.

Volition The act or power of willing or choosing.

Volkmann's canals Vascular channels in compact bone, not surrounded by concentric lamellae as are haversian canals.

Volkman's contractors Fibrosis, shortening and atrophy of muscles following ischemia.

Volley The discharge of a number of nerve stimuli in quick succession.

Volsella Forceps with one or more hooks at the end of each blade.

Volt The unit of electromotive force which when applied to a conductor with resistance of one ohm produces a current of one ampere.

Voltage Difference in potential expressed in volts.

Voltameter An instrument for measuring both volts and amperage.

Volume The space occupied by a substance.

v. expiratory reserve The, maximal amount of air that can be expelled after normal expiration

v. inspiratory reserve The maximal amount of air that can be inspired after end of normal inspiration.

v. mean corpuscular The mean volume of an average erythrocyte, 80-90 fentoliter.

v. minute Amount of air inspired in one minute.

v. packed cell The volume of packed RBCs in a centrifuged sample of blood. *SYN* — hematocrit, normal range—42 to 47%.

v. residual Volume of air remaining in the lungs after maximal expiration.

v. stroke Amount of blood ejected from ventricle per one beat.

v. tidal Volume of air inspired and expired in one normal respiratory cycle.

Voluntary muscle Any muscle whose contraction and relaxation is controlled by will. *SYN*–Stripped, Skeletal muscles.

Voluptuous Pleasures of senses.

Volvulus Twisting of bowel upon itself causing obstruction to lumen and even blood supply of the segment leading to necrosis.

Vomer A thin plate of vertical bone forming posterior part of nasal septum, articulating with ethmoid and sphenoid bones.

Vomitus Ejected material from stomach, the act of ejecting such material.

v. bilious Bile ejected in vomits.

v. coffee ground Blood mixed gastric content vomited as in bleeding peptic ulcer and erosive gastritis.

Vomiting The act of ejection of gastric contents through mouth.

Vomitus Material ejected by vomiting.

Von Gierke's disease Glycogen storage disease due to absence of glucose-6-phosphates resulting in hypoglycemia and acidosis.

Von Graefe's sign Failure of lid to roll downward on looking down as in thyrotoxicosis.

Von Jaksch's disease Symptom complex of severe anemia, hepatosplenomegaly, lymphocytosis, and lymphadenopathy.

Von Recklinghausen's disease 1. Neurofibromatosis. 2. Hemochromatosis 3. Generalized osteitis fibrosa cystica.

von-Willebrand's disease A congenital bleeding disorder due to factor VIII deficiency.

Voorhee's bag An inflatable rubber bag to dilate the cervix for inducing labour.

Voracious Having insatiable appetite.

Vortex A structure having whorled or spiral appearance.

v. of heart Apical portion of heart where the ventricular muscle takes a spiral turn.

Vorticose veins Four veins receiving all blood from choroid and emptying into posterior ciliary and superior ophthalmic veins.

Voyeurism Satisfaction obtained from observing nude persons or sexual activity of others.

V. synchronised intermittent mandatory (SIMV) Periodic assisted ventilation with positive pressure initiated by patient

Vuerometer Apparatus for measuring interpupillary distance.

Vulgaris Common or ordinary.

Vulnerate To wound.

Vulsellum A forcep with hook on each blade.

Vulnerable Susceptible to injury of any kind.

Vulva The external genital organ in female consisting of labia majora, labia minora, clitoris, vestibule and vaginal opening.

v. connivens A form of vulva where labia majora are in close opposition.

Vulvectomy Excision of vulva.

Vulvitis Inflammation of vulva.

Vulvovaginitis Inflammation of vulva and vagina; most commonly in diabetes.

W

Waardenburg syndrome A congenital pigmentary disorder with vitiligo, heterochromic irides, and often congenital deafness.

Wafer A flat vaginal pessary.

Waist The part of human body between trunk and hips.

Wakefulness Sleeplessness.

Wald cycle Metabolic cycle of breakdown and synthesis of rhodopsin.

Waldenstrom's disease Osteochondritis deformans juveniles.

Waldeyer's ring The lymphatic tissue encircling nasopharynx and oropharynx, consisting of two palatine tonsils, lingual and pharyngeal tonsils.

Walk Locomotion in upright posture.

Walking typhoid Typhoid fever with mild symptoms.

Wall The limiting material/substance of a cell, artery, vein, bladder.

Wallenberg's syndrome Occlusion of posterior inferior cerebellar artery syndrome manifest with dysphagia, cerebellar dysfunction, sensory-motor disturbances.

Wallerian degeneration Degeneration of nerve fiber along with myelin sheath. The neurilemma does not degenerate but forms a tube to guide growth of severed axons.

Wandering Not fixed, moving about.

Warburg apparatus A capillary manometer employed for O_2 consumption and CO_2 production studies.

Ward A large hospital room accommodating more than 4 patients.

Warfarin Anticoagulant drug (Cumadin).

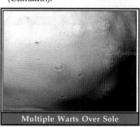
Multiple Warts Over Sole

Wart Hypertrophied epidermis due to papilloma virus infection.

Wasp A form of insects.

Wasp sting Injection of wasp venom into skin.

Wassermann reaction A complement fixation test for diagnosis of syphilis.

Waste Loss of strength; refuse no longer useful to the body; waste product.

Water bed A rubber bed filled partially with water to prevent bedsore formation.

Water hammer pulse Pulse marked by a forceful beat but sudden collapse.

Waterhouse-Friderichsen syndrome Acute adrenal insufficiency due to hemorrhage into its substance occurring in meningococcal infection.

Watson-Schwartz test A test used in acute porphyria to differentiate porphobilinogen from urobilinogen.

Watt Unit of electrical power, i.e. power produced by one ampere of current flowing with electromotive force of one volt.

Wave An undulating or vibrating motion; an oscillation seen in ECG, EEG or other graphic recordings.

w. 'a' A wave in Jugular venous pulse produced by atrial contraction and absent in atrial fibrillation.

w. 'c' A wave in jugular venous pulse that reflects closure of tricuspid valve.

w. excitation The excitatory impulse originating from SA node of heart and spreading to ventricles via A-V node.

w. pulse The ejection of blood into root of aorta that causes the impact to be transmitted along the arterial wall.

Wavelength The distance of a single wave cycle measured from top of one wave to top of next wave.

Wax Any substance of animal, plant or mineral origin consisting a mixture of high molecular weight fatty acids, high molecular weight monohydric alcohol, esters of fatty acids and alcohols and solid hydro carbons. Waxes are usually hard, brittle solid that become pliable on warming and melt on further heating.

Waxy cast Dense highly refractile urinary cast composed of amyloid material as in chronic renal disease.

Waxy degeneration 1. Amyloid degeneration 2. Zenker's degeneration.

Waxy flexibility In psychiatry, a form of stereotypy in which the patient maintains a posture in which he is placed with wax like rigidity for a much longer period than normally tolerable as in catatonic schizophrenia.

Wean To cease to suckle or breast milk substitution by other forms of nourishment.

Web A membrane extending across a space, e.g. esophageal web causing dysphagia.

Webbed Having a membrane or tissue connecting adjacent structures, e.g. toes of duck's feet.

Webbed neck A condition in which a thick triangular fold of loose skin extends from each lateral side of neck across the upper aspect of shoulder as in gonadal dysgenesis.

Weber-Christian disease Febrile, relapsing nodular non suppurative panniculitis.

Weber's glands Mucus glands at the lateral border of tongue.

Weber's palsy One side oculomotor palsy and contralateral spastic hemiplegia.

Weber's test A tuning fork test for unilateral deafness. A vibrating tuning fork is placed on middle of forehead. In conductive deafness the diseased ear perceives the vibrations better.

Wegener's syndrome Glomerulitis, vasculitis, granulomatous lesions of respiratory tract which respond to corticosteroids and cyclophosphamide.

Weil-Felix test Agglutination test for diagnosis of rickettsial diseases.

Weil's disease Leptospira ictero hemorrhagica.

Weitbrecht's ligament An oblique cord connecting ulna and radius.

Welt Skin elevation by allergy, lash or blow.

Wen A cyst resulting from sebaceous retention.

Wenckebach's phenomenon A form of incomplete heart block where there is progressive lengthening of P-R interval ending in a dropped beat.

Werdnig-Hoffmann disease Hereditary progressive infantile from muscular dystrophy resulting from degeneration of anterior horn cells. Wermer's syndrome multiple endocrine neoplasia.

Wernicke's encephalopathy Encephalopathy with memory deficit, ocular palsy, delirium associated with thiamine deficiency of chronic alcoholism.

Wernicke's syndrome Disorientation, memory loss and confabulation often due to old age.

Western blotting A technique for analyzing protein antigens and detecting small amount of antibodies as in test of AIDS.

Westphal-Edinger nucleus A parasympathetic nucleus rostral to motor nucleus of third nerve in midbrain whose efferent fibers innervate the ciliary muscles of eye.

Wet dream Nocturnal emission of semen.

Wharton's duct Duct of submandibular salivary gland opening by side of frenum linguae.

Wharton's jelly A gelatinous connective tissue constituent of umbilical cord.

Wheal An elevation of skin with white center and pale red periphery accompanied by itching as seen in urticaria, anaphylaxis, insect bite.

Wheel chair A chair with four wheels two small and two big for mobility of partially paralyzed patient or transporting sick.

Wheeze A whistling or sighing sound resulting from narrowing of airway.

Whinolalia Distorted nasal voice.

Whiplash injury Injury to cervical vertebra and adjacent soft tissues due to sudden jerking.

Whipple's disease Intestinal lipodystrophy characterized by abnormal pigmentation, fatty stool, arthritis, etc.

Whipworm Trichuris trichura.

Whirl To feel giddy, to revolve rapidly.

Whisky An alcoholic drink with ethyl alcohol content of 45-50%.

Whisper To speak in a low, soft voice.

Whistle A sound produced by blowing through pursed lips.

Whitfield ointment Benzoic acid + to salicylic acid, keratolytic, antifungal.

White line The midline (linea alba), of abdomen representing the white tendinous attachments of external oblique and transversus muscles.

White lotion Preparation of zinc sulphate and sulfurated potash.

White matter Part of central nervous system composed of myelinated nerve fibers.

Whitlow Suppurative inflammation involving pulp of finger or toe often extending to bone.

Whitmore's disease Melioidosis.

Whoop The inspiratory crowing sound following the cough paroxysm in whooping cough.

Whooping cough Acute infectious disease caused by *Bordetella pertussis*.

Whorl 1. A type of fingerprint 2. Spiral arrangement.

Widal test Agglutination test for diagnosis of typhoid and paratyphoid.

Will The mental faculty for control of one's actions, emotions, thoughts and deciding the actions.

Willi's circle An arterial arrangement at base of brain encircling the optic chiasma and hypophysis formed by internal carotids, anterior cerebrals, posterior cerebrals and basilar arteries.

Wilms' tumor Embryonic tumor of kidney occurring in children.

Wilson's disease Autosomal recessive hereditary disease due to disorder of copper metabolism with accumulation of copper in liver, kidney, brain and cornea producing cirrhosis of liver, brain degeneration and Kayser-Fleischer ring in cornea.

Wilson-Mikity syndrome Pulmonary dysmaturity syndrome seen in premature infants with dyspnea, cyanosis and multiple cystic changes in lungs.

Winckel's disease A disease of newborn with splenomegaly, hematuria, jaundice and convulsions.

Wind chill factor Heat loss from skin proportional to the speed of wind.

Window An aperture for admission of light and air.

w. oval The fenestra vestibuli.

w. round The fenestra cochlae.

Windpipe SYN—trachea.

Wine Fermented juice of any fruit with alcohol content of 1-5%.

Wing Any structure resembling wings of bird, e.g. greater and lesser wings of sphenoid.

Winking Jaw Involuntary simultaneous closure of the eyelids as the jaw is moved.

Winslow ligament The oblique popliteal ligament at back of knee.

Wintergreen oil Methyl salicylate used as counter irritant.

Wire Kirschner Steel wire placed through long bone for traction.

Wiring Gilmer Wire placed around opposing teeth for intermaxillary fusion.

Wirsung duct Pancreatic duct.

Wisdom tooth Third molar.

Wiskott-Aldrich syndrome Sex linked recessive disorder of immune function with impaired T and B cell activity, thrombocytopenia, eczema and propensity to infection.

Witche's milk Milk secreted from breast of newborn infant from stimulation by maternal LH.

Withdrawal syndrome Tachycardia, insomnia, hypotension etc., due to abrupt abstinence from alcohol and opiates in addicts.

Wolffian body An embryonic organ on each side of vertebral column, the mesonephros.

Wolffian duct Duct from meso-nephros to cloaca in fetus.

Wolff-Parkinson-White syndrome A cardiac rhythm disorder with short P-R interval, delta wave and propensity to supraventricular tachycardia.

Wolman's disease An inherited metabolic disease in infants with hepatosplenomegaly, adrenal calcification and foam cells in bone marrow.

Womb Uterus, the female reproductive organ for nourishing the fetus.

Wood alcohol Methyl alcohol distilled from wood is highly poisonous causing blindness.

Wood's light Ultraviolet light.

Wool fat Anhydrous lanolin obtained from sheep wool, used as base for ointment.

Woolsorter's disease Pulmonary anthrax.

Word blindness A form of aphasia where patient is unable to comprehend written words.

Word salad Use of words with no apparent meaning or relationship to each other as in schizophrenia.

Wormian bone Small irregular bones along cranial sutures.

Wound Break in continuity of skin or any tissue caused by trauma, infection.

w. incised Any sharp clean cut wound.

w. lacerated Wound with ragged unhealthy margins.

w. perforating The object causing the wound penetrates the skin, subcutaneous tissue.

w. puncture Wound made by sharp pointed instrument.

w. tunnel Wound with equal size entrance and exit points.

w. plasty Technique in plastic surgery to prevent contractures in straight line scars.

Wright's stain Combination of eosin and methylene blue to stain blood slides.

Wright's syndrome A neuromuscular syndrome caused by prolonged hyperabduction of arm leading to occlusion of subclavian artery and stretching of trunks of brachial plexus.

Wrinkles A furrow or ridge on skin.

Wrisberg's ganglion Ganglion of superficial cardiac plexus lying between aortic arch and pulmonary artery.

Wrisberg's cartilage The cuneiform cartilage of larynx.

Wrisberg's nerve A branch of facial nerve.

Wrist drop Inability to extend the wrist due to paralysis of radial nerve.

Writer's cramp Cramp affecting muscles of thumb and two adjacent fingers.

Wryneck *SYN* - Torticollis, due to spastic contraction of one or more neck muscles.

Wuchereria A genus of filarial worms.

w. bancrofti The causative agent of elephantiasis, spread by bite of culex mosquito.

w. malayi The causative agent of filariasis in south India.

Wylie's operation Shortening of round ligament of uterus for retroflexion in combating prolapse uterus.

X

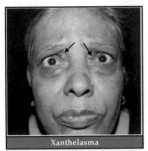
Xanthelasma

Xanthelasma Yellowish raised plaques occurring around eyelids resulting from lipid filled cells in the dermis.

Xanthine An intermediary product in transformation of adenine and guanine into uric acid.

Xanthine calculi Brown to red, hard and laminated calculi in urinary tract.

Xanthine oxidase A flavoprotein enzyme catalyzing oxidation of certain purines.

Xanthochromia Yellow discoloration of CSF due to hemolysis of RBC within it.

Xanthochroia Yellow discoloration of skin.

Xanthocyte A cell containing yellow pigment.

Xanthodont One with yellow teeth.

Xanthogranuloma A tumor having characteristics of both xanthoma and granuloma.

x. juvenile A skin disease present at birth or developing in early life with yellow, pink or orange papules comprising lipid filled histiocytes, inflammatory cells, and multinucleated vacuolated cells.

Xanthoma Flat, slightly elevated rounded plaque or nodule on the eyelids due to cholesterol accumulation.

Xanthomatosis Appearance of multiple xanthomas in skin due to cholesterol deposit within histiocytes and reticuloendothelial cells.

Xanthophyll The yellow pigment of egg yolk.

Xanthosis Yellow discoloration of skin in hypercarotinemia.

Xanthuria Excretion of excess of xanthine in urine.

X-chromosome The chromosome responsible for female sexual characteristic.

X-disease Poisoning caused by ingestion of nuts contaminated with aspergillus aflatoxin.

Xenobiotic An antibiotic not produced by body, hence foreign to body.

Xenograft Graft from one species to another *SYN*— heterograft.

Xenology Study of parasites, their relationship to each other.

Xenomenia Menstruation from a part other than vagina.

Xenon An inert gas whose radio-isotope (Xe^{133}) is used for photo-scintiscanning of lungs.

Xenophobia Abnormal fear for strangers.

Xenophthalmia Inflammation of eye caused by a foreign body.

Xenopsylla A genus of fleas whose

member X. cheopis is a vector for sylvatic plague, endemic typhus and *Hymenolepsis nana.*

Xerantic Causing dryness.

Xerasia Abnormal dryness and brittleness of hair.

Xerocyte An erythrocyte dehydrated thus appears to have pudled with half black and half white; seen in hereditary xerocytosis, an autosomal dominant trait

Xeroderma Roughness and dryness of skin.

x. pigmentosum Pigment discoloration, cutaneous atrophy and ulcers often causing death in infancy.

Xeroma Dry conjunctiva.

Xeromania Symptoms of menstruation in absence of menstrual flow.

Xerophagia Eating only of dry food.

Xerophthalmia Dry conjunctiva with keratinization as in vitamin A deficiency.

Xeroradiography A X-ray technique involving a dry process where selenium covered plates are altered by the X-ray producing the image.

Xerosis Abnormal dryness of skin and mucous membrane. Xerostomia Dryness of mouth due to poor salivary secretion.

X- linked Disease caused by genes located on X- chromosome e.g. hemophilia

Xilitol A five carbon sugar alcohol with sweetness similar to sucrose, hence used as artificial sweatner

Xiphisternum The pointed lower end of sternum.

Xiphoid Sword shaped.

Xiphoid process The lowest portion of sternum with a sword shaped cartilaginous process supported by bone.

X-ray An electromagnetic radiation in wavelength of 1-100 angstrom, produced by bombarding a tungsten target within vacuum tube by fast moving electrons.

Xylene Dimethyl benzene, used as a solvent and cleansing agent in microscopy.

Xylenol Dimethyl phenol, used in preparation of coaltar disinfectants.

Xylocaine Lidocaine, a local anaesthetic.

Xylometazoline A vasoconstrictor used in nasal decongestant drops.

Xylose A pentose sugar, non fermentable.

Xylulose A pentose sugar occurring in nature.

Xyrospasm Spasm of wrist and forearm muscles in professionals like barbers.

Xysma The flocculent pseudomembrane seen in diarrhea stool.

XYY male A super male with tall stature and tendency for criminal behavior.

Y

Yawning Deep inspiration with widely opened mouth induced by drowsiness, boredom.

Yaws Non-venereal spirochaetal disease caused by *Treponema per-tenue*.

y. cartilage The cartilage connecting pubis, ileum and ischium and extending into acetabulum.

y. chromosome The sex chromosome responsible for male sex.

Yeast Unicellular fungi of genus Saccharo myces. *S. cerevisiae* is a source of proteins and vitamin B complex.

Yellow body Corpus luteum.

Yellow fever An acute mosquito borne viral disease with fever, jaundice and hemorrhagic tendency.

Yellow spot 1. anterior end of vocal cord. 2. central point of retina, the sight of clearest vision.

Yersinia A genus of gram-negative bacteria.

y. entero colitica Producing mesenteric lymphadenitis and dysentery.

y. pestis Causative agent of plague.

y. pseudotuberculosis Produces pseudotuberculosis.

y. ligament The y shaped ligament on anterior capsule of hip joint

Yoga A system of beliefs and practices for union of self with supreme reality.

Yogurt A form of curdled milk by lactobacilli useful in patients with lactase deficiency.

Yohimbine A poisonous alkaloid having alpha-adrenergic blocking properties, often used as aphrodisiac and anti anginal agent.

Yolk The content of ovum.

y. sac Membranous sac surrounding food yolk in the embryo.

Young Helmoholtz theory Theory stating that retinal colour perception depends upon 3 different sets of fibers responsible for red, green and violet.

Young's rule The formula for calculating dose of a medicine for child from known adult dose, i.e. Age/ Age + 12 X adult dose.

Ytterbium Metallic element used in screens in radiography

Yttrium Metallic element used for radiotherapy of cancer

Z

Zahn's Line Transverse whitelines on thrombus.

Z axis Anteroposterior axis.

Z-disk A thin dark disk that transversely bisects I band of striated muscle fiber; actin filaments are attached to Z disk.

Z line A thin dark line that transversely bisects the clear zone of a muscle fiber; the distance between two z lines constitutes a sarcomere.

Zein A maize protein deficient in tryptophan and lysine.

Zenker degeneration A waxy hyaline degeneration of skeletal muscles in acute infectious diseases like typhoid fever.

Zenker's diverticula Herniation of mucous membrane of esophagus through a defect in its wall often swelling with food to cause esophageal obstruction.

Ziehl-Neelsen method A method for staining acid fast organisms like tubercle bacillus with boiled carbol fuschin followed by rinsing with alcohol.

Zieve's syndrome Transient hyperlipidemia, hemolytic anemia and jaundice following consumption of large amounts of alcohol.

Zinc A bluish white metal found as carbonate and silicate, astringent and antiseptic used in eye drops and as mineral supplement. Deficiency causes delayed ulcer healing, impaired epithelial growth, diminished fertility and acrodermatitis enteropathica. Commonly used salts are carbonate, chloride, oxide, stearate, sulfate and undecylenate.

Zinc-eugenol cement Used in dentistry for impression material, cavity liner, temporary restoration.

Zinc ointment 20% zinc oxide ointment for external application.

Zinn's ligament Connective tissue in eye to which recti are attached.

Zirconium A metallic element used as a white pigment in dental procelain.

Zollinger-Ellison syndrome Gastrin secreting tumors causing resistant peptic ulceration at unusual site; 60% of gastrinomas are malignant.

Zona 1. A bond or girdle 2. *SYN* - herpes zoster.

z. fasciculata The inner layer of adrenal cortex.

z. glomerulosa The outer layer of adrenal cortex.

z. pellucida Inner thick membranous covering of ovum.

z. reticularis The inner most layer of adrenal cortex.

Zonary placenta Placenta arranged like a broad ring around the chorion.

Zone An area or belt.

z- ciliary The peripheral part of the anterior surface of iris.

z. transitional That area of lens where the capsular epithelium changes into lens fibers.

Zonesthesia Constricting cord like sensation.

Zonule A small zone.

Zonular cataract Cataract where opacity is limited to certain layers of lens.

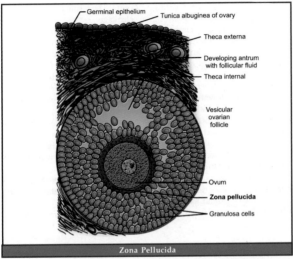

Zona Pellucida

Zonules of zin Suspensory ligament of the lens.

Zoogeny The development and evolution of animals.

Zoogony Animal breeding.

Zoology The science dealing with animal life.

Zoonoses Diseases communicable to man from animals.

Zoonotic Concerning zoonoses.

Zoophilism Abnormal love for animals.

Zoophobia Abnormal fear for animals.

Zoophyte Invertebrate animals resembling plants in growth and appearance.

Zoster *SYN*— Herpes zoster,

z. plasty A technique where *z* shaped incision is put to relieve tension in scar tissue; commonly employed in repair of cleft lip.

z. track A method of giving intramuscular injection to prevent reflux of injected material along the needle track.

Zygoma 1. The malar bone 2. The long arch joining zygomatic processes of temporal and malar bones.

Zygomaticoauricularis Muscle that draws pinna of ear forwards.

Zygomatic process 1. A thin projection from temporal bone at its squamous portion, articulating with zygomatic bone. 2. A strong prominent lateral projection from the supraorbital margin of the frontal bone articulating with maxillary process of zygomatic bone.

Zygomatic reflex When zygoma is percussed the lower jaw moves towards percussed side.

Zygomycosis A form of mycoses that predominantly affects the face, the lungs and paranasal sinuses with thrombosis of blood vessels and infarction, common to diabetics. *SYN* — mucormycosis.

Zygospore The spore resulting from union of two similar gametes, as in certain algae and fungi.

Zygote The fertilized ovum before cleavage.

Zymase An enzyme found in yeast, bacteria and plants that can convert carbohydrate into H_2O and CO_2 aerobically or ferment it to alcohol anaerobically.

Zyme An enzyme or ferment.

Zymogen The inactive precursor of an enzyme.

Zymology The science of fermentation.

Zymase An enzyme that changes a disaccharide into a monosaccharide.

Zymosis 1. Fermentation 2. Process by which infectious disease is supposed to develop.

Zymosterol A sterol from yeast.

Appendices

Appendix 1

Metric System Masses					
Scale	Table		Grams		Grains
Kilo	1 Kilogram	=	1000.0	=	15,432.35
Hecto	1 Hectogram	=	100.0	=	1,543.23
Deca	1 Decagram	=	10.0	=	154.323
Unit	1 Gram	=	1.0	=	15.432
Deci	1 Decigram	=	0.1		1.5432
Centi	1 Centigram	=	0.01	=	0.15432
Milli	1 Milligram	=	0.001		0.01543
Micro	1 Microgram	=	10^{-6}	=	15.432×10^{-6}
Nano	1 Nanogram	=	10^{-9}	=	15.432×10^{-9}
Pico	1 Picogram	=	10^{-12}	=	15.432×10^{-12}
Femto	1 Femtogram	=	10^{-15}	=	15.432×10^{-15}
Atto	1 Attogram	=	10^{-18}	=	15.432×10^{-18}

Arabic numbers are used with masses and measures, as 10 gm, or 3 ml, etc. Portions of masses and measures are usually expressed decimally. 10^{-1} indicates 0.1; 10^{-6} = 0.000001; etc.

Appendix 2

Prefixes and Multiples Used in SI			
Prefix	*Symbol*	*Power*	*Multiple or Portion of a Multiple*
tera	T	10^{12}	1,000,000,000,000
giga	G	10^9	1,000,000,000
mega	M	10^6	1,000,000
kilo	k	10^3	1,000
hecto	h	10^2	100
deca	da	10^1	10
unity			1
deci	d	10^{-1}	0.1
centi	c	10^{-2}	0.01
milli	m	10^{-3}	0.001
micro	μ	10^{-6}	0.000001
nano	n	10^{-9}	0.000000001
pico	p	10^{-12}	0.000000000001
femto	f	10^{-15}	0.000000000000001
atto	a	10^{-18}	0.000000000000000001

Appendix 3

Units of Length						
	Millimeters	*Centimeters*	*Inches*	*Feet*	*Yards*	*Meters*
1 mm =	1.0	0.1	0.03937	0.00328	0.0011	0.001
1 cm =	10.0	1.0	0.3937	0.03281	0.0109	0.01
1 in. =	25.4	2.54	1.0	0.0833	0.0278	0.0254
1 ft. =	304.8	30.48	12.0	1.0	0.333	0.3048
1 yd =	914.40	91.44	36.0	3.0	1.0	0.9144
1 m =	1000.0	100.0	39.37	3.2808	1.0936	1.0

1 μm = 1 micrometer = 0.001 millimeter   1 mm = 1000 μm
1 km = 1 kilometer = 1000 meters = 0.62137 statute mile
1 statute mile = 5280 feet = 1.609 kilometers
1 nautical mile = 6076.042 feet = 1852.276 meters

Appendix 4

Units of Volume (fluid or liquid)						
Milliliters		*US fluid Drams*	*Cubic Inches*	*US fluid Ounces*	*US fluid Quarts*	*Liters*
1 ml	= 1.0	0.2705	0.061	0.03381	0.00106	0.001
1 fl. ℥	= 3.697	1.0	0.226	0.125	0.00391	0.00369
1 cu. in.	= 16.3866	4.4329	1.0	0.5541	0.0173	0.01639
1 fl. ℥	= 29.573	8.0	1.8047	1.0	0.03125	0.02957
1 qt.	= 946.332	256.0	57.75	32.0	1.0	0.9463
1 L	= 1000.0	270.52	61.025	33.815	1.0567	1.0

1 gallon = 4 quarts = 8 pints = 3.785 liters
1 pint = 473.16 ml

Appendix 5

Units of Weight					
Grains		*Grams*	*Apothecaries Ounces*	*Avoirdupois Pounds*	*Kilograms*
1 gr	= 1.0	0.0648	0.00208	0.0001429	0.000065
1 gm	= 15.432	1.0	0.03215	0.002205	0.001
1 ℥	= 480.0	31.1	1.0	0.06855	0.0311
1 lb	= 7000.0	453.5924	14.583	1.0	0.45354
1 kg	= 15432.358	1000.0	32.15	2.2046	1.0

1 microgram (μg) = 0.001 milligram
1 mg = 1 milligram = 0.001 gm; 1000 mg = 1 gm
1 grain = 64.8 mg; 1 mg = 0.0154 grain

Appendix 6

Physical Constants of the Elements			
Element	*Symbol*	*Atomic Number*	*Approx. Relative Atomic Weight**
Actinium	Ac	89	(227)
Aluminum	Al	13	27.0
Americium	Am	95	(243)
Antimony	Sb	51	122
Argon	Ar	18	39.9
Arsenic	As	33	74.9
Astatine	At	85	(210)
Barium	Ba	56	137
Berkelium	Bk	97	(249)
Beryllium	Be	4	9.01
Bismuth	Bi	83	209
Boron	B	5	10.8
Bromine	Br	35	79.9
Cadmium	Cd	48	112
Calcium	Ca	20	40.1
Californium	Cf	98	(251)
Carbon	C	6	12.0
Cerium	Ce	58	140
Cesium	Cs	55	133
Chlorine	Cl	17	35.5
Chromium	Cr	24	52.0
Cobalt	Co	27	58.9
Copper	Cu	29	63.5
Curium	Cm	96	(247)
Dysprosium	Dy	66	162
Einsteinium	Es	99	(254)
Erbium	Er	68	167
Europium	Eu	63	152
Fermium	Fm	100	(253)
Fluorine	F	9	19.0
Francium	Fr	87	(223)
Gadolinium	Gd	64	157

Contd...

Contd...

Element	Symbol	Atomic Number	Approx. Relative Atomic Weight*
Gallium	Ga	31	69.7
Germanium	Ge	32	72.6
Gold	Au	79	197
Hafnium	Hf	72	178
Helium	He	2	4.00
Holmium	Ho	67	165
Hydrogen	H	1	1.01
Indium	In	49	115
Iodine	I	53	127
Iridium	Ir	77	192
Iron	Fe	26	55.8
Krypton	Kr	36	83.8
Lanthanum	La	57	139
Lawrencium	Lr	103	(257)
Lead	Pb	82	207
Lithium	Li	3	6.94
Lutetium	Lu	71	175
Magnesium	Mg	12	24.3
Manganese	Mn	25	54.9
Mendelevium	Md	101	(256)
Mercury	Hg	80	201
Molybdenum	Mo	42	95.9
Neodymium	Nd	60	144
Neon	Ne	10	20.2
Neptunium	Np	93	(237)
Nickel	Ni	28	58.7
Niobium	Nb	41	92.9
Nitrogen	N	7	14.0
Nobelium	No	102	(253)
Osmium	Os	76	190
Oxygen	O	8	16.0
Palladium	Pd	46	106'
Phosphorus	P	15	31.0
Platinum	Pt	78	195

Contd...

Contd...

Element	Symbol	Atomic Number	Approx. Relative Atomic Weight*
Plutonium	Pu	94	(242)
Polonium	Po	84	(210)
Potassium	K	19	39.1
Praseodymium	Pr	59	141
Promethium	Pm	61	(147)
Protactinium	Pa	91	231
Radium	Ra	88	(226)
Radon	Rn	86	(222)
Rhenium	Re	75	186
Rhodium	Rh	45	103
Rubidium	Rb	37	85.5
Ruthenium	Ru	44	101
Samarium	Sm	62	150
Scandium	Sc	21	45.0
Selenium	Se	34	79.0
Silicon	Si	14	28.1
Silver	Ag	47	108
Sodium	Na	11	23.0
Strontium	Sr	38	87.6
Sulfur	S	16	32.1
Tantalum	Ta	73	181
Technetium	Tc	43	(98.9)
Tellurium	Te	52	128
Terbium	Tb	65	159
Thallium	Tl	81	204
Thorium	Th	90	232
Thulium	Tm	69	169
Tin	Sn	50	119
Titanium	Ti	22	47.9
Tungsten	W	74	184
Unnilhexium	Uah	106	(263)
Unnilpentium	Unp	105	(262)
Unnilquadium	Unq	104	(264)
Unnilseptium	Uns	107	(262)
Uranium	U	92	238

Contd...

Contd...

Element	Symbol	Atomic Number	Approx. Relative Atomic Weight*
Vanadium	V	23	50.9
Xenon	Xe	54	131
Ytterbium	Yb	70	173
Yttrium	Y	39	88.9
Zinc	Zn	30	65.4
Zirconium	Zr	40	91.2

*The relative atomic mass values have been rounded off to three significant figures. Values for elements with no stable isotope are shown in parentheses and represent the most stable known isotopes.

Appendix 7

Phobias			
Fear of	*Condition*	*Fear of*	*Condition*
air	aerophobia	everything	panphobia, panopbobia, pantophobia
animals	zoophobia		
anything new	neophobia	excrement	coprophobia
bacilli	bacillophobia	eyes	ommatophobia
bearing a deformed child	teratophobia	failure	kakorrhaphiophobia
bees	apiphobia, melissophobia	fatigue	kopophobia
being buried alive	taphephobia	feathers	pteronophobia
birds	ornithophobia	fever	pyrexeophobia
blood	hematophobia, hemophobia	filth	mysophobia
		filth or odor, personal	automysophobia
blushing	ereuthrophobia	fire	pyrophobia
brain disease	meningitophobia	fish	ichthyophobia
bridges (crossing of)	gephyrophobia	floods	antlophobia
cats	ailurophobia, galeophobia	fog	homichlophobia
change or novelty	kainophobia	food	cibophobia, sitophobir
childbirth	tocophobia	forest	hylophobia
choking	pnigophobia	frogs	batrachophobia
cold or something cold	psychrophobia	ghosts	phasmophobia
color(s)	chromatophobia, chromophobia	giris	parthenophobia
		glare of light	photaugiaphobia
confinement	claustrophobia	glass	crystallophobia, hyalophobia
contamination or infection	molysmophobia	God	theophobia
corpses	necrophobia	gravity	barophobia
crowds	ochlophobia	hair	trichopathophobia
dampness	hygrophobia	heat	thermophobia
darkness	nyctophobia, scotophobia	height	acrophobia
dawn	eosophobia	hell	hadephobia, stygiophobia

Contd..

Contd...

Fear of	Condition	Fear of	Condition
daylight	phengophobia	heredity and hereditary disease	patroiophobia
death	thanatophobia		
definite, specific disease bathophobia	monopathophobia	high objects	
deformity	dysmorphophobia	or being on tall buildings	
depth	bathophobia	house, being in a	domatophobia oikophobia
developing a phobia	phobophobia		
dirt	mysophobia, rupophobia	ideas	ideophobia
disease	nosophobia, pathophobia	injury	traumatophobia
dogs	cynophobia	innovation	neophobia
dolls	pediophobia	insane, becoming	maniaphobia acarophobia,
drafts dust	anemophobia amathophobia	insects	entomophobia
eating	phagophobia	jealousy	zelophobia
electricity	electrophobis	justice	dikephobia
emptiness	kenophobia, cenophobia	knife or pointed objects	aichmophobia
error	hamartophobia	large objects	megalophobia
left	levophobia	rain or rain storm	ombrophobia
light	photophobia	rectum	proctophobia
lightning	astraphobia, astraphobia, keraunophobia	red	erythrophobia
		responsibility	hypengyophobia
		returning home	nostophobia
locked in, being	clithrophobia	light	dextrophobia
looked at, being	scopophobia	river	potamophobia

Contd...

Contd...

Fear of	Condition	Fear of	Condition
machinery	mechanophobia	robbers	harpaxophobia
men	androphobia	rod or instrument of punishment	rhabdophobia
many things	polyphobia	ruin	atephobia
marriage	gamophobia	sacred things	hierophobia
medicine	pharmacophobia		
metals	metallophobia	scabies	scabiphobia
mice	musophobia	school	school phobia
mirror and seeing oneself in	eisoptophobia, spectrophobia	scratches or being scratched	amychophobia
missiles	ballistophobia	sea	thalassophobia
moisture	hygrophobia	self	autophobia
money	chrematophobia	semen, loss of	spermatophobia
motion	kinesophobia	sex	genophobia
myths	mythophobia	sexual intercourse	coitophobia
naked body	gymnophobia	shock	hormephobia
name, hearing a certain	onomatophobia	sin	hamartophobia
needles	belonephobia	sinning	peccatiphobia
neglect or omission of duty	paralipophobia	sitting	thassophobia
night	noctiphobia, nyctophobia	sitting down	kathisophobia
northern lights	auroraphobia	skin disease	dermatosiophobia
novelty	kainophobia	skin lesion	dermatophobia
odor	olfactophobia, osmophobia osphresiophobia	skin of animals	doraphobia
		sleep	hypnophobia
Odor, Personal	bromidrosiphobia	small objects	microphobia, microbiphobia
open space	agoraphobia	smothering	pnigerophobia
overwork	ponophobia	snake	ophidiophobia
pain	algophobia, odynophobia	snow	chionophobia

Contd...

Contd...

Fear of	Condition	Fear of	Condition
parasites	parasitophobia	solitude or being alone	eremophobia
people	anthropophobia	sounds	acousticophobia
p	topophobia	sourness	acerophobia
pleasure	hedonophobia	speaking, talking	lalophobia
pointed objects	aichmophobia	spider	arachnophobia
poison	iophobia, toxicophobia	stairs	climacophobia
poverty	peniaphobia	standing or walking	stasibasiphobia
precipices	cremnophobia	standing up	stasiphobia
punishment	poinephobia	stars	siderophobia
rabies	cynophobia, lyssophobia	stealing	kleptophobia
railroad or train	siderodromophobia	stories	mythophobia
strangers	xenophobia	trichinosis	trichinophobia
street	agyiophobia	tuberculosis	phthisiophobia, tuberculophobia
string	linonophobia		
sunlight	heliophobia	vaccination	vaccinophobia
symbolism	symbolophobia	vehicle, being in	amaxophobia
syphillis	syphilophobia	venereal disease	cypridophobia
tapeworms	taeniophobia	voice, one's own	phonophobia
taste	geumaphobia	void	kenophobia
teeth	odontophobia	vomiting	emetophobia
thinking	phronemophobia	walking	basiphobia
thunder	astraphobia, brontophobia	water	hydrophobia
		weakness	asthenophobia
time	chronophobia	wind	anemophobia
touched, being	haphephobia, haptephobia	women	gynephobia
		words, hearing certain	onomatophobia
travel	hodophobia	work	ergasiophobia
trembling	tremophobia	writing	graphophobia

Appendix 8

Bones of the Skeleton

AXIAL (80 Bones)
- Head (29 Bones)
  - Cranial (8)
    - frontal — 1
    - parietal — 2
    - occipital — 1
    - temporal — 2
    - sphenoid — 1
    - ethmoid — 1
  - Facial (14)
    - maxilla — 2
    - mandible — 1
    - zygoma — 2
    - lacrimal — 2
    - nasal — 2
    - turbinate — 2
    - vomer — 1
    - palate — 2
  - Hyoid (1)
  - Auditory ossicles (6)
    - malleus — 2
    - incus — 2
    - stapes — 2
- Trunk (51 Bones)
  - Vertebrae (26)
    - cervical — 7
    - thoracic — 12
    - lumbar — 5
    - sacrum — 1
    - coccyx — 1
  - Ribs (24)
    - true rib — 14
    - false rib — 6
    - floating rib — 4
  - Sternum (1)

APPENDICULAR (126 Bones)
- Upper Extremities (64 Bones)
  - Arms and Shoulders (10)
    - clavicle — 2
    - scapula — 2
    - humerus — 2
    - radius — 2
    - ulna — 2
  - Wrists (16)
    - navicular or scaphoid — 2
    - lunate — 2
    - triquetrum — 2
    - pisiform — 2
    - trapezium — 2
    - trapezoid — 2
    - capitate — 2
    - hamate — 2
  - Hands (38)
    - metacarpal — 10
    - phalanx (finger bones) — 28
- Lower Extremities (62 Bones)
  - Legs and Hips (10)
    - innominate bone (a fusion of the ilium, ischium, and pubis-hip bone) — 2
    - femur — 2
    - tibia — 2
    - fibula — 2
    - patella (knee cap) — 2
  - Ankles (14)
    - astragaloid — 2
    - calcaneus (heel bone) — 2
    - scaphoid — 2
    - cuboid — 2
    - cuneiform, internal — 2
    - cuneiform, middle — 2
    - cuneiform, external — 2
  - Feet (38)
    - metatarsal — 10
    - phalanx (toe bones) — 28

Appendix 9

Psychomotor and Physical Development Birth to One Year					
		Physical Development			
		Length Range		Weight Range	
		in.	cm	lb	kg
Birth	boys	18¼ – 21½	46.4 – 54.4	5½ – 9¼	2.54 – 4.15
	girls	17¾ – 20¾	45.4 – 52.9	5¼ – 8½	2.36 – 3.81
1 Month	boys	19¾ – 23	50.4 – 58.6	7 – 11¾	3.16 – 5.38
	girls	19¼ – 22½	49.2 – 56.9	6½ – 10¾	2.97 – 4.92
3 Months	boys	22¼ – 25¾	56.7 – 65.4	9¾ – 16¼	4.43 – 7.37
	girls	21¾ – 25	55.4 – 63.4	9¼ – 14¾	4.18 – 6.74
6 Months	boys	25 – 28½	63.4 – 72.3	13¾ – 20¾	6.20 – 9.46
	girls	24¼ – 27¾	61.8 – 70.2	12¾ – 19¼	5.79 – 8.73
9 Months	boys	26¾ – 30¼	68.0 – 77.1	16½ – 24	7.52 – 10.93
	girls	26 – 29½	66.1 – 75.0	15½ – 22½	7.0 – 10.17
12 Months	boys	28¼ – 32	71.7 – 81.2	18½ – 26½	8.43 – 11.99
	girls	27½ – 31¼	69.8 – 79.1	17¼ – 24¾	7.84-11.24

Psychomotor Development

Birth Through	Ability to suck, swallow, gag, cry, and maintain eye contact with a person.
1st Month	The head needs to be supported. Loud noises may cause a startle reflex.
2nd Month	May turn to either side when on their backs; will follow moving objects; able to lift head but not for a sustained period; begin to smile, frown, and turn away.
3rd Month	Greater movement and vocal response to stimuli; notice own hands and suck on them; head will be steady while in a supported position.

Contd...

Contd...

4th and 5th Months	Able to lift head higher when lying on stomach; will reach for objects and may be able to encircle a bottle with both hands; may drool a lot; attempt to put all kinds of objects in mouth.
6th-9th Months	Develop ability to grasp and pick up food; are able to pull themselves up to a sitting position and eventually will crawl; they begin to make noises that sound like words and to recognize certain words; will play peek-a-boo.
9th-11th Months	Develop ability to handle food and to drink from a cup; may imitate sounds and say certain words; crawl by pulling body along with arms, and pull themselves to a standing position; they will point at objects and throw things; they want to feed themselves and to help with dressing and undressing; they will walk while holding a person's hand.
12th Month	Can eat food alone and drink from a cup with assistance; able to move around easily, and crawl up stairs, and out of crib.

Appendix 10

Size, Weight, and Capacity of Various Organs and Parts of the Adult Body ♂ male ♀ female

Description	Size	Weight	Capacity
Adrenal gland	5 cm high 3 cm across 1 cm thick	5.0 gm	
Bladder	12 cm in diameter		50 ml (when moderately full)
Blood volume			♂ 4680 ml ♀ 3400 ml
Brain		♂ 1240-1680 gm ♀ 1130-1570 gm	
Ear, external canal	2.5 cm long (from concha)		
Esophagus	23-25 cm		
Eye	23.5 mm vertical diameter 24 mm antero-posterior diameter		
Fallopian tube	10 cm		
Gallbladder	7-10 cm long 3 cm wide		30-50 ml
Heart	12 × 8-9 × 6 cm	♂ 280-340 gm ♀ 230-280 gm	
Intestines — small	Quite variable 6-7 meters long		
Intestines — large	1.5 meters long		
Intestines — vermiform appendix	2-20 cm long Average 9 cm		

Contd...

Contd...

Description	Size	Weight	Capacity
Intestines—			
rectum	12 cm long		
Kidney	11 cm long	♂ 150 gm	
	6 cm broad	♀ 135 gm	
	3 cm thick		
Larynx	o 44 × 43 × 36 mm		
	o 36 × 41 × 26 mm		
Liver		♂ 1.4-1.8 kg	6500 cc
		♀ 1.0-2.5 kg	
Lung		Rt. 625 gm	
		Lt. 565 gm	
Ovaries	6 × 3-4 × 1-2 mm	50 mg	
Pharynx	12.5 cm long		
Prostate	2 × 4 × 3 cm	8 gm	
Skeleton		Average adult	
		male, 4957 gm	
Skull		Average	♂ 406 ml
		(without teeth),	♀ 207 ml
		642 gm	
Spinal cord	42-45 cm long	30 gm	
Spleen	12 × 7 × 3-4 cm	150 gm	
		Range 80-300 gm	
		Decreases wilh age	
Stomach	Quite variable		Quite variable
	25 cm long		1500 ml
	10 cm wide		
Testes	4-5 × 2.5 × 3.0 cm	10.5-14 gm	
Thoracic duct	38-45 cm long		
Thymus		Newborn,	
		10.9 gm	
		10-15 yr,	
		29.5 gm	
		20-25 yr,	
		18.6 gm	

Contd...

Contd...

Description	Size	Weight	Capacity
Thyroid	Each lobe 5 × 3 × 2 cm	30 gm total	
Trachea	11 cm long 2-2.5 cm in diameter		
Ureter	28-34 cm long		
Urethra	♂ 17.5-20 cm long ♀ 4 cm long		
Uterus	7.5 × 5.0 × 2.5 cm	30-40 gm (nonpregnant)	
Vagina	Anterior wall length 7.5 cm Posterior wall length 9.0 cm		

Appendix 11

Composition of Whole Milk		
	Human Milk	*Cow's Milk*
Water	87–88%	85–88%
Minerals	0.2%	0.8%
Protein	1.1%	3.3%
Fat	3.8%	3.7%
Sugar (lactose, carbohydrate)	6.5–7.0%	4.8%
Sodium	7 mEq/liter	25 mEq/liter
Potassium	14 mEq/liter	35 mEq/liter
Calories	22 kcal/oz	20 kcal/oz

Appendix 12

Colors of Indicators of pH			
	Color		
	Toward Acid	*Toward Alkali*	*Range of pH*
Methyl yellow	Red	Yellow	2.9 – 4.0
Congo red	Blue	Red	3.0 – 5.2
Methyl orange	Red	Yellow	3.1 – 4.4
Methyl red	Red	Yellow	4.2 – 6.2
Litmus	Red	Blue	4.5 – 8.3
Bromcresol purple	Yellow	Purple	5.2 – 6.8
Bromothymol blue	Yellow	Blue	6.0 – 7.6
Phenol red	Yellow	Red	6.8 – 8.4
Phenolphthalein	Colorless	Pink	8.2 – 10.0

Appendix 13

Incubation and Isolation Periods in Common Infections		
Infection	*Incubation Period*	*Isolation of Patient*
AIDS	Serological evidence in several months. Clinical development of signs and symptoms may require years. Approx. half of infected patients will have developed clinical signs and symptoms by 11 years post infection	Blood and body fluid precautions. Private room if personal hygiene habits are poor
Brucellosis	Highly variable, usually 5-21 days; may be months	None
Chickenpox	2-3 weeks	1 week after appearance of vesicles
Cholera	A few hours to 5 days	Enteric precautions
Common cold	12 hr to 3 days	None
Diphtheria	Usually 2 to 5 days	Until two cultures from nose and throat, taken at least 24 hr apart, are negative; cultures to be taken after cessation of antibiotic therapy
Dysentery, amebic	From a few days to several months, commonly 2-4 weeks	None
Dysentery, bacillary (shigellosis)	1-7 days	As long as stools remain positive
Encephalitis, mosquito-borne	5-15 days	None
Giardiasis	Variable; median 7-10 days	Enteric precautions
Gonorrhea	2-7 days; may be longer	No sexual contact until cured
Hepatitis A	Variable, 15-50 days; mean about 30 days	Enteric precautions until 1 week after onset of jaundice
Hepatitis B	Variable, usually 45-180 days; mean 60-90 days	Blood and body fluid precautions until antibodies to virus disappear

Contd...

Contd...

Infection	Incubation Period	Isolation of Patient
Hepatitis C	15–64 days	As for hepatitis A
Influenza	1–3 days	As practical
Legionella	2–10 days	None
Malaria	12 days *for Plasmodium falciparum*; 14 days for *P. vivax, P. ovale*; 30 days for *P. malariae*	Protect from mosquitoes
Measles (rubeola)	8–13 days from exposure to onset of fever; 14 days until rash appears	From diagnosis to 7 days after appearance of rash; strict isolation from children under 3 yrs
Meningitis, meningococcal	2–10 days	Until 24 hr after start of chemotherapy
Mononucleosis, infectious	4–6 weeks	None; disinfect articles soiled with nose and throat discharges
Mumps	2–3 weeks	Until the glands recede
Paratyphoid fevers	1–3 weeks for fever; 1–10 days for gastroenteritis	Until 3 stools are negative
Pneumonia, pneumococcal	Believed to be 1-3 days	Until 24 hr after administration of antibiotics
Poliomyelitis	3–35 days	1 week from onset
Puerperal fever, streptococcal	1–3 days	Transfer from maternity ward
Rabies	Usually 2–8 weeks; occasionally only 10 days	Strict for duration of illness; danger to attendants
Rubella (German measles)	16–18 days with range of 23 days	None, but avoid contact with nonimmune pregnant women
Salmonellosis	6–72 hr; usually 12–36 hr	Until stool cultures are salmonella-free on two consecutive specimens collected not less than 24 hr apart

Contd...

Contd...

Infection	Incubation Period	Isolation of Patient
Scabies	2–6 weeks before onset of itching in patients without previous infections; 1–4 days after re-exposed	Excuse patient from school or work until day after treatment
Scarlet fever	1–3 days	7 days; may be terminated in 24 hr
Smallpox	8–17 days	Strict; in screened hospital wards until all scabs have disappeared
Syphilis	10 days – 10 weeks; usually 3 weeks	In noncooperative patients, it should be enforced until surface lesions are healed
Tetanus	4 days–3 weeks	None
Toxic shock syndrome	Unknown but may be as brief as several hours	None
Trachoma	5–12 days	Until lesions disappear, but usually not practical
Tuberculosis	4–12 weeks to demonstrable primary lesion or significant tuberculin reactions	Variable, depending on conversion of sputum to negative after specific therapy and on ability of patient to understand and carry out personal hygiene methods
Tularemia	2–10 days	None
Typhoid fever	Usually 1–3 weeks	Until 3 cultures of feces and urine are negative. These should be taken not earlier than 1 month after onset
Typhus fever	7–14 days	None
Whooping cough	Usually 1 week	For 3 weeks after onset of spasmodic cough

Appendix 14

Exercise: Energy Required*	
Calories Required per Hour of Exercise	*Activity⁺*
80	Sitting quietly, reading
200	Golf with use of powered cart
250	Walking 3 miles/hr (4.83 km/hr); housework; light industry; cycling 6 miles/hr (9.7 km/hr)
330	Heavy housework; walking 3.5 miles/hr (5.6 km/hr) cycling 6 miles/hr (9.7 km/hr); golf, carrying own bag; tennis, doubles; ballet exercises
400	Walking 5 miles/hr (8 km/hr); cycling 10 miles/hr (16.1 km/hr); tennis, singles; water skiing
500	Manual labor; gardening; shoveling
660	Running 5.5 miles/hr (8.9 km/hr); cycling 13 miles/hr (20.9 km/hr); climbing stairs; heavy manual work
1020	Running 8 miles/hr (12.9 km/hr); climbing stairs with 30-pound (13.61 kg) load

*These estimates are approximate and can serve only as a general guide. They are based on an average person who weighs 160 pounds (72.58 kg).
⁺Energy requirements for swimming are not provided because of the variables such as temperature of the water, whether the water is fresh or salt, buoyancy of the individual, and whether the water is calm or not.

Appendix 15

Nutrition Ready Reckoner for International Foods

	Calories (Kcal)	Proteins (g)	Fats (g)	Carbo-hydrates (g)	Fibre (g)	Calcium (mg)	Iron (mg)	Caro-tene (mcg)	Retinol (mcg)	Vit B1 (mg)	Vit B2 (mg)	Niacin (mg)	Vit C (mg)	Serving Portion
BEVERAGES														
Hot tea	34	0.6	1.0	5.7	0.0	31.0	0.0	0.0	7.00	0.01	0.01	0.0	0	1 Tea cup
Instant coffee	149	1.0	13.3	6.3	0.0	31.0	0.0	0.0	7.00	0.01	0.01	0.0	0	1 Tea cup
Cold coffee (with Cream)	279	3.9	17.0	27.7	0.0	144.0	0.3	487.0	183.00	0.06	0.23	0.1	2	1 Tall glass
Banana milk Shake	228	6.2	7.5	33.8	0.0	223.0	0.5	40.0	101.00	0.11	0.37	0.4	7	1 Tall glass
Mango milk Shake	237	6.2	7.7	35.6	0.8	227.0	1.3	2067.0	608.00	0.15	0.41	9.0	16	1 Tall glass
Lemonade	107	0.3	0.3	25.7	0.5	21.0	0.1	0.0	0.00	0.01	0.00	0.0	12	1 glass
BREAKFAST CEREALS														
Cracked wheat Porridge	292	10.0	10.4	39.7	2.5	296.0	1.5	152.0	39.00	1.29	0.49	1.3	5	1 bowl
Oat meal Porridge	217	6.6	6.6	32.8	2.0	154.0	1.0	70.0	18.00	0.80	0.26	0.3	2	1 bowl
Cornflakes with milk	291	9.8	10.8	38.7	1.2	290.0	0.9	157.0	41.00	1.28	0.48	0.6	5	1 bowl

Contd...

Contd...

	Calories (Kcal)	Proteins (g)	Fats (g)	Carbo-hydrates (g)	Fibre (g)	Calcium (mg)	Iron (mg)	Caro-tene (mcg)	Retinol (mcg)	Vit B1 (mg)	Vit B2 (mg)	Niacin (mg)	Vit C (mg)	Serving Portion
EGGS														
Boiled egg	87	6.7	6.7	0.0	0.0	25.0	0.7	300.0	180.00	0.05	0.20	0.1	0	1 Egg
Poached egg	87	6.7	6.7	0.0	0.0	25.0	0.7	300.0	180.00	0.05	0.20	0.1	0	1 Egg
Fried egg	160	6.7	14.8	0.0	0.0	25.0	0.7	620.0	260.00	0.05	0.20	0.1	0	1 Egg
Scrambled egg	172	6.7	15.8	0.8	0.0	57.0	0.7	620.0	267.00	0.06	0.22	0.1	0	1 Egg
Baked egg	124	6.7	10.8	0.0	0.0	25.0	0.7	460.0	220.00	0.05	0.20	0.1	0	1 Egg
Fluffy omelette	160	6.7	14.8	0.0	0.0	25.0	0.7	620.0	260.00	0.05	0.20	0.1	0	1 Egg
Cheese and Mushroom omelette	308	12.9	27.1	3.0	0.0	182.0	1.3	780.0	373.00	0.09	0.42	1.5	1	1 Egg
SOUPS														
Minestrone soup	90	1.4	5.2	9.4	1.2	43.0	0.7	491.0	123.00	0.07	0.03	0.5	17	1 Bowl
Chicken sweet	322	25.5	13.5	24.6	6.0	23.0	2.6	10.7	93.00	0.21	0.34	8.6	6	1 Bowl
Corn soup														
French onion Soup	208	4.8	11.6	21.1	2.4	102.0	0.8	321.0	110.00	0.08	0.05	0.6	8	1 Bowl
Tomato soup	82	2.1	4.5	8.3	2.3	101.0	1.3	862.0	216.00	0.25	0.21	0.8	55	1 Bowl
Green pea soup	186	9.0	6.4	23.1	2.2	70.0	1.9	375.0	109.00	0.28	0.08	1.1	11	1 Bowl
Spinach soup	561	3.9	8.9	116.2	5.9	81.0	1.5	5902.0	1475.00	0.06	0.27	0.08	29	1 Bowl
Mixed vegetable soup	146	3.3	9.2	12.5	1.4	124.0	0.9	779.0	225.00	0.11	0.16	0.6	23	1 Bowl
Cream with tomato Soup	245	5.4	16.6	18.5	2.3	180.0	1.5	984.0	287.00	0.32	0.25	1.0	45	1 Bowl

Contd

Contd...

	Calories (Kcal)	Proteins (g)	Fats (g)	Carbo-hydrates(g)	Fibre (g)	Calcium (mg)	Iron (mg)	Caro-tene (mcg)	Retinol (mcg)	Vit B1 (mg)	Vit B2 (mg)	Niacin (mg)	Vit C (mg)	Serving Portion
Cream with spinach soup	307	8.5	23.2	16.0	5.1	200.0	2.2	6214.0	1644.0	0.20	0.52	0.9	32	1 Bowl
Cream with carrot soup	250	4.6	16.2	21.5	2.0	172.0	1.4	1935.0	531.00	0.17	0.17	0.9	6	1 Bowl
Cream with Mixed vegetable soup	263	7.5	13.4	28.0	3.2	179.0	2.0	1160.0	331.00	0.33	0.24	1.5	45	1 Bowl
Cream with mushroom soup	308	6.6	22.4	19.9	0.7	136.0	1.5	554.0	189.00	0.13	0.41	2.9	6	1 Bowl
Hot and Sour Soup	181	11.2	9.3	13.2	1.6	65.0	2.8	86.0	22.00	0.22	0.25	23	6	1 Bowl
CEREALS														
Boiled rice	277	6.0	0.8	61.4	3.6	8.00	2.6	2.0	0.40	0.17	0.13	3.1	0	1
Beans and macaroni	352	12.1	16.8	38.0	3.7	243.0	2.2	673.0	242.00	0.20	0.20	1.5	40	1 Plate
Spaghetti bolognese	346	14.6	14.9	38..3	33.0	174.0	3.2	867.0	236.00	0.28	0.21	4.8	30	1 shallow dish
Chicken chowmein	542	31.4	24.2	49.6	3.9	104.0	5.6	9.8	333.00	0.39	0.36	8.1	59	1 shallow dish

Contd

Contd...

Calories	Proteins (Kcal)	Fats (g)	Carbo-hydrates (g)	Fibre (g)	Calcium (mg)	Iron (mg) (mcg)	Caro-tene (mcg)	Retinol (mcg)	Vit B1 (mg)	Vit B2 (mg)	Niacin (mg)	Vit C (mg)	Serving Portion
MEATS													
Shepherd's Pie	486	23.8	34.5	20.0	2.2	206.0	3.5	339.0	98.00	0.31	0.18	9.2	15	1 Bowl
Roast chicken	297	25.3	21.8	0.0	0.0	18.0	2.0	334.0	166.00	0.13	0.20	10.0	0	1 Bowl
Chilli chicken	464	27.3	35.5	8.8	1.9	46.0	3.1	222.0	135.00	0.35	0.31	10.9	50	1 Bowl
Chicken sweet and sour	420	27.0	33.3	3.1	0.8	39.0	2.7	270.0	181.0	0.28	0.35	10.6	30	1 Bowl
Fried fish with chips	443	26.3	26.2	25.4	2.2	307.0	3.3	165.0	94.00	0.09	0.11	0.9	9	1 Bowl
Fish in coconut milk	371	27.0	17.1	27.2	3.2	150.0	3.2	4.0	1.00	0.06	0.03	0.5	7	1 Bowl
Prawn curry	342	30.1	19.9	10.5	2.7	509.0	9.3	3.0	0.80	0.05	0.18	7.5	4	1 Bowl
Crispy baked Fish	390	32.3	15.1	31.2	4.1	461.0	4.1	496.0	153.00	0.13	0.13	1.3	16	1 Bowl
VEGETABLES													
Egg Curry	314	15.5	17.6	23.3	2.8	85.0	2.8	483.0	237.00	0.38	0.25	1.2	21	1 Bowl
Stuffed Tomatoes	233	6.0	15.6	17.1	2.8	138.0	1.5	829.0	228.00	0.27	0.08	1.1	41	2 Tomatoes
Stuffed okra	132	2.3	10.2	7.7	5.9	79.0	0.5	62.0	16.00	0.08	0.12	0.7	16	1 Bowl
Roast Potatoes	191	2.4	5.0	34.0	3.8	15.0	0.8	228.0	57.00	0.15	0.01	1.8	26	1-2 Potatoes
Stuffed Baked Potato	334	7.1	18.8	34.0	3.8	33.0	1.3	698.0	248.00	0.19	0.16	1.8	26	1-2 Potatoes

Contd...

Contd...

	Calories (Kcal)	Proteins (g)	Fats (g)	Carbo-hydrates(g)	Fibre (g)	Calcium (mg)	Iron (mg)	Caro-tene (mcg)	Retinol (mcg)	Vit B1 (mg)	Vit B2 (mg)	Niacin (mg)	Vit C (mg)	Serving Portion
Creamed spinach	429	21.4	29.8	18.8	9.3	458.0	3.5	11812.0	3195.00	0.25	1.00	1.4	58	1 Small Bowl
Creamed spinach and mushrooms	363	13.4	25.8	19.2	7.1	366.0	2.9	8692.0	2284.00	0.23	0.90	3.5	45	1 Bowl
SALADS														
Russian Salad	959	19.7	85.6	27.5	3.3	100.0	3.8	879.0	333.00	0.38	0.33	5.4	39	1 Small Bowl
Beetroot and egg salad	366	8.9	30.8	13.4	3.6	62.0	2.1	300.0	180.00	0.12	0.29	0.6	15	1 Small Bowl
Tossed Green salad	153	1.5	12.2	9.2	2.0	50.0	0.9	225.0	57.00	0.18	0.04	0.5	43	1 Small Bowl
Cucumber and yogurt salad	29	1.3	1.3	2.9	1.0	53.0	0.5	10.0	4.00	0.04	0.05	0.2	6	1 Small Bowl
French dressing	722	0.0	80.0	0.4	0.0	1.0	0.0	0.0	0.00	0.00	0.00	0.01	1	3/4 Cup
Mayonnaise	1220	7.1	131.8	1.3	0.0	56.0	1.4	380.0	229.00	0.08	0.26	0.1	4	1 Cup
Mayonnaise without eggs	886	7.7	90.1	11.0	0.0	288.0	0.5	139.0	36.00	1.20	0.46	0.3	6	1 Cup
DESSERTS														
Vanilla ice Cream	288	2.3	22.9	18.2	0.0	90.0	0.2	415.0	139.00	0.03	0.14	0.1	0	1 Ice Cream Cup

Contd

Contd...

	Calories (Kcal)	Proteins (g)	Fats (g)	Carbo-hydrates (g)	Fibre (g)	Calcium (mg)	Iron (mg)	Carotene (mcg)	Retinol (mcg)	Vit B1 (mg)	Vit B2 (mg)	Niacin (mg)	Vit C (mg)	Serving Portion
Strawberry ice cream	288	2.3	22.9	18.2	0.0	90.0	0.2	415.0	139.00	0.03	0.14	0.1	0	1 Ice Cream Cup
Chocolate ice cream	288	2.3	22.9	18.2	0.0	90.0	0.2	415.0	139.00	0.03	0.14	0.1	0	1 Ice Cream Cup
Fruit ice cream	323	2.6	23.0	26.5	0.3	95.0	0.4	832.0	246.00	0.05	0.16	0.3	5	1Sundae Glass
Cold lemon	534	6.9	41.9	32.3	0.4	41.0	0.8	1000.0	355.00	0.05	0.20	0.1	8.8	1 Souffle Dish
Souffle cold orange	594	7.8	42.0	46.2	1.5	64.0	1.2	2656.0	769.00	0.05	0.20	0.1	45	1 Souffle Dish
Souffle cold pineappple	525	6.7	42.0	30.00	0.0	25.0	0.7	1000.0	355.00	0.00	0.20	0.1	0	1 Souffle Dish
Souffle cold vanila	536	7.3	42.7	30.6	0.0	57.0	0.7	1000.0	362.00	0.06	0.20	0.1	0.2	1 Souffle Dish
Souffle cold chocolate	536	7.3	42.7	30.6	0.0	57.0	0.7	1000.0	362.00	0.06	0.20	0.1	0.2	1 Souffle Dish
Souffle bread and butter pudding	222	7.4	11.3	22.7	1.0	124.0	0.7	316.0	177.00	0.08	0.27	0.2	2	1 Small Plate

Contd